The Vulva

EDITED BY

C. Marjorie Ridley
MA, BM, BCh, FRCP
Honorary Consultant and Senior Lecturer
St John's Institute of Dermatology
Guy's and St Thomas' Trust
St Thomas' Hospital, London

AND

Sarah M. Neill
MB, ChB, FRCP
Honorary Consultant and Senior Lecturer
St John's Institute of Dermatology
Guy's and St Thomas' Trust
St Thomas' Hospital, London;
and Consultant Dermatologist
St Peter's Hospital, Chertsey, Surrey

SECOND EDITION

b
Blackwell
Science

Editorial Offices:
Osney Mead, Oxford OX2 0EL
25 John Street, London WC1N 2BL
23 Ainslie Place, Edinburgh EH3 6AJ
350 Main Street, Malden
MA 02148 5018, USA
54 University Street, Carlton
Victoria 3053, Australia
10, rue Casimir Delavigne
75006 Paris, France

Other Editorial Offices:
Blackwell Wissenschafts-Verlag GmbH
Kurfürstendamm 57
10707 Berlin, Germany

Blackwell Science KK
MG Kodenmacho Building
7–10 Kodenmacho Nihombashi
Chuo-ku, Tokyo 104, Japan

First published 1975
(by Churchill Livingstone)
Second edition 1999

Set by Excel Typesetters Co., Hong Kong
Printed and bound in Spain
by Mateu Cromo

A catalogue record for this title
is available from the British Library

ISBN 0-632-04768-2

Library of Congress
Cataloging-in-publication Data

The vulva/edited by
C. Marjorie Ridley and Sarah M. Neill.
p. cm.
ISBN (invalid) 0-632-04768-2
1. Vulva—Diseases.
2. Vagina—Diseases.
I. Ridley, Constance Marjorie.
II. Neill, Sarah Mary
[DNLM: 1. Vulva. 2. Vulvar
Diseases.
WP 200 V991 1998]
RG261.V85 1998
618.1′6—dc21
DNLM/DLC
for Library of Congress 98-23209
CIP

DISTRIBUTORS

Marston Book Services Ltd
PO Box 269
Abingdon, Oxon OX14 4YN
(*Orders*: Tel: 01235 465500
Fax: 01235 465555)

USA
Blackwell Science, Inc.
Commerce Place
350 Main Street
Malden, MA 02148 5018
(*Orders*: Tel: 800 759 6102
781 388 8250
Fax: 781 388 8255)

Canada
Login Brothers Book Company
324 Saulteaux Crescent
Winnipeg, Manitoba R3J 3T2
(*Orders*: Tel: 204 837-2987)

Australia
Blackwell Science Pty Ltd
54 University Street
Carlton, Victoria 3053
(*Orders*: Tel: 3 9347 0300
Fax: 3 9347 5001)

For further information on
Blackwell Science, visit our website:
www.blackwell-science.com

The Vulva

EN ceste figure sont demonstrez les Membres estant en la femme, quant a la situatiõ, liaison,&entremeslure. A.demõstre la partie de la veine du foye,autremẽt dicte,caué. BB.les veines seminales,elles sont de coleur blanchastre: par ces vaines est iecte la semence. CC.sont les veines,les qlles embrassent l'amarri,ou matrice.DD.les couillõs de la femme. F.l'amarri,matrice.la portiere.GG.les cornes de la matrice.H.lentree deans la matrice,ou l'orifice interieux. I. le col de la matrice,aultremẽt,la partie honteuse.KK.le tronc de la veine du foye,caué.plante par les cuisses au bas du genou. LL.cest le tronc de la plus grãde artere dicte aorte,a cause qu'elle est la source de toutes les aultres Arteres. M.monstre la veisie. Q Q. petiz conduictz par ou passe l'ourine en la vessie,dictz en grec vriteres . P P.Les reins,ou roignõs,OO,les veines descendãt aux roignõs de couleur blãchatre.

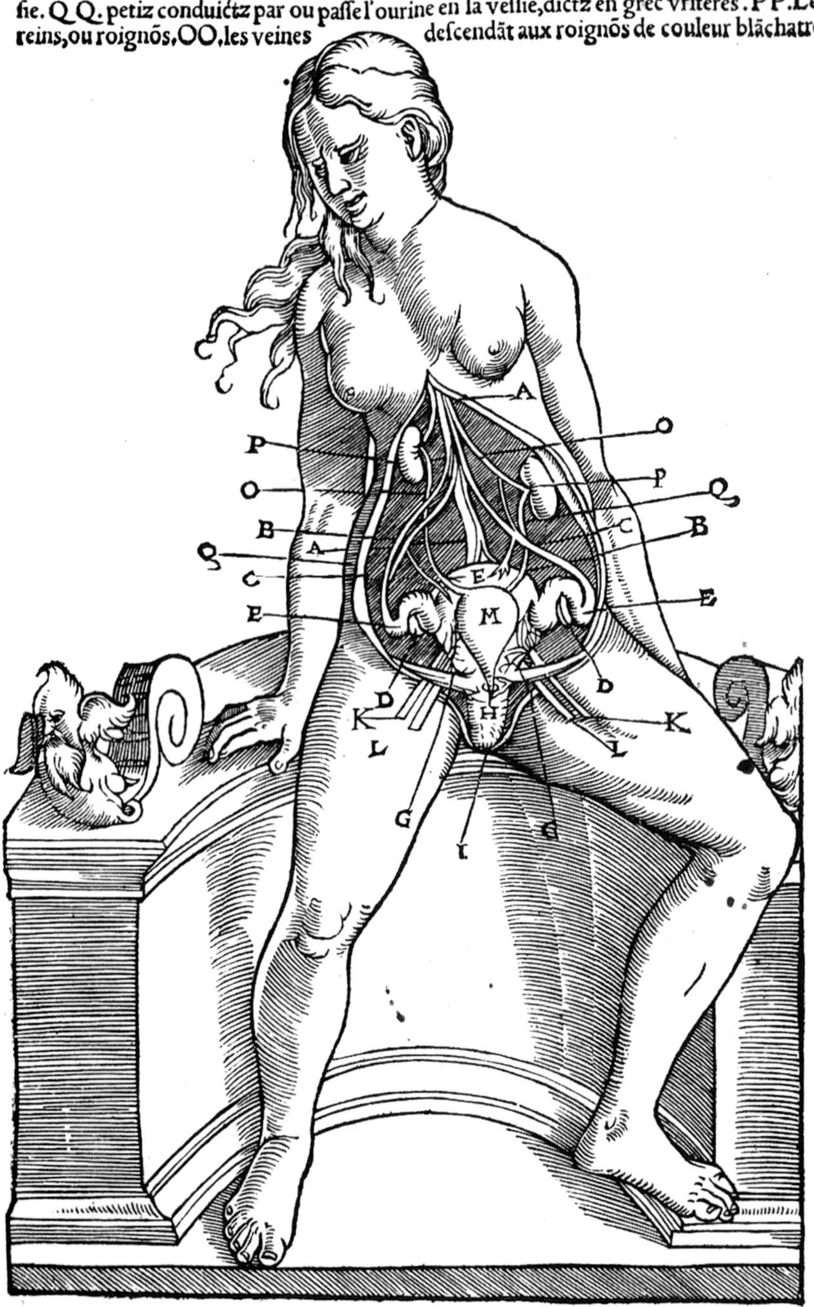

IN HAC FIGVRA GENERATIONIS MEMBRA IN muliebri sexu quo ad situm & colligantiam demonstrantur. A. pars venæ cauæ est. BB.venæ seminales candidæ. CC.venæ vterum amplexantes. EE.inuolucrum ex seminarijs venis & arterijs constans. DD.mulieris testiculi. F. matrix siue vterus. GG.cornua matricis. H.orificium matricis interius. I.collum matricis,pudibunda. KK.venæ cauæ truncus in crura implantatus. LL.arteriæ aortæ truncus est.M,vesica.QQ vreteres.PP.renes.OO.venæ albæ renales.

FRONTISPIECE: *Seated female showing viscera. Walter Herman Ryff (fl. 1539). From the original in the Wellcome Library by courtesy of the Trustees.*

Contents

List of contributors

John J. Bradley
MB, BS, FRCP, FRCPsych, DPM
Emeritus Consultant Psychiatrist, Camden and Islington CHS NHS Trust, 112 Hampstead Road, London NW1 2LT and Honorary Senior Lecturer, University College, London WC1E 6BT

C. Hilary Buckley
MD, FRCPath
Reader in Gynaecological Pathology, Department of Reproductive Pathology, St Mary's Hospital for Women and Children, Whitworth Park, Manchester M13 0JH

Harold Fox
MD, FRCPath, FRCOG
Emeritus Professor of Reproductive Pathology, Department of Pathological Sciences, Stopford Building, University of Manchester, Manchester M13 9PT

John M. McLean
MB, BS, BSc, MD
Formerly Senior Lecturer in Anatomy, University of Manchester, Manchester M13 9PT

John M. Monaghan
MB, FRCS(Ed.), FRCOG
Senior Lecturer in Gynaecological Oncology, Queen Elizabeth Hospital, Sheriff Hill, Gateshead, Tyne and Wear NE9 6SX

Sarah (Sallie) M. Neill
MB, ChB, FRCP
Honorary Consultant and Senior Lecturer, St John's Institute of Dermatology, Guy's and St Thomas' Hospital Trust, Lambeth Palace Row, London SE1 7EH; Consultant Dermatologist, St Peter's Hospital, Chertsey, Surrey KT16 OPZ

J. David Oriel
MD
Formerly Consultant Physician in Genitourinary Medicine, University College and Middlesex School of Medicine, 5 University Street, London WC1 6JJ

Bernard J. Paniel
Professor of Obstetrics and Gynaecology, Centre Hospitalier Intercommunal de Créteil, Service de Gynécologie Obstétrique, 40 Avenue de Verdun, 94000 Créteil, France

C. Marjorie Ridley
MA, BM, BCh, FRCP
Honorary Consultant and Senior Lecturer, St John's Institute of Dermatology, Guy's and St Thomas' Trust, St Thomas' Hospital, Lambeth Palace Road, London SE1 7EH

Preface

The contents of this new, expanded, multi-author edition range over embryology and development, anatomy and physiology, history, general aspects of management, infections, non-infective cutaneous conditions, pain problems, psychiatric disorders, cysts and non-neoplastic swellings, non-epithelial and epithelial tumours, and surgical procedures applicable to benign and malignant conditions.

The general expansion and considerable revision of content, and the inclusion of new chapters, are, in our opinion, justified by the great increase of interest in vulval disease which has become apparent in the last few years.

There have been significant changes in thought as well as many scientific advances during this period. The relevant material, however, remains scattered in the literatures of the several disciplines involved. This latest edition of *The Vulva* attempts to collate the existing information on the subject and to note its interrelations. We hope that the result will be to facilitate the multidisciplinary cooperation which is so vital in the study and management of vulval disease.

There is of necessity some overlap between the chapters, but we believe that there are no important discrepancies in the views of our contributors.

The book is directed towards those specialists in dermatology, genitourinary medicine, gynaecology and pathology who are involved with vulval problems. It is intended to be a repository of information, interpretation and guidance on management rather than simply an illustrated text; it aims to offer to the reader material which, as a coherent whole, is not readily available elsewhere.

Acknowledgements

We thank all our contributors for their cooperation and hard work. Our thanks go also to the colleagues who have allowed us to use their photographs; that is, those who helped with previous editions and now also Miss Betty Mansell and Dr Jennifer Salisbury.

We are very grateful to the editorial staff of Blackwell Science for their great help and forbearance; in particular to Rebecca Huxley, Dr Stuart Taylor, Audrey Cadogan and Victoria Oddie.

We are indebted to the publishers for permission to use photographs previously published in the following books:

A Colour Atlas of Diseases of the Vulva (1992) (eds Ridley, C.M., Oriel, J.D. & Robinson, A.J.). Chapman and Hall Medical, London.

Dewhurst, J. (1980) *Practical Pediatric and Adolescent Gynecology*. Marcel Dekker, New York.

Haines and Taylor, Textbook of Obstetrical and Gynaecological Pathology (1987) (ed. Fox, H.), 3rd edn. Churchill Livingstone, Edinburgh.

Haines and Taylor, Textbook of Obstetrical and Gynaecological Pathology (1995) (eds Fox, H. & Wells, M.), 4th edn. Churchill Livingstone, New York.

Ricci, J. (1943) *The Genealogy of Gynaecology*, 2000 B.C.–1800 A.D. Blakiston, Philadelphia.

Ridley, C.M. (1975) *The Vulva*. Major Problems in Dermatology, No. 5. W.B. Saunders Co., Philadelphia.

Sawday, J. (1995) *The Body Emblazoned*. Routledge, London.

Chapter 1: Embryology and congenital anomalies of the vulva

J.M. McLean

Initially the embryonic pelvis or tail fold contains only the hindgut, which terminates at the cloacal membrane. Subsequently the urorectal septum divides the hindgut and cloacal membrane into the ventral or anterior urogenital sinus and genital membrane and the dorsal or posterior terminal gastrointestinal tract and anal membrane. At a later stage the female reproductive tract develops within the urorectal septum and in doing so incorporates part of the urogenital sinus and body wall elements associated with the genital membrane. Thus, the pelvis eventually accommodates parts of the urinary, reproductive and gastrointestinal systems, all of which communicate with the exterior at the pelvic outlet. That part of the pelvic outlet caudal to the pelvic floor is the anatomical perineum, which is divided by a line joining the ischial tuberosities into an anterior urogenital triangle and a posterior anal triangle. The anal triangle, bounded by the sacrotuberous ligaments, contains the anal canal and ischiorectal fossae. The urogenital triangle, contained within the subpubic arch, is occupied by the vulva.

Although the critical events in the embryogenesis and organogenesis of the female reproductive tract are genetically determined, the subsequent processes of differentiation are also crucial to the development of the urinary system and terminal part of the gastrointestinal system. Thus, congenital abnormalities of the female reproductive tract, including the vulva, may occur in isolation or in association with urinary or gastrointestinal abnormalities. Some of the aetiological factors responsible for abnormal or ambiguous human sexual development have now been established. This information has helped rationalize the medical management of affected individuals. In addition, these 'experiments of nature' have provided much information concerning the biological mechanisms underlying normal sexual development.

Embryology and development

Human life and development begin at fertilization when the spermatozoon and ovum fuse to form the zygote or conceptus. Each of the participating gametes contributes more than a million genetic units to the single-cell zygote in an arrangement unique to that human being. The normal haploid set of 23 chromosomes in each gamete yields a zygote with the diploid set of 46 chromosomes. Six days after fertilization the conceptus begins the process of implantation in the endometrium, which establishes a relationship with the mother essential to its survival. The first 8 weeks of gestation constitute the embryonic period during which the essential form of the human infant is established. Indeed the crucial events of human development occur during the first quarter of gestation. Thereafter maturation and growth occur and continue post-partum, throughout childhood and into adulthood.

Because development is a continuous process, various means have been used to identify and tabulate the progression of events during normal human embryogenesis. Franklin Mall, the founder of the Department of Embryology at the Carnegie Institution in Washington, was the first to introduce staging into human embryology. His observations, and those of George Streeter, his successor at the Carnegie Institution, form the basis upon which the first 8 weeks of human development are described in 23 Carnegie stages. Alternatively, embryonic length or age may be used as a means of identifying the developmental stage. Generally the crown–rump length of larger embryos and all fetuses should be stated in preference to, or at least in addition to, the supposed age (O'Rahilly & Muller 1987) but in this account the reference point will be the post-ovulatory age, i.e. the length of time since the last ovulation, related when appropriate, to the Carnegie stage. Since ovulation and fertilization are closely related in time the post-ovulatory interval is an adequate measure of embryonic age. Embryonic age, length and stage are all interrelated. Age, however, conveys an immediate meaning, since it is a familiar yardstick, but it must be recognized that prenatal ages are only as useful as postnatal ages, since they are reference points for the usual pattern or range of developmental events.

Fertilization

At ovulation the oocyte has a diameter of 100 µm and is enclosed by the zona pellucida, a non-cellular envelope, 16–18 µm thick (Allen *et al.* 1930), which is thought to be produced by the follicular cells (O'Rahilly & Muller 1987). Each female gamete begins its first meiotic division during intrauterine life and completes it at ovulation while its second meiotic division is only completed if fertilization occurs (Uebele-Kallhardt 1978). Carnegie stage 1 of embryogenesis begins with the entry of the fertilizing spermatozoon into the oocyte and ends with the first mitotic division of the zygote. The female gamete's protracted reduction division delivers 23 X chromosomes to the newly formed zygote, which also receives 23 X or 23 Y chromosomes from the male gamete. The resulting chromosomal complement or karyotype of the zygote is either 46XX or 46XY and thus its genetic or chromosomal sex is established. The importance of the first cleavage division is that it heralds the onset of Carnegie stage 2 of human embryogenesis. After *in vivo* fertilization the first cleavage division takes place some time between 24 and 30 hours after fertilization (Hertig 1968), whereas after *in vitro* fertilization it occurs some 22 to 40 hours after insemination (Bolton & Braude 1987).

SEX CHROMOSOMES

While studying spermatogenesis in the insect *Pyrrochoris apterus* the German cytologist Henking (1891) observed one of the chromosomes to remain undivided. This chromosome was therefore present in only half of the spermatozoa produced by the adult male insect. When it was later suggested (McClung 1902) that this chromosome might have a sex-determining role, it had already been designated the X chromosome (McClung 1899) and so it has remained. Thus, the male *Pyrrochoris apterus* with only one sex chromosome is XO and the female with two sex chromosomes is XX. Stevens (1905) subsequently noted a variant of the two types of spermatozoa. In the common mealworm beetle *Tenebrio molitor* she observed that spermatozoa had either 10 large chromosomes or nine large chromosomes and a single small chromosome. Since adult female cells possessed 20 large chromosomes and adult male cells one small and 19 large chromosomes, she suggested that the character of the spermatozoon determined the sex of the progeny. About the same time Wilson (1906) made identical observations and referred to the small chromosome as the Y chromosome. Thus, in *Drosophila melanogaster*, so beloved of geneticists, males are XY and females XX. The Y chromosome, however, was not considered to have any male-determining function, since, in *Drosophila*, flies with XXY chromosomes are normal fertile females while those with XO chromosomes are sterile males (Bridges 1916). Indeed the chromosomal constitution of the human male was thought to be XO (von Winiwarter 1912, Oguma & Kihara 1923) until the Y chromosome was demonstrated in man (Painter 1924).

Before the introduction of modern cytological techniques, observations on human chromosomes were not wholly reliable. With the use of dividing cells in tissue culture, however, Tjio and Levan (1956) established the human diploid number of chromosomes as 46. This was confirmed by Ford and Hamerton (1956), who also provided unequivocal evidence of the presence of an X and a Y chromosome in human male cells. These new techniques not only established the normal male and female sex chromosome constitutions, they also revealed a number of sex chromosome abnormalities associated with familiar clinical syndromes. The XXY sex chromosome pattern in Klinefelter's syndrome (Jacobs & Strong 1959) and the XO pattern in Turner's syndrome (Ford *et al.* 1959) suggested that, contrary to the situation in *Drosophila*, the human Y chromosome was male determining and the number of X chromosomes had no major effect on the process of sex determination.

SEXUAL DIFFERENTIATION AND DETERMINATION

Procreation by sexual means allows an infinite range of genetic variation, the opportunity of its unique expression and its subsequent conservation for future generations. Sex exists partly because of its powerful evolutionary advantages, although it is far from clear why there are only two sexes in vertebrates (Austin *et al.* 1981). Gonochorism, whereby males and females develop as separate individuals, may arise by the operation of environmental factors such as temperature in reptiles or host size in nematodes (Bull 1981). It is generally, although not unanimously, accepted that environmental sex determination was the first and primitive mechanism for producing two sexes and that this was later replaced by the XX/XY genotypic mechanism (Witschi 1929, Ohno 1967, Mittwoch 1971, 1975). The majority of mammalian species conform to the XY male/XX female system with the Y chromosome being male determining (Vorontsov 1973). In contrast the sex chromosome pattern in birds is ZZ male/ZW female with the W chromosome being female determining (Owen 1965). Reference to sex-determining chromosomes draws attention to the problem of distinguishing between determination and differentiation during embryogenesis. Determination describes events that irrevocably commit cells to a certain course of development, and differentiation describes the processes whereby these cells achieve this development. Since the sex of an individual is established at fertilization this may be regarded as the definitive act of determination with all that follows being processes of embryonic differentiation.

This is a sequential process whereby the genetic or chromosomal sex of the zygote determines the gonadal sex of the embryo, which itself regulates the differentiation of the internal and external genital apparatus and hence the sexual phenotype of the individual. At puberty the development of secondary sexual characteristics reinforces the phenotypic manifestations of the sexual dimorphism, which achieves its biological fulfilment in successful procreation. Both male and female embryos possess the same indifferent gonadal and genital primordia, which have an inherent tendency to feminize unless there is active interference by masculinizing factors. An ovary differentiates unless the indifferent embryonic gonad becomes a testis under the influence of 'a battery of genes on the Y chromosome . . . and certain genes on other chromosomes' (Mittwoch & Burgess 1991). Female differentiation of the internal and external sexual organs occurs in the absence of a testis whether or not ovaries are present. The sexual dimorphism that results from sexual differentiation in placental mammals is mediated by the testis and its secretions. Furthermore this male differentiation takes place in an environment of high oestrogen and progestogen concentrations. By contrast, in birds it is the W chromosome of the heterogametic female (ZW) that imposes ovarian differentiation on the indifferent gonad, and the ovarian secretions that induce feminization of the internal and external sexual organs. The homogametic avian zygote develops the male phenotype in the absence of any hormonal stimulus (Mittwoch 1981).

In humans, these differentiating processes are regulated by at least 30 specific genes located on sex chromosomes or autosomes that act through a variety of mechanisms, including organizing factors, sex steroid and peptide secretions and specific tissue receptors (Grumbach & Conte 1992).

Early embryogenesis

Progress in assisted human reproduction and parliamentary legislation (Human Fertilization and Embryology Act 1990) have focused attention on the early stages of human embryogenesis. The events of this period are critically important for the subsequent development of all organ systems including the genitourinary and terminal gastrointestinal systems.

Carnegie stage 1 embraces the process of fertilization in which the human zygote, with its XX or XY sex chromosome constitution, is conceived in the distal third of the uterine tube (Croxatto & Ortiz 1975). Carnegie stage 2 extends from the two-cell embryo, through the dissolution of the zona pellucida, to the appearance of the fluid-filled segmentation cavity, which identifies the blastocyst and enables embryonic and trophoblastic cells to be specifically identified (Fig. 1.1). Carnegie stage 3 is the period of development during which the blastocyst normally lies free within the female reproductive tract. The embryo subsequently adheres to, penetrates and is eventually buried within the endometrium during the process of implantation, which extends from the sixth to the 12th post-ovulatory day and embraces Carnegie stages 4 and 5 (O'Rahilly & Muller 1987). During this period the outer envelope of cytotrophoblast, forming the wall of the blastocyst, generates syncytiotrophoblast on its external surface (Enders 1965, Tao & Hertig 1965) and extraembryonic mesoderm on its internal surface (Hertig & Rock 1949). The syncytiotrophoblast, cytotrophoblast and extraembryonic mesoderm together form the chorion (Fig. 1.2a).

The primitive amniotic cavity develops some $7\frac{1}{2}$ days after fertilization (Blechschmidt 1968, Luckett 1973) and its floor forms the primary ectoderm (Fig. 1.2b). The primary endoderm is probably formed from ectoderm by cells that migrate around the blastocoelic cavity (Heuser & Streeter 1941) and enclose the yolk sac. The ectoderm covering the floor of the amniotic cavity and the endoderm

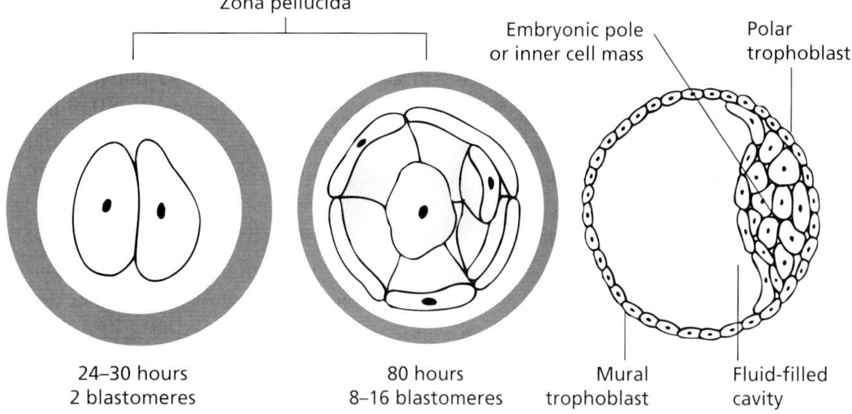

Fig. 1.1 The conceptus is enclosed within an acellular envelope, the zona pellucida. After the formation of the blastocyst and dissolution of the zona pellucida the characteristic fluid-filled cavity, the embryonic pole or inner cell mass and the mural trophoblast can be identified.

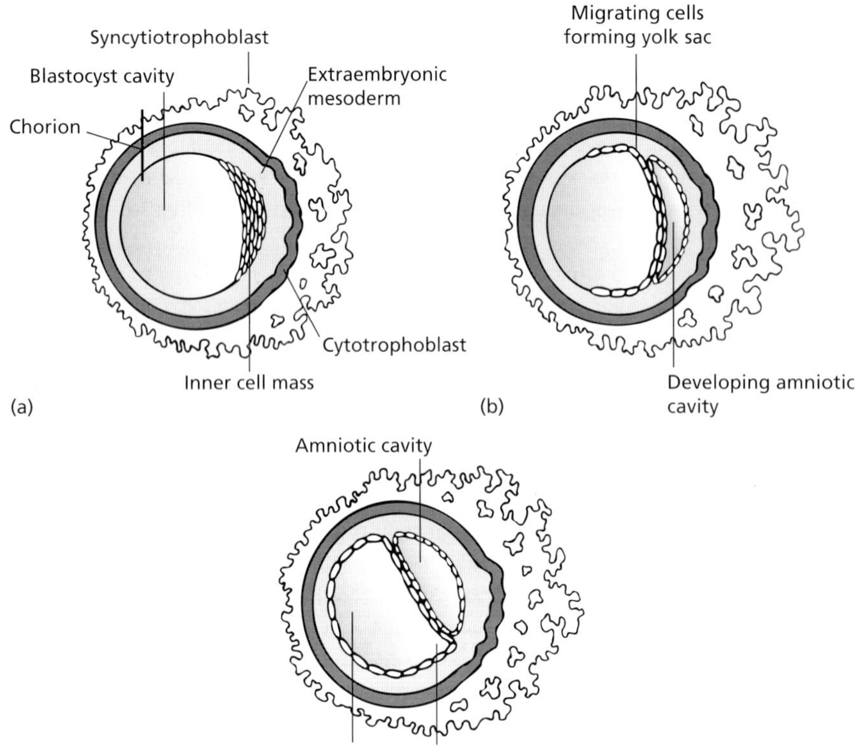

Fig. 1.2 The conceptus continues to differentiate forming (a) the chorion, (b) the amniotic cavity and (c) the yolk sac. The area of contact between the amniotic cavity and yolk sac is the bilaminar embryonic disc.

forming the roof of the yolk sac, together in apposition, establish the bilaminar embryonic disc (Fig. 1.2c). A projection of the yolk sac endoderm into the extraembryonic mesoderm forms the allantoic diverticulum and its location identifies the caudal end of the bilaminar embryonic disc and the site of the body stalk (Fig. 1.2c).

During the 13th, 14th and 15th post-ovulatory days (Carnegie stage 6) several significant events occur within the conceptus, one of which is the formation of the primitive streak (Fig. 1.3a) lying caudally in the midline of the embryonic disc (Heuser & Streeter 1941). The primitive streak subsequently generates intraembryonic mesoderm, which migrates through the bilaminar embryonic disc, in the plane between ectoderm and endoderm (Fig. 1.3b), and converts it into a trilaminar disc. Two areas of ectoderm–endoderm apposition remain: the cloacal membrane immediately caudal to the primitive streak, and the buccopharygneal membrane, immediately rostral to the notochord, which itself extends from the rostral end of the primitive streak (Fig. 1.3b). At the same time, the intraembryonic coelom, the forerunner of the pericardial, pleural and peritoneal cavities, is being formed within the intraembryonic mesoderm (Fig. 1.4).

Carnegie stage 9, from the 19th to the 21st day, heralds the onset of that phase of embryogenesis dominated by the formation of the neural plate and the longitudinally running neural ridges (Figs 1.5 & 1.6). During the next 5 days the neural ridges fuse and the primitive neural tube is buried in the underlying mesoderm (Fig. 1.6d).

The growth of the nervous system initially produces a simple dorsal convexity and ventral concavity (Fig. 1.7a). Eventually the portion of the embryo that accommodates the neural tube attains maximum dorsal convexity (Fig. 1.7b) and the once rostral and caudal portions of the embryo are so displaced ventrally that the neural tube is freed from their constraining influences. Unimpeded, the neural tube extends rostrally and caudally, overriding the now ventrally displaced original rostral and caudal regions of the embryonic disc, which are therefore inverted and reversed in the formation of the head and tail folds (Fig. 1.7c). Neural tube closure and growth has also effected significant folding in the transverse plane, producing the lateral folds (Fig. 1.6d). This process of flexion reorientates the primitive embryonic tissues and structures and establishes new relationships between them, which are essential to subsequent development. The endoderm of the dorsal part of the yolk sac is drawn into the ventral concavity of the embryo and is subdivided into foregut, midgut and hindgut. The hindgut is caudal to the rostral limit of the allantoic diverticulum and also dorsal and rostral to the cloacal membrane (Fig. 1.8a). The intraembryonic mesoderm in the midembryo region (Fig. 1.8b) is subdivided into paraxial mesoderm, lateral mesoderm and intermediate mesoderm. The paraxial mesoderm surrounds the neural

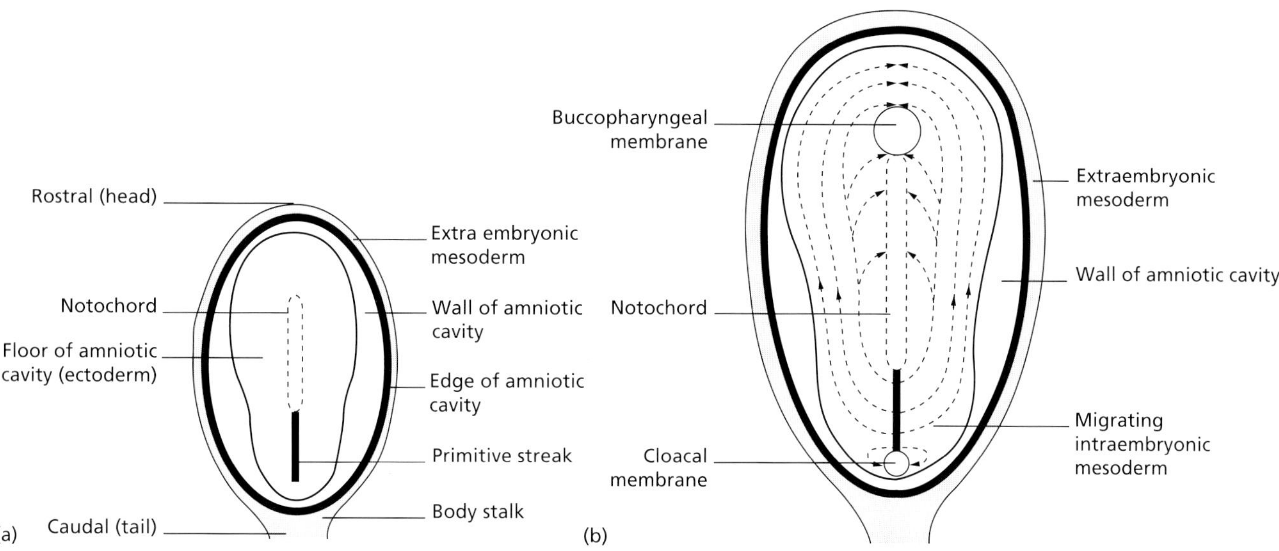

Fig. 1.3 (a) A diagrammatic view of the floor of the amniotic cavity, the dorsal surface of the bilaminar embryonic disc, revealing the primitive streak and notochord. (b) Intraembryonic mesoderm, generated by the primitive streak and interposed between the floor of the amniotic cavity and roof of the yolk sac, converts the bilaminar embryonic disc into a trilaminar disc. The buccopharyngeal and cloacal membranes remain bilaminar.

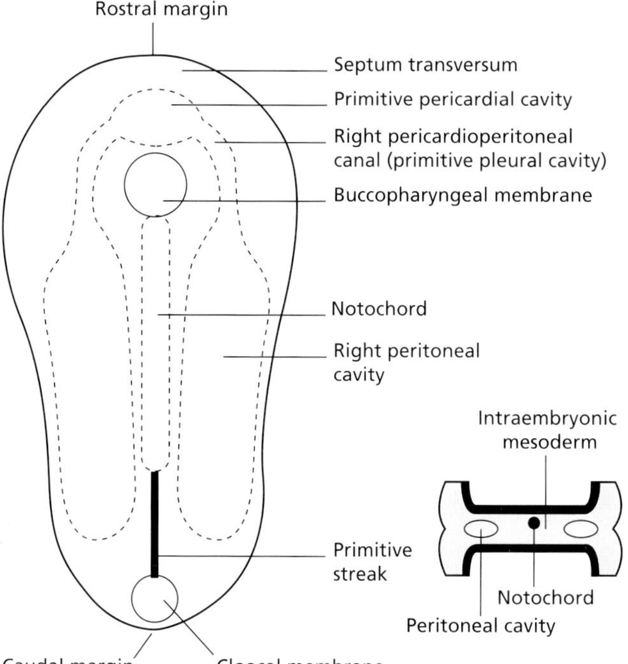

Fig. 1.4 The intraembryonic coelom forms within the intraembryonic mesoderm of the trilaminar embryonic disc.

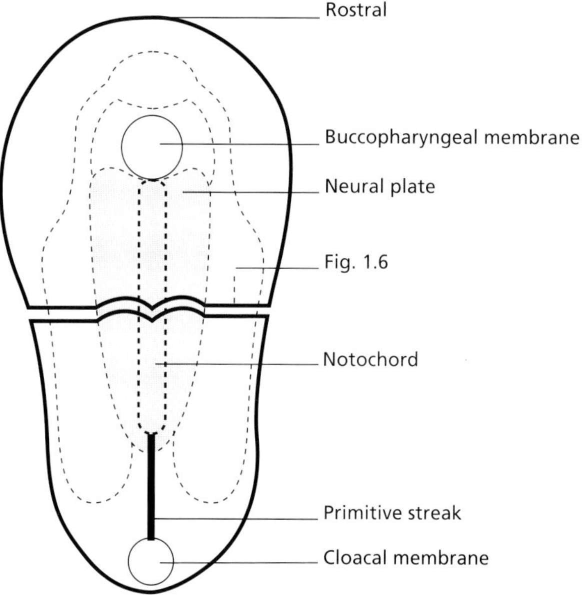

Fig. 1.5 The ectoderm on the dorsal surface of the trilaminar embryonic disc overlying the notochord forms the neural plate.

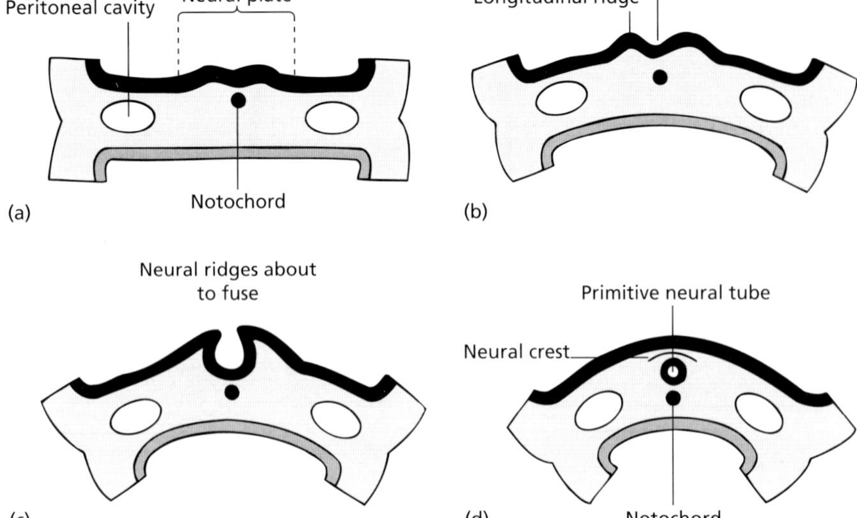

Fig. 1.6 (a) A midline longitudinal groove appears in the neural plate ectoderm. (b) The neural groove deepens with elevation of the neural ridges. (c) The neural ridges approximate and fuse to form the neural tube. (d) As the neural tube is enclosed by the intraembryonic mesoderm the trilaminar embryo folds in the transverse plane displaying a dorsal convexity and ventral concavity.

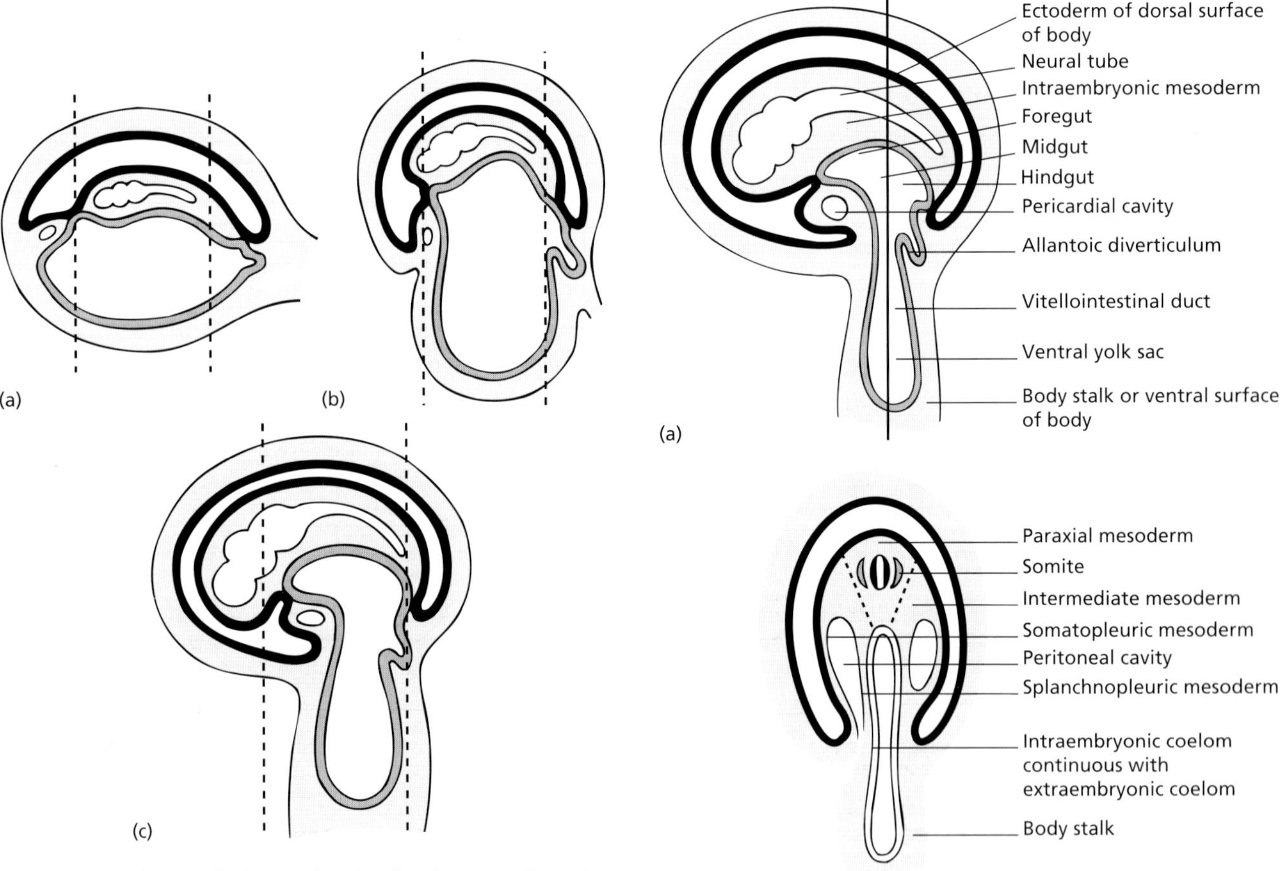

Fig. 1.7 (a) As the neural tube is enclosed within the intraembryonic mesoderm it lengthens, and expands rostrally, causing a dorsal convexity and ventral concavity. (b) Further growth of the neural tube increases this curvature in the longitudinal plane, (c) with the eventual formation of the head and tail folds.

Fig. 1.8 (a) A midline section of the embryo after formation of the head and tail folds. (b) A transverse section of the midembryo region after formation of the lateral folds.

tube and is the site of somite formation. The lateral mesoderm, so named because of its location in the flat trilaminar embryo, is carried ventrally by the formation of the lateral folds. The lateral mesoderm accommodates the primitive peritoneal cavity, which divides it into splanchnopleuric mesoderm, associated with endoderm and destined to form the visceral muscle of the gut derivatives, and somatopleuric mesoderm, associated with ectoderm and destined to participate in the formation of the body wall. The intermediate mesoderm lies between the paraxial and lateral mesoderm. It is within the intermediate mesoderm that important elements of the genitourinary system develop.

The indifferent embryo

The intermediate mesoderm extends the length of the body cavity (Fig. 1.9). It is lateral and ventral to the paraxial mesoderm and adjacent to the midline dorsal mesentery of the gut tube, which is itself being formed at this time (Keith 1948). At the caudal limit of the intraembryonic coelom or primitive peritoneal cavity the intermediate mesoderm is in continuity with the mesoderm investing the terminal or cloacal portion of the hindgut (Fig. 1.9). Change and differentiation are continuous during organogenesis and several events are taking place during the same time period and are relevant to more than one system. In particular, some of the events involved in the development of the urinary system, reproductive system and terminal part of the digestive system are interrelated and interdependent.

THE URORECTAL SEPTUM

The hindgut appears about the 20th post-ovulatory day, during Carnegie stage 9 (O'Rahilly & Muller 1987) and is established during the process of flexion as that part of the primitive yolk sac enclosed within the tail fold of the embryo. In this situation the hindgut lies caudal to the rostral limit of the allantoic diverticulum and dorsal and rostral to the cloacal membrane (Fig. 1.10a). The mesoderm at the rostral limit of the allantoic diverticulum extends dorsally then caudally, in line with the curvature of the tail fold, dividing the hindgut into ventral and dorsal parts. As the division proceeds, the two parts of the hindgut remain in continuity with each other caudal to the advancing mesoderm of the urorectal septum (Fig. 1.10b). The mesoderm reaches the cloacal membrane at 30–32 days (O'Rahilly 1977) as the Carnegie stage moves from 13 to 14 (O'Rahilly & Muller 1987). As the urorectal septum fuses with the cloacal membrane, the embryonic hindgut is completely divided into the ventral (anterior) urogenital sinus and dorsal (posterior) rectum (Fig. 1.10c). The formation of the urorectal septum transforms the caudal part of the

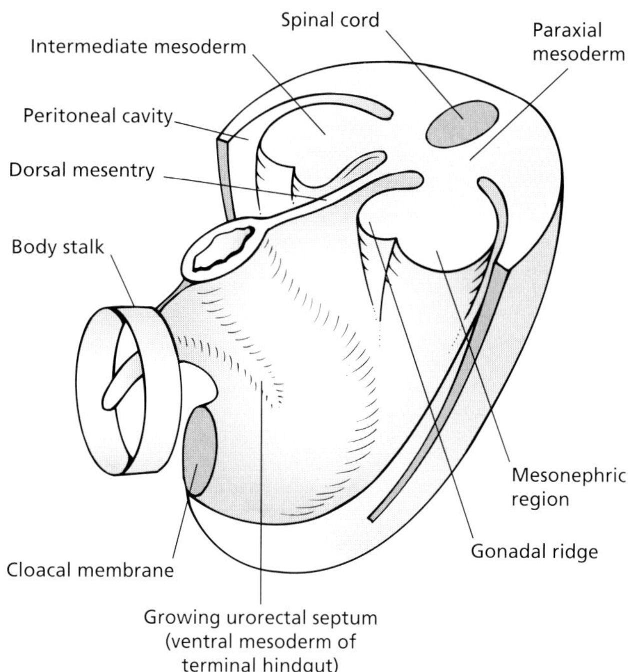

Fig. 1.9 The caudal half of the embryo showing the gonadal ridge and mesonephric region of the intermediate mesoderm, which, at its caudal limit, is continuous with the mesoderm investing the hindgut.

embryo. In the future pelvis the block of mesoderm, interposed between the dorsal gut tube and the ventral urogenital sinus, is in direct continuity across the side wall of the gut tube with the intermediate mesoderm (Fig. 1.11). Indeed the caudal limit of the intermediate mesoderm 'runs into' the urorectal septum (Fig. 1.11).

THE MESONEPHRIC DUCTS

The first indication of the urinary system in the human embryo appears at 22 days with the formation of the nephrogenic cord within the intermediate mesoderm (O'Rahilly & Muller 1992). Nephrogenic vesicles arising from the nephrogenic cord are medially associated with branches of the dorsal aorta. Laterally they remain associated with the nephrogenic cord, which acquires a lumen at 26 days and forms the mesonephric duct (O'Rahilly & Muller 1992). The mesonephric vesicles open into the mesonephric duct as it extends caudally through the intermediate mesoderm. Skirting the gastrointestinal hindgut the bilateral mesonephric ducts enter the developing urorectal septum to reach the posterior (dorsal) surface of the urogenital sinus, still incompletely divided from the rectum. The mesonephric ducts open into the urogenital sinus at 28 days during Carnegie stage 13 (O'Rahilly 1977). Thereafter the urorectal septum completes the separation of the urogenital sinus from the rectum. The functioning

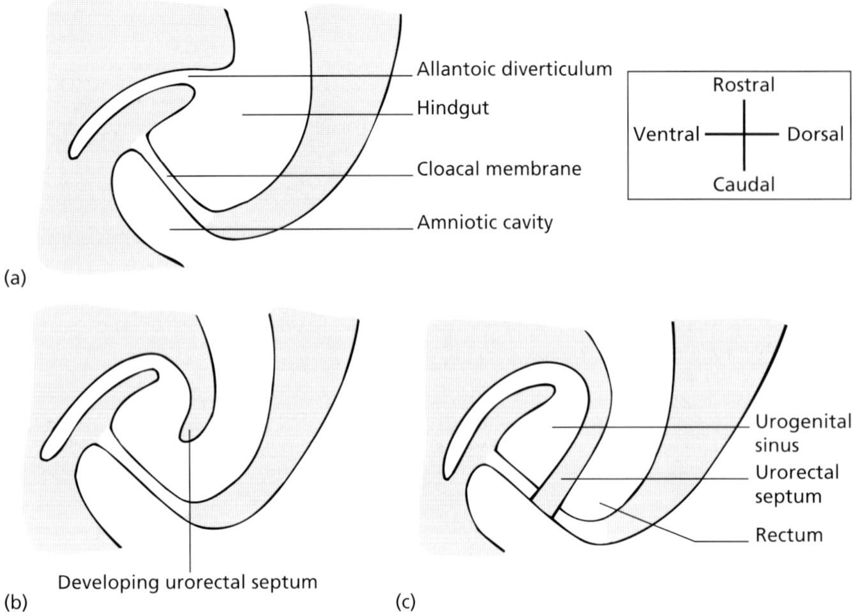

Fig. 1.10 (a) The primitive hindgut is enclosed within the embryonic tail fold. (b) The developing urorectal septum grows dorsally and caudally from the rostral limit of the allantoic diverticulum. (c) The fusion of the urorectal septum with the cloacal membrane divides the hindgut into urogenital sinus and rectum.

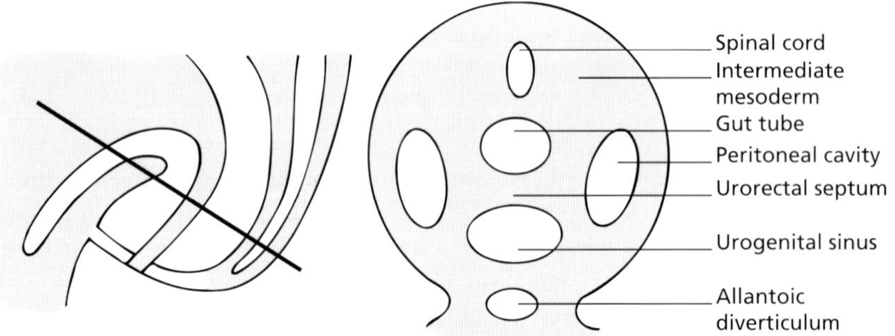

Fig. 1.11 A transverse section through the embryonic pelvis demonstrates the continuity of the intermediate mesoderm with the mesoderm of the urorectal septum.

mesonephros produces an increase in pressure in the closed urogenital sinus, which ruptures the ventral part of the cloacal membrane and allows the urogenital sinus to communicate with the amniotic cavity (Ludwig 1965).

In 1759, Caspar Friedrich Wolff, in a publication concerned with the embryology of the chick, described a symmetrical pair of paravertebral swellings as being the precursors of the kidneys. Later Rathke (1825) referred to these areas in which the mesonephros was developing as 'Wolffian bodies after Wolff'. The term Wolffian was subsequently used by other investigators to describe the duct and vesicles of the mesonephros (Stephens 1982). The mesonephros has only a transient renal function in the human embryo but its excretory duct is crucial to the subsequent development of the kidney. As the urorectal septum reaches the cloacal membrane at 30–32 days, the caudal end of each mesonephric duct, having already opened into the urogenital sinus, gives origin to a ureteric bud and itself begins to be incorporated into the posterior wall of the urogenital sinus (Keith 1948). The portion of each mesonephric duct incorporated into the urogenital sinus subsequently forms the trigone of the bladder and the posterior wall of the urethra (Fig. 1.12). The ureteric bud arising from the mesonephric duct ascends the duct's path of descent and acquiring a lumen eventually forms the collecting system and ureter of the ipsilateral kidney. As the ureteric bud appears, intermediate mesoderm condenses at its growing end to form the metanephric cap (Fig. 1.12c) within which nephrons develop. The mesonephros achieves its maximum size and maximum excretory function in the human embryo at 42 days (Potter & Osathanondh 1966). At the same stage of development nephrons appear in the metanephric cap (Kissane 1974) and begin to function at 50 days (Potter & Osathanondh 1966). Thereafter the metanephros begins to take over the excretory function of the mesonephros and the mesonephric vesicles begin to degenerate.

THE PARAMESONEPHRIC DUCTS

Johannes Muller (1830), in a publication concerned with genital development, described a cord (of cells) on the outer

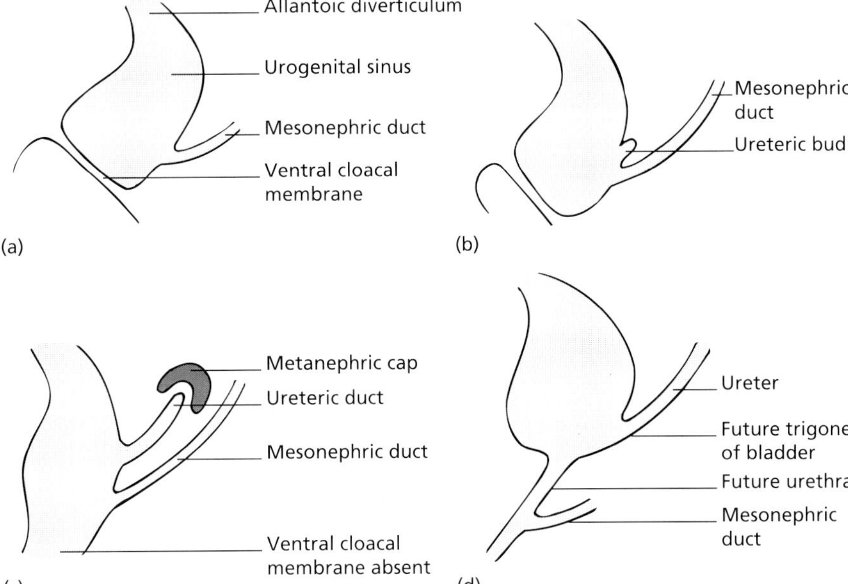

Fig. 1.12 (a) The mesonephric duct, within the urorectal septum, opens into the urogenital sinus. (b) The caudal limit of the mesonephric duct gives origin to the ureteric bud. (c) The metanephric cap forms at the growing end of the ureteric bud or duct. (d) The mesonephric duct gives origin to the ureter and forms the trigone of the bladder and the posterior wall of the urethra.

aspect of the Wolffian body that was much thinner than the Wolffian cord. He concluded that, although the two cords were either attached or adjacent to each other, they were 'two quite different things'. These Mullerian ducts are now referred to as the paramesonephric ducts and they appear in the human embryo at about 40 days. Each duct is initially observed as a thickening and invagination of the coelomic epithelium on the lateral aspect of the intermediate mesoderm at the cephalic end of the mesonephros (Felix 1912, Faulconer 1951). The site of the invagination later becomes the abdominal ostium of the uterine tube with its associated fimbriae. The precursor of each paramesonephric duct extends caudally as a solid rod of cells in the intermediate mesoderm, in close association with, and initially lateral to, the mesonephric duct. The mesonephric duct has been shown experimentally both to induce the paramesonephric duct (Didier 1973a,b) and to guide its descent (Gruenwald 1941); indeed the growing caudal tip of the paramesonephric duct lies within the basement membrane of the mesonephric duct (Frutiger 1969). As the paramesonephric cord of cells continues its descent, a lumen appears in its cranial portion, which is in continuity with the intraembryonic coelom. This lumen extends caudally behind the growing tip of the paramesonephric cord converting it into a duct. During descent the paramesonephric ducts pass ventral to the mesonephric ducts and, coming into close association with one another, reach the posterior aspect of the urogenital sinus within the urorectal septum (Fig. 1.13). Indeed as soon as the two paramesonephric ducts come into contact they begin to fuse even before their growing ends reach the urogenital sinus (Koff 1933). The external surface of their medial walls, initially in apposition, begin to fuse and eventually the duct lumina are separated only by a median septum (O'Rahilly 1977). At 49 days, before the paramesonephric ducts reach the urogenital sinus, a tubercle appears on the internal aspect of its posterior wall between the openings of the mesonephric ducts. This tubercle is not formed by the paramesonephric ducts but identifies the site at which the common paramesonephric duct fuses with the posterior wall of the urogenital sinus at 56 days (Glenister 1962, Josso 1981).

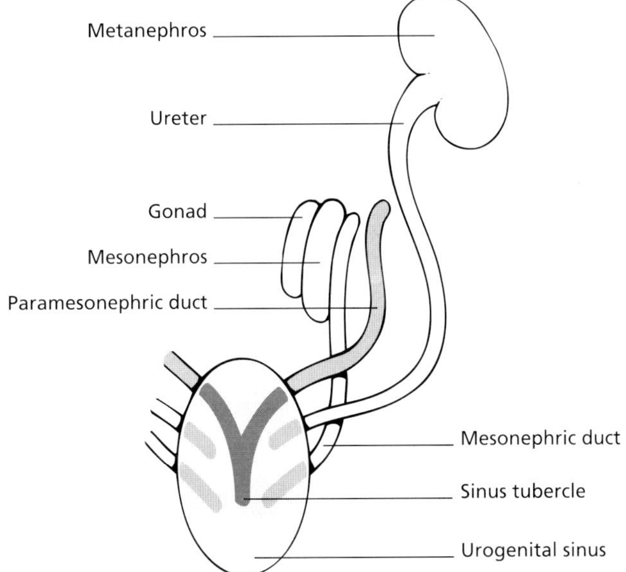

Fig. 1.13 The indifferent human embryo possesses mesonephric and paramesonephric ducts. The terminal paramesonephric ducts fuse within the urorectal septum and reach the urogenital sinus at the sinus tubercle situated between the openings of the two mesonephric ducts.

PRIMORDIAL GERM CELLS

Perhaps the most significant event of early embryogenesis is the separation of a clone of gonia or primordial germ cells, subsequently capable of mitosis and meiosis, from the pool of somatic cells capable only of mitosis. In the female mammal these gonia also retain two functional X chromosomes in contrast to the somatic cells, which possess only one functional X chromosome (Lyon 1974). Although Hertig *et al.* (1958) identified possible gonia 'stuffed with glycogen' within the yolk sac endoderm of the allantoic diverticulum in a 13-day embryo, they are unmistakably present in the allantoic diverticulum and adjacent parts of the yolk sac in 17–20-day embryos (Jirasek 1977).

From this location the primordial germ cells migrate (Figs 1.9 & 1.14a) through the mesoderm surrounding the hindgut and into the dorsal mesentery (Hardisty 1978). The destination of these migrating cells is the medial aspect of the intermediate mesoderm adjacent to the mesonephros (Fig. 1.9) and they begin to reach this area in the human embryo at 35 days (Jirasek 1971). The mechanisms that initiate and direct the migration of the gonia to the future gonad are unknown.

THE INDIFFERENT GONAD

The area to which the primordial germ cells migrate is referred to as the indifferent gonad until gonadal sex is established. At 35 days the indifferent gonad begins to be formed on the medial aspect of the mesonephros by the invasion of that area of the intermediate mesoderm by three other cell types: the primordial germ cells, cells from the overlying coelomic epithelium and the cells from the adjacent mesonephros. All four cell types are probably essential to the proper differentiation of the gonad (Byskov 1981).

Germ cells are the *sine qua non* of a functional gonad; yet their absence, achieved by experimental means in rat embryos, does not wholly suppress the formation of the gonad (Merchant 1975). In normal circumstances the primordial germ cells, having entered the mesoderm of the indifferent gonad, undergo rapid mitotic proliferation. Before the gonads are established as testes or ovaries the pattern of germ-cell proliferation is similar in both sexes.

The basal lamina of the somatic coelomic epithelium overlying the medial aspect of the intermediate mesoderm in the region of the mesonephros is incomplete, and dividing epithelial cells readily invade the underlying mesoderm. The proliferating ceolomic epithelial cells at the cranial end of the mesonephros condense to form the primordium of the cortex (Crowder 1957). Just caudal to this adrenal area is the gonadal mesoderm. The epithelial adrenal cells link up with other cells originating from the mesonephros to establish the urogenital connection (Brambell 1956). These events occur between day 35 and day 42 (Jirasek 1977) and establish the main features of the indifferent gonad.

EMERGENT GONADAL SEX

Until approximately 42 days of gestation, male and female embryos are indistinguishable morphologically (Fig. 1.15). At this stage there are 300–1300 primordial germ cells within the indifferent gonads destined to become either spermatogonia or oogonia. The close association between the gonad and adrenal at this early stage of development

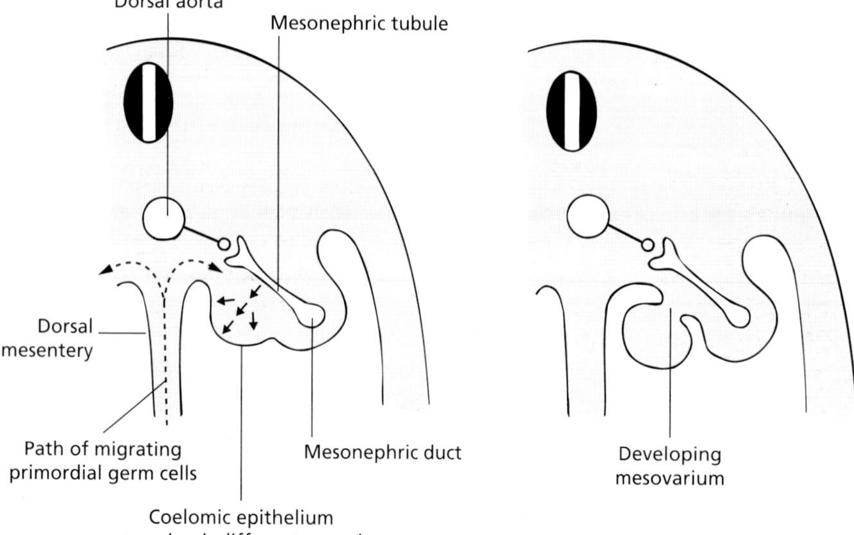

Fig. 1.14 A transverse section showing (a) the invasion of the indifferent gonad by mesonephric cells and primordial germ cells and (b) the developing mesovarium.

can result in adrenal cells being sequestered in the gonad and maintaining their function in the mature ovary or testis (Grumbach & Conte 1992).

The transformation of the indifferent gonad into an embryonic testis occurs in 43–49-day embryos during Carnegie stage 18 (Jirasek 1977). After differentiation of the testes, Leydig cells become evident at 56 days. Their numbers increase, are maximal between 90 and 120 days, decline thereafter and disappear shortly after birth (Mancini *et al.* 1963). Testosterone production, which is directly related to the number of Leydig cells in the testes (Zondek & Zondek 1979), begins at 56 days and reaches a peak towards midgestation (Siiteri & Wilson 1974). In addition to testosterone, the developing testes secrete another hormone as predicted by Jost (1947). This anti-Mullerian hormone (AMH) is synthesized by Sertoli cells (Blanchard & Josso 1974), which appear in the differentiating testes at 60 days (Jirasek 1977). AMH secretion begins and continues until puberty when its serum concentration declines (Hudson *et al.* 1990). The initial role of AMH during early gestation is to cause paramesonephric duct regression while the ducts remain responsive to the hormone's action (Josso *et al.* 1977). Thereafter AMH is thought to be involved in the process of testicular descent and the suppression of male germ-cell meiosis (Josso & Picard 1986).

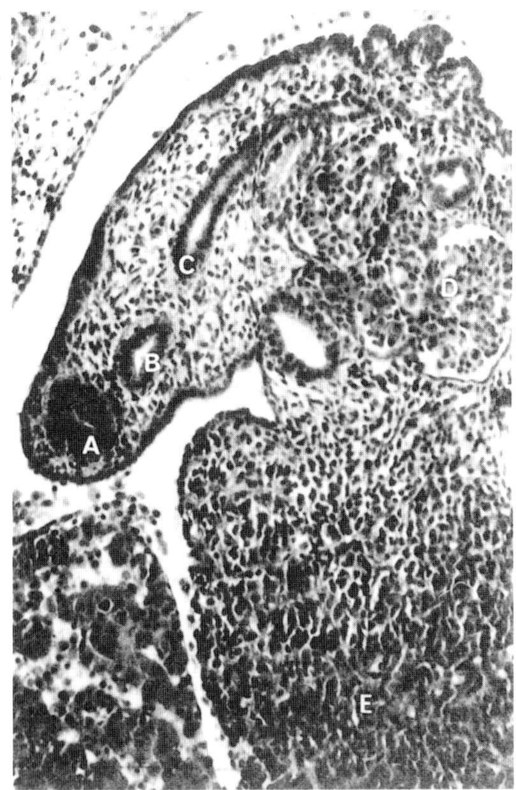

Fig. 1.15 A transverse section of the right side of the upper abdomen of a 42-day embryo showing: A, the pararamesonephric duct with a barely discernible lumen; B, the mesonephric duct; C, a mesonephric tubule; D, the mesonephros; E, the gonad. (H & E × 325.)

The transformation of the indifferent gonad into an embryonic ovary occurs gradually in 45–55-day embryos during Carnegie stages 18–22 (Jirasek 1977). An indifferent gonad with germ cells in meiosis is an ovary since meiotic division does not occur in the testes until puberty. The stage of ovarian development at which meiosis begins varies between species (Grinsted & Aagesen 1984). In the human embryo, germ cells are distributed evenly throughout the gonad and their entry into meiosis follows the early stages of ovarian differentiation. The onset of meiosis begins at the centre of the ovary (Waldeyer 1870) and is said to occur in the human embryo at 56–60 days (Jirasek 1977), although other investigators maintain that meiosis does not occur until 70–84 days (Baker 1963). This discrepancy probably results from difficulty in identifying the earliest stages of the first meiotic division. The first germ cells to enter meiosis and form follicles are those which made first contact with the mesonephric-derived cells (Byskov 1975). It has been shown in mouse and sheep ovaries that granulosa cells originate from mesonephric tissue (Zamboni *et al.* 1979). In the human ovary, follicles begin to form sometime between 12 weeks (Gondos & Hobel 1973) and 16 weeks (Jirasek 1977) of gestation. About this stage of development there is some evidence of steroidogenesis by interstitial cells (Resko 1977, Block 1979) but no evidence of steroid secretion by the developing human ovary (Reyes *et al.* 1973).

Mechanisms of gonadal differentiation

As indicated earlier, investigation of patients with numerical abnormalities of the sex chromosomes has shown the Y chromosome to be extremely potent in inducing testicular differentiation (Ford *et al.* 1959, Jacobs & Strong 1959).

THE Y CHROMOSOME

All chromosomes have a constriction at some point along their length, termed the centromere, and this point is fixed for each chromosome. The centromere, which itself has specific functions, divides the chromosome into a short arm, p, and a long arm, q. The terminal portion of each arm is referred to as either pter or qter. The technique of Giemsa banding applied to human chromosomes produces a specific pattern of light and dark bands, which allows each individual chromosome to be identified. These chromosomal bands are numbered sequentially from the centromere to the terminal portion of each arm. Variations of this technique will demonstrate 350–850 bands per haploid set of chromosomes with each band representing approximately $5–10 \times 10^6$ base pairs (bp) of DNA. Since genes vary in DNA content from 10^3 bp for α-globin to more than 2×10^6 bp for Duchenne muscular dystrophy, a single band may represent either a few or many individual genes (Gelehrter & Collins 1990).

Within populations of phenotypically normal men, Y chromosomes exhibit significant differences in length (Bishop *et al.* 1962) and DNA content (Wall & Butler 1989). The length of the Y chromosome (Fig. 1.16) varies with race (Cohen *et al.* 1966) and between individuals of the same race (Lin *et al.* 1976). This characteristic of the Y chromosome is considered to be an excellent familial marker since it is transmitted from father to son (Genest *et al.* 1970). The variation in length of the Y chromosome occurs because of deletions from Yq and in particular from the distal heterochromatic segment. Since such deletions are not associated with any phenotypic effects it has been assumed that this segment, which is composed of highly repetitive DNA sequences, is genetically inactive (Grumbach & Conte 1992).

Two further regions on the Y chromosome have been identified. One, at the distal end of Ypter, recombines with the comparable region of Xpter during meiosis. Since the meiotic behaviour of these regions resembles that of autosomal chromosomes they are referred to as the pseudoautosomal regions of the sex chromosomes (Burgoyne 1982). The other, between the pseudoautosomal region and the heterochromatic portion of Yq, has been designated the sex-specific region, within which there are a number of functional genes. Cytogenetic analyses of tissues from 46XX males and 46XY females indicated that testicular development was dependent upon the DNA sequence just proximal to the pseudoautosomal region of Yp (Page 1986). Within this sequence two genes were subsequently identified, the ZFY (zinc finger Y) gene (Page *et al.* 1987) and the more distal SRY (sex-determining region Y) gene (Sinclair *et al.* 1990). Other genes present, or considered to be present, within the sex-specific region of the Y chromosome include, on Yq, one controlling histocompatibility Y (H-Y) antigen expression (Simpson *et al.* 1987) and another affecting spermatogenesis (Buhler 1980) and, on Yp, one controlling the expression of serological H-Y antigen (Wolf 1988) and another preventing the stigmata of Turner's syndrome (Grumbach 1979).

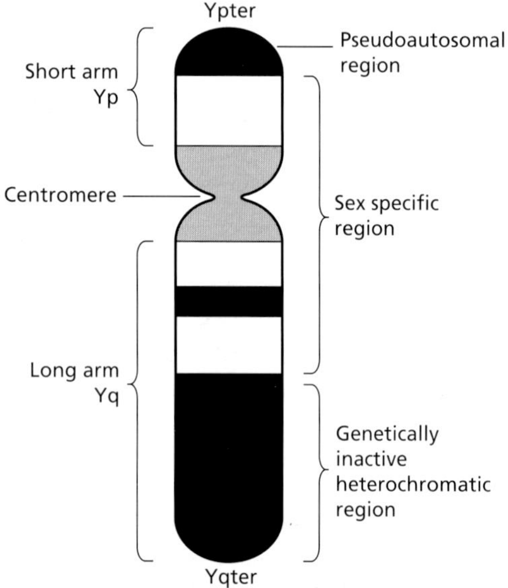

Fig. 1.16 A diagrammatic representation of a Giemsa-banded Y chromosome with the terminal portion of the short arm identified as Ypter and that of the long arm as Yqter.

Since sex determination is essentially testis differentiation (Grumbach & Conte 1992), with ovarian differentiation occurring only in the absence of a testis inducer, the search for the gene that initiates and controls testis differentiation has focused on the Y chromosome and a number of candidate genes have been proposed.

The H-Y gene

Following the identification of antibodies to H-Y antigen in the sera of female mice after rejection of male skin grafts (Goldberg *et al.* 1971), anti-H-Y serum was generated in female mice or rats by repeated injections of male spleen cells. Such antisera were used to assay H-Y antigen expression on target cells. These tests demonstrated that the H-Y antigen was invariably associated with the heterogametic sex in a wide variety of species and led to the suggestion that it was the product of the testis-determining factor that induced differentiation of the heterogametic gonad (Wachtel *et al.* 1975).

Following further experiments it was proposed that the Y chromosome possessed a locus or loci that either coded for H-Y antigen or regulated its expression (Wachtel & Ohno 1979) and that testicular differentiation would always be associated with the expression of H-Y antigen regardless of sexual phenotype or apparent karyotype (Wachtel & Koo 1981). However, it was subsequently shown that some XX phenotypic male mice with testes were H-Y antigen negative (McLaren *et al.* 1984, Goldberg 1988) indicating that the testis-determining factor on the Y chromosome was separate and distinct from the H-Y genes. This separation was confirmed when some 46XX men with testes were shown to be H-Y antigen negative (Simpson *et al.* 1987) and some 46XY women were H-Y antigen positive (Wachtel 1983, Simpson *et al.* 1987). These observations demonstrated that the H-Y genes do not encode products that initiate testicular differentiation.

The ZFY gene

Since XX males possess translocated Y chromosomal DNA on one of their X chromosomes (Affara *et al.* 1986) and XY females show comparable deletions from their Y chromosomes (Disteche *et al.* 1986) the testis-determining factor was presumed to be within the relevant DNA sequences. Page *et al.* (1987) cloned a 140-kilobase (kb) sequence of DNA that was present in an XX male and absent from an XY female. Within this region they found a conserved sequence of DNA which, when cloned, hybridized to male and female DNA of a number of species but had an extra band present in male DNA. This male-specific DNA sequence on Yp was thought to encode a zinc finger protein and was called the ZFY gene. Page *et al.* (1987) proposed that the ZFY gene was the primary sex-determining signal on the Y chromosome.

The case against ZFY being the testis-determining factor emerged in subsequent studies (Erickson & Verga 1989, Mardon & Page 1989). However, the crucial evidence against ZFY being the testis-determining factor was that some XX men do not have detectable ZFY despite having other Y chromosomal DNA sequences (Palmer *et al.* 1989).

The SRY gene

The four ZFY-negative XX males described by Palmer *et al.* (1989) had a 35-kb Y-specific translocation on one of their X chromosomes. This translocated sequence is normally located adjacent to the pseudoautosomal region of Yp, distal to the sequence within which ZFY is situated. A 2.1-kb sequence, 8 kb from the pseudoautosomal boundary, was subsequently cloned and shown to be conserved in a variety of species (Sinclair *et al.* 1990). This sequence, termed the sex-determining region of the Y chromosome or SRY gene, is thought to be present in all XX males and absent from all XY females. SRY encodes a DNA binding protein and has a counterpart on the mouse Y chromosome, the Sry gene, which is expressed at the appropriate stage of murine testis differentiation and may be gonad specific (Gubbay *et al.* 1990). Further evidence in support of SRY being the testis-determining factor was obtained from the transfer of the Sry gene to pronucleate mouse embryos. These experiments yielded eight Sry-positive XX fetuses and three Sry-positive XX adults, of which two fetuses and one adult exhibited testicular development, while the other two adults were fertile females (Koopman *et al.* 1991). This evidence, the authors suggest, is sufficient to indicate that Sry is the only Y-linked gene required for male development and they proposed Sry as the testis-determining factor.

Nevertheless, doubts remain as to the validity of this proposal. Apart from the failure of a testis to differentiate in the majority of the Sry-positive transgenic XX mice generated by Koopman *et al.* (1991), clinical reports indicate that a correctly sequenced SRY gene on an intact Y chromosome in an XY individual does not guarantee testicular differentiation (Berta *et al.* 1992, Lobaccaro *et al.* 1993).

Reviewing this issue Mittwoch (1992) argued that the hypothesis of a single dominant Y chromosomal gene being capable of determining functional testicular differentiation is not supported by the available evidence. In patients with Klinefelter's syndrome there is a sevenfold increase in the incidence of undescended testis and a much greater increase in the incidence of other congenital abnormalities, while adults have abnormal Leydig cells and reduced testosterone levels (Ratcliffe *et al.* 1979, Robinson *et al.* 1979). In males with more than two X chromosomes the pathological changes associated with a single supernumerary X chromosome are exacerbated; Leydig cells may be entirely absent (Fryns *et al.* 1983) and major malformations and severe mental retardation have been reported (de Grouchy & Turleau 1982). The evidence indicates that the dominant effect of the Y chromosome on male sexual development is attenuated in the presence of supernumerary X chromosomes resulting in sterility and hypogonadism. Comparable attenuation is evident in males with autosomal trisomies (Stearns *et al.* 1960, Sylvester & Rundle 1962).

The use of recombinant DNA technology has shown XX males to be divisible into two groups: those with Y-derived DNA sequences on one of their X chromosomes and those who apparently lack such Y chromosomal DNA (Ferguson-Smith *et al.* 1990). A comparison of the phenotypes of the Y-negative XX males (Ferguson-Smith *et al.* 1990) with those in whom the SRY sequence is present (Palmer *et al.* 1989) demonstrates similar deficiencies of masculinization. Since XX males and true hermaphrodites sometimes coexist in the same pedigree (Skordis *et al.* 1987, Abbas *et al.* 1990), the possibility exists that these two conditions represent different stages of the same spectrum of disordered sexual development. In true hermaphroditism the commonest gonadal pattern is a unilateral ovotetis with either an ovary or a testis contralaterally. In the remainder of reported cases there is an ovary on one side and a testis on the other, or there are bilateral ovotestes (van Niekerk 1981). The karyotype of such patients may be 46XX, 46XX/46XY or 46XY; they have ambiguous genitalia and possess both mesonephric (Wolffian) and paramesonephric (Mullerian) derivatives (Grumbach & Conte 1992). The possible causes of true hermaphroditism include chimerism, sex-chromosomal mosaicism, Y-to-autosome or Y-to-X chromosome translocation or mutation of either X-linked or autosomal genes involved in sexual differentiation (Grumbach & Conte 1992). Mittwoch (1992) considers that XX males are not a natural clinical entity, but are to be regarded as a subset of intersexual individuals who are not overtly hermaphrodite and whose phenotypes are nearer the male than the female distribution. She considers that the dogma of a single testis-determining factor lacks biological validity since the available evidence indicates that the development of male fertility requires the presence of multiple Y chromosomal genes and a single X chromosome which operate together in an appropriate genetic background.

Ovarian differentiation

The observations presented in the previous section suggest that ovarian differentiation is a passive event which occurs in the absence of testicular differentiation. It has, however, been known for some time that two functional X chromosomes are normally required for ovarian differentiation in the human embryo (Ford *et al.* 1959). In individuals with a 45X karyotype (Turner's syndrome) the germ cells rarely survive meiosis, follicular formation usually fails and the resulting streak gonads are sterile and devoid of endocrine activity (Carr *et al.* 1968). However, almost 25% of girls with Turner's syndrome show some pubertal development, and 2–5% have spontaneous menses due to residual ovarian function (Saenger 1996). As an interesting corollary to these observations it is well established that an XO chromosomal constitution in the mouse does not prevent the development of fertile functioning ovaries (Cattanach 1962). The occurrence of familial XX gonadal dysgenesis, transmitted as an autosomal recessive trait, also suggests that autosomal genes are essential for human ovarian organogenesis (Grumbach & Conte 1992). It is possible that a counterpart to the testis-determining factor exists in the female and that it determines ovarian differentiation.

THE X CHROMOSOME

The human X chromosome represents about 5% of the total DNA content of the haploid genome and is rich in structural genes encoding protein products involved in a diverse array of housekeeping and specialized functions (Handel & Hunt 1992). Some of these genes have a critical influence on both male and female sexual development while others, more than 130, are unrelated to sexual development (Grumbach & Conte 1992).

The X chromosome (Fig. 1.17) has a pseudoautosomal region at the end of its short arm, Xpter, homologous to that at Ypter (Burgoyne 1982). Immediately proximal to this pseudoautosomal region are a number of genes that are also represented on the Y chromosome. These include STS, the gene for steroid sulphatase (Yen *et al.* 1987), ZFX, the zinc finger gene of the X chromosome (Schneider-Gadicke

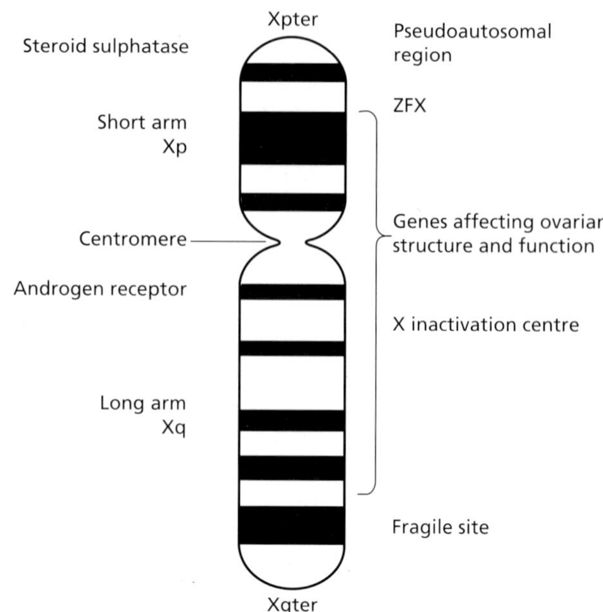

Fig. 1.17 A diagrammatic representation of a Giemsa-banded X chromosome with the terminal portion of the short arm identified as Xpter and that of the long arm as Xqter. The loci of some X-linked genes are shown.

et al. 1989), a gene that affects the expression of H-Y antigen (Wolf 1988) and others that prevent short stature and many of the somatic abnormalities associated with the syndrome of gonadal dysgenesis (Ferguson-Smith 1965, Grumbach 1968). In some 46XX patients with gonadal dysgenesis, deletions from either Xp or Xq or from both indicate that genes located on both arms of the X chromosome are involved in ovarian differentiation and maturation (Ferguson-Smith 1965, Krauss *et al.* 1987).

Numerous other genes are located on Xq. These include, in the distal part, the fragile X gene (Yu *et al.* 1991) associated with mental retardation and macro-orchidism, first described by Lubs (1969), and, in the paracentromeric region, the androgen receptor protein (Meyer *et al.* 1975) and the gene for X inactivation.

X chromosome inactivation

Any dosage differences between the sexes for this chromosome, i.e. XX, XY, suggests a compensation mechanism to avoid the effects of aneuploidy. This phenomenon was studied in *Drosophila* and the term 'dosage compensation' was introduced to describe the mechanism that allows normal development (Muller *et al.* 1931). In female mammals, dosage compensation is achieved by inactivation of one X chromosome (Lyon 1961). At some stage, therefore, in the early development of the female mammalian embryo, one of the X chromosomes in each cell is inactivated so that the effective dosage of X-linked genes is equivalent in males and females. This random inactivation is fixed for each cell and its progeny and each female becomes a cell mosaic of paternally and maternally active X chromosomes.

In somatic cells, however, inactivation does not involve the entire X chromosome. Since partial synapsis of the X and Y chromosomes was evident during meiotic prophase in numerous mammalian species, including humans (Solari 1974), it was argued that the pairing regions of Xp and Yp possessed homologous genes. Furthermore it was assumed that both groups were functional in the somatic cells of XX and XY individuals; otherwise XO individuals would not demonstrate any somatic defects (Burgoyne 1981). Thus, the pseudoautosomal regions of Xp and Yp were identified (Burgoyne 1982). Nevertheless, the genes of the pseudoautosomal region are not alone in escaping inactivation (Brown & Willard 1990).

When an X chromosome is disrupted by a translocation, only one of the two resulting segments is inactivated. This suggests that the process of inactivation requires the presence of an inactivation centre from which a signal spreads to affect those genes in physical continuity with it (Lyon 1993). Nevertheless, some human X chromosomal genes do not appear to respond to this signal since they escape inactivation. Because these genes are in inactivated regions, with inactivated genes on either side of them, the spreading signal must run through them and they must in some way either resist it or undergo reactivation (Lyon 1993). Observation of the behaviour of different X chromosome translocations has allowed the inactivation centre to be mapped to Xq13 of the human chromosome (Brown *et al.* 1991). A gene has been cloned from this region, and from the comparable region of the mouse X chromosome, which has the unique property of being expressed from the inactive, but not from the active, X chromosome (Lyon 1993). It has recently been confirmed that this is the Xist gene (Penny *et al.* 1996).

Various observations of preimplantation development in a number of mammalian species, including humans (Park 1957), indicate that X inactivation does not occur until the blastocyst stage or later. The absence of any dosage compensation during this early phase of embryogenesis must be of some functional significance in view of the potentially lethal effect of aneuploidy in mammals. The onset of X inactivation at the blastocyst stage appears to coincide with the differentiation of trophoblast, ectoderm and endoderm. Various observations suggest (Ohno *et al.* 1961, 1962, Teplitz & Ohno 1963, Ohno 1964), and it is generally accepted that inactivation does occur in primordial germ cells but that reactivation follows when the oogonia reach the gonadal mesoderm. Several studies of X-linked gene expression in human and mouse oocytes are consistent in demonstrating activity of both X chromosomes in each oocyte (Gartler & Cole 1981).

Ovarian development

One of the distinguishing features of the developing gonads is the rapid proliferation of primordial germ cells by mitosis, followed in the ovary by their entry into meiosis. Meiosis is essential to gametogenesis and consists of two cell divisions. The first, a specialized reduction division, is followed by the second, which is a modified mitotic division. During the reduction division, genetic material is exchanged between the original maternal and paternal chromosomes of each homologous pair. This exchange enables meiosis, at its completion, to generate genetically unique gametes. Meiosis I begins during intrauterine life and is completed at ovulation some 15–45 years later. Meiosis II occurs only at fertilization.

GONADAL INDUCTION

The transformation of the indifferent gonad into an embryonic ovary occurs gradually in 45–55-day embryos during Carnegie stages 18–22 (Jirasek 1977). The early fetal stage is defined by Jirasek (1977) as extending from the end of the embryonic period until the completion of the 16th week of gestation. During the first week of this early fetal period, oogonia at the centre of the gonad enter meiosis. The onset of meiosis rapidly extends peripherally to reach oogonia at the surface of the ovary. No differences have been observed in the structure of the early fetal ovaries from 45X and 46XX individuals. Normal meiotic oocytes in the early fetal ovaries of 45X individuals suggest that the presence of two X chromosomes is not necessary for the beginning of meiosis (Jirasek 1977).

The late fetal stage begins at the completion of the 16th week of gestation (Jirasek 1977). Primary follicles, which begin to form in the fetal ovary after the 16th week, are characterized by an oocyte, completely surrounded by a single layer of follicular cells and separated from the follicular cells of adjacent primary follicles by connective tissue. Oocytes that are incompletely surrounded by follicular cells degenerate. The formation of primary follicles requires the presence of two normal X chromosomes, since all the oocytes in 45X individuals degenerate because the envelope of follicular cells is incomplete (Jirasek 1977).

The fetus achieves legal viability at 24 weeks of gestation. At this stage some of the ovarian follicles consist of growing occytes surrounded by several layers of cuboidal granulosa cells. The stroma surrounding these growing follicles becomes organized into a cellular theca interna and a fibrous theca externa. Towards the end of gestation some of these compact, multilayered, growing follicles become vesicular and cells of the associated theca interna demonstrate a well-developed smooth endoplasmic reticulum and contain 3β-hydroxysteroid dehydrogenase. These growing vesicular follicles degenerate and disappear from the ovary within 6 months of birth and are not normally again present until the onset of puberty (Jirasek 1977).

During the early fetal stage, the ovaries contain 5 million primordial germ cells, oogonia and oocytes (Witschi 1962) and some 7 million at 20 weeks of gestation (Baker 1963). Their numbers decline thereafter and about 5 million germ cells degenerate before, or at, the primary follicle stage, during the remainder of gestation. This process continues after birth and it has been estimated that only 400 000 oocytes remain in the ovaries at the onset of puberty. Since no more than 400 of these will be ovulated during a woman's reproductive life, 99.9% degenerate and disappear in follicular atresia (Jirasek 1977).

Genital duct differentiation

At the end of the embryonic period, the fetus has gonads that are recognizable as either testes or ovaries, but possesses both mesonephric and paramesonephric duct systems (see Fig. 1.15). Subsequent sexual differentiation of these ducts is governed by fetal testicular hormones (Jost 1947), which cause regression of the paramesonephric ducts and further development of the mesonephric ducts. In the female fetus the absence of testicular hormones allows regression of the mesonephric ducts and development of the paramesonephric ducts.

MALE DIFFERENTIATION

Paramesonephric duct

In the human male fetus paramesonephric duct regression begins in that part of the duct adjacent to the caudal pole of the testis at 56–60 days (Jirasek 1977). Once initiated, regression extends caudally and cranially and is complete at 70 days (Jirasek 1971). The inhibitory effect of the fetal testes on paramesonephric duct development is not caused by testosterone, since experimentally induced high testosterone levels have no effect on paramesonephric ducts in the castrated male rabbit fetus (Jost 1947). The inhibitory substance, a glycoprotein termed anti-Mullerian hormone (AMH), is produced by fetal Sertoli cells (Blanchard & Josso 1974, Price, 1979), which are first identified in the human testes at 60 days (Jirasek 1977). AMH is capable of causing paramesonephric duct regression for only a very limited time during intrauterine life. Unless its action is initiated at the end of the embryonic period and rapidly completed, the paramesonephric ducts become resistant to any inhibitory effect of AMH (Josso *et al.* 1977). Persistence of paramesonephric ducts has been observed in otherwise normal human males and in some animals (Jost 1965, Josso 1979). This abnormality is X linked (Sloan & Walsh 1976) and may be due to a defect in AMH production or a block to its action. The gene coding for human AMH production has been localized to the short arm of chromosome 19 (Cohen-Haguenauer *et al.* 1987).

Although the mechanism of action of AMH on the paramesoneprhic ducts is unclear the morphological appearances indicate dissolution of the basal membrane and mesodermal condensation around the duct (Josso & Picard 1986). The fetal and postnatal testes continue to produce AMH until puberty (Hudson *et al.* 1990) and although its role during this period is unknown, it may be involved in the process of testicular descent (Hutson 1985) and the suppression of male germ-cell meiosis (Josso & Picard 1986). Postnatally, granulosa cells also secrete AMH (Ueno *et al.* 1989) resulting in serum concentrations in pubertal girls and women that are similar to those in men (Gustafson *et al.* 1992).

Mesonephric duct

The second aspect of male differentiation is the integration of the mesonephric duct into the genital system after it has completed its excretory function with the mesonephric kidney. The persistence of the mesonephric duct and its incorporation into the genital system of the male fetus is referred to as stabilization of the duct and is testosterone dependent. Mesonephric ducts removed from testicular influence by castration or explantation regress unless testosterone is administered exogenously or added to the culture medium (Jost 1947, Price & Pannabecker 1959). Testosterone production by the Leydig cells of the human testis begins at 56 days (Siiteri & Wilson 1974) and stabilization of the mesonephric ducts occur between 56 and 70 days in synchrony with the degeneration of the paramesonephric ducts (Price *et al.* 1975). Testosterone secretion by the fetal testis is controlled by maternal chorionic gonadotrophin, which binds to fetal testicular cells (Hudson & Burger 1979). Stabilization of the mesonephric ducts is brought about by testosterone, not by dihydrotestosterone since the undifferentiated mesonephric ducts lack 5α-reductase, the enzyme necessary to generate dihydrotestosterone (Siiteri & Wilson 1974).

Mesonephric ducts in young female embryos can be stabilized by exposure to testosterone before the end of the 'critical period' for sex differentiation. In humans this critical period embraces the end of embryogenesis and the beginning of early fetal life, after which exposure of the female fetus to testosterone does not prevent the degeneration of the mesonephric ducts (Josso 1981).

FEMALE DIFFERENTIATION

At the time of apparent male differentiation in the XY fetus, the comparable undifferentiated structures in the XX fetus are already irreversibly committed to female organogenesis. Female organogenesis involves stabilization of the paramesonephric ducts and regression of the mesonephric ducts.

Paramesonephric duct

At the end of the embryonic period the caudal segments of the two paramesonephric ducts have fused within the urorectal septum (O'Rahilly 1977).

Uterine tube. The upper segment of each paramesonephric duct develops fimbria at its cephalic end and subsequently forms the uterine tube. The transverse lie of the uterine tubes is established by the descent of the ovary (Fig. 1.18). As descent occurs the ipsilateral uterine tube and ovary are juxtaposed and cellular exchange takes place between them (O'Rahilly 1977). The uterotubal junction is demarcated by an abrupt increase in the diameter of the uterine segment. These changes occur progressively during the first half of intrauterine life and at term the uterine tube in the human infant is very well developed (Josso 1981).

Uterus. In the female embryo as soon as the paramesonephric ducts come into apposition within the urorectal septum and begin to fuse the uterus is being formed. At 63 days Hunter (1930) refers to the fused paramesonephric ducts as the uterus and identifies the body and the cervix by the presence of a constriction between them. The genital canal is established at 80 days when resorption of the median septum completes the fusion of the paramesonephric ducts (Koff 1933). The genital canal continues to lengthen by further fusion of the paired paramesonephric ducts at its cephalic end and by continued growth of its caudal end (O'Rahilly 1977). This growing caudal end, at its point of contact with the posterior wall of the urogenital sinus, is involved in additional cellular proliferation, which is essential to the development of the vagina.

The cervix, which forms the caudal two-thirds of the fetal uterus (Pryse-Davies & Dewhurst 1971), is generally believed to be of paramesonephric origin (Koff 1933, Forsberg 1965, Witschi 1970). It has, however, been claimed that its mucous membrane is derived from the urogenital sinus (Fluhmann 1960) but the exact contribution of para-

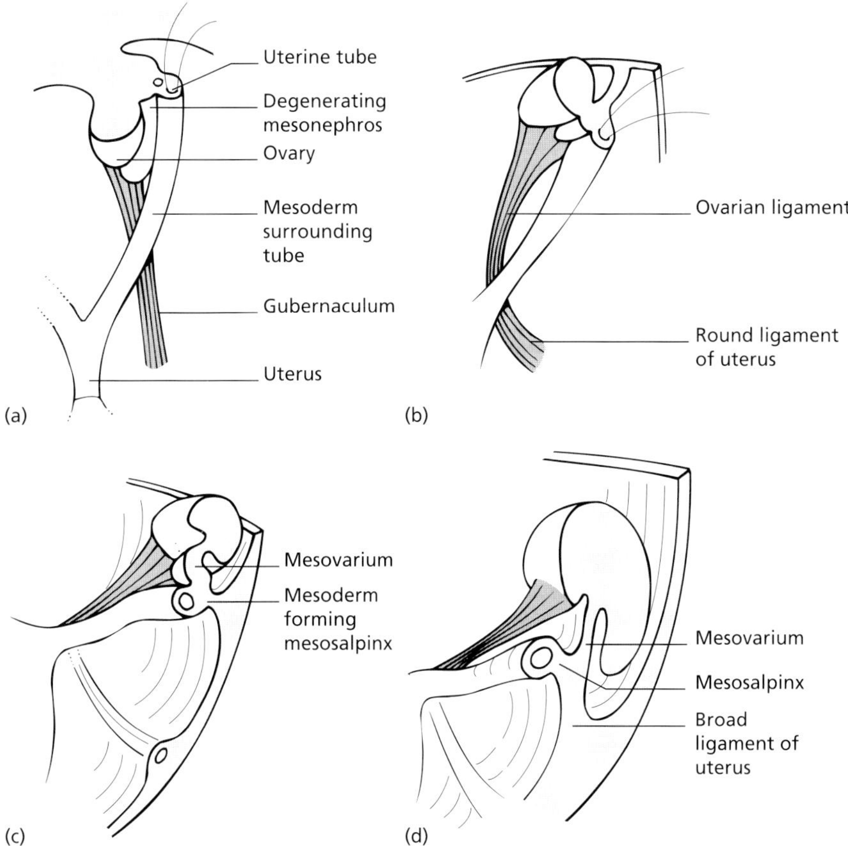

Fig. 1.18 Sequential stages in the descent of the ovary into the pelvis.

mesonephric and sinus tissue to the cervix remains uncertain (Davies & Kusama 1962). About the 17th week cervical glands appear (Koff 1933) and the future os is identifiable (Bulmer 1957). It has been variously reported that at 22 weeks the cervical canal is lined with stratified squamous epithelium with an entropion present (Eida 1961), while from 22 weeks to term the squamocolumnar junction is said to be situated some distance external to the os producing the congenital ectropion (Davies & Kusama 1962). The cervical epithelium of the newborn is described as stratified or pseudostratified columnar epithelium (Davies & Kusama 1962). Around the 19th week the corpus begins to differentiate into layers of mucosa, muscle and serosa (Hunter 1930, Witschi 1970) and approximately a week later glands begin to form in the simple columnar epithelium (Koff 1933). A well-marked fundus is apparent at 26 weeks and 'the change in the form of the upper limit of the uterus from a V-shaped notch to a convex curve . . . is due to the general thickening of its walls, brought about by the growth and development of muscle tissue' (Hunter 1930). At birth the endometrium is lined by a low columnar or cuboidal epithelium (Fluhmann 1960) and the endometrium itself may resemble either the proliferative or the secretory mucosa of the adult (Song 1964).

Vagina. For many years the conflicting opinions expressed concerning the development of the vagina were of little more than academic interest. Since the early 1970s, however, many publications have associated the occurrence of cervical and vaginal ridges, vaginal adenosis, ectropion and clear-cell carcinoma of the vagina in young adult females with prenatal exposure to diethylstilboestrol (Greenwald *et al.* 1971, Herbst *et al.* 1971, 1972, 1974, Fetherston *et al.* 1972, Hill 1973, Pomerance 1973, Barber and Sommers 1974). The drug was considered to have had a teratogenic effect on the developing lower genital tract. Uterine synechiae and hypoplasia in 60% of exposed females indicates that the teratogen also affects the upper genital tract (Kaufman *et al.* 1977). In addition, some 20% of exposed males demonstrate some abnormality of their reproductive tracts such as epididymal cysts, hypoplastic testes, cryptorchidism and spermatozoal deficiencies (Gill *et al.* 1976). It has been variously suggested that the vagina develops solely from the paramesonephric ducts (Felix 1912), the mesonephric ducts (Forsberg 1973), the urogenital sinus (Bulmer 1957, Fluhmann 1960), or from a combination of paramesonephric and mesonephric tissue (Witschi 1970), paramesonephric and sinus tissue (Koff 1933, Agogue 1965), or mesonephric and sinus tissue (Forsberg 1973) with the relative contributions of each tissue being an additional matter for controversy (O'Rahilly 1977). The following account of the development of the vagina is derived largely from O'Rahilly (1977).

At 49 days, before the paramesonephric ducts reach the urogenital sinus, a tubercle appears on the internal aspect of its posterior wall between the openings of the two mesonephric ducts. This is the sinus tubercle which identifies the site at which the fused paramesonephric ducts make contact (Fig. 1.19a) with the posterior wall of the urogenital sinus at 56 days (Glenister 1962, Josso 1981). The fusion of the paramesonephric ducts is complete at 80 days with the formation of the genital canal. The growing caudal end of the canal impinges on the posterior wall of the uro-

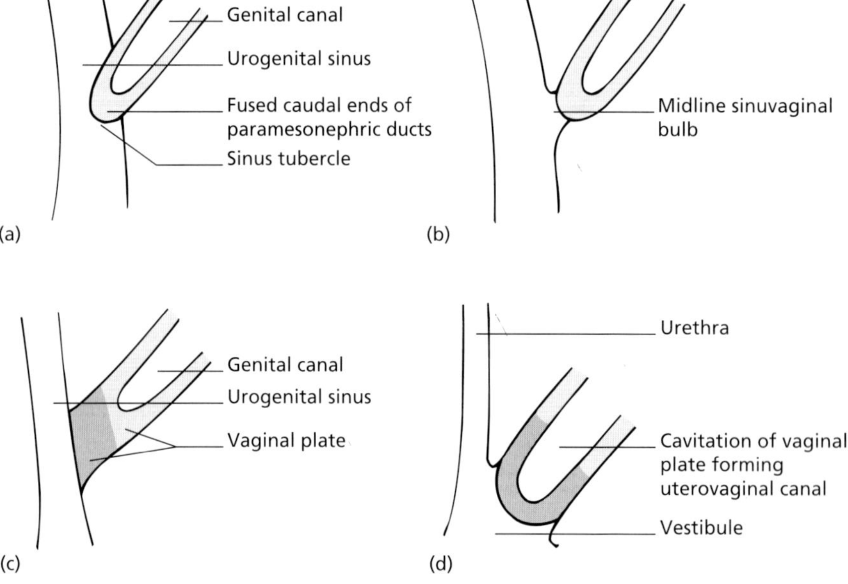

Fig. 1.19 (a) The fused paramesonephric ducts form the genital canal, the solid caudal end of which abuts on the posterior wall of the urogenital sinus at the sinus tubercle. (b) Cellular proliferation of the sinus epithelium generates the sinuvaginal bulbs, which displace the genital canal dorsally. (c) Further cellular proliferation converts the sinuvaginal bulbs into solid tissue projections, which participate in the formation of the vaginal plate. (d) Extensive caudal growth of the vaginal plate brings its lower surface into the primitive vestibule.

genital sinus and induces additional cellular proliferation. At 87 days three dorsal projections of the posterior wall of the urogenital sinus are identified, one in the midline and one on either side (Fig. 1.19b). These projections, or sinuvaginal bulbs, are probably of sinus origin (Koff 1933, Bulmer 1957), although other authors dispute this. Proliferation of the lining epithelium of these sinuvaginal bulbs converts them into solid tissue projections at 95 days. Together these projections displace the original genital canal in a dorsal direction (Fig. 1.19c). The solid sinuvaginal outgrowth and the solid caudal end of the genital canal together form the vaginal plate (Fig. 1.19c). The vaginal plate is recognizable between 87 and 95 days and its formation is complete at 19 weeks. Desquamation of cells from the vaginal plate precedes the formation of the vaginal lumen (O'Rahilly 1977).

The establishment of the vaginal plate is followed immediately by extensive growth caudally (Figs 1.19d & 1.20) so that by the 16th week the vaginal rudiment approaches the cloacal vestibule (Witschi 1970). It has long been assumed that lengthening of the uterovaginal canal was achieved by cephalic extension, whereas Witschi (1970) maintains that 'the lower end of the vagina is sliding down the urethra to its separate opening'. At this stage the sinus element and the paramesonephric element are equally represented in the uterovaginal canal. At approximately 14 weeks the uterovaginal canal has a cephalic dilatation representing the corpus and a cervical dilatation, which marks the region of the vaginal fornices (Koff 1933). The transition from pseudostratified columnar to stratified squamous epithelium observed at 17 weeks is considered to identify the cervicovaginal junction (Bulmer 1957, Davies & Kusama 1962).

The cervix is generally considered to be of paramesonephric origin (Koff 1933, Forsberg 1965, Witschi 1970) but Fluhmann (1960) claimed its mucous membrane to be of sinus origin and this indeed may be so. It has been suggested that the cervix and the upper segment of the vagina is initially lined by paramesonephric tissue, which subsequently degenerates to be replaced by sinus tissue. In explanation of the teratogenic effect of diethylstilboestrol it has been further suggested that the drug prevents this degeneration and replacement and adversely affects the persisting paramesonephric tissue (Ulfelder & Robboy 1976). Certainly the occurrence of upper genital tract abnormalities associated with prenatal exposure to diethylstilboestrol (Kaufmann *et al.* 1977) supports these suggestions.

Cavitation of the vaginal plate, according to the various authorities cited by O'Rahilly (1977), is complete at about the midpoint of gestation, with the uterovaginal canal then having access to the exterior. However, it has since been shown that at 14 weeks the vagina, uterus and uterine tubes have a continuous lumen accessible by intravaginal injection of a rapidly setting silicon liquid (Terruhn 1980). At approximately 17 weeks the high oestrogen levels in the maternal circulation began to influence the fetal vagina although there is no evidence of an oestrogen response in

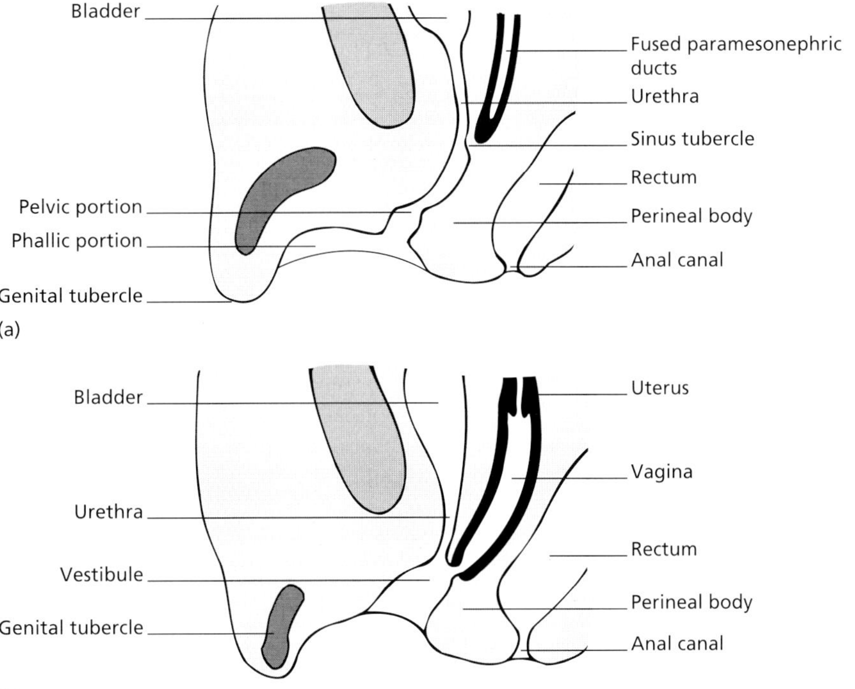

Fig. 1.20 (a) The fused paramesonephric ducts abut on the posterior surface of the urogenital sinus at the sinus tubercle. Above the sinus tubercle the urogenital sinus forms the bladder and urethra while below the tubercle it is divided into pelvic and phallic portions. (b) After the formation of the vaginal plate its extensive caudal growth transfers the vaginal opening into the vestibule.

the uterine corpus (Witschi 1970). In the newborn the stratified squamous epithelium of the vagina shows evidence of a marked oestrogen response. The site of the junction between the cervical and vaginal epithelia is variable and there is a range of normal appearance.

Oestrogens appear to have no role in the normal development of the paramesonephric ducts in the female, since castration (Jost 1947), or explantation to steroid-free culture media (Picon 1969), is followed by normal differentiation. However, in some experimental animals oestrogen has been shown to modify paramesonephric organogenesis, and oestrogen receptors have been demonstrated in the paramesonephric ducts of late fetal rats (Somjen *et al.* 1976) and guinea pigs (Pasqualini *et al.* 1976).

Mesonephric duct

As the urorectal septum reaches the cloacal membrane at 30–32 days the caudal end of the mesonephric duct, having already opened into the urogenital sinus, gives origin to the ureteric bud and begins to be incorporated into the posterior wall of the urogenital sinus (Keith 1948). The portion of each duct incorporated into the urogenital sinus subsequently forms the trigone of the bladder and the posterior wall of the urethra (see Fig. 1.12). At 30–32 days cells from cephalic mesonephric vesicles invade the coelomic epithelium on the medial aspect of the adjacent intermediate mesoderm (see Fig. 1.14a) to induce the formation of the indifferent gonad (Wartenberg 1982). Meanwhile the mesonephric vesicles and ducts provide a functional excretory system for the developing embryo. This role begins to be taken over by the metanephric kidney before the end of embryogenesis and in the female fetus the mesonephric system then becomes redundant. It has, however, been suggested that the mesonephric ducts contribute to the formation of the uterine wall (Witschi 1970) and that their caudal ends are involved in vaginal organogenesis (Forsberg 1965).

Towards the end of embryogenesis the mesonephric vesicles begin to degenerate together with the mesonephric ducts. The lumen of the mesonephric duct is obliterated at 75 days and only remnants persist at 105 days (Josso 1981). A number of mesonephric derivatives may be located in the adult female. A constant finding is the epoophoron associated with the ovary and derived from the cephalic mesonephric duct and adjacent vesicles (Duthie 1925). A more caudal portion of the mesonephros may be encountered in the broad ligament as the paroophoron while remnants of the terminal mesonephric duct may persist lateral to the uterus and vagina or incorporated into the cervix (O'Rahilly 1977, Buntine 1979). Adjacent to the lower genital tract such remnants are referred to as Gartner's ducts.

Development of the external genitalia

UROGENITAL SINUS

The urorectal septum divides the hindgut into the urogenital sinus anteriorly and the terminal portion of the gastrointestinal tract posteriorly (see Fig. 1.10c). This subdivision is completed at 30–32 days, but at 28 days the growing ends of the mesonephric ducts, within the urorectal septum, open into the posterior aspect of the developing urogenital sinus. Immediately the terminal mesonephric ducts give origin to the ureteric buds and are themselves incorporated into the urogenital sinus (see Fig. 1.12). This incorporation separates the mesonephric ducts and ureters, and at 49 days the mesonephric ducts terminate in the urogenital sinus on either side of the sinus tubercle (see Fig. 1.13). Cranial to the sinus tubercle the urogenital sinus is referred to as the vesicourethral canal and from it arise the bladder, the whole of the female urethra and the intramural and prostatic parts of the male urethra (Jirasek 1977). The portion of the urogenital sinus caudal to the sinus tubercle continues to be referred to as the urogenital sinus and is subdivided into pelvic and phallic portions (see Fig. 1.20a).

PERINEUM

At the completion of flexion, about day 24, the anterior limit of the extensive cloacal membrane abuts on the base of the umbilical cord. On either side of the cloacal membrane just below the umbilical cord are the paired primordia of the genital tubercle (Fig. 1.21a). During the next few days retraction of the anterior end of the cloacal membrane from the base of the umbilical cord allows formation of an anterior body wall caudal to the umbilicus. The paired primordia of the genital tubercle fuse.

Extending posteriorly from the base of the tubercle on either side of the cloacal membrane are the cloacal folds, lateral to which are the genital swellings (Fig. 1.21b). At 30–32 days the urorectal septum reaches the cloacal membrane and divides it into an anterior genital membrane and a posterior anal membrane. The anterior component of each cloacal fold becomes the genital fold and the posterior component the anal fold (Fig. 1.21c). The genital membrane ruptures soon afterwards, due to the increasing pressure associated with the functional mesonephric kidney (Ludwig 1965), as also does the anal membrane (Jirasek 1977) (Fig. 1.22a). After the rupture of the genital membrane the phallic portion of the urogenital sinus is limited anteriorly by the underside of the genital tubercle. The genital tubercle elongates and is referred to as a phallus. This indifferent state, when phenotypic sex cannot be determined from the appearance of the external genitalia, lasts until day 63 (Jirasek 1977).

MASCULINIZATION OF THE EXTERNAL GENITALIA

In the normal male fetus masculinization begins between 63 and 70 days with the lengthening both of the phallus and the anogenital distance (Jirasek *et al.* 1968). The genital folds fuse carrying the opening of the phallic portion of the urogenital sinus to the base of the phallus. Thereafter the cavernous urethra, enveloped in its spongy tissue, is completely closed and its opening is carried to the distal end of the phallus. These changes are completed by 84–98 days and during the same period the genital swellings fuse in the midline to form the scrotum (Jirasek 1977).

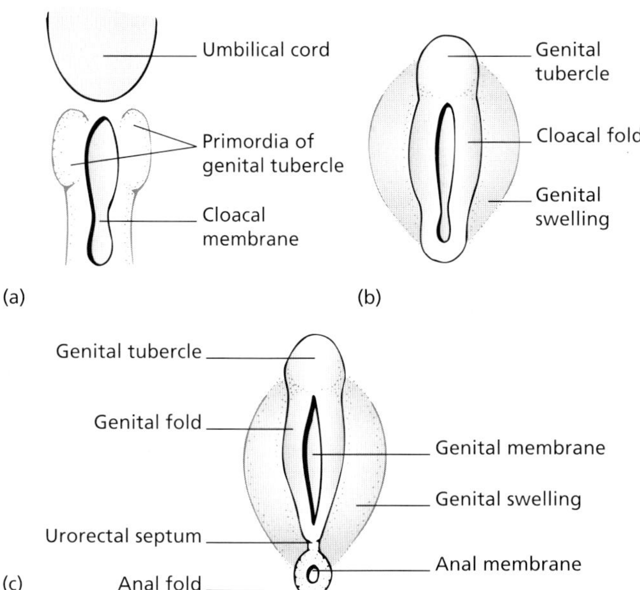

Fig. 1.21 (a) The paired primordia of the genital tubercle lie immediately caudal to the umbilical cord. (b) Migration of tissue towards the midline from both sides separates the umbilical cord and cloacal membrane, causes fusion of the primordia to form a midline genital tubercle and establishes bilateral cloacal folds and genital swellings. (c) Fusion of the urorectal septum with the cloacal membrane separates an anterior genital region from a posterior anal region.

FEMINIZATION OF THE EXTERNAL GENITALIA

In the normal female fetus feminization begins at between 63 and 77 days, when the phallus, without lengthening, bends caudally (Jirasek 1977). During this period the anogenital distance remains unchanged, there is no fusion of the genital folds and the phallic portion or the urogenital sinus remains open. Sometime between 14 weeks (Terruhn 1980) and 20 weeks (O'Rahilly 1977) the vagina opens into the pelvic portion of the urogenital sinus converting it into the vaginal vestibule (Fig. 1.22b). During the second half of gestation the urethral and vaginal openings separate. As they do so the phallus becomes the clitoris, being incorporated within the fused anterior ends of the genital folds, which become the labia minora. The genital swellings, lateral to the labia minora, become the labia majora and are continuous with the future mons pubis, anterior to the clitoris.

MECHANISM OF DIFFERENTIATION

Testosterone is the only steroid hormone produced by the fetal gonad at the time of sexual differentiation (Wilson & Siiteri 1973, Siiteri & Wilson 1974) and it enters its target cells by diffusion. In cells possessing the enzyme 5α-reductase, testosterone is converted to dihydrotestosterone (DHT); otherwise it remains as testosterone. Within the cell, the androgen, either as testosterone or DHT, is bound by a specific high-affinity cytosol protein receptor. The androgen–receptor complex is activated and translocated to the nucleus where it initiates gene transcription. After

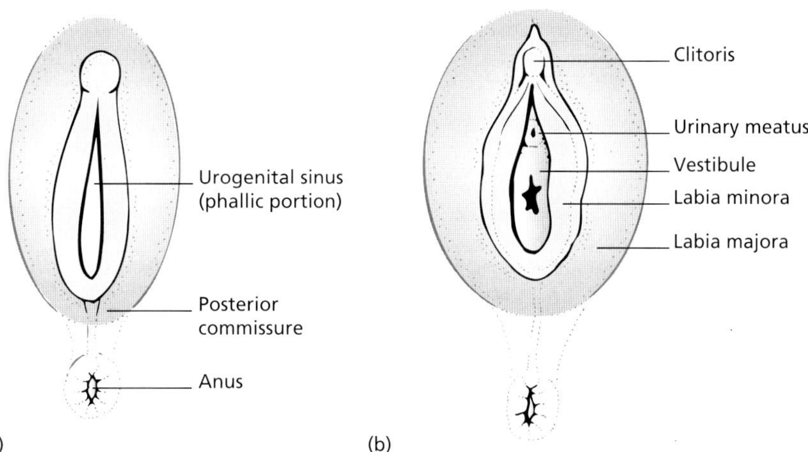

Fig. 1.22 (a) The genital and anal membranes rupture. (b) In the female fetus the urogenital sinus remains open as caudal growth of the vaginal plate brings the urethral and vaginal openings into this region converting it into the vestibule.

transcription and processing of the messenger RNA, the specific RNA within the cytoplasm is involved in the synthesis of new androgen-induced proteins (Liao 1978).

The synthesis of the androgen cytosol protein receptor is regulated by genes at the X-linked Tfm locus (Ohno 1977). Therefore both sexes possess the cellular apparatus for androgen action with the limiting factor being the plasma concentration of testosterone. Male differentiation of the mesonephric ducts is testosterone dependent since the undifferentiated ducts lack the enzyme 5α-reductase (Wilson & Lasnitzki 1971, Siiteri & Wilson 1974). In contrast male differentiation of the urogenital sinus and external genitalia is DHT dependent, and 5α-reductase is present in these tissues, in both sexes, before sexual differentiation begins (Wilson & Lasnitzki 1971, Wilson 1973).

In the female fetus the absence of testosterone allows the mesonephric ducts to degenerate and enables the urogenital sinus and external genitalia to follow their inherent tendency and differentiate according to the female phenotype. In the male fetus any defect that prevents the effective action of androgen will impair masculinization of the internal and/or external organs of reproduction. Failure to synthesize the cytosol protein receptor prevents the action of testosterone on the mesonephric ducts and of DHT on the urogenital sinus and the external genitalia. This receptor defect causes complete or incomplete androgen insensitivity, as observed in the testicular feminization syndromes (Morris 1953). Failure to synthesize 5α-reductase prevents the conversion of testosterone to its intracellular metabolite DHT, which is necessary for the virilization of the urogenital sinus and external genitalia (Imperato-McGinley *et al.* 1974). This enzyme defect, transmitted as an autosomal recessive (Simpson *et al.* 1971(b), Peterson *et al.* 1979), causes the clinical syndrome first described by Novakowski and Lenz (1961) in which patients have female external genitalia in association with normal testes and male internal reproductive organs.

The external genitalia of the human male fetus are completely masculinized by 84–98 days (Jirasek 1977). If a female fetus is exposed to significant androgen levels before the end of this period of development complete external virilization will occur (Grumbach and Ducharme 1960), while lower levels or later exposure will produce various forms of incomplete virilization.

Congenital anomalies

The sex of the newborn is established from the appearance of the external genitalia but occasionally this may not be possible because of their ambiguous nature. In such circumstances, despite parental anxiety, sex should not be assigned on the basis of approximation to male or female phenotype. Such assignment must await careful examination of the pudenda, karyotyping to establish chromosomal complement and if necessary full endocrine and cytogenetic investigations. These latter procedures may be necessary since the genital appearances of an undermasculinized male, a masculinized female and a hermaphrodite are essentially similar (Dewhurst, 1980). Some of these abnormalities are known to be caused by genetic defects while others are caused by endogenous or exogenous factors which influence development at certain critical periods of embryogenesis. There are also certain conditions of abnormal sexual differentiation in which the apparent sex of the infant, assigned on the basis of pudendal phenotype, will not accord with the chromosomal, gonadal or genital duct sex of the child. In such cases the associated problems will not present until adolescence or later. In addition there are a number of readily recognizable structural defects involving the lower female genital tract and external genitalia in which the cause is unknown.

Ambiguous external genitalia

In infants, children or adults in whom the external genitalia are not characteristic of male or female phenotype there are a number of possible presentations. Almost all such individuals, however, possess a phallus enlarged to a varying degree with a small opening on its ventral surface, at its base or on the perineum, through which urine is voided. A second opening or depression may be identified more posteriorly, while on either side of the midline virilization, ranging from rugose labia majora-like structures to scrotal sacs, may be seen (Dewhurst 1980). A structural classification of such conditions is possible since comparable anatomical findings occur in a variety of clinical syndromes. However, the following classification, adapted from Grumbach and Conte (1992) and Simpson (1982), is preferred. It is based upon aetiological mechanisms and clinical syndromes and comprises three main groups:

1 disorders of gonadal differentiation;
2 female pseudohermaphroditism;
3 male pseudohermaphroditism.

DISORDERS OF GONADAL DIFFERENTIATION

Ovarian dysgenesis

Approximately 50% of all patients with ovarian dysgenesis have a chromosomal complement of 45X; a further 25% have sex chromosomal mosaicism without a structural chromosomal abnormality (45X/46XX; 45X/46XY) while the remainder have either a structurally abnormal X or Y chromosome or no detectable chromosomal abnormality (Simpson 1982).

45X Turner's syndrome. Only a small number of 45X embryos survive intrauterine life (Boue *et al.* 1975, Cockwell *et al.* 1991). At birth the genital ducts and external genitalia are entirely female although clitoral enlargement may occasionally be present (Grumbach & Conte 1992). The ovaries, located in their normal anatomical positions, consist mainly of fibrous stroma and are termed streak gonads. Nevertheless, secondary sexual development does occur in some 25% of 45X individuals, 2–5% menstruate (Saenger 1996) and very occasionally they bear children (King *et al.* 1978, Kohn *et al.* 1980). Patients with Turner's syndrome are of short stature and exhibit a range of somatic abnormalities including webbing of the neck, coarctation of the aorta and renal anomalies. Also associated with the condition is a predisposition to develop diabetes mellitus (Engel & Forbes 1965).

It has since been shown (Kocova *et al.* 1993, Kocova & Trucco 1994) that the sex-determining region of the Y chromosome (SRY gene) was present in six of 18 patients with Turner's syndrome who had no detectable Y chromosome in their karyotype. This finding further confirms the thesis of Mittwoch (1992) that the presence of a single dominant Y chromosomal gene is incapable of determining functional testicular differentiation. However, Kocova and colleagues express the concern that the presence of Y chromosomal material may increase the risk of gonadal neoplasia.

45X/46XX mosaicism and X chromosome abnormality. This form of mosaicism is the most common cause of ovarian dysgenesis after Turner's syndrome. Such patients usually exhibit fewer of the somatic abnormalities associated with Turner's syndrome, their phenotype is invariably female and some may menstruate and even be fertile. One gonad may be of the streak type and the contralateral gonad a normal or hypoplastic ovary; alternatively, both ovaries may be either normal or hypoplastic (Grumbach & Conte 1992).

45X/46XY mosaicism and Y chromosome abnormality. A highly diverse phenotype is encountered in 45X/46XY mosaicism since the presence of a Y-bearing cell line may induce some testicular differentiation. Such individuals may appear typically male or female or may possess ambiguous external genitalia with varied genital duct development. In a series of 60 patients with 45X/46XY mosaicism, two-thirds were reared as females (Zah *et al.* 1975). Several cases of structural abnormality of the Y chromosome have been reported (Davis 1981). The affected individuals are phenotypic females with bilateral streak gonads who remain sexually immature.

46XX, 46XY. Gonadal dysgenesis may occur in association with apparently normal 46XX or 46XY karyotypes. These individuals are phenotypically female but have streak gonads and remain sexually immature. The 46XX form of gonadal dysgenesis appears to be inherited as an autosomal recessive condition (Simpson *et al.* 1971(b)). The genetic heterogeneity of this form of gonadal dysgenesis is evidenced by its occurrence in some families in association with neurosensory deafness, which may also afflict otherwise normal male siblings (Pallister & Opitz 1979). The 46XY form of gonadal dysgenesis is again a genetically heterogeneous syndrome, being associated with deletions and/or mutations involving the Y chromosome (Blagowidow *et al.* 1989) and/or the X chromosome (Scherer *et al.* 1989). Clitoral enlargement is not uncommon but the most important aspect of this condition is the increased incidence of gonadal neoplasms (Simpson 1982). Bilateral gonadectomy is therefore indicated as a prophylactic measure (Dewhurst 1980, Grumbach & Conte 1992). In all forms of ovarian dysgenesis oestrogen replacement therapy is recommended at 12–13 years of age eventually to be cycled monthly with progesterone (Grumbach & Conte 1992).

True hermaphroditism

True hermaphrodites possess both ovarian and testicular tissue, with an ovary on one side and a testis on the other or, more commonly, with ovotestes situated bilaterally or unilaterally (Grumbach & Conte 1992). The differentiation of the genital tract, the appearance of the external genitalia and the development of secondary sexual characteristics are variable. Although the external genitalia are often ambiguous (Fig. 1.23), three-quarters of reported cases have been reared as males because of the size of the phallus (van

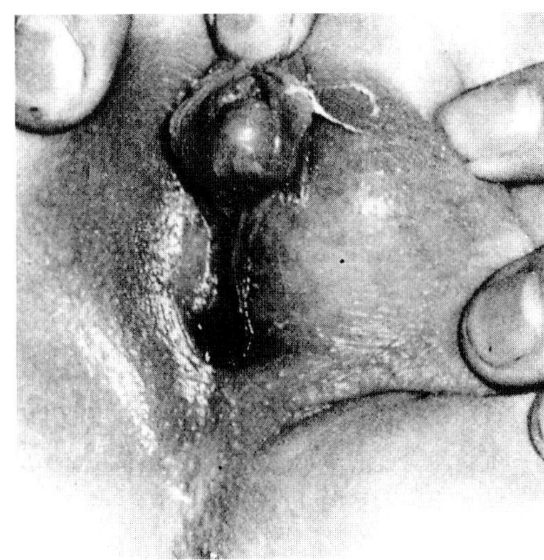

Fig. 1.23 External genitalia of a true hermaphrodite.

Niekerk 1976). Despite the tendency to rear these patients as males the majority of their gonads exhibit oocytes but not spermatozoa, a uterus is almost invariably present and 60% of them have a 46XX karyotype; indeed four 46XX true hermaphrodites have become pregnant (Tegenkamp *et al.* 1979). The remaining 40% of true hermaphrodites in van Niekerk's 1976 review were equally distributed between 46XY karyotypes, 46XX/46XY chimeras and sex-chromosome mosaics.

Gonadal agenesis

These patients have a 46XY karyotype but do not possess any gonadal tissue. The condition, variously termed the 'the XY gonadal agenesis syndrome' (Sarto & Opitz 1973) or the 'testicular regression syndrome' (Coulam 1979), is characterized by the presence of ambiguous genitalia in association with hypoplastic Mullerian and Wolffian derivatives. A small phallus, ill-developed labia majora and fusion of the labioscrotal folds are features of the external genital appearance (Sarto & Opitz 1973). The frequent association of somatic anomalies suggests a possible teratogen.

FEMALE PSEUDOHERMAPHRODITISM

Female pseudohermaphrodites are 46XX individuals with normal ovaries, normal Mullerian duct derivatives and atypical female external genitalia. The clitoris is enlarged, labial fusion produces a variable vaginal orifice and the urethral opening may not be distinct from the vagina. The external genitalia of the male fetus are completely masculinized by 84–98 days (Jirasek 1977). If a female fetus is exposed to significant androgen levels, in the presence of 5α-reductase, before the end of this period of development, complete virilization will occur (Grumbach & Ducharme 1960), while lower levels or later exposure will produce various forms of incomplete virilization. The source of the virilizing influence may be fetal, maternal or exogenous.

Fetal

Congenital adrenal hyperplasia accounts for most of the cases of female pseudohermaphroditism and approximately half of all patients with ambiguous external genitalia. There are several types of congenital adrenal hyperplasia and all are transmitted as an autosomal recessive trait (Laue & Rennert 1995). The common denominator in all types is impaired cortisol formation due to an enzyme defect on the steroid biosynthetic pathway. Depressed cortisol synthesis produces hypersecretion of adrenocorticotrophic hormone (ACTH) through the negative-feedback mechanism and consequent hyperplasia of the adrenal cortex. There are essentially two types of enzyme defect. The first, caused by 21-hydroxylase deficiency or 11β-hydroxylase deficiency, limits cortisol production and diverts the synthetic pathway towards overproduction of adrenal androgens and androgen precursors. The second, caused by 3β-ol-dehydrogenase deficiency or 17α-hydroxylase deficiency, limits cortisol production and also impairs the synthesis of sex steroids by the gonads and adrenals.

21-hydroxylase deficiency. Since the adrenal begins to function during the third month of intrauterine life, excessive production of adrenal androgens will virilize the fetal female external genitalia (Fig. 1.24). Several forms of 21-hydroxylase deficiency exist, some of which are associated with sodium depletion and are therefore life threatening in the neonatal period. All deficiency states result from a mutant autosomal recessive gene, located on chromosome 6, which is closely linked to the human leucocyte antigen (HLA) locus (Dupont *et al.* 1977). Linkage to the HLA locus permits antenatal diagnosis (Simpson 1982) and the possibility of pharmacological suppression of the fetal adrenal gland *in utero*. Such intervention, beginning at the 10th week of gestation, with dexamethasone administration to the mother, was not harmful to the fetus (Evans *et al.*

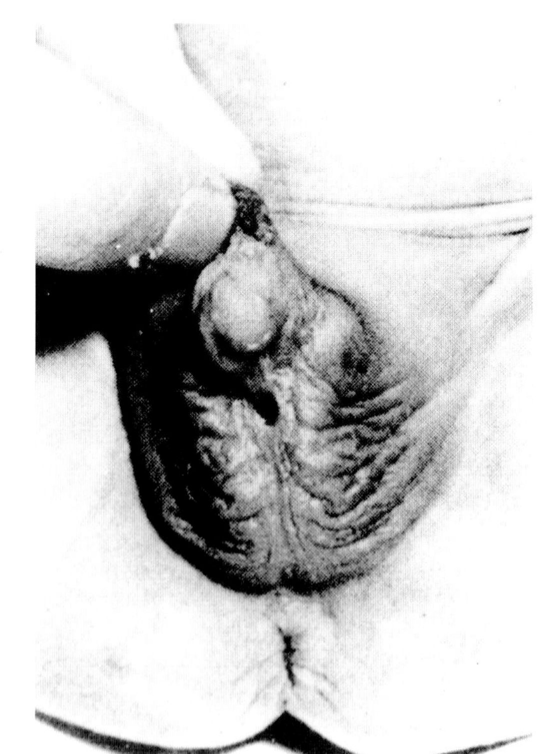

Fig. 1.24 External genitalia of a female child with congenital adrenal hyperplasia.

1985). In affected individuals adrenal hormone supplementation is required post-natally.

11β-hydroxylase deficiency. This enzyme deficiency is less common than 21-hydroxylase deficiency. It is associated with overproduction of androgens and mineralocorticoids, which cause virilization of the female fetus and hypertension in both sexes (Sinaiko 1996). Affected males appear normal at birth and the diagnosis may not be made until signs of precocious puberty develop (Laue & Rennert 1995). Sodium depletion does not usually occur in association with this defect.

3β-ol-dehydrogenase deficiency. With this enzyme defect the only androgen synthesized is dehydroepiandrosterone (DHEA), which is relatively weak. Females with this deficiency are less virilized than females with 21- or 11β-hydroxylase deficiencies. In fact DHEA is such a weak androgen that males with 3β-ol-dehydrogenase deficiency may fail to masculinize fully (Simpson 1982) and be left with varying degrees of hypospadias (Laue & Rennert 1995).

17α-hydroxylase deficiency. Females with this enzyme defect have normal female external genitalia at birth but show no secondary sexual development at puberty (Simpson 1982).

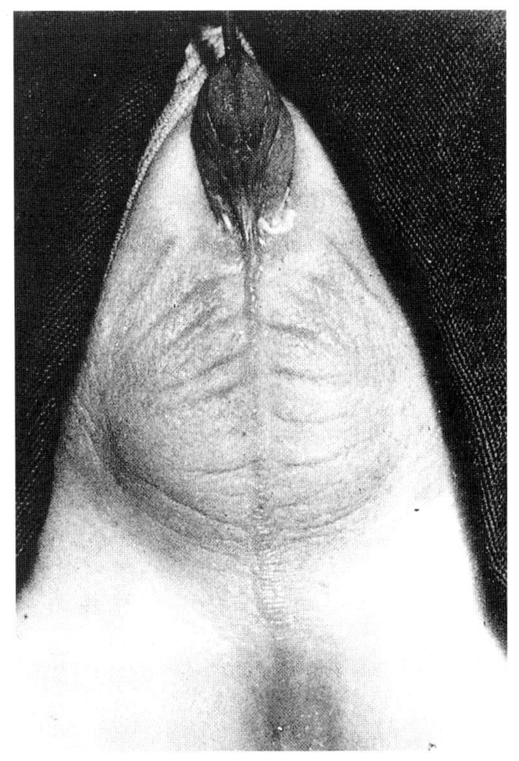

Fig. 1.25 Marked virilization of a female child caused by maternal androgen therapy during early pregnancy.

Maternal

In rare instances, virilization of the female fetus may occur if the mother is suffering from certain ovarian or adrenal tumours or has unrecognized congenital adrenal hyperplasia. The absence of virilization in the mother does not exclude a maternal source since the level of androgen required to virilize the external genitalia of the early female fetus is much less than would be required to have a virilizing effect on the adult female (Kai *et al.* 1979).

Exogenous

Virilization of the external genitalia of female infants has been frequently observed following maternal ingestion of testosterone or synthetic progestational agents during the first trimester of pregnancy (Grumbach & Ducharme 1960, Wilkins 1960, Dewhurst & Gordon 1984, Reschini *et al.* 1985). Administration of such agents between the eighth and 12th week of gestation causes marked virilization (Fig. 1.25), while later in pregnancy their use causes clitoral enlargement (Fig. 1.26). These agents, as well as stilboestrol, were often prescribed in the past for women with habitual or threatened abortion. Although exposure to stilboestrol during intrauterine life is known to cause malfor-

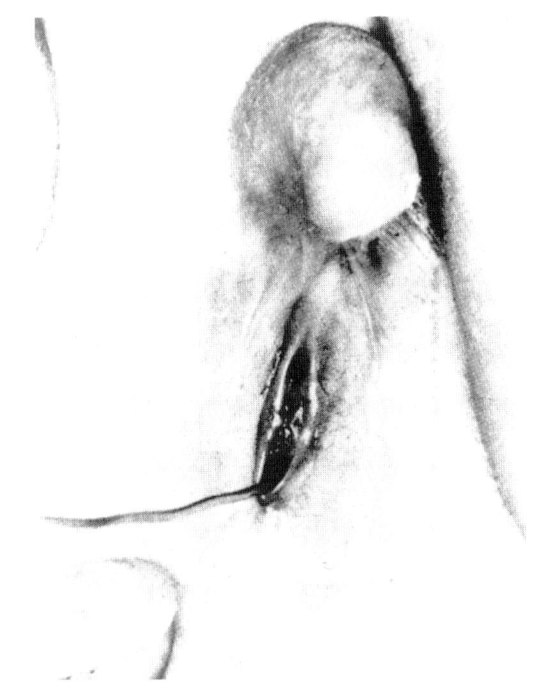

Fig. 1.26 Partial virilization of a female child caused by maternal androgen therapy during pregnancy.

mations in the reproductive tracts of both sexes and an increased incidence of cervical and vaginal neoplasia (Herbst *et al.* 1972, 1974), it has also been shown to cause female pseudohermaphroditism (Bongiovani *et al.* 1959). Intrauterine exposure to danazol (Danocrine, Chronogyn), a carbon 17-alkylated derivative of ethinyltestosterone used in the treatment of endometriosis, has also been associated with the occurrence of female pseudohermaphroditism (Rosa 1984, Shaw & Farquhar 1984).

Ambiguous genitalia in both male and female infants, in association with other congenital malformations, has been reported following maternal use of cocaine during pregnancy (Chasnoff *et al.* 1988).

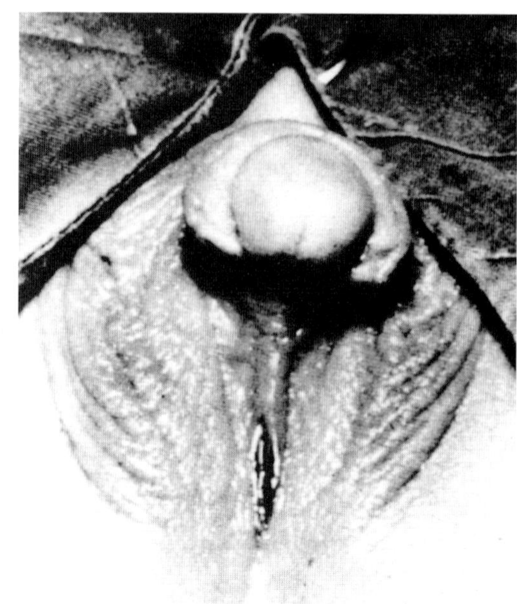

Fig. 1.27 External genitalia of an incompletely masculinized male child in whom there was partial testicular failure.

MALE PSEUDOHERMAPHRODITISM

In male pseudohermaphroditism the testes, which are always present, are unable to effect complete masculinization of the genital ducts and external genitalia. This functional defect can occur at any of several stages in the masculinization process and will therefore produce varying degrees of the female phenotype.

Lack of testicular response to gonadotrophin

Production of testosterone by the Leydig cells of the fetal testes is essential for Wolffian duct stabilization and masculinization of the external genitalia. An individual with Leydig-cell agenesis or a receptor abnormality rendering Leydig cells unresponse to gonadotrophins has female external genitalia, no Wolffian derivatives and, because of AMH production by Sertoli cells, absent Mullerian derivatives (Berthezene *et al.* 1976, Brown *et al.* 1978). Such individuals have ectopic testes and exhibit no secondary sexual characteristics with the approach of adulthood. When the defect involves Leydig-cell hypoplasia or partial responsiveness to gonadotrophins, masculinization of the external genitalia is incomplete (Fig. 1.27). Familial studies of this condition indicate that it is transmitted as an autosomal recessive trait (Saldanha *et al.* 1987).

Any defect in the Sertoli-cell response to gonadotrophins, or a lack of responsiveness by the Mullerian ducts to AMH, results in the presence of internal female organs of reproduction in otherwise normal males.

Enzyme defects in testosterone biosynthesis

A number of familial enzymatic defects in testosterone biosynthesis have been identified, each of which disturbs one of the various reactions required for the conversion of cholesterol to testosterone (Grumbach & Conte 1992). There are essentially two types of enzyme defect. The first involves enzymes affecting both glucocorticoid and sex steroid biosynthesis, while the second involves enzymes principally concerned with testosterone biosynthesis in the testes. Patients affected by the first type of enzyme defect will require adrenal hormone therapy throughout life and those with either type of defect will require appropriate sex steroid therapy at puberty depending on the degree of surgical intervention and the sex of rearing.

Each of these enzyme defects is inherited as an autosomal or X-linked recessive trait. In general their effect is to produce external genitalia ranging from the normal female appearance to that of a hypospadic male. Mullerian duct derivatives are invariably absent but a blind-ending vaginal pouch is common in affected individuals. The Wolffian duct derivatives may be normal or hypoplastic while the testes are usually ectopically situated. Pubertal masculinization may be a major problem in some of these conditions when the child, because of the appearance of the external genitalia, has been raised as a girl (Fig. 1.28).

Defects in androgen-dependent target tissue

Effective biosynthesis of testosterone is essential, but not sufficient, for full masculinization of the 46XY fetus. Male differentiation of the external genitalia is effected by DHT, produced from testosterone by the enzyme 5α-reductase. The action of testosterone on the Wolffian ducts and of

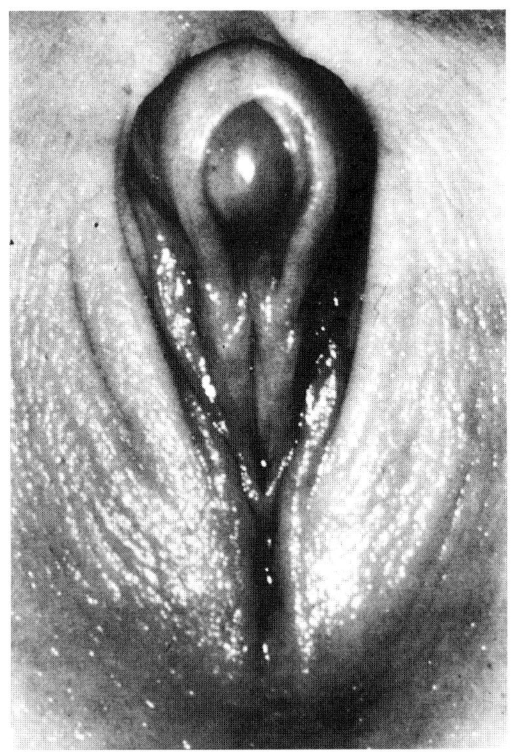

Fig. 1.28 External genitalia of an XY child reared as a girl.

DHT on the external genitalia is dependent on a specific intracellular cytosol protein receptor, which, after binding the androgen, is activated to initiate gene transcription, which achieves the masculinizing effect (Liao 1978).

Androgen receptor and post-receptor defects. The synthesis of the androgen cytosol protein receptor is regulated by genes at the Tfm locus on the X chromosome (Ohno 1977). Failure to synthesize the receptor or activate the receptor–androgen complex effectively blocks the androgen's masculinizing role. Such receptor defects cause complete or incomplete androgen insensitivity, typical of the testicular feminization syndrome (Morris 1953).

In the complete androgen insensitivity syndrome, 46XY males are phenotypically female and possess a blind vaginal pouch. They develop female secondary sexual characteristics at puberty but fail to menstruate since Mullerian duct derivatives are absent. The Wolffian duct derivatives are also absent or vestigial while the testes are intra-abdominal or situated in the labial or inguinal regions (Grumbach & Conte 1992). The incomplete syndrome presents in a variety of forms due to decreased numbers of cytosol androgen receptors in the target tissues (Griffin *et al.* 1976).

5α-reductase deficiency. This familial type of male pseudohermaphroditism was first reported by Novakowski and Lenz (1961), who described it as 'pseudovaginal perineoscrotal hypospadias'. Affected individuals at birth had a clitoris-like hypospadic phallus, a bifid scrotum and a urogenital sinus opening on the perineum. Further investigation showed a 46XY karyotype, normally differentiated ectopic testes, male internal ducts and no Mullerian derivatives. This abnormality of sexual development, transmitted as an autosomal recessive trait (Simpson *et al.* 1971(a), Peterson *et al.* 1979), was later shown to be due to an absence of 5α-reductase from the external genital tissue. Failure to synthesize 5α-reductase prevents the conversion of testosterone to DHT, which is now known to be necessary for the masculinization of the external genitalia (Imperato-McGinley *et al.* 1974). Perhaps the most striking but as yet unexplained phenomenon associated with this condition is the masculinization that occurs at puberty: the voice deepens, muscle mass increases, the phallus enlarges, the bifid scrotum becomes rugose and pigmented while the enlarging testes descend into the labioscrotal folds (Grumbach & Conte 1992).

Structural defects

Various abnormalities may arise in the genital system, as in other systems, due to inherent defects of development, migration, canalization and fusion. The interdependence during development of the reproductive, urinary and terminal gastrointestinal systems causes some genital defects to be associated with renal, rectal or anal anomalies. Numerous attempts have been made to classify the various structural abnormalities that may affect the female genital tract but none has been entirely satisfactory because of the complexity of the permutations that may be encountered, the lack of knowledge concerning the basic mechanisms involved and the fact that a single anomaly may represent the end-point of different mechanisms (Fox 1995). In this account brief reference will be made to abnormalities of the upper reproductive tract in so far as they effect the lower reproductive tract.

UPPER REPRODUCTIVE TRACT

Absence of the uterine tubes without associated uterine abnormalities is very rare (Warkany 1971). Partial absence or atresia of a tube, with or without the presence of tubal diverticula has been reported, the latter form of isolated abnormality being associated with tubal pregnancy (McNally 1926). Absence of the uterus is common in some disorders of gonadal differentiation and in male pseudohermaphroditism but it may occur in otherwise normal females in whom the Mullerian ducts have failed to develop. More often, however, there is unilateral Mullerian duct development and this type of anomaly is associated with renal agenesis (Frost 1958). Fusion defects of the Mullerian ducts can cause abnormalities ranging from a bicornuate uterus with various degrees of cervical and vaginal septation to the formation of two uteri and two vaginae. In some of these latter cases there has been duplication of the vulva, urethra and bladder (Warkany 1971).

Congenital or later prolapse of the uterus is not uncommon in the female spina bifida infant, when the protrusion between the labia minora exhibits a cervical opening. The cause of this condition is thought to be paralysis of the pelvic floor musculature arising as a consequence of the neural tube defect (Torpin 1942).

LOWER REPRODUCTIVE TRACT

Vaginal agenesis

The absence of a vagina forms part of the presenting clinical picture in some patients with male or female pseudohermaphroditism. Agenesis of the vagina, however, may occur in 46XX females who are not pseudohermaphrodites. Total vaginal agenesis is usually found in association with tubal and uterine agenesis, presumably as a consequence of complete Mullerian aplasia. Occasionally the upper reproductive tract is normal and functional and the vaginal agenesis has resulted from a partial Mullerian defect or because the vaginal plate has failed to form or cavitate. In a survey of 167 women with total vaginal agenesis, one-third had associated renal tract defects while others had skeletal abnormalities (Evans *et al.* 1981). The authors of this study suggest familial transmission, the variable expression of an underlying recessive trait or the action of a teratogen as the most likely cause of this condition, in which the average age at presentation was 16 years. In some patients with vaginal agenesis a very shallow vaginal opening may be present and when this is associated with a rudimentary upper reproductive tract it is referred to as the Rokitansky–Kuster–Hauser syndrome (Simpson 1982).

Vaginal atresia

In this condition the urogenital sinus fails to form the inferior portion of the vagina. The lower vagina is replaced by fibrous tissue above which there is a normal reproductive tract (Simpson 1976).

Vaginal septa

Transverse vaginal septa are said to be located at the junction of the upper third and lower two-thirds of the vagina (Simpson 1976). The probable cause of transverse vaginal septa formation is the failure of either the Mullerian or urogenital sinus contributions to the vagina to cavitate completely. This aetiology would therefore cause transverse septa to form at any level in the vagina. In the Amish community this abnormality is inherited as an autosomal recessive trait (McKusick *et al.* 1964). Patients with transverse vaginal septa may present at puberty with retained menstrual products or alternatively with a continuous vaginal discharge.

A longitudinal vaginal septum may present in the midline as the result of a fusion defect in the Mullerian system and will be associated with abnormalities of the upper reproductive tract. More usually longitudinal septa are formed by aberrant cellular proliferation; they can occur in any plane and are rarely associated with clinical problems.

Imperforate hymen

This is commonly caused by the failure of the central epithelial cells of the hymenal membrane to degenerate. However, this condition may arise as the result of an inflammatory reaction in the hymen after birth. The majority of cases are identified with the onset of puberty.

Vaginal cysts

In the neonatal period vaginal cysts may be found posterior to the urethral meatus. These cysts arise from the anterior or lateral walls of the vagina at the introitus and usually rupture spontaneously (Warkany 1971). Occasionally one or more of these cysts may enlarge and obstruct the urethra. These cysts are thought to be inclusions from the urogenital sinus epithelium and may persist asymptomatically into adulthood (Robboy *et al.* 1978). Certainly mucous cysts are found in the same location, interior to the labia minora and external to the hymen, in about 3% of adults attending a vulvar clinic (Friedrich & Wilkinson 1973). In addition the Wolffian ducts, which degenerate in the female, leave caudal remnants in the lateral walls of the vagina. These remnants may undergo cystic degeneration, when they are termed Gartner's cysts.

EXTERNAL GENITALIA

Various abnormalities of the vulva are caused by disturbances of sexual differentiation, which lead to an ambiguous appearance of the external genitalia. Other vulvar defects, such as duplication, occur in association with abnormalities of the upper reproductive tract and urinary system. Congenital anomalies of the vulva that occur in isolation involve the clitoris and the labia.

Clitoris

The clitoris may be absent (Falk & Hyman 1971), probably as a result of the genital tubercles remaining hypoplastic or failing to fuse. It is, however, more likely that failure of the genital tubercles to fuse will be interpreted as duplication of the clitoris. Enlargement occurs in the rare genetically determined condition of lipoatrophic diabetes (Lawrence–Seip syndrome) (Burton & Cunliffe 1992).

Labia minora

Hypertrophy and/or an asymmetry of the labia minora may occur without demonstrable aetiology or in some cases may be attributable to, for example, neurofibromatosis (Friedrich & Wilkinson 1985). True hypoplasia of the labia minora occurs infrequently, and may be a sign of defective steroidogenesis.

Fusion of the labia minora may occur in association with defective sexual differentiation but it may also be observed in the neonatal period or in infancy as a result of inflammatory adhesion.

VULVAL AND URINARY SYSTEM ABNORMALITIES

Kidney

Bilateral renal agenesis is a lethal congenital malformation (Potter 1946) and in the female is frequently associated with deformation of the external genitalia, absence of the uterus and vagina and abnormalities of other systems (Potter 1965).

Unilateral renal agenesis, which is compatible with a long and active life, may be associated with malformation of the external genitalia. The incidence of genital anomalies in unilateral renal agenesis is about 40% in females and 12% in males (Warkany 1971).

Ureter

The ureteric bud arises from the Wolffian (mesonephric) duct. It is eventually separated from the Wolffian duct as the latter structure is incorporated into the urogenital sinus to form the trigone of the bladder and urethra. Failure of dissociation between the ureteric bud and Wolffian duct in the female will allow the ureteric orifice to be located at any site along the caudal remnant of the Wolffian duct (Gartner's duct). Vaginal drainage of the ectopic ureter occurs because of secondary rupture of Gartner's duct into the vagina (Weiss *et al.* 1984).

Bladder

Exstrophy of the bladder is caused by a failure of the subumbilical portion of the anterior abdominal wall to meet in the midline above the genital tubercles. The genital tubercles remain as paired primordia and the anterior wall of the bladder is either partially or totally absent. This condition may therefore exist as incomplete or complete bladder exstrophy and is always associated with epispadias and other abnormalities of the external genitalia. A more severe form of this structural defect is cloacal exstrophy, in which the urorectal septum fails to divide the hindgut, and the abdominal wall deficit gives access not only to the bladder but also to the terminal gastrointestinal tract (Diamond & Jeffs 1985). In comparison with the urinary and/or intestinal abnormalities those of the external genitalia may seem minor. However, these conditions may now be surgically repaired and it is important to refashion the external genitalia in accordance with the chromosomal and gonadal sex of the infant in so far as this is possible (Dewhurst 1980).

Urethra

Congenital abnormalities of the urethra occur predominantly in the male. Those that occur in females have a lower incidence than in males. In duplication of the urethra, a cause of urinary incontinence in the female, the accessory urethra usually arises from the trigone and opens onto the anterior wall of the vagina (Williams 1958). Mild forms of epispadias may occur in the female giving rise to disturbance of bladder control and urinary incontinence. In this condition the urethral opening lies deep to the mons veneris between two clitoral elements (Williams 1958). Hypospadias, when it occurs in the female, does so in association with female pseudohermaphroditism. In both epispadias and hypospadias, the female urethra is congenitally short (Burbige & Hensle 1985). Meatal stenosis is uncommon in the female but may simulate bladder neck obstruction (Warkany 1971). Prolapse of urethral mucosa occurs only in the female (Capraro *et al.* 1970). Urethral cysts may develop in Skene's glands, which open at the termination of the urethra. Inadequate drainage or infection will cause recurrent urinary symptoms. Finally, an ectopic ureter may open into the urethra.

These various urethral abnormalities may present as urinary incontinence, although lesser degrees of incontinence may cause constant vulval wetness and skin irritation. They are all amenable to surgical repair.

VULVAL AND INTESTINAL ABNORMALITIES

In the female an imperforate anus or anal stenosis may be

associated with a variety of abnormalities of the genital tract and vulva (Hall *et al.* 1985). An ectopic bowel opening may be found in the vagina or elsewhere in the perineum. When a rectovaginal fistula is formed there are often urinary tract abnormalities present also.

VULVAL MAMMARY TISSUE

The number of mammary glands is determined by the average number of young delivered with each pregnancy. During embryogenesis paired thickenings of ectoderm descend the ventral body wall, on either side of the midline, from the base of the forelimb bud to the medial aspect of the hindlimb bud. The caudal two-thirds of these 'milk lines' disappears in the human and the breast primordia are restricted to the thoracic region. Persistence of the most caudal elements of the milk lines in the human will therefore involve the labia majora. Recently, however, the presence of milk lines has been disputed (Chapter 8).

References

Abbas, N.E., Toublanc, J.E., Boucekkine, C. *et al.* (1990) A possible common origin of Y negative human XX males and XX true hermaphrodites. *Human Genetics* **84**, 356–360.

Affara, W.A., Ferguson-Smith, M.A., Tolmie, J. *et al.* (1986) Variable transfer of Y specific sequences in XX males. *Nucleic Acids Research* **14**, 5375–5387.

Agogue, M. (1965) Dualité embryologique du vagin humain et origine histologique de sa muqueuse. *Gynécologie et Obstétriques* **64**, 407–414.

Allen, E., Pratt, J.P., Newell, Q.U. & Bland, L.J. (1930) Human tubal ova: related early corpora lutea and uterine tubes. *Contributions to Embryology* **22**, 45–76.

Austin, C.R., Edwards, R.G. & Mittwoch, U. (1981) Introduction. In: *Mechanisms of Sex Differentiation in Animals and Man* (eds C.R. Austin & R.G. Edwards), pp. 1–54. Academic Press, London.

Baker, T.G. (1963) A quantitative and cytological study of germ cells in human ovaries. *Proceedings of the Royal Society of London Series B* **158**, 417–433.

Barber, H.R.K. & Sommers, S.C. (1974) Vaginal adenosis, dysplasia and clear-cell adenocarcinoma after diethylstilboestrol treatment in pregnancy. *Obstetrics and Gynecology* **43**, 645–682.

Berta, P., Morin, D., Poulat, F. *et al.* (1992) Molecular analysis of the sex-determining region from the Y chromosome in two patients with Frasier syndrome. *Hormone Research* **37**, 103–106.

Berthezene, F., Forest, M.G., Grimaud, J.A., Clanstrat, B. & Mornex, R. (1976) Leydig cell agenesis; a cause of male pseudo-hermaphroditism. *New England Journal of Medicine* **295**, 969–972.

Bishop, A., Blank, C.E. & Hunter, H. (1962) Heritable variation in the length of the Y chromosome. *Lancet* **ii**, 18–20.

Blagowidow, N., Page, D.C. & Huff, D. (1989) Ullrich–Turner syndrome in an XY female fetus with deletion of the sex determining portion of the Y chromosome. *American Journal of Medical Genetics* **34**, 159–162.

Blanchard, M.G. & Josso, N. (1974) Source of the anti-Mullerian hormone synthesised by the fetal testes. *Paediatric Research* **8**, 968–971.

Blechschmidt, E. (1968) *Vom Ei zum Embryo*. Deutsche Verlags-Austalt, Stuttgart.

Block, E. (1979) Fetal gonadal endocrine activity and reproductive tract differentiation. *Contributions to Gynecology and Obstetrics* **5**, 21–37.

Bolton, V.N. & Braude, P.R. (1987) Development of the human preimplantation embryo. In: *Current Topics in Developmental Biology*, Vol. 23. *Recent Advances in Mammalian Development* (eds A.A. Moscona & A. Monroy), pp. 93–114. Academic Press, London.

Bongiovani, A.M., DiGeorge, C. & Grumbach, M.M. (1959) Masculinisation of the female infant associated with estrogen therapy alone during gestation. *Journal of Clinical Endocrinology and Metabolism* **19**, 1004–1010.

Boue, J., Boue, A. & Lazar, P. (1975) Retrospective and prospective epidemiological studies of 1500 karyotyped spontaneous human abortions. *Teratology* **12**, 11–16.

Brambell, F.W.R. (1956) Ovarian changes. In: *Marshall's Physiology of Reproduction*, Vol. 1 (ed. A.S. Parkes), pp. 397–544. Longmans Green, London.

Bridges, C.B. (1916) Non-disjunction as proof of the chromosome theory of heredity. *Genetics* **1**, 1–52.

Brown, C.J. & Willard, H.F. (1990) Localisation of a gene that escapes inactivation to the X chromosome proximal short arm: implications for X inactivation. *American Journal of Human Genetics* **46**, 273–279.

Brown, C.J., Lafreniere, R.G., Powers, V.E. *et al.* (1991) Localisation of the X inactivation centre in the human chromosome in Xq 13. *Nature* **349**, 82–84.

Brown, D.M., Markland, C. & Dehner, L.P. (1978) Leydig cell hypoplasia: a cause of male pseudohermaphroditism. *Journal of Clinical Endocrinology and Metabolism* **46**, 1–7.

Buhler, E.M. (1980) A synopsis of the human Y chromosome. *Human Genetics* **55**, 145–175.

Bull, J.J. (1981) Evolution of environmental sex determination from genotypic sex determination. *Heredity* **47**, 173–184.

Bulmer, D. (1957) The development of the human vagina. *Journal of Anatomy* **91**, 490–509.

Buntine, D.W. (1979) Adenocarcinoma of the uterine cervix of probable Wolffian origin. *Pathology* **11**, 713–718.

Burbige, K.A. & Hensle, T.W. (1985) Surgical management of urinary incontinence in girls with congenitally short urethra. *Journal of Urology* **133**, 67–71.

Burgoyne, P.S. (1981) The genetics of sex in development. In: *Basic Reproductive Medicine*, Vol. 1. *Basis and Development of Reproduction* (eds D. Hamilton & F. Naftolin), pp. 1–31. MIT Press, Cambridge.

Burgoyne, P.S. (1982) Genetic homology and crossing over in the X and Y chromosomes of mammals. *Human Genetics* **61**, 85–90.

Burton, J.L. & Cunliffe, W.J. (1992) The subcutaneous fat. In: *A Textbook of Dermatology* (eds R.H. Champion, J.L. Burton & F.J.G. Ebling), p. 2157, 5th edn. Blackwell Scientific Publications, Oxford.

Byskov, A.G. (1975) The role of the rete ovarii in meiosis and follicle formation in the cat, mink and ferret. *Journal of Reproduction and Fertility* **45**, 201–209.

Byskov, A.G. (1981) Gonadal sex and germ cell differentiation. In: *Mechanisms of Sex Differentiation in Animals and Man* (eds

C.R. Austin & R.G. Edwards), pp. 145–164. Academic Press, London.

Capraro, V.J., Bayonet-Rivera, N.P. & Magoss, I. (1970) Vulvar tumors in children due to prolapse of urethral mucosa. *American Journal of Obstetrics and Gynecology* **108**, 572–575.

Carr, D.H., Haggar, R.A. & Hart, A.G. (1968) Germ cells in the ovaries of XO female infants. *American Journal of Clinical Pathology* **49**, 521–526.

Cattanach, B.M. (1962) XO mice. *Genetic Research* **3**, 487–490.

Chasnoff, I.J., Chisum, G.M. & Kaplan, W.E. (1988) Maternal cocaine use and genitourinary tract malformations. *Teratology* **37**, 201–204.

Cockwell, A., MacKenzie, M., Youings, S. & Jacobs, P. (1991) A cytogenetic and molecular study of a series of 45X fetuses and their parents. *Journal of Medical Genetics* **28**, 152–155.

Cohen, M.M., Shaw, M.W. & McLuer, J.W. (1966) Racial differences in the length of the Y chromosome. *Cytogenetics* **5**, 34–52.

Cohen-Haguenauer, O., Picard, J.Y., Mattei, M.G. *et al.* (1987) Mapping of the gene for anti-mullerian hormone to the short arm of human chromosome 19. *Cytogenetics and Cellular Genetics* **44**, 2–6.

Coulam, C.B. (1979) Testicular regression syndrome. *Obstetrics and Gynecology* **53**, 44–49.

Crowder, R.E. (1957) Development of the adrenal gland in man, with special reference to origin and ultimate location of cell types and evidence in favour of the 'cell migration' theory. *Contributions to Embryology* **36**, 195–210.

Croxatto, H.B. & Ortiz, M.E.S. (1975) Egg transport in the Fallopian tube. *Gynecologic Investigation* **6**, 215–225.

Davies, J. & Kusama, H. (1962) Developmental aspects of the human cervix. *Annals of the New York Academy of Science* **97**, 534–550.

Davis, R.M. (1981) Localisation of male determining factors in men. *Journal of Medical Genetics* **18**, 161–195.

de Grouchy, J. & Turleau, C. (1982) *Clinical Atlas of Human Chromosomes*, 2nd edn. Wiley, New York.

Dewhurst, J. (1980) *Practical Pediatric and Adolescent Gynecology*. Marcel Dekker, New York.

Dewhurst, J. & Gordon, R.R. (1984) Fertility following change of sex: a follow up. *Lancet* **ii**, 1461–1462.

Diamond, D.A. & Jeffs, R.D. (1985) Cloacal exstrophy: a 22 year experience. *Journal of Urology* **133**, 779–782.

Didier, E. (1973a) Recherches sur la morphogenèse du canal de Muller chez les oiseaux. I. Étude descriptive. *Wilhelm Roux Archives* **172**, 271–286.

Didier, E. (1973b) Recherches sur la morphogenèse du canal de Muller chez les oiseaux. II. Étude expérimentale. *Wilhelm Roux Archives* **172**, 287–302.

Disteche, C.M., Cassanova, M., Saal, H. *et al.* (1986) Small deletions of the short arm of the Y chromosome in 46XY females. *Proceedings of the National Academy of Sciences USA* **83**, 7841–7844.

Dupont, B., Oberfield, S.E., Smithwick, E.M., Lee, T.D. & Levine, L.S. (1977) Close genetic linkage between HLA and congenital adrenal hyperplasia (21-hydroxylase deficiency). *Lancet* **ii**, 1309–1312.

Duthie, G.M. (1925) An investigation of the occurrence, distribution and histological structure of the embryonic remains in the human broad ligament. *Journal of Anatomy* **59**, 410–431.

Eida, T. (1961) Entwicklungsgeschichtliche Studien uber der Verschiebung der Epithelgrenze an der Portio vaginalis cervicis. *Yokohama Medical Bulletin Supplement* **12**, 54–63.

Enders, A.C. (1965) Formation of syncytium from cytotrophoblast in the human placenta. *Obstetrics and Gynecology* **25**, 378–386.

Engel, E. & Forbes, A.P. (1965) Cytogenic and clinical findings in 48 patients with congenitally defective or absent ovaries. *Medicine* **44**, 135–164.

Erickson, R.P. & Verga, V. (1989) Is zinc finger Y the sex-determining gene? *American Journal of Human Genetics* **45**, 671–674.

Evans, M.I., Chrousos, G.P., Mann, D.W. *et al.* (1985) Pharmacological suppression of the fetal adrenal gland *in utero*. *Journal of the American Medical Association* **253**, 1015–1020.

Evans, T.N., Poland, M.L. & Boving, R.L. (1981) Vaginal malformations. *American Journal of Obstetrics and Gynecology* **141**, 910–920.

Falk, H.C. & Hyman, A.B. (1971) Congenital absence of clitoris: a case report. *Obstetrics and Gynecology* **38**, 269–271.

Faulconer, R.J. (1951) Observations on the origin of the Mullerian groove in human embryos. *Contributions to Embryology* **34**, 159–164.

Felix, W. (1912) The development of the urogenital organs. In: *Manual of Human Embryology* (eds F. Keibel & F.P. Mall), pp. 752–979. Lippincott, Philadelphia.

Ferguson-Smith, M.A. (1965) Karyotype–phenotype correlations in gonadal dysgenesis and their bearing on the pathogenesis of malformations. *Journal of Medical Genetics* **2**, 142–155.

Ferguson-Smith, M.A., Cooke, A., Affara, M.A., Boid, E. & Tolmie, J.L. (1990) Genotype–phenotype correlation in XX males and their bearing on current theories of sex determination. *Human Genetics* **84**, 198–202.

Fetherston, W.C., Meyers, A. & Speckhard, M.E. (1972) Adenocarcinoma of the vagina in young women. *Wisconsin Medical Journal* **71**, 87–93.

Fluhmann, C.F. (1960) The developmental anatomy of the cervix uteri. *Obstetrics and Gynecology* **15**, 62–69.

Ford, C.E. & Hamerton, J.L. (1956) The chromosomes of man. *Nature* **178**, 1020–1023.

Ford, C.E., Jones, K.W., Polani, P.E., de Almeida, J.C. & Briggs, J.H. (1959) A sex chromosome anomaly in a case of gonadal dysgenesis (Turner's syndrome). *Lancet* **i**, 711–713.

Forsberg, J.G. (1965) Origin of vaginal epithelium. *Obstetrics and Gynecology* **25**, 787–791.

Forsberg, J.G. (1973) Cervicovaginal epithelium: its orgin and development. *American Journal of Obstetrics and Gynecology* **115**, 1025–1043.

Fox, H. (1995) Congenital malformations of the female genital tract. In: *Haines and Taylor Obstetrical and Gynaecological Pathology*, Vol. 1 (eds H. Fox & M. Wells), pp. 41–50. Churchill Livingstone, London.

Friedrich, E.G. & Wilkinson, E.J. (1973) Mucous cysts of the vulvar vestibule. *Obstetrics and Gynecology* **42**, 407–414.

Friedrich, E.G. & Wilkinson, E.J. (1985) Vulvar surgery for neurofibromatosis. *Obstetrics and Gynecology* **65**, 135–138.

Frost, I.F. (1958) Case report of a patient with a true unicornuate uterus with unilateral renal agenesis. *American Journal of Obstetrics and Gynecology* **75**, 210–212.

Frutiger, P. (1969) Zur Fruhentwicklung der Ductus paramesenephrici und des Mullerschen Hugels beim Memschen. *Acta Anatomica* **72**, 233–245.

Fryns, J.P., Kleczkowska, A. & van den Berghe P. (1983) The X chromosome and sexual development. In: *Cytogenetics of the*

Mammalian X Chromosome, part B. *X Chromosome Anomalies and their Clinical Manifestations* (ed. A.A. Sandberg), pp. 115–126. Liss, New York.

Gartler, S.M. & Cole, R.E. (1981) Mammalian X-chromosome inactivation. *Mechanisms of Sex Differentiation in Animals and Man* (eds C.R. Austin & R.G. Edwards), pp. 113–143. Academic Press, London.

Gelehrter, T.D. & Collins, F.S. (1990) *Principles of Medical Genetics*. Williams and Wilkins, Baltimore.

Genest, P., Laberge, C., Poty, J., Gagne, R. & Bouchard, M. (1970) Transmission d'un petit 'y' durant onze générations dans une lignée familiale. *Annales Génétique* **13**, 233–238.

Gill, W.B., Schumacher, G.F.B. & Bibbo, M. (1976) Structural and functional abnormalities in the sex organs of male offspring of mothers treated with diethylstilboestrol. *Journal of Reproductive Medicine* **16**, 147–152.

Glenister, T.W. (1962) The development of the utricle and of the so called 'middle' or 'median' lobe of the human prostate. *Journal of Anatomy* **96**, 443–455.

Goldberg, E. (1988) H-Y antigens and sex determination. *Philosophical Transactions of the Royal Society of London (Biology)* **322**, 72–81.

Goldberg, E.H., Boyse, E.A., Bennett, D., Scheid, M. & Carswell, E.A. (1971) Serological demonstration of H-Y (male) antigen on mouse sperm. *Nature* **232**, 478–480.

Gondos, B. & Hobel, C.J. (1973) Interstitial cells in the human fetal ovary. *Endocrinology* **93**, 736–739.

Greenwald, P., Barlow, J.J., Nasca, P.C. & Burnett, W.S. (1971) Vaginal cancer after maternal treatment with synthetic estrogens. *New England Journal of Medicine* **285**, 390–392.

Griffin, J.E., Punyashthiti, K. & Wilson, J.D. (1976) Dihydrotestosterone binding by cultured human fibroblasts. *Journal of Clinical Investigation* **57**, 1342–1351.

Grinsted, J. & Aagesen, L. (1984) Mesonephric excretory function related to its influence on differentiation of fetal gonads. *The Anatomical Record* **210**, 551–556.

Gruenwald, P. (1941) The relation of the growing Mullerian duct to the Wolffian duct and its importance for the genesis of malformations. *Anatomical Record* **81**, 1–19.

Grumbach, M.M. (1968) Male reproductive tract development, anatomy, physiology and disorders. In: *The Biologic Basis of Pediatric Practice* (ed. R.E. Cooke), pp. 1058–1081. McGraw-Hill, New York.

Grumbach, M.M. (1979) Genetic mechanisms of sexual development. In: *Genetic Mechanisms of Sexual Development* (eds H.L. Vallet & I.H. Porter), pp. 33–74. Academic Press, New York.

Grumbach, M.M. & Conte, F.A. (1992) Disorders of sex differentiation. In: *Williams' Textbook of Endocrinology*, 8th edn (eds J.D. Wilson & D.W. Foster), pp. 853–951. Saunders, Philadelphia.

Grumbach, M.M. & Ducharme, J.R. (1960) The effects of androgens on fetal sexual development, androgen-induced female pseudohermaphroditism. *Fertility and Sterility* **11**, 157–180.

Gubbay, J., Collignon, J., Koopman, P. *et al.* (1990) A gene mapping to the sex-determining region of the mouse Y chromosome is a member of a novel family of embryonically expressed genes. *Nature* **346**, 245–250.

Gustafson, M.L., Lee, M.M., Scully, R.E. *et al.* (1992) Mullerian inhibiting substance as a marker for ovarian sex-cord tumor. *New England Journal of Medicine* **326**, 466–471.

Hall, R., Fleming, S., Gysler, M. & McLorie, G. (1985) The genital tract in female children with imperforate anus. *American Journal of Obstetrics and Gynecology* **151**, 169–171.

Handel, M.A. & Hunt, P.A. (1992) Sex-chromosome pairing and activity during mammalian meiosis. *Bioessays* **14**, 817–822.

Hardisty, M.W. (1978) Primordial germ cells and the vertebrate germ line. In: *The Vertebrate Ovary* (ed. R.E. Jones), pp. 1–45. Plenum Press, New York.

Henking, H. (1891) quoted by Emery A.E.H. (1974) *Elements of Medical Genetics*, 3rd edn. Churchill Livingstone, Edinburgh.

Herbst, A.L., Ulfelder, H. & Pozkanzer, D.C. (1971) Adenocarcinoma of the vagina: association of maternal stilboestrol therapy with tumor appearance in young women. *New England Journal of Medicine* **284**, 878–881.

Herbst, A.L., Kurman, R.J. & Scully, R.E. (1972) Vaginal and cervical abnormalities after exposure to stilboestrol *in utero*. *Obstetrics and Gynecology* **40**, 287–298.

Herbst, A.L., Robboy, S.J., Scully, R.E. & Poskanzer, D.C. (1974) Clear-cell adenocarcinoma of the vagina and cervix in girls: analysis of 170 registry cases. *American Journal of Obstetrics and Gynecology* **119**, 713–724.

Hertig, A.T. (1968) *Human Trophoblast*. Thomas, Springfield, Illinois.

Hertig, A.T. & Rock, J. (1949) Two human ova of the previllous stage, having a developmental age of about eight and nine days respectively. Carnegie Institution of Washington Publication 583. *Contributions to Embryology* **33**, 169–186.

Hertig, A.T., Adams, E.C., McKay, D.G. *et al.* (1958) A thirteen day human ovum studied histochemically. *American Journal of Obstetrics and Gynecology* **76**, 1025–1043.

Heuser, C.H. & Streeter, G.L. (1941) Development of the macaque embryo. Carnegie Institution of Washington Publication 525. *Contributions of Embryology* **29**, 15–55.

Hill, E.C. (1973) Clear cell carcinoma of the cervix and vagina in young women. A report of six cases with association of maternal stilbestrol therapy and adenosis of the vagina. *American Journal of Obstetrics and Gynecology* **116**, 470–484.

Hudson, B. & Burger, H.G. (1979) Physiology and function of the testes. In: *Human Reproduction Physiology*, 2nd edn (ed. R.P. Shearman), pp. 73–96. Blackwell Scientific Publications, Oxford.

Hudson, P.L., Douglas, I., Donahoe, P.K. *et al.* (1990) An immunoassay to detect human mullerian inhibiting substances in males and females during normal development. *Journal of Clinical Endocrinology and Metabolism* **70**, 16–22.

Hunter, R.H. (1930) Observations on the development of the human female genital tract. *Contribution to Embryology* **22**, 91–108.

Hutson, J.M. (1985) A biphasic model for the hormonal control of testicular descent. *Lancet* **ii**, 419–421.

Imperato-McGinley, J., Guerrero, L., Gauther, T. & Peterson, R.E. (1974) Steroid 5a reductase deficiency in man: an inherited form of male pseudo-hermaphroditism. *Science* **186**, 1213–1215.

Jacobs, P.A., Strong, J.A. (1959) A case of human intersexuality having a possible XXY sex determining mechanism. *Nature* **183**, 302–303.

Jirasek, J.E. (1971) Development of the genital system in human embryos and fetuses. In: *Development of the Genital System and Male Pseduohermaphroditism* (ed. M.M. Cohen), pp. 3–23. Johns Hopkins Press, Baltimore.

Jirasek, J.E. (1977) Morphogenesis of the genital system in the human. In: *Morphogenesis and Malformation of the Genital System* (eds R.J. Blandau & D. Bergsma), pp. 13–39. Liss, New York.

Jirasek, J.E., Raboch, J. & Uher, J. (1968) The relationship between the development of the gonads and external genitals in human fetuses. *American Journal of Obstetrics and Gynecology* **101**, 830–833.

Josso, N. (1979) Development and descent of the fetal testes. In: *Cryptorchidism* (eds J.R. Bierich & A. Giarola), pp. 7–20. Academic Press, London.

Josso, N. (1981) Differentiation of the genital tract: stimulators and inhibitors. In: *Mechanisms of Sex Differentiation in Animals and Man* (eds C.R. Austin & R.G. Edwards), pp. 165–203. Academic Press, London.

Josso, N. & Picard, J.Y. (1986) Anti-mullerian hormone. *Physiological Reviews* **66**, 1038–1090.

Josso, N., Picard, J.Y. & Tran, D. (1977) The anti-mullerian hormone. In: *Morphogenesis and Malformations of the Genital System* (eds R.J. Blandau & D. Bersma), pp. 59–84. Liss, New York.

Jost, A. (1947) Recherches sur la différenciation sexuelle de l'embryon de Lapin. *Archives d'Anatomie Microscopique et Morphologie Expérimental* **36**, 271–315.

Jost, A. (1965) Gonadal hormones in the sex differentiation of the mammalian fetus. In: *Organogenesis* (eds R.L. de Haan & H. Ursprung), pp. 611–628. Holt Reinhart and Wilson, New York.

Kai, H., Nose, O. & Iida, Y. (1979) Female pseudohermaphroditism caused by maternal congenital adrenal hyperplasia. *Journal of Paediatrics* **95**, 418–420.

Kaufman, R.H., Binder, G.L., Grav, P.M. Jr & Adam E. (1977) Upper genital tract changes associated with exposure *in utero* to diethylstilbestrol. *American Journal of Obstetrics and Gynecology* **128**, 51–56.

Keith, A. (1948) *Human Embryology and Morphology*, 6th edn. Arnold, London.

King, C.R., Magenis, E. & Bennett, S. (1978) Pregnancy and the Turner Syndrome. *Obstetrics and Gynecology* **52**, 617–624.

Kissane, J.M. (1974) Development of the kidney. In: *Pathology of the Kidney*, 2nd edn (ed. R.H. Hepinstall), pp. 51–68. Little, Brown, Boston.

Kocova, M. & Trucco, M. (1994) Centromere of Y chromosome in Turner's syndrome. *Lancet* **343**, 925–926.

Kocova, M., Siegel, S.F., Wenger, S.L., Lee, P.A. & Trucco, M. (1993) Detection of Y chromosome sequences in Turner's syndrome by Southern blot analysis of amplified DNA. *Lancet* **342**, 140–143.

Koff, A.K. (1933) Development of the vagina in the human fetus. *Contributions to Embryology* **24**, 59–90.

Kohn, G., Yarkonis, S. & Cohen, M.M. (1980) Two conceptions in a 45X woman. *American Journal of Medical Genetics* **5**, 339–343.

Koopman, P., Gubbay, J., Vivian, N., Goodfellow, P. & Lovell-Badge, R. (1991) Male development of chromosomally female mice transgenic for Sry. *Nature* **351**, 117–121.

Krauss, C.M., Turksoy, N., Atkins, L. *et al.* (1987) Familial premature ovarian failure due to an interstitial deletion of the long arm of the X chromosome. *New England Journal of Medicine* **317**, 125–131.

Laue, L. & Rennert, O.M. (1995) Congenital adrenal hyperplasia: molecular genetics and alternative approaches to treatment. *Advances in Pediatrics* **42**, 113–143.

Liao, S. (1978) Molecular actions of androgens. In: *Biochemical Actions of Hormones*, Vol. 4 (ed. G. Litwack). Academic Press, New York.

Lin, C.C., Gedeon, M.M., Griffith, P. *et al.* (1976) Chromosome analysis on 930 consecutive newborn children using quinacrine fluorescent bonding technique. *Human Genetics*, **31**, 315–328.

Lobaccaro, J.M., Medlej, R., Berta, P. *et al.* (1993) PCR analysis and sequencing of the Sry sex determining gene in four patients with bilateral congenital anorchia. *Clinical Endocrinology* **38**, 197–201.

Lubs, H.A. (1969) A marker X chromosome. *American Journal of Human Genetics* **21**, 231–234.

Luckett, W.P. (1973) Amniogenesis in the early human and rhesus monkey embryos. *Anatomical Record* **175**, 375 (abstract).

Ludwig, W. (1965) Uber die Beziehungen der Kloakenmembran zum Septum urorectale beimenschlichen Embryonen von 9 bis 33 mm SSL 2. *Anatomische Entwicklung* **124**, 401–413.

Lyon, M.F. (1961) Gene action in the X chromosome of the mouse (*Mus musculus* L). *Nature* **190**, 372–373.

Lyon, M.F. (1974) Mechanisms and evolutionary origins of variable X chromosome activity in mammals. *Proceedings of the Royal Society of London Series B* **187**, 243–268.

Lyon, M.F. (1993) Epigenetic inheritance in mammals. *Trends in Genetics* **9**, 123–128.

McClung, C.E. (1899) A peculiar nuclear element in the male reproductive cells of insects. *Zoology Bulletin* **2**, 187–197.

McClung, C.E. (1902) The accessory chromosome—sex determinant? *Biology Bulletin* **3**, 43–84.

McKusick, V.A., Bauer, R.L., Koop, C.E. & Scott, R.B. (1964) Hydrometrocolpos as a simply inherited malformation. *Journal of the American Medical Association* **159**, 813–816.

McLaren, A., Simpson, E., Tomonari, K. *et al.* (1984) Male sexual differentiation in mice lacking H-Y antigen. *Nature* **312**, 552–555.

McNally, F.P. (1926) The association of congenital diverticula of the Fallopian tube with tubal pregnancy. *American Journal of Obstetrics and Gynecology* **12**, 303–318.

Mancini, R.E., Vilar, O., Lavieri, J.C., Andrada, J.A. & Heinrich, J.J. (1963) Development of the Leydig cells in the normal human testis. *American Journal of Anatomy* **112**, 203–210.

Mardon, G. & Page, D.C. (1989) The sex-determining region of the mouse Y chromosome encodes a protein with a highly acidic domain and 13 zinc fingers. *Cell* **56**, 765–770.

Merchant, H. (1975) Rat gonadal and ovarian organogenesis. *Developmental Biology* **44**, 1–21.

Meyer, W.J., Migeon, B.R. & Migeon, C.J. (1975) Locus on the human X chromosome for dihydrotestosterone receptor and androgen insensitivity. *Proceedings of the National Academy of Science USA* **72**, 1469–1472.

Mittwoch, U. (1971) Sex determination in birds and mammals. *Nature* **231**, 432–434.

Mittwoch, U. (1975) Chromosomes and sex differentiation. In: *Intersexuality in the Animal Kingdom* (ed. R. Reinboth). Springer-Verlag, Berlin.

Mittwoch, U. (1981) Whistling maids and crowing hens—hermaphroditism in folklore and biology. *Perspectives in Biology and Medicine* **24**, 595–606.

Mittwoch, U. (1992) Sex determination and sex reversal: genotype, phenotype, dogma and semantics. *Human Genetics* **89**, 467–479.

Mittwoch, U. & Burgess, A.M.C. (1991) How do you get sex? *Journal of Endocrinology* **128**, 329–331.

Morris, J.M. (1953) The syndrome of testicular feminisation in male pseudohermaphrodites. *American Journal of Obstetrics and Gynecology* **65**, 1192–1211.

Muller, H.J., League, B.B. & Offerman, C.A. (1931) Effects of dosage changes of sex-linked genes and the compensatory effects of other gene differences between male and female. *Anatomical Record (Suppl.)* **51**, 110 (abstract).

Muller, J. (1830) *Bildungsgeschichte der Genitalien aus anatomischen Untersuchangen an Embryonen des Menschen und der Thiere*. Arnz, Dusseldorf.

Novakowski, H. & Lenz, W. (1961) Genetic aspects in male hypogonadism. *Recent Progress in Hormone Research* **17**, 53–95.

Oguma, K. & Kihara, H. (1923) Études des chromosomes chez l'homme. *Archives de Biologie (Paris)* 33, 493–516.

Ohno, S. (1964) Life history of female germ cells in mammals. In: *Proceedings of the Second International Conference of Congenital Malformations*, pp. 36–40.

Ohno, S. (1967) *Sex Chromosomes and Sex Linked Genes*. Springer-Verlag, Berlin.

Ohno, S. (1977) Testosterone and cellular response. In: *Morphogenesis and Malformation of the Genital System* (eds R.J. Blandau & D. Bergsma), pp. 99–106. Liss, New York.

Ohno, S., Kaplan, W.D. & Kinosita, R. (1961) X chromosome behaviour in germ and somatic cells of *Rattus norvegicus*. *Experimental Cell Research* **22**, 535–544.

Ohno, S., Klinger, H.P. & Atkin, N.B. (1962) Human oogenesis. *Cytogenetics* **1**, 42–51.

O'Rahilly, R. (1977) The development of the vagina in the human. In: *Morphogenesis and Malformation of the Genital System* (eds R.J. Blandau & D. Bergsma), pp. 123–136. Liss, New York.

O'Rahilly, R. & Muller, F. (1987) *Developmental Stages in Human Embryos*. Carnegie Institution of Washington, Washington DC.

O'Rahilly, R. & Muller, F. (1992) *Human Embryology and Teratology*. Wiley, New York.

Owen, J.J.T. (1965) Karyotype studies on *Gallus domesticus*. *Chromosoma* **16**, 601–608.

Page, D.C. (1986) Sex reversal: deletion mapping of the male-determining function of the human Y chromosome. *Cold Spring Harbor Symposium on Quantitative Biology* **51**, 229–235.

Page, D.C., Mosher, R. & Simpson, E.M. (1987) The sex-determining region of the human Y chromosome encodes a finger protein. *Cell* **51**, 1091–1104.

Painter, T.S. (1924) The sex chromosomes of man. *American Naturalist* 58, 506–524.

Pallister, P.D. & Opitz, J.M. (1979) The Perrault syndrome; autosomal recessive ovarian dysgenesis with non-sex-linked sensorineural deafness. *American Journal of Medical Genetics* **4**, 239–246.

Palmer, M.S., Sinclair, A.H., Berta, P. *et al.* (1989) Genetic evidence that Zfy is not the testis determining factor. *Nature* **342**, 937–939.

Park, W.W. (1957) The occurrence of sex chromatin in early human or macaque embryos. *Journal of Anatomy* **91**, 369–373.

Pasqualini, J.R., Sumida, C., Gelly, C. & Nguyen, B.L. (1976) Specific 3H-estradiol binding in the fetal uterus and testes of guinea pig. *Journal of Steroid Biochemistry* **7**, 1031–1038.

Penny, G.D., Kay, G.F., Sheardown, S.A., Rastan, S. & Brockdorff, N. (1996) Requirement for Xist in X chromosome inactivation. *Nature* **379**, 131–137.

Peterson, R.E., Imperato-McGinley, J., Gautier, T. & Sturla, E. (1979) Hereditary steroid 5a reductase deficiency. In: *Genetic Mechanism of Sexual Development* (eds H.L. Vallet & I.H. Porter), pp. 149–174. Academic Press, New York.

Picon, R. (1969) Action du testicule fétal sur le développement *in vitro* des canaux de Muller chez le rat. *Archives d'Anatomie et Microscopie* **58**, 1–19.

Pomerance, W. (1973) Post-stilboestrol secondary syndrome. *Obstetrics and Gynecology* **42**, 12–18.

Potter, E.L. (1946) Bilateral renal agenesis. *Journal of Paediatrics* **29**, 68–76.

Potter, E.L. (1965) Bilateral absence of ureters and kidneys. A report of 50 cases. *Obstetrics and Gynecology* **25**, 3–12.

Potter, E.L. & Osathanondh, V. (1966) Normal and abnormal development of the kidney. In: *The Kidney* (eds F.K. Mostofi & D.E. Smith), pp. 1–16. Williams & Wilkins, Baltimore.

Price, D. & Pannabecker, R. (1959) Comparative responsiveness of homologous sex ducts and accessory glands of fetal rats in culture. *Archives of Anatomy and Microscopy* **48**, 223–244.

Price, D., Zaaijer, J.J.D., Ortiz, E. & Brinkmann, A.O. (1975) Current views on embryonic sex differentiation in reptiles, birds and mammals. *American Zoology* **15**, 173–195.

Price, J.M. (1979) The secretions of mullerian inhibiting substance by cultured isolated Sertoli cells of the neonatal calf. *American Journal of Anatomy* **156**, 147–158.

Pryse-Davies, J. & Dewhurst, C.J. (1971) The development of the ovary and uterus in the fetus, newborn and infant: a morphological and enzyme histological study. *Journal of Pathology and Bacteriology* **103**, 5–25.

Ratcliffe, S.G., Axworthy, D. & Ginsborg, A. (1979) The Edinburgh study of growth and development in children with sex chromosome abnormalities. *Birth Defects* **15**, 243–260.

Rathke, M.H. (1825) Quoted by Stephens (1982).

Reschini, E., Giustina, G., D'Alberton, A. & Candiani, G.B. (1985) Female pseudohermaphroditism due to maternal androgen administration: 25 year follow up. *Lancet* **i**, 1226.

Resko, J.A. (1977) Fetal hormones and development of the central nervous system in primates. *Advances in Sex Hormone Research* **3**, 139–168.

Reyes, F.I., Winter, J.S.D. & Faiman, C. (1973) Studies on human sexual development 1. Fetal gonadal and adrenal sex steroids. *Journal of Clinical Endocrinology and Metabolism* **37**, 74–78.

Robboy, S.J., Ross, J.S., Prat, J., Keh, P.C. & Welch, W.R. (1978) Urogenital sinus origin of mucinous and ciliated cysts of the vulva. *Obstetrics and Gynecology* **51**, 347–351.

Robinson, A., Lubs, H.A., Nielsen, J. & Sorenson, K. (1979) Summary of clinical findings: profiles of children with 47XXY, 47XXX, 47XYY karyotypes. *Birth Defects* **15**, 261–266.

Rosa, F.W. (1984) Virilization of the female fetus with maternal danazol exposure. *American Journal of Obstetrics and Gynecology* **149**, 99–100.

Saenger, P. (1996) Turner's Syndrome. *New England Journal of Medicine* **335**, 1749–1754.

Saldanha, P.H., Arnhold, I.J.P. & Mendonca, B.B. (1987) A clinico-genetic investigation of Leydig cell hypoplasia. *American Journal of Medical Genetics* **26**, 337–344.

Sarto, G.E. & Opitz, J.M. (1973) The XY gonadal agenesis syndrome. *Journal of Medical Genetics* **10**, 288–293.

Scherer, G., Shempp, W. & Baccichetti, C. (1989) Duplication of an Xp segment that includes the Zfx locus causes sex inversion in man. *Human Genetics* **81**, 291–294.

Schneider-Gadicke, A., Beer-Romero, P., Brown, L.G. *et al.* (1989) Zfx has a gene structure similar to Zfy, the putative human sex determinant, and escapes X inactivation. *Cell* **57**, 1247–1258.

Shaw, R.W. & Farquhar, J.N. (1984) Female pseudohermaphroditism associated with danazol exposure *in utero*. *British Journal of Obstetrics and Gynaecology* **91**, 386–389.

Siiteri, P.K. & Wilson, J.D. (1974) Testosterone formation and metabolism during male sexual differentiation in the human embryo. *Journal of Clinical Endocrinology and Metabolism* **38**, 113–125.

Simpson, E., Chandler, P., Goulmy, E. *et al.* (1987) Separation of the genetic loci for H-Y antigen and testis determination on the Y chromosome. *Nature* **326**, 876–878.

Simpson, J.L. (1976) *Disorders of Sexual Differentiation.* Academic Press, New York.

Simpson, J.L. (1982a) Abnormal sexual differentiation in humans. *Annual Review of Genetics* **16**, 193–224.

Simpson, J.L., New, M., Peterson, R.E. & German, J. (1971a) Pseudovaginal periscrotal hypospadias in sibs. *Birth Defects* **7**, 196–200.

Simpson, J.L., Christakos, A.C., Horwith, M. & Silverman, F.S. (1971b) Gonadal dysgenesis in individuals with apparently normal chromosomal complements. *Birth Defects* **7**, 215–228.

Sinaiko, A.R. (1996) Hypertension in children. *New England Journal of Medicine* **335**, 1968–1973.

Sinclair, A.H., Berta, P. & Palmer, M.S. (1990) A gene from the human sex-determining region encodes a protein with homology for a conserved DNA-binding motif. *Nature* **346**, 240–244.

Skordis, N.A., Stetka, D.G., MacGillivray, M.H. & Greenfield, S.P. (1987) Familial 46XX males co-existing with familial 46XX true hermaphrodites in the same pedigree. *Journal of Paediatrics* **110**, 244–248.

Sloan, W.R. & Walsh, P.C. (1976) Familial persistent Mullerian duct syndrome. *Journal of Urology* **115**, 459–461.

Solari, A.J. (1974) The behaviour of the XY pair in mammals. *International Review of Cytology* **38**, 273–317.

Somjen, G.J., Kaye, A.M. & Linder, H.R. (1976) Demonstration of 8-S-cytoplasmic oestrogen receptor in rat mullerian duct. *Acta Biochemica and Biophysica* **428**, 787–791.

Song, J. (1964) *The Human Uterus: Morphogenesis and Embryological Bases for Cancer.* Thomas, Springfield, Illinois.

Stearns, P.E., Droulard, K.E. & Sahhar, F.H. (1960) Studies bearing on fertility of male and female mongoloids. *American Journal of Mental Deficiency* **65**, 37–41.

Stephens, T.D. (1982) The Wolffian ridge: history of a misconception. *Isis* **73**, 254–259.

Stevens, N.M. (1905) Studies in spermatogenesis with special reference to the accessory chromosome. *Carnegie Institution Washington Publication* **36**, 1–32.

Sylvester, P.E. & Rundle, A.T. (1962) Endocrinological aspects of mental deficiency. Maturation status of adult males. *Journal of Mental Deficiency Research* **6**, 87–92.

Tao, T.W. & Hertig, A.T. (1965) Viability and differentiation of human trophoblast in organ culture. *American Journal of Anatomy* **116**, 315–327.

Tegenkamp, T.R., Brazzell, J.W., Tegenkamp, I. & Labidi, F. (1979) Pregnancy without benefit of reconstructive surgery in a bisexually active true hermaphrodite. *American Journal of Obstetrics and Gynecology* **135**, 427–428.

Teplitz, R. & Ohno, S. (1963) Postnatal induction of oogenesis in the rabbit. *Experimental Cell Research* **31**, 183–189.

Terruhn, V. (1980) A study of impression moulds of the genital tract of female fetuses. *Archives of Gynecology* **229**, 207–217.

Tjio, J.H. & Levan, A. (1956) The chromosome number of man. *Hereditas* **42**, 1–6.

Torpin, R. (1942) Prolapsus uteri associated with spina bifida and club feet in newborn infants. *American Journal of Obstetrics and Gynecology* **43**, 892–894.

Uebele-Kallhardt, B.M. (1978) *Human Oocytes and their Chromosomes.* Springer-Verlag, Berlin.

Ueno, S., Takahashi, M., Manganaro, T.F., Ragin, R.C. & Donahoe, P.K. (1989) Cellular localisation of mullerian inhibiting substance in the developing rat ovary. *Endocrinology* **124**, 1000–1006.

Ulfelder, H. & Robboy, S.J. (1976) Embryologic development of human vagina. *American Journal of Obstetrics and Gynecology* **126**, 769–776.

van Niekerk, W.A. (1976) True hermaphroditism. An analytic review with a report of 3 new cases. *American Journal of Obstetrics and Gynecology* **126**, 890–907.

van Niekerk, W.A. (1981) True hermaphroditism. In: Josso, N. (ed). The intersex child. *Pediatric and Adolescent Endocrinology*, vol. 8. Karger, Basel, pp. 80–99.

von Winiwarter, H. (1912) Études sur la spermatogenèse humaine. *Archives de Biologie* **27**, 91–188.

Vorontsov, N.N. (1973) The evolution of sex chromosomes. In: *Cytotaxonomy and Vertebrate Evolution* (eds A.B. Chiarelli & E. Capanno), pp. 619–657. Academic Press, London.

Wachtel, S.S. (1983) *H-Y Antigen and the Biology of Sex Determination.* Grune and Stratton, New York.

Wachtel, S.S. & Koo, G.C. (1981) H-Y antigen in gonadal differentiation. In: *Mechanisms of Sex Differentiation in Animals and Man* (eds C.R. Austin & R.G. Edwards), pp. 255–299. Academic Press, London.

Wachtel, S.S. & Ohno, S. (1979) The immunogenetics of sexual development. *Progress in Medical Genetics* **3**, 109–142.

Wachtel, S.S., Ohno, S., Koo, G.C. & Boyse, E.A. (1975) Possible role for H-Y antigen in the primary determination of sex. *Nature* **257**, 235–236.

Waldeyer, W. (1870) *Eierstock und Ei.* Enzelmann, Leipzig.

Wall, W.J. & Butler, L.J. (1989) Classification of Y chromosome polymorphisms by DNA content and C-banding. *Chromosoma* **97**, 296–300.

Warkany, J. (1971) *Congenital Malformations.* Year Book Medical Publishers, Chicago.

Wartenberg, H. (1982) Development of the early human ovary and role of the mesonephros in the differentiation of the cortex. *Anatomy and Embryology* **165**, 253–280.

Weiss, J.P., Duckett, J.W. & Snyder, H.M. (1984) Single unilateral vaginal ectopic ureter: is it really a rarity? *Journal of Urology* **132**, 1177–1179.

Wilkins, L. (1960) Masculinisation of female fetus due to use of orally given progestins. *Journal of the American Medical Association* **172**, 1028–1032.

Williams, D.L. (1958) Urology in childhood. In: *Encyclopaedia of Urology*, Vol. XV. Springer-Verlag, Berlin.

Wilson, E.B. (1906) Studies on chromosomes III. The sexual differences of the chromosome groups, with some considerations on the determination and inheritance of sex. *Journal of Experimental Zoology* **3**, 1–40.

Wilson, J.D. (1973) Testosterone uptake by the urogenital tract of the rabbit embryo. *Endocrinology* **92**, 1192–1199.

Wilson, J.D. & Lasnitski, I. (1971) Dihydrotestosterone formation in fetal tissues of the rabbit and rat. *Endocrinology* **89**, 659–668.

Wilson, J.D. & Siiteri, P.K. (1973) Developmental pattern of testosterone synthesis in the fetal gonad of the rabbit. *Endocrinology* **92**, 1182–1191.

Witschi, E. (1929) Studies on sex differentiation and sex determination in amphibians. *Journal of Experimental Zoology* **54**, 157–223.

Witschi, E. (1962) Embryology of the ovary. In: *The Ovary* (eds H.G. Gray & D.E. Smidt), pp. 1–10. Williams & Wilkins, Baltimore.

Witschi, E. (1970) Development and differentiation of the uterus. In: *Prenatal Life* (ed. H.C. Mack), pp. 11–35. Wayne State University Press, Detroit.

Wolf, U. (1988) Sex inversion as a model for the study of sex determination in vertebrates. *Philosophical Transactions of the Royal Society of London (Biology)* **322**, 97–107.

Wolff, C.F. (1759) *Theoria generationis* quoted by Adelman H.B. (1966) *Marcello Malphigi and the Evolution of Embryology*. Cornell University Press, New York.

Yen, P.H., Allen, E., Marsh, B. *et al.* (1987) Cloning and expression of steroid sulfatase cDNA and the frequent occurrence of deletions in STS deficiency: implications for X–Y interchange. *Cell* **49**, 443–454.

Yu, S., Pritchard, E., Kramer, E. *et al.* (1991) Fragile X genotype characterised by an unstable region of DNA. *Science* **252**, 1179–1181.

Zah, W., Kalderon, A.E. & Tucci, J.R. (1975) Mixed gonadal dysgenesis. *Acta Endocrinologica (Suppl.)* **197**, 1–39.

Zamboni, L., Mauleon, P. & Bezard, T. (1979) The role of the mesonephros in the development of the sheep fetal ovary. *Annals of Biology, Biochemistry and Biophysics* **19**, 1153–1178.

Zondek, L.H. & Zondek, T. (1979) Observations on the determination of fetal sex in early pregnancy. *Contributions to Gynecology and Obstetrics* **5**, 91–108.

Chapter 2: Anatomy and physiology of the vulva

J.M. McLean

The perineum is that part of the pelvic outlet caudal to the pelvic diaphragm. It is divided into an anterior urogenital triangle and a posterior anal triangle. The vulva lies principally within the urogenital triangle but extends beyond it to overlie the pubic symphysis and adjacent parts of the pubic bones while the anal canal and ischiorectal fossae are wholly accommodated within the anal triangle. Embryologically the perineum is a junctional zone being derived from body wall ectoderm, hindgut endoderm and the intervening mesoderm surrounding the original cloacal membrane. The perineum is therefore not simply an area of skin; it forms an essential part of the female genital tract, urinary tract and gastrointestinal tract. Although the elements of the genital, urinary and gastrointestinal tracts within the perineum are distinct and separate structures, their anatomical location within the perineum determines their functional interrelationship and shared vulnerability to certain pathological conditions. Indeed changing patterns of sexual behaviour indicate that the female anal canal has assumed a sexual function, since in one clinic 33% of female patients with perianal condylomata acuminata reported anal penetration on a regular basis (Jensen 1985).

The pelvic floor

The pelvic floor, or pelvic diaphragm, is a sheet of muscle slung around the midline urethra, vagina and anal canal. The muscles of the pelvic floor, ischiococcygeus, iliococcygeus and pubococcygeus, should be regarded as one morphological entity. Their linear origin, from the white line overlying the obturator fascia on the side wall of the pelvis, extends from the ischial spine posteriorly to the pubic bone anteriorly. From this bilateral linear origin the muscles reach their midline insertion into the sacrum, coccyx, anococcygeal raphe and perineal body, forming a gutter-shaped pelvic floor, which slopes downwards and forwards (Fig. 2.1).

The ischiococcygeus muscle arises from the ischial spine and is inserted into the fifth sacral vertebra and the coccyx. Iliococcygeus and pubococcygeus arise in linear continuity from the ischial spine to the body of the pubis. The iliococcygeus arises from the posterior half of the fibrous linear origin and, overlying the pelvic surface of ischiococcygeus, it is inserted into the coccyx and anococcygeal raphe. This raphe is the interdigitation of muscle fibres from the right and left sides and it extends from the tip of the coccyx to the anorectal junction.

The pubococcygeus arises from the anterior half of the fibrous linear origin and from the posterior surface of the body of the pubis. The muscle fibres arising from the fibrous linear origin sweep backwards on the pelvic surface of iliococcygeus to be inserted into the anococcygeal raphe. Those fibres arising from the pubic bone form a muscle sling around the anorectal junction, which produces a forward angulation of the junction. This part of pubococcygeus is referred to as puborectalis and it lies beneath the anococcygeal raphe and intermingles with the deep part of the external anal sphincter. The most medial fibres arising from the pubis form a muscle sling around the vagina. This part of pubococcygeus is the sphincter vaginae and behind the vagina its fibres intermingle with the fibromuscular tissue of the perineal body. The midline gap between the medial edges of the sphincter vaginae is occupied by the pubovesical ligaments and the deep dorsal vein of the clitoris.

The nerve supply of the pelvic diaphragm is from the lumbosacral plexus (S2, 3, 4). The main functions of the pelvic diaphragm are to support the pelvic viscera and to assist in the maintenance of continence when intra-abdominal pressure is raised during episodes of coughing, sneezing and muscular effort. The posterior midline portion of the pelvic diaphragm is an important component of the post-anal plate (Smith & Wilson 1991) upon which the terminal rectum rests.

The anal triangle

The anal canal

The anorectal junction, lying at the level of the pelvic floor, is angled forward by the puborectalis muscle. The anal canal is about 4 cm long and extends from the anorectal

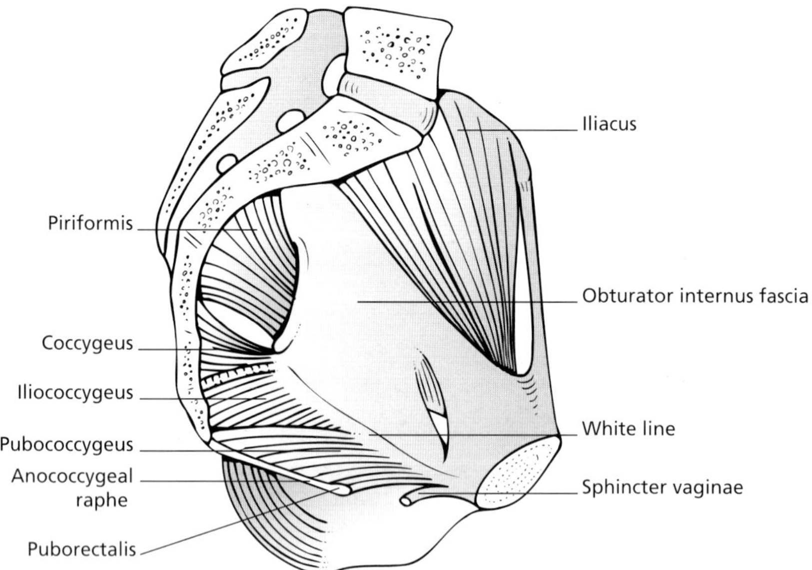

Fig. 2.1 The muscles of the pelvic walls and pelvic floor.

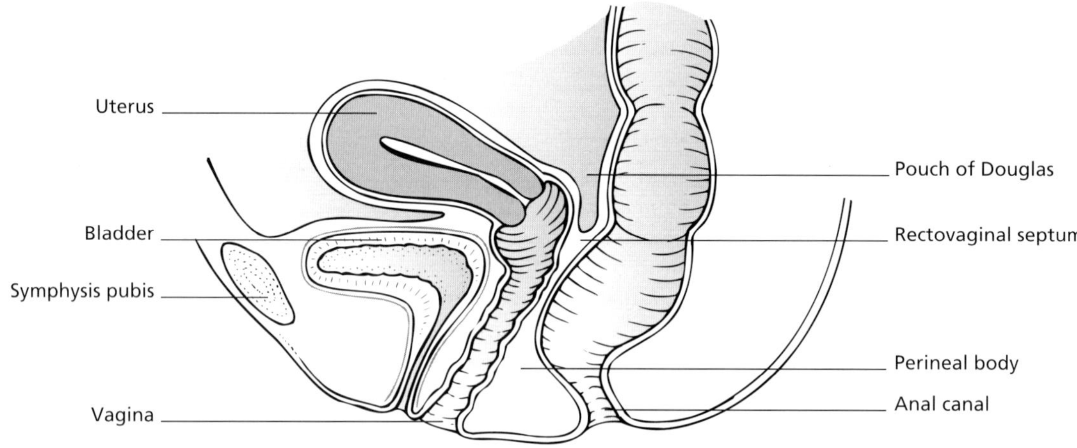

Fig. 2.2 A midline section through the pelvis and perineum.

junction downwards and backwards to the anal orifice. Posteriorly the fibromuscular anococcygeal raphe tethers the anal canal to the coccyx. Anteriorly it is separated from the lower vagina by another fibromuscular mass, the perineal body (Fig. 2.2), while laterally it is related to the ischiorectal fossae. The whole length of the anal canal, however, is enclosed in sphincter muscles, which normally keep it closed.

The lining of the anal canal is said to reflect its dual embryological origin from hindgut endoderm and body wall ectoderm. Certainly in the upper two-thirds, or hindgut portion, the mucosa is thrown into several longitudinal folds termed anal columns. Each column contains a terminal radical of the superior rectal artery and vein, the largest ones being in the left lateral, right posterior and right anterior quadrants. These are the principal sites of internal haemorrhoid formation. The lower ends of the anal columns are linked by short crescentic folds of mucosa, the anal valves (Fig. 2.3). An anal valve may be torn during defecation and such a tear may result in an anal fissure. Above the anal valves are the anal sinuses, recesses in the mucosa of the anal wall, which may retain faecal matter. Opening into the anal sinuses are anal glands, which, extending superiorly and inferiorly, penetrate deeply into the anal wall. This anatomical arrangement may result in anal gland infection and abscess formation. Below the anal valves, or pectinate line, is a transitional zone limited inferiorly by Hilton's white line, which identifies the lower border of the internal anal sphincter. The short segment of anal canal below the transitional zone is lined with skin, which possesses sweat and sebaceous glands.

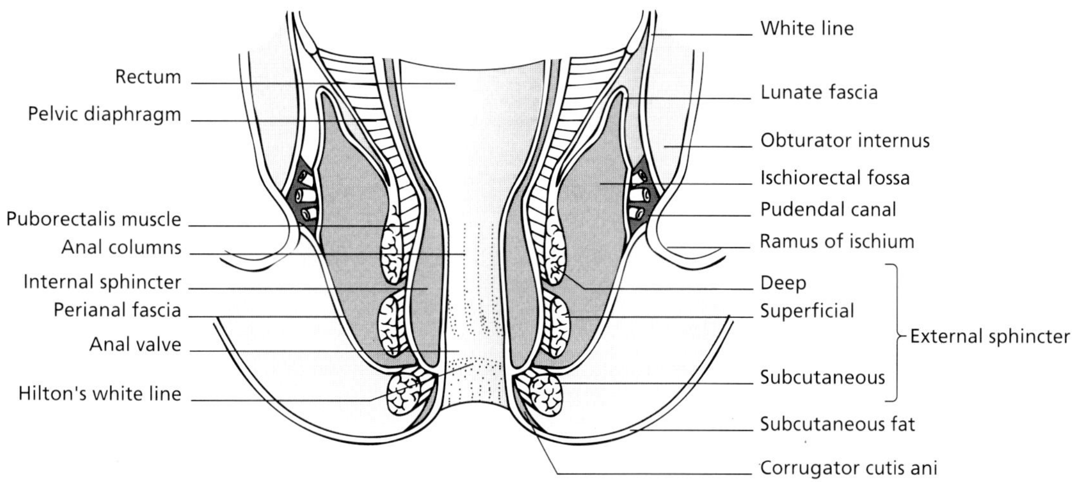

Fig. 2.3 A coronal section through the anal canal and ischiorectal fossa.

There are two separate anal sphincters, one internal and the other external. The internal sphincter of smooth muscle surrounds the upper two-thirds of the anal canal. It is the thickened lower end of the inner, circular muscle layer of the gut tube and is innervated by the autonomic nervous system via the rectal component of the pelvic plexus. The longitudinal layer of gut muscle becomes fibrous as it descends the anal canal and eventually fuses with the anal wall below the internal sphincter. The external anal sphincter surrounds the entire length of the anal canal, being separated from the internal sphincter by the fibrous continuation of the longitudinal muscle layers of the gut. The external sphincter is usually described as having subcutaneous, superficial and deep parts (Fig. 2.3). The subcutaneous part surrounds the lowest portion of the anal canal and lies in the same vertical plane as the internal sphincter. It is separated from the rest of the external sphincter by the perianal fascial layer, which is reflected from Hilton's white line to the lateral wall of the ischiorectal fossa. The superficial or middle part of the external sphincter forms an elliptical loop around the anal canal, being attached to the tip of the coccyx posteriorly and the perineal body anteriorly. The deep part of the muscle surrounds the commencement of the anal canal and blends with the puborectalis muscle laterally and posteriorly. Anteriorly it fills the gap between the two halves of the puborectalis muscle in front of the anorectal junction and blends with the deep perineal muscles. The integrity of this part of the external sphincter is essential to continence, which may be jeopardized if tissue injury during parturition extends into the anterior wall of the anal canal. The corrugator cutis ani muscle is formed by thin slips of smooth muscle, which radiate from the anal canal into the perianal skin. It is part of panniculus carnosus, as is the dartos muscle in the labia majora and platysma in the neck, and is not part of the external sphincter.

The arterial supply to the endodermal hindgut portion of the anal canal is by the terminal branches of the superior rectal artery while its ectodermal lower part is supplied by the inferior rectal branch of the internal pudendal artery. The muscular wall of the canal is supplied by the middle rectal branch of the internal iliac artery. The venous drainage follows the arterial supply and the anal canal is therefore a site of portal systemic venous anastomosis. The lymphatic vessels also follow the arterial supply to the para-aortic and internal iliac lymph nodes, but the terminal anal canal drains to the superficial inguinal nodes.

The autonomic nervous system supplies the upper part of the anal canal, which, although relatively insensitive to pain, is responsive to distension. The lower part of the anal canal is supplied by the inferior haemorrhoidal branch (S3, 4) of the pudendal nerve (S2, 3, 4) and it is very sensitive to pain. The deep and subcutaneous parts of the external sphincter muscle are supplied by the inferior haemorrhoidal branch of the pudendal nerve while the perineal branch of the fourth sacral nerve supplies the superficial part.

The ischiorectal fossa

This wedge-shaped space fills the lateral part of the anal triangle and extends forwards into the urogenital triangle. Its lateral wall is formed by the obturator fascia overlying the lower part of obturator internus muscle. Medially the two fossae are separated by the anococcygeal body, a fibromuscular mass extending to the skin from the anococcygeal raphe, and by the anal canal and perineal body. The pelvic diaphragm forms the roof of the fossa and the perianal fascia its floor. Each fossa is occupied by loose fatty areolar tissue and together they provide dead space for expansion of the anal canal during defecation (Fig. 2.3).

The perianal fascia extends from the anal canal to the lower margin of the lateral wall of the ischiorectal fossa, where it splits to form the pudendal canal. Below the perianal fascia lies the subcutaneous perianal space. The lunate fascia is a continuation of the perianal fascia, extending up the lateral wall of the ischiorectal fossa, medially across its roof and fading out as it descends the medial wall.

The pudendal nerve (S2, 3, 4) and internal pudendal vessels leave the pelvis through the greater sciatic foramen below piriformis. Turning forwards immediately, the vessels around the tip of the ischial spine and the nerve around the sacrospinous ligament, they enter the lesser sciatic foramen. In doing so they reach the ischiorectal fossa, in which they run forward, on its lateral wall, within the pudendal canal to gain the urogenital triangle. As the neurovascular bundle proceeds through the ischiorectal fossa, the inferior rectal vessels and inferior haemorrhoidal nerve arise and arch over the lunate fascia to reach the midline structures that they supply. The inferior haemorrhoidal nerve (S3, 4) supplies afferent fibres to the terminal part of the anal canal and the perianal skin and efferent fibres to two-thirds of the external anal sphincter. Since both vessels and nerves arch upwards from their origin on the lateral wall, incisions into the ischiorectal fossa do not endanger them. As it enters the urogenital triangle the pudendal nerve divides into the perineal nerve and dorsal nerve of the clitoris, while the internal pudendal vessels also break up into a number of branches to supply the clitoris and perineum.

The urogenital triangle

The urogenital triangle is contained within the subpubic arch.

The urogenital diaphragm

The urogenital diaphragm (Fig. 2.4) is a strong, fibrous membrane, attached to the pubic rami, which divides the urogenital triangle into deep and superficial perineal pouches. The urogenital diaphragm is often referred to as the perineal membrane or triangular ligament and it is deficient at three sites in the midline. An apical opening, situated just below the pubic symphysis, transmits clitoral vessels and nerves from the deep to the superficial perineal pouch, while the urethra and vagina enter the superficial pouch more posteriorly.

The deep perineal pouch

The deep perineal pouch is bounded above by the pelvic floor and pubovesical ligaments and below by the urogenital diaphragm. On either side lie the pubic rami while posteriorly it is continuous with the ischiorectal fossae. Emerging from each ischiorectal fossa the pudendal nerve gives origin to the perineal nerve, which divides into deep and superficial branches, and the dorsal nerve of the clitoris. In the same way the internal pudendal artery gives off a perineal branch, which supplies the perineal body and superficial structures, before entering the deep perineal pouch with the deep branch of the perineal nerve and the dorsal nerve of the clitoris. As the artery traverses the deep pouch it gives off branches that pierce the urogenital diaphragm to reach the erectile tissue of the vestibule in the superficial perineal pouch and it then divides into deep and superficial arteries to supply the clitoris. Passing through the deep perineal pouch, in the midline, are the urethra and vagina. The vessels and nerves pass forwards on either side of the urethra and vagina. The clitoral branches leave the deep perineal pouch through the apical opening in the urogenital diaphragm. The deep pouch also contains voluntary

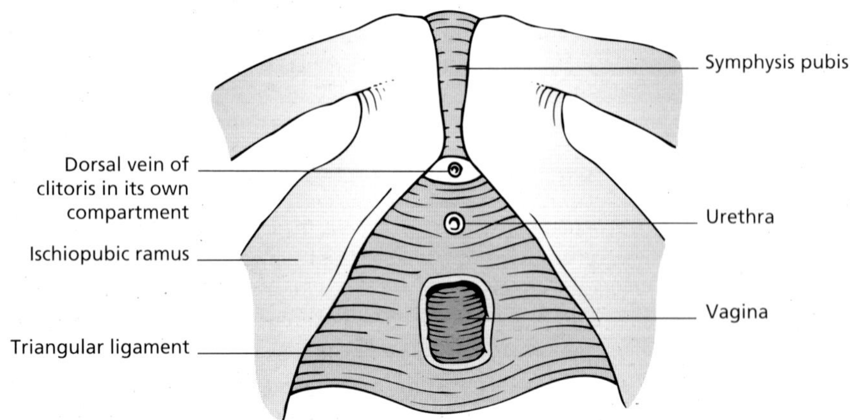

Fig. 2.4 The urogenital diaphragm.

muscle fibres, some of which surround the urethra and vagina while others run transversely into the perineal body behind the vagina.

The urethra

The female urethra is 4 cm long. From the internal urethral orifice it runs downwards and forwards behind the symphysis pubis embedded in the anterior wall of the vagina. After passing through the pelvic floor and perineal membrane it ends at the external urethral orifice, anterior to the vaginal opening, a variable distance behind the glans clitoridis. The urethra is fixed at its origin by the pubovesical ligaments, throughout its length by the anterior wall of the vagina and as it enters the perineum by the perineal membrane.

The walls of the urethra, which are normally in apposition, present longitudinal epithelial folds on their inner aspect. One of these folds, on the posterior wall, is termed the urethral crest since it projects into the lumen rendering it crescentic in cross-section (Fig. 2.5). The urethra possesses an inner epithelial lining supported by a loose vascular lamina propria, and a peripherally situated muscle coat consisting of an outer layer of striated muscle, the external urethral sphincter and an inner layer of smooth muscle.

The striated muscle of the urethra is quite distinct and separate from the pelvic floor musculature. The fibres of this external urethral sphincter are arranged in a circular and an oblique fashion. In the middle third the striated muscle completely surrounds the urethra, although the posterior element, between the urethra and vagina, is relatively thin. In the proximal and distal thirds of the urethra the obliquely arranged fibres leave the posterior urethral wall deficient of striated muscle. The thickness of the external urethral sphincter in the female is less than that of the male but its constituent fibres are able to exert tone upon the urethral lumen over prolonged periods, especially in its middle third (Gosling *et al.* 1983). The smooth muscle of the urethra extends throughout its length and consists of slender muscle bundles, the majority of which are arranged obliquely or longitudinally, although a few on the outer aspect are circularly disposed and blend with the striated muscle of the external urethral sphincter. The urethral smooth muscle is continuous proximally with the detrusor muscle of the bladder and distally with the subcutaneous tissue at the external urethral meatus (Gosling *et al.* 1983).

The lamina propria of the female urethra contains glands and many thin-walled veins, which give it the appearance of erectile tissue, the corpus spongiosum urethrae. The glandular tissue is predominantly found in the lower third of the urethra. Groups of these glands, on either side of the urethra, possess common ducts, which open on the lateral aspect of the external urethral orifice. These ducts are known as paraurethral or Skene's ducts and they may be the site of infection. The proximal urethral epithelium is transitional and continuous with that of the bladder, while distally and throughout most of its length it is non-cornifying stratified squamous in type (Fig. 2.6). The external urethral meatus opens onto the vestibule.

The blood supply, nerve supply and lymphatic drainage of the pelvic urethra are the same as those for the bladder neck. The perineal urethra is supplied by the pudendal vessels and nerves, and the voluntary muscle of the external urethral sphincter is supplied by the perineal branch of the

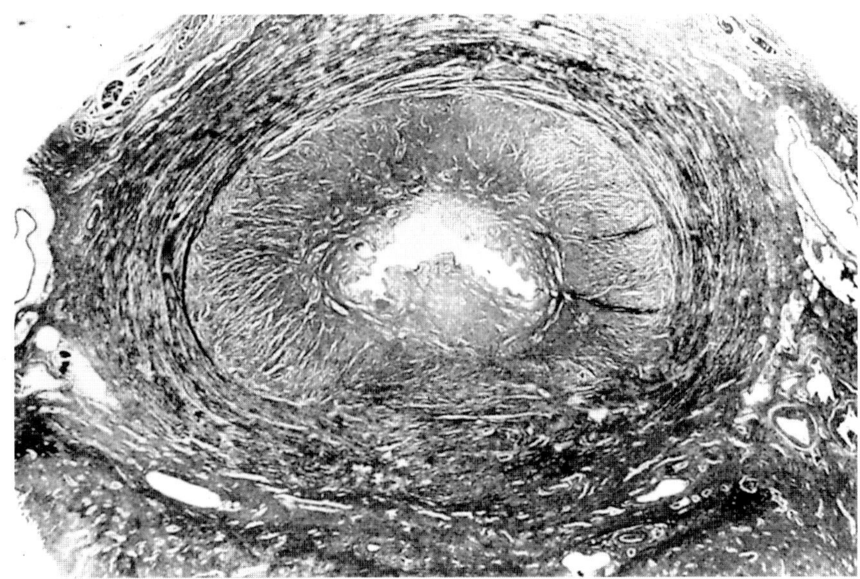

Fig. 2.5 A transverse section through the midportion of the urethra showing the posterior urethral crest.

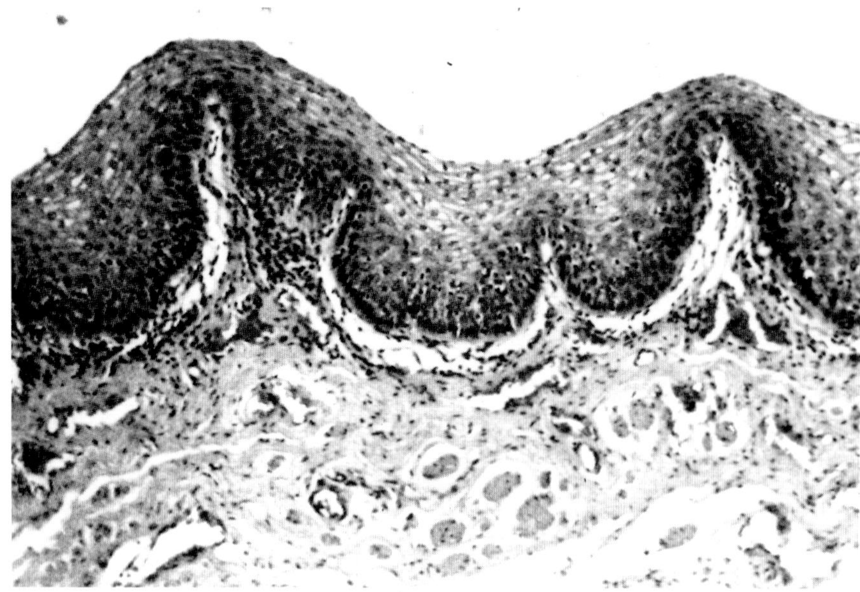

Fig. 2.6 Non-cornifying stratified squamous epithelium lining most of the urethra.

pudendal nerve. The lymphatic drainage of the perineal urethra is to the inguinal nodes.

The cervix uteri

The cervix uteri is an important structure in the female reproductive tract and its secretions have a profound effect upon the vulva. The cervix comprises one-third of the uterine length, being about 2.5 cm long and its inferior portion projects into the vault of the vagina. This anatomical arrangement divides the cervix into supravaginal and vaginal segments. The supravaginal cervix lies below the uterovesical pouch of peritoneum anteriorly and is firmly adherent to the trigone of the bladder. As the ureter approaches the upper angle of the trigone it lies some 2 cm lateral to the supravaginal cervix (Fig. 2.7). At a slightly higher level, the uterine artery, in the base of the broad ligament, begins its ascent of the lateral margin of the uterus. Posteriorly the supravaginal cervix is covered with peritoneum, which extends on to the posterior vaginal wall, before sweeping backwards to the rectum to form the rectouterine pouch. The vaginal cervix usually projects downwards and backwards into the vaginal vault. It is bounded by a deep posterior vaginal fornix, a shallow anterior fornix and by lateral fornices of intermediate depth. On its lower surface is a circular aperture, the external os, which gives entry to the cervical canal and the uterine cavity (see Fig. 2.2).

The uterine cavity is divisible into the cavity of the body and the cervical canal. The cervical canal is continuous above with the cavity of the body through the internal os, and below with the vagina through the external os. The upper third of the cervix is the isthmus uteri; it dilates and is taken up into the corpus uteri as it enlarges during pregnancy.

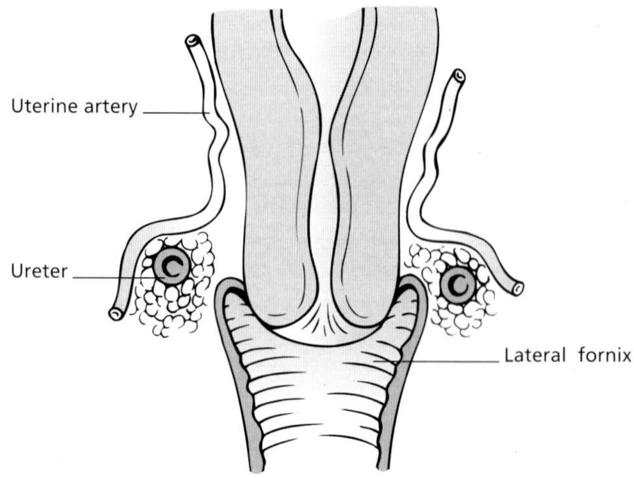

Fig. 2.7 A diagrammatic view of the relationships between the uterine artery, ureter and lateral vaginal fornix.

The uterine artery arises directly or indirectly from the anterior division of the internal iliac artery. The artery and the accompanying veins and nerves constitute the neurovascular pedicle, which, enclosed within the fascia of the pelvic floor, forms the lateral or transverse cervical ligament, often termed the cardinal ligament. As the uterine artery approaches the cervix it divides into an ascending branch, which supplies the body and fundus of the uterus as well as the uterine tube, and a descending branch, which supplies the cervix and upper vagina.

The veins of the corpus, cervix and vagina drain to the uterovaginal venous plexus formed, lateral to the cervix, in the base of the broad ligament. This venous plexus communicates anteriorly with the vesical plexus and posteriorly with the rectal plexus. It drains laterally across the pelvic floor in a number of venous channels that surround the artery and are enclosed with it in the lateral cervical ligament. On the lateral pelvic wall the uterine veins open into the internal iliac veins.

The majority of lymphatics leaving the fundus and upper part of the corpus pass into the upper part of the broad ligament. Here they join lymphatics from the tube and ovary and, travelling with the gonadal vessels, they reach the para-aortic nodes at the level of the second lumbar vertebra. A minority of lymphatics from the fundus, together with some from the uterine tube and ovary, accompany the round ligament of the uterus and drain to the superficial inguinal nodes. The round ligament lies within the broad ligament and runs from the uterotubal junction to enter the deep (internal) inguinal ring. As the round ligament traverses the inguinal canal, fibres leave it to fuse with the canal's fibrous and muscular walls and the remnant emerges from the superficial (external) inguinal ring to fuse with the labium majus. The round ligament may be accompanied by a peritoneal diverticulum, the canal of Nuck, into the inguinal canal. The lymphatics from the lower part of the body and cervix pass laterally in the base of the broad ligament, in the company of the uterine artery, to reach the nodes alongside the internal iliac vessels. Some of these lymph vessels, however, turn upwards on the lateral pelvic wall and drain to the external iliac nodes (Way 1977). Although unusual, umbilical metastasis by lymphatic spread has been reported in a patient with squamous carcinoma of the cervix (Daw & Riley 1982).

Nerve fibres accompany the vessels as they penetrate the walls of the corpus, cervix and vagina. There is general agreement that almost all of the motor fibres to uterine muscle are sympathetic while afferent innervation of the corpus is sympathetic and of the cervix is parasympathetic (Swash 1991).

The cervix exhibits two forms of epithelium: the vaginal surface is covered with stratified squamous epithelium while the cervical canal is lined by columnar epithelium in which there are numerous mucus-secreting cells. The squamocolumnar junction may occur at the external os but more often there is a transformation zone of variable extent situated around the external os, the nature and development of which is described by Singer (1995). The daily cervical mucus secretion varies from 600 mg at midcycle to 20–60 mg during other phases of the menstrual cycle (Elstein & Chantler 1991). At midcycle the main function of cervical mucus is to facilitate the entry of spermatozoa into the upper reproductive tract while at other times its function is to act as a barrier between the vagina and the upper reproductive tract. This barrier function of cervical mucus is effected by its physical character and by its content of specific immunoglobulins. Unfortunately the presence of an intrauterine contraceptive device allows the normally sterile upper reproductive tract to be colonized by vaginal bacteria (Sparkes *et al.* 1981) and frequently results in increased cervical mucus secretion. Any increase in such secretion as a consequence of genital infection, a large cervical eversion or an excessive physiological response will produce vulval symptoms and signs.

The vagina

The vagina, a fibromuscular tube which gives access to the cervical canal and uterine cavity from the perineum, ensheathes the penis during sexual intercourse and is the birth canal for the emergent infant. These two functions of the vagina demand that it can constrict or be constricted and also dilate.

From its opening between the labia minora the adult vagina extends some 7–10 cm upwards and backwards, to be attached around the periphery of the cylindrical cervix uteri, at some distance above its lower margin. As the vagina ascends from the perineum into the pelvis its long axis forms a right angle with the long axis of the normal anteverted uterus. The cervix therefore projects downwards and backwards into the upper vagina. The circumferential vaginal attachment is achieved by the posterior wall of the vagina being some 2 cm longer than the anterior wall. For ease of description the part of the vaginal cavity surrounding the cervix is divided into anterior, posterior and lateral fornices. The deep posterior fornix is continuous, via the lateral fornices on either side of the cervix, with the shallow anterior fornix. The anterior and posterior walls of the undistended vagina are in contact with each other throughout most of their length, giving the vagina a crescentic or H-shaped appearance in cross-section.

The vagina is related anteriorly to the base of the bladder and to the urethra, which is embedded in its anterior wall. Posteriorly the upper part of the vaginal wall is covered with peritoneum. Below the rectouterine pouch the posterior vaginal wall is directly related to the ampulla of the rectum, while in the perineum the fibromuscular perineal body separates if from the anal canal (see Fig. 2.2). The upper vagina gives attachment to the uterosacral ligaments posteriorly, the cardinal or transverse ligaments laterally, and the base of the bladder anteriorly, which itself is supported by the pubovesical ligaments. As the vagina passes through the pelvic floor the most medial fibres of pubococcygeus blend with its walls to form a supporting muscular sling. Below the pelvic floor the vagina is supported by the urogenital diaphragm, the perineal body and the perineal musculature. Thus, the vagina has three compartments: an upper, which is above the pelvic floor and related to the rectum; a middle, which traverses the pelvic floor and urogenital diaphragm; and a lower, which is in the perineum (Blaustein 1982). Diseases such as infections, haematomas and tumours spread somewhat differently from these three compartments (Schmidt 1995).

The vagina has an outer adventitial coat of fibroelastic tissue by which it is bound to the urethra and anchored to the pelvic walls by the pelvic ligaments. The intermediate coat of circular and longitudinal smooth muscle is intermingled with striated muscle from the pelvic floor. Between the muscular and inner epithelial layers is a layer of loose fibroelastic tissue in which there is an extensive network of venous channels. When distended, this network converts the vaginal walls into erectile tissue and is the probable source of vaginal secretion during sexual intercourse (Smith & Wilson 1991). The inner aspect of the vagina is lined with non-cornifying stratified squamous epithelium. The basal generative layer of this epithelium is overlain by rounded cells rich in glycogen, which are the source of the glycogen-containing squames shed into the vaginal lumen. The glycogen content of the vaginal epithelium is oestrogen dependent.

The outer wall of the vagina accommodates the vascular, lymphatic and nerve plexuses that supply it. The vaginal artery may arise from the internal iliac artery or one of its branches, most commonly the internal pudendal artery (Hollinshead 1971). The uterine artery supplies a descending branch to the upper vagina and there is frequently a vaginal branch from the middle rectal artery. The lower vagina is supplied by branches of the internal pudendal artery. These vessels anastomose with each other in or on the vaginal walls. Vessels from the right and left sides anastomose to form unpaired, midline, anterior and posterior azygos arteries. The base of the bladder also receives an arterial supply from this vaginal plexus. The veins of the vagina drain to the uterovaginal plexus, which itself communicates with the vesical and rectal venous plexuses. These venous plexuses drain principally to the internal iliac veins. The lymphatic drainage of the upper two-thirds of the vagina is with the cervix uteri to the internal iliac or external iliac lymph nodes. The lower third of the vagina drains with the rest of the perineum to the superficial inguinal nodes.

The superficial perineal pouch

The superficial perineal pouch lies below the urogenital diaphragm. Attached to the lateral margins of the undersurface of the urogenital diaphragm and to the ischiopubic rami are the crura of the clitoris, each of which is covered by the ischiocavernosus muscle. These crura extend forward as the corpora cavernosa, which fuse at the subpubic angle to form the body of the clitoris. The clitoral body is attached to the pubic symphysis by a suspensory ligament. Between each clitoral crus and the vaginal opening lies the erectile tissue of the vestibular bulb, also attached to the urogenital diaphragm. These bulbs extend forwards beyond the urethra where they fuse to form a slender band of erectile tissue, which is situated on the ventral surface of the clitoris. The vestibular bulbs are covered by the bulbospongiosus muscles, which extend from the perineal body, around the vagina and urethra, to the clitoris. Just behind the vestibular bulbs, also lying on the urogenital diaphragm, are the greater vestibular glands of Bartholin, which open into the vestibule on its lateral aspect. Lying transversely across the base of the urogenital triangle at the posterior margin of the superficial perineal pouch are the superficial transverse perineal muscles (Fig. 2.8). The superficial perineal pouch therefore contains the structural elements of the female external genitalia, which, with their skin covering, exhibit the external appearance characteristic of the vulva.

The vulva

In common with all other parts of the female reproductive tract the vulva is a target organ for the female sex hormones (Omsjo *et al.* 1984). Although it is insufficient to consider the vulva solely from a dermatological perspective, it is nevertheless covered by a specialized area of skin that undergoes significant change at puberty, during sexual intercourse, pregnancy and labour, at the menopause and during the postmenopausal period. The vulva consists of the mons pubis, the labia majora and minora, the vestibule of the vagina, the hymen, the greater vestibular glands of Bartholin, the clitoris with its prepuce and frenulum, the bulbs of the vestibule and the external urethral orifice. Simple inspection will allow only the mons pubis, the labia majora, the margins of the labia minora, the perineal body and the anus to be seen (Fig. 2.9). Adequate exposure of the vulva requires the separation of the labia majora and minora (Fig. 2.10).

Mons pubis

The mons pubis or mons veneris becomes an identifiable structure at puberty with the deposition of subcutaneous fat and the appearance of pubic hair. In the adult female it forms a prominent cushion of hair-bearing skin and subcutaneous fat overlying the pubic symphysis. Although the character of pubic hair varies with ethnic background, its distribution rarely extends more than 2 cm beyond the upper limit of the genitofemoral folds (Lunde 1984). This pattern of distribution produces the horizontal upper margin of female pubic hair.

The mons pubis overlies the pubic symphysis and it has now been established that in countries with very inadequate

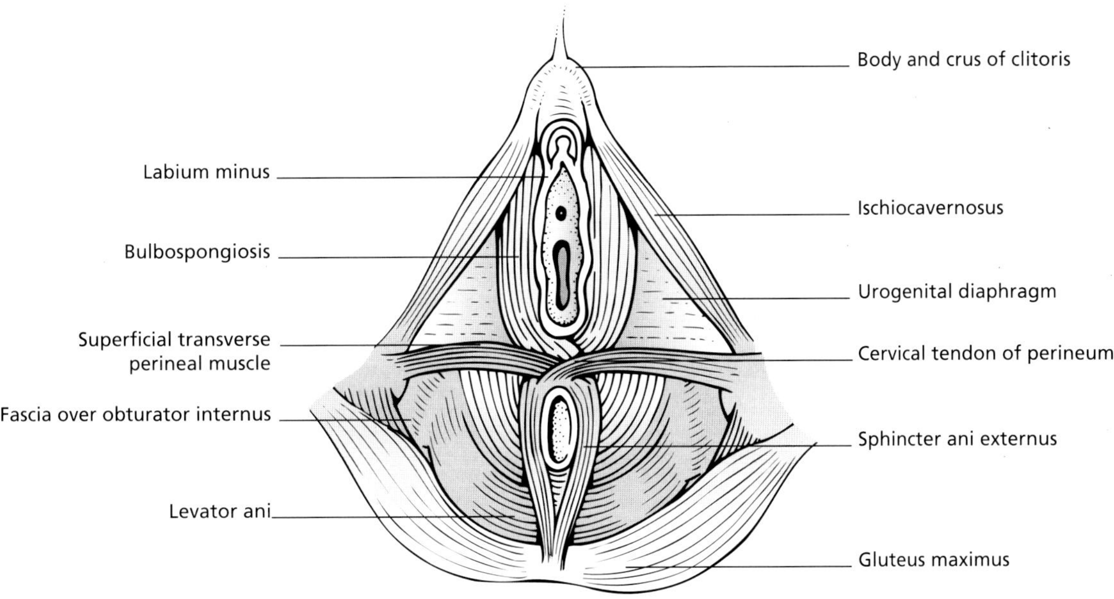

Fig. 2.8 The superficial structures of the perineum.

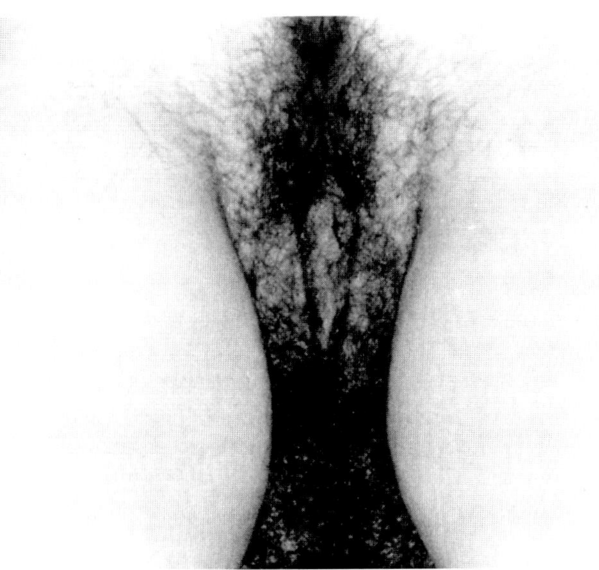

Fig. 2.9 The vulva without separation of the labia.

health care provision symphysectomy is a much safer intervention during obstructed labour than caesarean section. When a caesarean section is delayed or inexpertly done the sequelae may include various fistulae draining to the vulva (van Roosmalen 1991).

Labia majora

The labia majora are two cutaneous folds that form the lateral boundaries of the pudendal cleft. They originate from the mons pubis anteriorly and merge with the perineal body posteriorly. After puberty the deposition of subcutaneous fat within the labia majora produces a greater degree of prominence and the presence of pigmentation and hair on their lateral surfaces establishes them as well-defined structures. Their lack of definition posteriorly is partially due to an absence of subcutaneous fat from the perineal body and the extension of pigmented and hair-bearing skin to surround the anal opening. The lateral surfaces of the labia majora are adjacent to the medial surfaces of the thighs and are separated from them by a deep groove. The medial surfaces of the labia majora, which are hairless and possess numerous sebaceous glands, may be in contact with each other or separated by the protrusion of the labia minora.

The size of the labia majora varies with age, ethnic origin and parity (Krantz 1977). While asymmetry is not uncommon and is usually of no significance it has been reported as a presenting sign in neurofibromatosis (Friedrich & Wilkinson 1985). After the menopause the labia majora become less prominent. This is associated with a thinning of labial hair due to loss of hair follicles with increasing age (Barmann *et al.* 1969) and a reduction of pigmentation. Conversely pregnancy or the use of anovulatory drugs may cause hyperpigmentation of the labia majora in the sexually mature woman (Parker 1981).

Labia minora

The labia minora are two thin folds of hairless skin, devoid of subcutaneous fat, which are situated between the labia majora on either side of the vaginal and urethral openings.

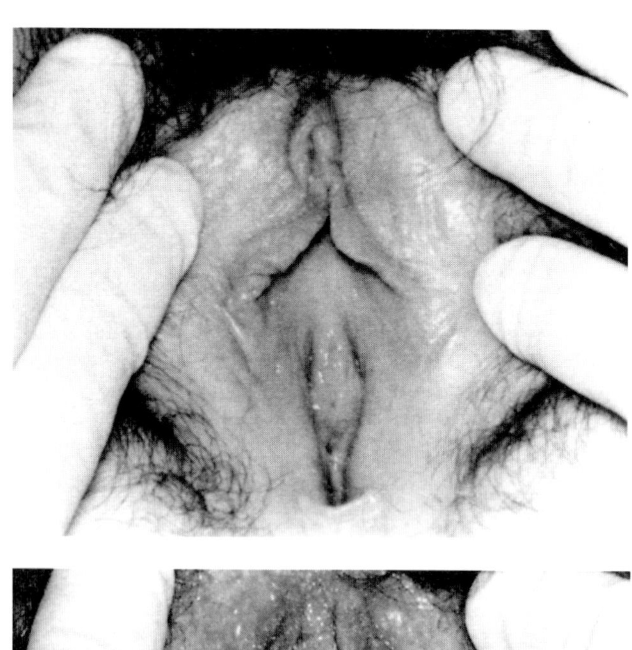

(a)

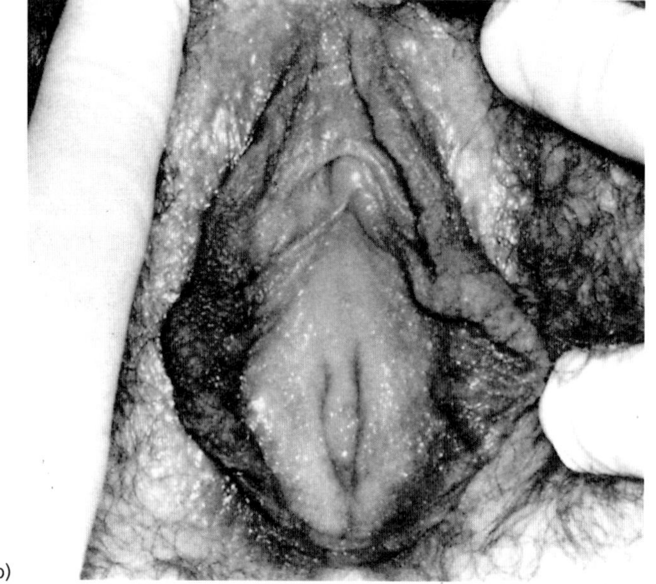

(b)

Fig. 2.10 (a, b) Adequate exposure of the vulva by separation of the labia majora and minora. Note the variable form of the labia minora.

The labia minora are separated from the labia majora by interlabial furrows in which the normal secretions from the adjacent skin surfaces may accumulate in the absence of adequate hygiene. Anteriorly the labia minora divide into lateral and medial parts. The lateral parts unite anterior to the clitoris, in a fold of skin overhanging the glans clitoridis to form the prepuce of the clitoris. The medial parts unite on the undersurface of the clitoris to form its frenulum. This anterior division of the labia minora in relation to the clitoris is variable (Fig. 2.10). Posteriorly the labia minora fuse to form a transverse fold behind the vaginal opening. This fold, the frenulum of the labia or fourchette, is broken at parturition.

Hypertrophy of the labia minora may be present at birth, be produced intentionally in certain tribal groups or occur as the result of certain sexual practices. Such hypertrophy may be associated with local irritation, discomfort in walking and sitting, problems of personal hygiene or coital difficulty. Surgical removal of excess labial tissue, leaving the clitoris and fourchette intact, is recommended in such patients (Baruchin & Cipollini 1986). The sequelae of female circumcision as practised in some cultures may cause serious functional disturbance, which should not occur after simple labial reduction.

The skin of the labia minora is smooth and pigmented, the pigmentation becoming obvious during adolescence. Being devoid of adipose tissue the labia minora are composed mainly of elastic fibres and blood vessels and possess a rich innervation. The arrangement of blood vessels within the labia minora forms erectile tissue comparable to that in the penile corpus spongiosus, their embryological counterpart in the male. During sexual excitation the blood supply to the labia minora is increased and causes not only a change in colour but also significant enlargement, sufficient to induce a minimal degree of traction on the clitoris.

The vestibule

The vestibule extends anteroposteriorly from the frenulum of the clitoris to the fouchette and laterally from the hymenal ring to Hart's line on each labium minus. Localized within the vestibule are the openings of the vagina, urethra, the ducts of Bartholin's glands and the minor vestibular glands. That part of the vestibule between the vaginal orifice and the frenulum of the labia minora forms a shallow depression termed the vestibular fossa or fossa navicularis.

Hymen

The junction of the vestibule with the vagina is identified by the presence of the hymen or its remnants. The hymen is normally a thin, incomplete membrane of connective tissue, which is easily ruptured. Routine use of tampons and/or regular coitus will reduce the hymen to a series of small irregular deviations around the vaginal opening termed carunculae myrtiformes. Occasionally the hymen may be a rigid structure and will prevent sexual intercourse. Alternatively during coitus a rigid hymen may tear into the vaginal wall and cause severe bleeding.

Bartholin's glands

Bartholin's glands, the eponymous description of the greater vestibular glands, are situated deeply within the posterior parts of the labia majora. Each gland lies just inferior and lateral to the bulbocavernosus muscle and is normally not palpable. The glandular secretion is clear, mucoid and alkaline and is increased during sexual arousal. Krantz (1977) maintains that these glands 'undergo involution, shrink in size and become atrophic after the thirtieth year of life'. Nevertheless they may be the site of infection or cyst formation at any age. Bartholin's glands are lobulated and contain multiple acini grouped around the termination of each of the many branching ducts. The acini are lined with cuboidal epithelium and the ducts with stratified transitional epithelium (Kaufman 1981). The main duct of each Bartholin's gland passes deep to the labium minus to open at the lateral margin of the vagina just behind the midpoint and superficial to the hymenal ring. Argentaffin cells have been described in the epithelial lining of the Bartholin duct system predominantly in the transitional epithelium of the main excretory duct (Fetissof *et al.* 1985). The same investigators also observed these endocrine cells in the paraurethral glands and, as in Bartholin's glands, they were distributed randomly among the layers of the transitional epithelium.

Minor vestibular glands

The structure of these glands is comparable to that of the greater vestibular glands. They were present in nine of 19 post-mortem examinations of young women, in numbers varying from one to more than 100, with the average being two to 10, and their commonest location was around the fourchette (Robboy *et al.* 1978). The openings of their ducts are visible to the naked eye.

Anogenital 'sweat' glands

Recently a previously undescribed gland has been discovered in the anogenital area (van der Putte 1991). These glands are found predominantly in the interlabial sulci of the vulva and have distinctive morphological, histological and histochemical features. The glands cannot be categorized as eccrine, apocrine or mammary glands, although they may share some of their morphological features. Interestingly, similar glands have been described in association with hidradenoma papilliferum and on the labia minora of post-mortem specimens (Woodworth *et al.* 1971).

The morphology of the glands ranges from a simple wide duct with a few small diverticula to a complicated, convoluted tubular system. Most glands, however, consist of a coiled duct with diverticular extensions at irregular intervals along its length. Some of the diverticula are short and acinar whilst others are more duct-like and have their own acini. Occasionally some of the glands reach a complexity that gives them a lobular appearance reminiscent of the mammary glands of the breast. The glands all have a straight excretory duct that opens directly onto the skin surface. The anogenital glands extend deep into the dermis, twice as deeply as the eccrine or apocrine glands. The glands are lined by simple columnar epithelium that rests on a thin layer of myoepithelium; this extends into the straight excretory duct until a short distance from the surface where the columnar epithelium gives way to non-cornifying, stratified squamous epithelium without a myoepithelial layer. The columnar cells have oval nuclei and a small to moderate amount of cytoplasm with a cytoplasmic 'snout' at the luminal side. There is some variation in the histology seen in these glands in relation to the different degrees of morphological complexity. Ultrastructurally these glands have features that are unique and not seen in other tubular cutaneous glands (van der Putte 1993).

The clitoris

The clitoris is a specialized structure covered with a stratified squamous epithelium that is thinly cornified. No sebaceous, apocrine or sweat glands are present (Friedrich & Wilkinson 1982). The body of the clitoris is situated in the midline, at the apex of the vulval cleft. The manner of its formation, from the crura and the vestibular bulbs, has already been described when considering the superficial perineal pouch. The whole of the clitoris is composed of erectile tissue and as such is the homologue of the penis. Although uncommon, persistent priapism of the clitoris may occur. Its delayed spontaneous resolution in a fit, parous 36-year-old woman some 9 days after normal marital intercourse has been described (Melville & Harrison 1985). These authors acknowledge that the use of an α-adrenergic agonist, as described by Brindley (1984) for the treatment of priapism in the male, might have achieved an earlier resolution of the problem. Lozano and Castenada (1981) described a case secondary to neoplastic embolism in the corpora cavernosa. The distal portion, or glans clitoridis, can be exposed by upward displacement of the prepuce. Those elements of the labia minora that form the prepuce and frenulum of the clitoris are generously endowed with sebaceous glands, and some mucus-secreting glands are also present.

Bulbs of the vestibule

As already indicated, these erectile tissue masses participate in the formation of the clitoris. Each bulb lies in the superficial perineal pouch adjacent to the lateral wall of the vagina. It is attached to the inferior surface of the urogenital diaphragm by the overlying bulbospongiosus muscle. Thus, the bulbar erectile tissue embraces the vaginal opening and during sexual arousal its engorgement narrows the vaginal introitus.

The external urethral meatus

The external urethral orifice lies between the vagina and the clitoris. Although always in the midline its exact location is variable. Its orifice is usually recognizable but on occasions may be hidden by prolapsing flaps of urethral mucosa.

Vulval skin

The epidermis of the vulval skin and its appendages—hair, sebaceous and sudoriferous glands—are developed from ectoderm. The dermis is developed from mesoderm.

The primitive epidermis is established about the eighth day when ectoderm differentiates within the developing embryo. At this stage the epidermis is a single layer of cells but during the course of the subsequent 3 weeks specific features of the epidermis develop that set it apart from other epithelia in the body (Holbrooke 1983). A second outer layer develops, the periderm, beneath which the primitive epidermis begins the process of stratification. When keratinization occurs at the end of the sixth month, with the formation of the stratum corneum, the periderm is sloughed into the amniotic fluid (Lind *et al.* 1969). Cells that are shed from the stratum corneum combine with sebaceous secretions to form the vernix caseosa, which protects the skin from the amniotic fluid and persists until birth (O'Rahilly & Muller 1992).

Three cell types invade the developing epidermis during the first 6 months of intrauterine life. Melanocytes, derived from neural crests (Niebauer 1968), and Langerhans cells, derived from mesoderm (Breathnach & Wyllie 1965), are present at the end of the third month, while Merkel cells, the origin of which is uncertain, are present by the sixth month (Breathnach 1971).

With the exception of the palms of the hands and the soles of the feet the dermal–epidermal junction is flat in all parts of the body until hair and glandular primordia descend from the epidermis into the dermis. Primary hair follicles begin to form during the third month of gestation and the process proceeds in a craniocaudal manner (Pinkus 1958). Secondary follicles form in close association with the primary follicles and it is thought that the full complement of hair follicles is present at birth (Ebling 1968). Sebaceous glands arise as buds mostly from the hair follicles (O'Rahilly & Muller 1992). They begin to appear during the fourth month and differentiation of the primordial cells into sebum-producing cells proceeds rapidly (Holbrooke 1983). The development and function of sebaceous glands before birth and in the neonatal period is thought to be regulated by maternal androgens and endogenous fetal steroids (Solomon & Esterly 1970). At birth the glands are large and well developed over the entire body and display the same regional variation in size as is seen in the adult. Post-natally they involute and remain quiescent until puberty. Eccrine sweat glands appear during the third month of prenatal life and their ducts are open to the skin surface by the sixth month. Although eccrine sweat glands are innervated as soon as they develop (Montagna 1960) the premature infant usually shows an absent or limited sweating response (Sinclair 1972). The number of sweat glands, like hair follicles, seems to be complete at birth (Pinkus 1910). The apocrine glands do not develop until the sixth month of intrauterine life. It has been suggested that apocrine gland primordia develop in association with each hair follicle but regress in all areas except the areola, axilla, scalp, eyelids, external auditory meatus, umbilicus and anogenital region (Serri *et al.* 1962, Hashimoto 1970). Apocrine gland activity begins during the last trimester but ceases soon after birth (Montagna & Parakkal 1974).

The formation of the dermis is induced by the epidermis and its intrinsic components originate from mesoderm during the second month of embryonic life. The matrix of the dermis is formed by the structural proteins collagen and elastin while the mesodermal cells form fibroblasts, macrophages, melanoblasts and mast cells. The organization of the dermis is progressive throughout gestation and is not complete until some months after birth. Essential for epidermal function is the process of vascularization and innervation, which proceeds *pari passu*. The development of the cutaneous appendages is determined by the dermis.

The epidermis

The epidermis is a stratified squamous epithelium that varies in thickness in different regions of the body. In stained vertical sections its lower border, at the dermal–epidermal junction, presents an undulating appearance due to the epidermal or rete ridges. Histologically the epidermis is described in four layers (MacKie 1984):

1 a basal layer, or stratum germinativum, the lower border of which rests on the basal lamina;
2 a spinous or prickle-cell layer, which forms the bulk of the epidermis;
3 a granular layer;
4 a horny layer or stratum corneum.

This descriptive approach is advantageous because of the variations that occur in the prominence of the different layers in different regions. It must not, however, obscure an appreciation of the progressive differentiation that occurs as a single cell line, the keratinocyte, moves upwards through the various layers to form the tough, protective, flexible outer surface of the skin. A section of epidermis from the labia majora, stained with haematoxylin and eosin (Fig. 2.11), shows a classical basal layer of columnar

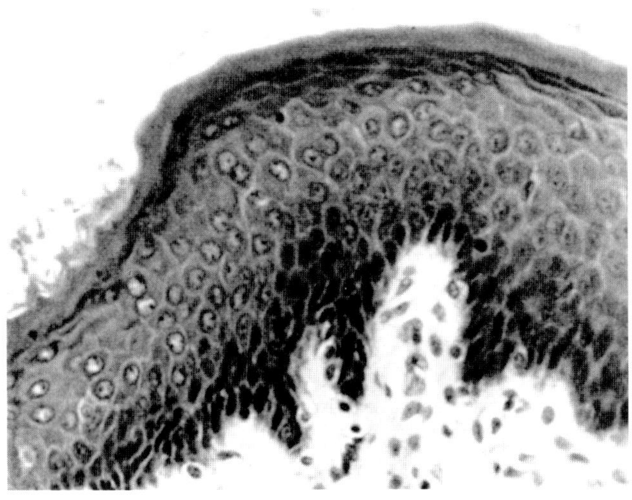

Fig. 2.11 Epidermis from the labium majus showing darkly stained cells in the basal layer above which are lighter-stained polygonal cells in the thicker spinous layer. At the surface the granular layer is composed of flatter cells, above which is an inconspicuous horny layer. (H & E.)

shaped, darkly staining cells. Immediately above the basal layer are the larger polygonal cells of the spinous layer. The cells of this layer are much less basophilic than those of the basal layers and consequently appear more lightly stained. In this particular section a distinct variation in the thickness of the spinous layer is evident. As the keratinocytes ascend the epidermis they become flatter and broader, deeply staining keratohyaline granules appear in their cytoplasm and they establish the granular layer. Above the granular layer an abrupt change occurs, the cells become anucleate and the horny layer is formed.

The epidermis of the labia majora, labia minora and the frenulum of the clitoris is of the type illustrated in Fig. 2.11 in which both the granular and horny layers are relatively inconspicuous. The epithelium on the inner aspects of the labia minora is still cornified but towards the lower part it merges with the vestibule, which is covered in non-cornified stratified squamous epithelium, i.e. a mucous epithelium. Hart's line (Fig. 2.12) may be clearly seen with the naked eye in some patients marking this transition from cornified to non-cornified epithelium.

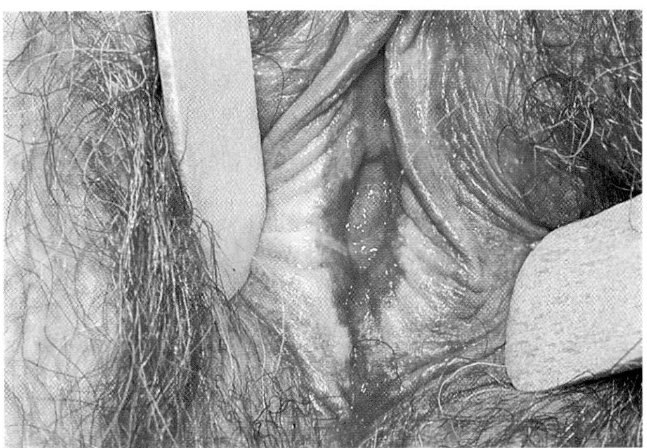

Fig. 2.12 Hart's line.

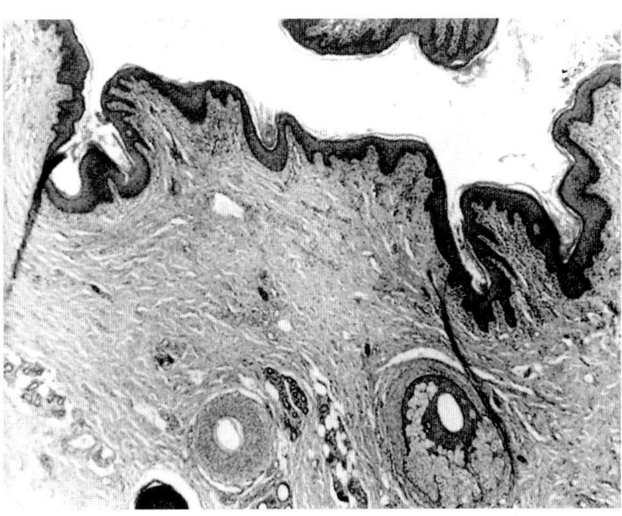

Fig. 2.13 A section of skin from the labium majus showing hair, hair follicles, sebaceous glands, apocrine glands and eccrine sweat glands. (H & E.)

EPIDERMAL DERIVATIVES

The mons pubis, the lateral and exposed aspects of the labia majora and the perianal area are covered with hair-bearing skin. The hair follicle, the hair, the sebaceous gland, the arrectores pilorum muscle and the apocrine glands form a distinct functional unit throughout these areas of the perineal skin. In addition eccrine sweat glands are present and all of these features are usually seen in sections of the labia majora (Fig. 2.13).

The inner aspects of the labia majora, the whole of the labia minora and the frenulum and prepuce of the clitoris are covered with non-hair-bearing skin. These areas of skin are richly provided with sebaceous glands, which open directly onto the skin (Fig. 2.14). Because these sebaceous glands are not associated with hair follicles they frequently form tiny elevations visible on the skin surface, which are referred to as Fordyce's spots. These areas are devoid of apocrine glands and indeed eccrine glands are rarely seen (Fig. 2.15).

EPIDERMAL SYMBIONTS

This term is used to describe three cell types—melanocytes,

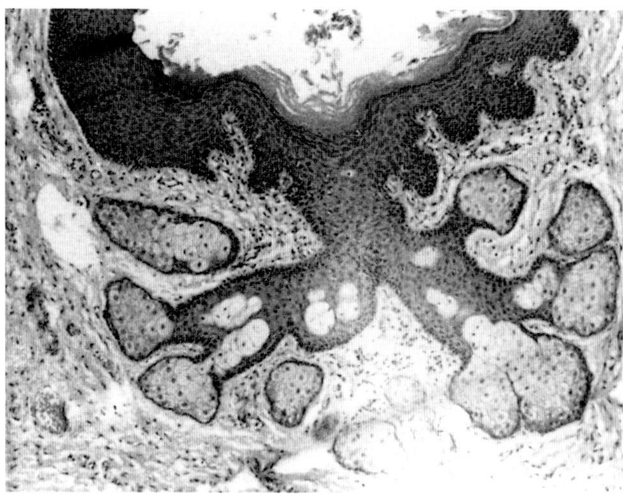

Fig. 2.14 A section of skin from the labium minus showing sebaceous glands opening directly on to the skin. (H & E.)

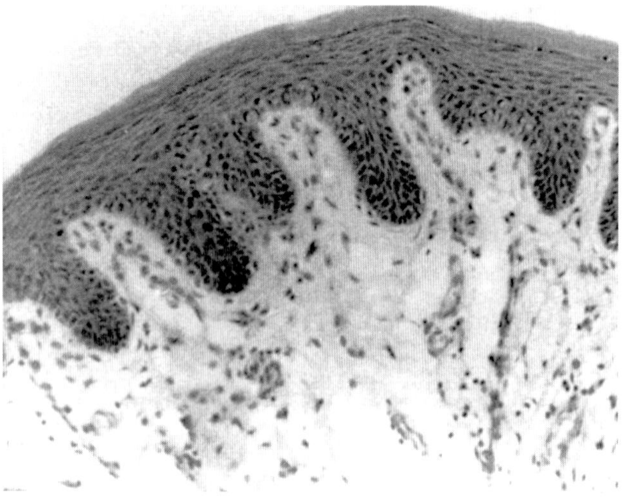

Fig. 2.15 A section of skin from the labium minus showing melanocytes, rounded cells with clear cytoplasm, in the basal layer of the epidermis and a vascular dermis. (H & E.)

Langerhans and Merkel cells—within the epidermis, for which there is evidence of reciprocal supportive function (MacKie 1984).

Melanocytes

Melanocytes are cells of neural crest origin that specialize in the production of melanin pigments, and they are situated mainly in the epidermis. In haematoxylin- and eosin-stained paraffin sections they appear as rounded cells with clear cytoplasm (Fig. 2.15). From this strategic location in the basal layer of the epidermis each melanocyte communicates via dendritic processes with 36–40 keratinocytes (Jimbow *et al.* 1991). It is claimed that keratinocytes exert a controlling influence upon melanocytes, both inducing their dendritic morphology and regulating their proliferation so as to maintain a stable and consistent keratinocyte/melanocyte ratio (Herlyn & Shih 1994). Indeed, although melanocyte numbers show some regional variation they are normally present in a ratio of between 1 : 10 and 1 : 5 of the epidermal basal keratinocytes (Hu 1981). Melanocytes convert the amino acid tyrosine to melanin pigments within the melanosomes, which are membrane-bound organelles. Through the melanocytes' dendritic extensions these melanosomes are transferred to keratinocytes (Jimbow *et al.* 1993). It is generally assumed that the main purpose of this transfer within the 'epidermal melanin unit' is the protection of keratinocyte DNA from damage by ultraviolet radiation and certain toxins (Slominski *et al.* 1993). From matched sites, dark and light skinned people have comparable numbers of melanocytes per unit area of skin. The colour of black skin is produced by the increased quantity of melanin pigment synthesized and its dispersal as melanin granules amongst the adjacent basal cells.

It is now recognized that melanocytes have a considerably wider range of secretory activity than that involved in melanin transfer. Human melanocytes are capable of secreting a number of signal molecules. The potential skin targets for these secretory products are keratinocytes, lymphocytes, fibroblasts, Langerhans cells, mast cells and endothelial cells, all of which express receptors for several of these secretory products (Slominski *et al.* 1993). Hormones profoundly influence human melanocyte activity, although their precise action at the cellular level is obscure. There is also a marked regional variation in the sensitivity of melanocytes to specific hormones. Thus, during pregnancy oestrogens and progestogens stimulate increased melanogenesis in the areola, nipples and perineum, and to a lesser extent in the face and midline of the anterior abdominal wall. Facial hyperpigmentation of pregnancy usually diminishes after delivery but it is likely to recur with subsequent pregnancies. The facial hyperpigmentation associated with anovulant contraceptives is accentuated by exposure to ultraviolet light and may not resolve completely after they are discontinued (Parker 1981).

Langerhans cells

Langerhans cells were named after Paul Langerhans, who discovered them in 1865 while staining sections of human skin with gold chloride. They are found in the epidermis and also in lymph nodes, thymic epithelium and bronchial mucosa (Chu & Jaffe 1994). Epidermal Langerhans cells were once thought to be 'effete' melanocytes (Medawar

1953) but are now known to be bone-marrow-derived dendritic cells, present in all layers of the epidermis. They have an important role in the immune system (Rowden *et al.* 1977), being one of the most potent antigen-presenting cells in the body (Austyn 1987).

Within the skin Langerhans cells represent 1–2% of the epidermal cell population and are located mainly in the suprabasal area. They have been observed in different phases of a cell cycle, which is of 16.3 days' duration, sufficient to renew the entire epidermal Langerhans cell population by local proliferation (Czernielewski & Demarchez 1987). In normal human skin Langerhans cells are present at a density of about 1.6×10^5 cells per square millimetre of epidermis. Each cell possesses five to nine dendrites, which extend out in the same horizontal plane. With their dendrites Langerhans cells cover 25% of the surface area of the skin (Yu *et al.* 1992). More specifically a quantitative study of healthy tissue has shown the distribution of Langerhans cells to be 19 per 100 basal squamous cells in the vulva, 13 per 100 basal squamous cells in the cervix and six per 100 basal squamous cells in the vagina (Edwards & Morris 1985).

Using transmission electron microscopy Langerhans cells can be identified by the presence of Birbeck granules (Birbeck *et al.* 1961) but they are more often visualized by light microscopy, using either the gold chloride method or various histochemical or immunological techniques. These latter techniques exploit the fact that Langerhans cells express a number of phenotypic markers, the most important of which are class II major histocompatibility complex (MHC)-encoded molecules and the CD1a complex (Kapsenberg *et al.* 1990). MHC molecules are essential to antigen presentation and they exist as either class I or class II molecules. Langerhans cells in common with all nucleated cells express MHC class I molecules, but in non-pathological states they are the only epidermal cells expressing MHC class II molecules (Rowden *et al.* 1977) and they express all three subtypes: human leucocyte antigen (HLA)-DR, -DP and -DQ (Teunissen 1992). The MHC molecules bind antigen and the antigen–MHC molecule complex expressed on the surface of the antigen-presenting cell is recognized by and interacts with the T-cell receptor of T lymphocytes. This interaction is accompanied by the binding of T-cell surface molecules CD4 and CD8 with MHC class II and MHC class I molecules, respectively. This in turn initiates T-lymphocyte activation, which results in cellular proliferation and the production of several lymphokines (Golub & Green 1991). MHC class I molecules are thought to be engaged in the presentation of endogenously derived antigens while MHC class II molecules are engaged in the presentation of foreign antigens. The CD1 family is a group of non-polymorphic membrane glycoproteins and CD1a has considerable homology to MHC class I molecules (Bisland & Milstein 1991) and it has been suggested that CD1a may be directly involved in immunological reactions. The T-cell surface marker CD4 has also been reported by several investigators as being expressed by Langerhans cells (Teunissen 1992). Since CD4 is a binding site for the human immunodeficiency virus (HIV), the Langerhans cell is a possible target for HIV infection and HIV proliferation (Tschachler *et al.* 1987).

The immunological function of Langerhans cells involves the activation of T lymphocytes, which circulate freely through the skin. Such activation is essential in any immune response initiated at the surface of the body. Immunological responses of this type are particularly important at the squamous epithelial surfaces of the female genital tract since they are exposed to a whole range of potentially harmful bacteria, viruses and fungi as well as the antigens of the ejaculate. Particularly important in this context is the oncogenic human papilloma virus. Indeed reports suggest that the papilloma virus may induce changes in Langerhans cells in the cervix (Morris *et al.* 1983, Tay *et al.* 1987a,b) and skin (Gatter *et al.* 1984).

Although much of the research on Langerhans cells has concentrated on their role in the immune system there is some evidence from experimental animals that they may also be involved in the control of keratinization (MacKie 1984). The interdependence of the skin and the immune system is further supported by the increasing evidence that keratinocytes perform a significant role in the post-thymic maturation of T lymphocytes (Patterson & Edelson 1982).

Merkel cells

These cells, first described by Merkel in 1875, are found throughout the skin, situated singly or in clusters in the basal layer of the epidermis. Not only do their dendritic cytoplasmic processes surround adjacent keratinocytes (Winkelmann 1977) but their cell bodies are intimately associated with contiguous nerve fibres (Winkelmann & Breathnach 1973). It had been generally assumed that because of their histochemical characteristics Merkel cells belonged to the so-called 'amine-precursor uptake and decarboxylation' (APUD) group of cells and were therefore of neural crest origin (Pearse 1969). However, observations on human fetal skin transplanted on to nude mice indicate that Merkel cells arise *in situ* and are derived from epithelial cells (Moll *et al.* 1990). Immunohistochemical studies have shown that Merkel cells in humans, as well as in many other species, contain vasoactive intestinal polypeptide (VIP) (Gould *et al.* 1985). The precise role of Merkel cells in the skin is obscure but it has been suggested that they function as paracrine regulators of surrounding epidermal and adnexal structures in a manner comparable with their gastrointestinal and bronchopulmonary APUD counterparts (Gould *et al.* 1985). Malignant neoplasms of epidermal Merkel cells may occur (see Chapter 10).

The dermis

The dermis is divisible into papillary and reticular parts. The papillary dermis projects upwards into the rete ridges and is composed of fine collagen fibres, running at right angles to the surface, together with reticular and elastic fibres. This fibre arrangement supports vascular and lymphatic channels as well as nerve terminals. The reticular dermis lies below the papillary dermis and is composed of coarse collagen fibres lying parallel with the surface. Accompanying the collagen fibres are thicker elastic fibres that prevent the dermal collagen from being overstretched. The vascular and lymphatic plexuses that drain the papillary dermis lie within the reticular dermis, which also contains the nerve fibres associated with the papillary nerve terminals.

BLOOD SUPPLY

The arterial supply of the perineum is provided bilaterally by branches of the internal iliac and femoral arteries. The internal pudendal artery, a branch of the internal iliac artery, leaves the pelvis through the greater sciatic notch below the piriformis muscle (see Fig. 2.1). Lying on the tip of the ischial spine it turns forwards through the lesser sciatic foramen to enter the anal triangle posteriorly. Within the anal triangle it runs forwards on the side wall of the ischiorectal fossa enclosed by the fascia of the pudendal canal. During its course through the ischiorectal fossa it gives off the inferior rectal artery, which arches over the fascial roof of the fossa to reach and supply the anococcygeal raphe, anal canal and perineal body. Entering the urogenital triangle the internal pudendal artery gives off the perineal branch to the perineal body and the structures situated more posteriorly in the superficial perineal pouch. The parent artery enters the deep perineal pouch and supplies the erectile tissue of the vestibule, by perforating branches into the superficial perineal pouch, and the clitoris by way of its deep and superficial terminal branches. The latter vessel reaches the body of the clitoris by entering the superficial perineal pouch through the apical deficit in the urogenital diaphragm.

Within the femoral triangle the femoral artery gives off the superficial and deep external pudendal arteries. The superficial external pudendal artery pierces the deep fascia of the thigh anteriorly, to overlie the round ligament of the uterus. It runs medially to supply the mons pubis and labia of the vulva. The deep external pudendal artery pierces the deep fascia of the thigh medially to enter the labia of the vulva. Within the superficial perineal pouch the terminal branches of the internal and external pudendal arteries anastamose with one another.

The venous drainage of the perineum is similarly arranged and eventually reaches the femoral and internal iliac veins. The internal iliac veins drain a rich venous plexus in the pelvic floor, which, at least in part, drains all the pelvic viscera. Thus, the venous drainage of the terminal gastrointestinal tract is partially to the pelvic plexus but principally to the portal system via the superior rectal and thence the inferior mesenteric vein. The pelvic venous plexus therefore provides a portal systemic anastomosis and portal hypertension predisposes to distension and even thrombosis of the pelvic, rectal, vaginal and vulval veins. Vulvovaginal varices, however, are most common during pregnancy although they may occur in patients with endometriosis, pelvic inflammatory disease or pelvic tumours. Since many women develop vulval varices during the first trimester of pregnancy the underlying cause is probably not obstructive but hormonal and indeed progesterone is known to cause increased venous distensibility (Gallagher 1986). In the non-pregnant patient, particularly those using anovulant contraceptives, vulval varices may undergo cyclic change during the menstrual cycle (Gallagher 1986).

LYMPHATIC DRAINAGE

Lymphatic capillaries arise in the extracellular tissue spaces and form larger channels, which drain to the regional lymph nodes. Efferent vessels leave these regional lymph nodes and the lymph passes through a series of intermediate lymph nodes before returning to the blood via the thoracic duct. Although the lymphatic system forms an essential part of the vascular and immune systems the clinical relevance of regional lymph drainage is in the management of patients with malignant disease.

The regional lymph nodes of the perineum are situated in the groin at the base of the femoral triangle. These superficial lymph nodes subsequently drain to deep nodes in the pelvis and ultimately to para-aortic nodes on the posterior abdominal wall. Any midline structure, and especially an anatomical region as well defined as the perineum, has bilateral lymphatic drainage. Thus, the lymphatic drainage of either labium minus is to both the ipsilateral and contralateral superficial lymph nodes (Iversen & Aas 1983). Although the lymphatic drainage of the vulva is regularly reviewed, this account is derived principally from Way (1977).

The femoral triangle is a gutter-shaped depression below the groin, with its apex situated medially and inferiorly. Its base is formed by the inguinal ligament, the lower free aponeurotic margin of the external oblique muscle of the anterior abdominal wall. The inguinal ligament extends from the anterior superior spine of the iliac bone laterally to the tubercle on the body of the pubic bone medially. Inferiorly the inguinal ligament gives attachment to the fascia lata, the deep fascia of the thigh. Midway between the pubic symphysis and the anterior iliac spine the external iliac artery becomes the femoral artery as it enters the femoral triangle deep to the inguinal ligament and the fascia lata. As the external iliac vessels enter the femoral triangle they create a short downward extension of the abdominal fascia, the femoral sheath, which encloses the femoral vessels, with the femoral artery lying lateral to the vein. Medial to the femoral vein is that portion of the femoral sheath termed the femoral canal. The long saphenous vein ascends the leg in the superficial fascia and at the medial end of the inguinal ligament passes through the saphenous opening in the fascia lata to enter the femoral vein. The regional lymph nodes of the perineum are arranged in two groups at the base of the femoral triangle. A variable number of lymph nodes lie transversely in the superficial fascia of the thigh, immediately below the medial two-thirds of the inguinal ligament. Another more vertically disposed group lie adjacent to the termination of the long saphenous vein and are referred to as the superficial femoral or subinguinal lymph nodes. This latter group, varying from three to 20 in number, are arranged on both the medial and lateral aspects of the long saphenous vein. Those on the lateral side send efferent lymphatics, through the saphenous opening, to the external iliac group of deep lymph nodes. The superficial lymph nodes of the femoral triangle communicate freely with one another and drain the whole of the perineum, including the lower thirds of the urethra, vagina and anal canal.

The external iliac lymph nodes are described with reference to their relationship with the external iliac vessels. The medial group of three to six nodes lie on the medial side of the commencement of the external iliac vein. Some of these nodes, as many as three, may be located in the femoral triangle medial to the femoral vein, and in this situation they are referred to as the deep femoral nodes. If all three are present the lower one is situated just below the junction of the great saphenous and femoral veins, the medial node in the femoral canal and the uppermost node is known as the node of Cloquet or Rosenmuller. This latter gland is frequently missing (Borgno *et al.* 1990). The anterior group is inconstant and when present comprises no more than three nodes lying in the sulcus between the external iliac artery and vein. The lateral group of two to five nodes lies on the lateral side of the external iliac artery. The nodes of the external iliac group communicate freely with one another and with the obturator node. This large constant node, so named because of its proximity to the obturator nerve, lies below the external iliac vessels on the side wall of the pelvis and probably belongs to the external iliac group.

The efferent lymphatics from the external iliac group drain to the common iliac nodes situated on the lateral side of the common iliac artery. The external and common iliac nodes drain, either directly or indirectly, the lower limb, the lower anterior abdominal wall, the perineum and some of the pelvic viscera. Many small nodes lie close to each pelvic viscus and these drain into the numerous nodes embedded in the extraperitoneal tissue on the walls of the pelvis. These pelvic nodes are situated alongside the branches of the internal iliac artery and many groups are named according to the vessels with which they are associated. Such classifications, however, are not helpful since the nodes are so widely scattered that extensive stripping of the pelvic walls is necessary to identify them. All lymphatics from the pelvis eventually drain to the para-aortic nodes.

INNERVATION

The perineum has both somatic and autonomic innervation and in each there are sensory and motor components. Since the future perineum is the most caudal part of the developing embryo, its somatic innervation is from the most caudal segmental spinal levels S1, 2, 3, 4. The lower abdominal wall, however, is formed by the migration of body wall tissue into the area between the umbilicus and genital tubercles. Thus, the nerve supply of the perineal area anteriorly is supplemented by input from the upper lumbar segments, i.e. L1, 2. The autonomic or visceral innervation of the perineum is entirely from the most caudal elements of both the sympathetic and parasympathetic systems. The sympathetic outflow from and input to the central nervous system are restricted to the region between the first thoracic and second lumbar levels of the spinal cord. The sympathetic innervation of the perineum is located therefore at L1, 2. It reaches the perineum via post-ganglionic grey rami communicantes, arising from the first two lumbar and all four sacral ganglia of the sympathetic trunks. These fibres are distributed with the first and second lumbar segmental nerves and the first, second, third and fourth sacral segmental nerves. In addition, other sympathetic fibres from L1, 2 leave the sympathetic trunk as the hypogastric nerves (lumbar splanchnics, presacral nerves) and descend into the pelvis to be associated with the autonomic pelvic plexuses, which are distributed with the blood vessels. The parasympathetic outflow from and input to the central nervous system consist of cranial and caudal portions. The cranial portion is associated with four of the cranial nerves while the caudal portion is associated with the second and third, or third and fourth sacral segments of the spinal cord as the nervi erigentes. These nerves together with the hypogastric sympathetic nerves form the autonomic pelvic plexuses.

The cutaneous innervation of the perineum conveys all modalities of common sensation—touch, pain, itch, warmth and cold, as well as complex sensations such as wetness. In addition these cutaneous nerves carry postganglionic sympathetic nerves that are motor to sweat glands, pilomotor units and the adventitia of the microvasculature. No parasympathetic fibres participate in this cutaneous innervation (Odland 1983), which is provided by the terminal or perineal branches of several nerves. The anterior part of the perineum is supplied by two nerves that emerge from the superficial inguinal ring just above the body of the pubic bone. These are the ilioinguinal nerve (L1) and the genital branch (L2) of the genitofemoral nerve (L1, 2). The lateral aspect of the perineum, more posteriorly, is supplied by the perineal branch (S1) of the posterior cutaneous nerve of the thigh (S1, 2, 3). The remainder of the cutaneous innervation of the perineum is supplied by the pudendal nerve (S2, 3, 4) and the perineal branch of the fourth sacral nerve. This latter nerve supplies the skin of the anal margin. The pudendal nerve enters the ischiorectal fossa, close to the tip of the ischial spine on the medial side of the pudendal artery. Running anteriorly on the lateral wall of the ischiorectal fossa it gives rise to the inferior haemorrhoidal nerve, which arches over the roof of the fossa to reach the midline, where it supplies the terminal part of the anal canal and the perianal skin. The pudendal nerve then divides into the perineal branch, which supplies the rest of the perineal skin, and the dorsal nerve of the clitoris, which supplies the anterior labia minora and the glans clitoridis.

These sacral spinal nerves also supply motor innervation to the muscles of the perineum. The pudendal nerve, through its inferior haemorrhoidal branch, supplies the deep and subcutaneous parts of the external anal sphincter and through its perineal branch the muscles of both deep and superficial perineal pouches, as well as the anterior part of the levator ani muscle and the sphincter urethra. The remainder of the levator ani muscle and the superficial part of the external anal sphincter are supplied by the perineal branch of the fourth sacral nerve. Damage to the pudendal nerves may cause loss of muscle tone in the pelvic floor and be associated with problems of incontinence.

The sensory components of the parasympathetic innervation of the perineum mediate the sensation of distension from the anal canal and vagina while its motor component is responsible for the vascular engorgement of vaginal erectile tissue.

Changes in the vulva and vagina throughout life

The changes that are clinically recognizable in the vulva and vagina throughout life are undoubtedly hormonally dependent, since they correlate well with the onset of both puberty and the menopause. During reproductive life additional cyclic changes occur in the female reproductive tract as a result of sequential alterations in ovarian hormone secretion. These changes may be transiently interrupted by pregnancy, which creates its own unique hormonal environment, or by short-term use of anovulant drugs. The principal hormones involved in these changes are oestrogens and progestogens, although the ovary also secretes small amounts of the male sex hormones. Specialized receptors for these steroid hormones have been identified in the female reproductive tract and perineum but the mechanisms of the actions of oestrogen and progesterone at cellular and tissue level are not entirely clear.

Birth to puberty

During the first few weeks of life the reproductive tract of the female infant is responsive to the sex steroids which she has received transplacentally from her mother. The effects of these hormones are entirely physiological and may be evident for about 4 weeks or so (Dewhurst 1980). During this period the infant's vagina will be lined with a stratified squamous epithelium rich in glycogen as a direct effect of the maternal oestrogen (Fig. 2.16). There will often be an obvious vaginal discharge, which in some cases will be bloodstained as the result of the infant's endometrium breaking down as oestrogen levels begin to fall. The external appearance of the vulva during this neonatal period also reflects the effect of the passively transferred oestrogens (Fig. 2.17). Breast development occurs to some extent in infants of both sexes but will disappear, as do the vulval signs, around the fourth post-natal week.

Thereafter the vaginal epithelium loses its stratification and glycogen and becomes much thinner (Fig. 2.18). These conditions persist until the young girl begins to produce her own oestrogen at puberty. During the prepubertal period the absence of glycogen from the vaginal epithelium restricts the action of lactobacilli, present within 24 hours of birth (Marshall & Tanner 1981), in the acidification of the vaginal environment. The resultant neutrality or alkalinity of the vaginal secretions renders all young girls vulnerable to vulvovaginitis and the possibility of lower urinary tract infections.

Puberty is an ill-defined period of time in the life of each individual during which secondary sexual characteristics are being developed. It is also a time when many other physical and psychological changes are taking place. The most important observation concerning the events of puberty is their variability. This applies not only to the age at which they begin but also to the time taken for them to be completed and occasionally the sequence in which they

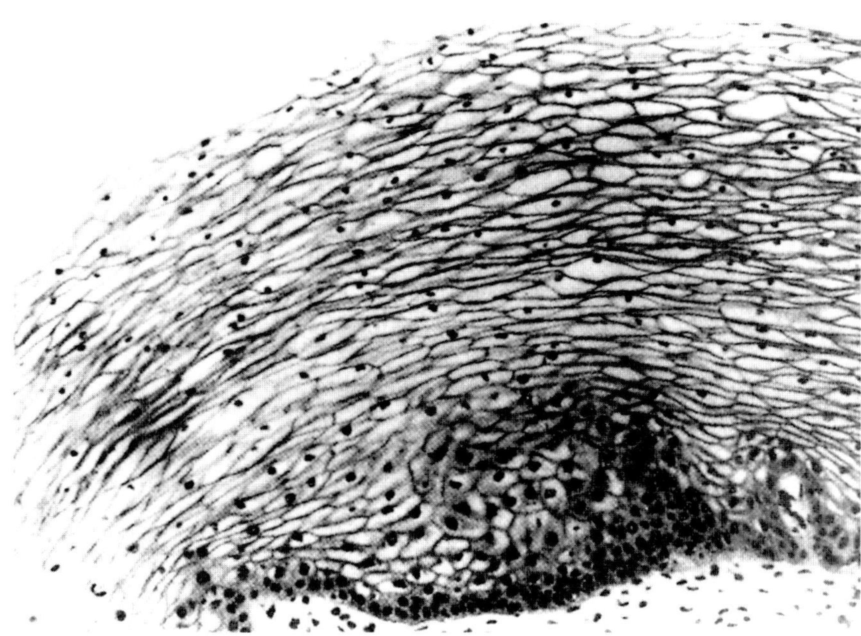

Fig. 2.16 A section from the vagina of a newborn infant showing many layers of cells in the squamous epithelium.

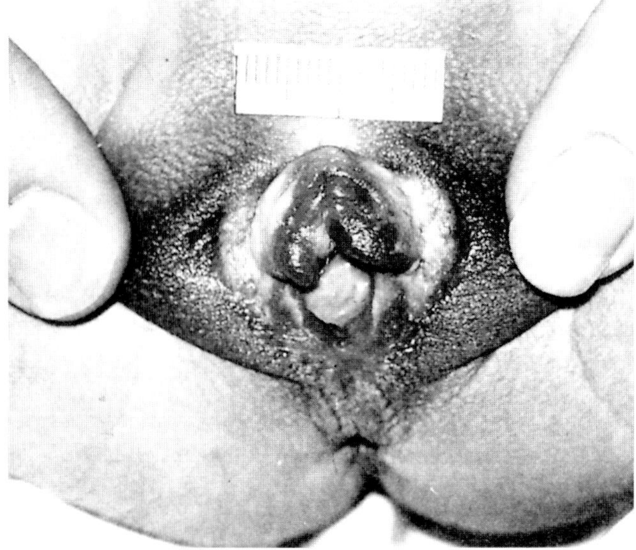

Fig. 2.17 The external genitalia in a newborn female infant.

appear. The physical changes associated with puberty in the female are breast development, the appearance of pubic and axillary hair, increase in height and the onset of menstruation.

Breast development has been described in five stages (Tanner 1962):

Stage 1 is the infantile state, which persists from the time that the effects of maternal oestrogen have regressed until the changes of puberty begin.

Stage 2 is the 'bud' stage, during which the breast tissue appears as a small mound beneath an enlarged areola. This is the first sign of pubertal change in the breast.

Stage 3 establishes a small adult breast with a continuous rounded contour.

Stage 4 is associated with further enlargement of the nipple and areola to produce a secondary projection above the contour of the remainder of the breast.

Stage 5 is the typical adult breast with smooth, rounded contour, the secondary projection present in the preceding stage having disappeared.

The first signs of breast development may occur at any age from 8 years onwards and it is unusual for it not to have begun by 13 years of age. Some girls never show a typical stage 4, passing directly from stage 3 to 5, while others persist in stage 4 until the first pregnancy or beyond (Marshall & Tanner 1981). Premature breast development seems to occur more often in Afro-Caribbean girls than in any other ethnic group. The enlargement may occur as early as 4–5 years of age but is not accompanied by other evidence of puberty or signs of endocrine disease (Black 1985).

The development and growth of pubic hair is also described in five stages (Tanner 1962), although during stage 1 there is no pubic hair. In stage 2 sparse hair appears on the labia majora and on the mons pubis in the midline. There is an increase in quantity and coarseness of the hair, particularly on the mons pubis during stage 3. Further increase occurs during stage 4 such that only the upper lateral corners of the usual triangular distribution are deficient. Stage 5 describes the normal adult pubic hair

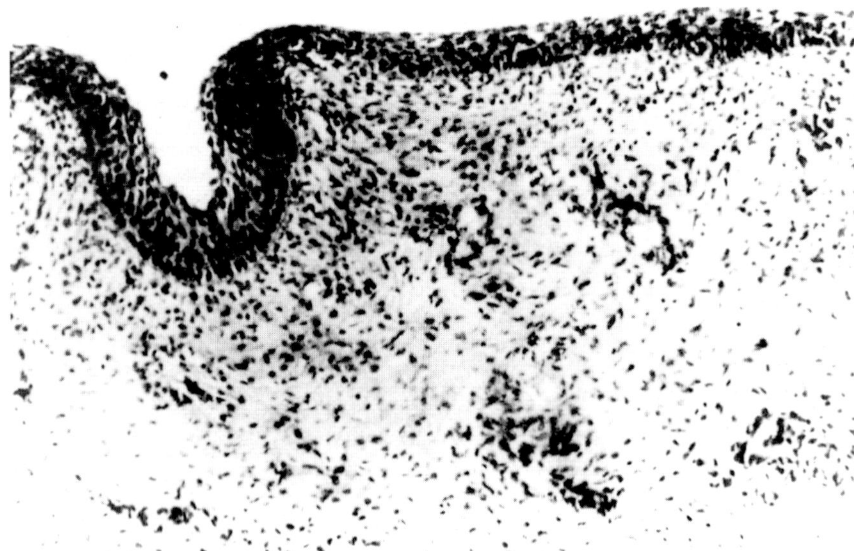

Fig. 2.18 A section from the vagina of a prepubertal female showing a thin epithelial layer.

pattern with its extension from the labia on to the medial aspects of the thighs. The adult distribution of pubic hair is usually attained between 12 and 17 years of age.

Axillary hair growth is described in three stages: from a stage at which it is absent, through an intermediate stage to full development.

The apocrine glands of the axilla and vulva begin to function at about the time that axillary and pubic hair appear. At the same time the sebaceous glands of the general body skin become more active. The growth of any individual is dictated by a number of factors and Marshall and Tanner (1969) have found that most adolescent girls achieve maximum growth rate between their 10th and 14th birthdays.

Menarche occurs near the end of the sequence of changes characteristic of puberty. In the UK the average age of the menarche is 13.0 years with a standard deviation of approximately 1 year. Thus, 95% of the adolescent female population have the menarche between their 11th and 15th birthdays (Marshall & Tanner 1981). It is very unusual for a girl to menstruate before her breasts have reached stage 3 and 25% of girls do so while actually in this stage. The majority of girls, however, begin to menstruate while they are in stage 4 of breast development but, in about 10% of girls, menarche is delayed until their breasts have reached stage 5 (Marshall & Tanner 1981). It is not possible to define the maximum interval that may be allowed after the attainment of stage 5 before it can be assumed that the menarche will not occur. The assessment of skeletal age in these circumstances can be helpful, since a bone age in excess of 14.5 'years' is frequently indicative of primary amenorrhoea (Marshall & Tanner 1981). Menarche is not related to the attainment of a particular body weight and it is unlikely that it has any direct relationship to the relative amounts of water, fat, bone or muscle present in the individual (Billewicz *et al.* 1976, Faust 1977, Marshall 1978).

During the 2 years preceding the menarche the ovaries increase in size. There is an increase in the number of enlarging follicles, although they subsequently regress. This follicular development is associated with increasing levels of oestrogen production, which is responsible for the cytological changes evident in the vaginal epithelium. As oestrogen secretion increases, the vaginal epithelium thickens and intracellular glycogen appears. The vagina begins to lengthen and this process continues until after the menarche. During the immediate pre-menarchal period the uterine cervix increases in size and develops its adult shape. The cervical canal lengthens and the cervical glands become active. It is during this phase of development that the vaginal fluid increases in quantity and regains its acidity, with a pH of between 4 and 5. At about the same time fat deposition increases the size of the labia majora and the prominence of the mons pubis. The labial skin becomes rugose, the clitoris increases in size and the urethral orifice becomes more obvious. Coincidentally the vestibular glands of Bartholin become active and the hymenal orifice increases in diameter.

The reproductive years

In addition to ovarian steroids and pituitary gonadotrophins it is now known that hypothalamic releasing factors, other ovarian hormones and numerous growth factors regulate intraovarian events and the female reproductive system (Carr 1992). Ovulation, however, is the significant event of the ovarian cycle and it occurs approximately midway between two successive episodes of menstruation. During the pre-ovulatory or follicular phase of the cycle, oestrogen secretion increases to reach a peak before ovulation. Oocyte release probably occurs as a result of coincident surges in the secretion of luteinizing hormone and follicle-stimulating hormone. During the post-ovulatory or luteal phase of the ovarian cycle, progesterone, from the corpus luteum, is the predominant hormone, while oestrogen secretion is sustained at a level below that of the pre-ovulatory peak. These cyclic changes in ovarian hormone secretion influence the female reproductive tract so as to create the appropriate environment for internal fertilization and implantation of the embryo.

UTERUS

During the pre-ovulatory phase of the cycle, the effect of oestrogen on the endometrium is to stimulate mitotic activity and thereby regenerate the endometrial lining, to replace that shed during the previous menstrual flow. After ovulation the endometrium becomes progressively more vascular under the influence of progesterone. These hormones induce cyclic changes in both the quantity and quality of the mucus secreted by the endocervical glands, which are significant in interpreting the vulval signs of ovarian function. Mucus production is oestrogen dependent and is therefore usually minimal immediately after menstruation. As the pre-ovulatory surge of oestrogen production approaches, the secretion of mucus increases and qualitatively it becomes transparent, more viscous and more elastic. These characteristics are maximal just before ovulation when oestrogen secretion is maximal (Ross & Van de Wiele 1981, Elstein & Chantler 1991). Women interpret these changes as a sensation of vulval 'wetness' (Etcheparebord *et al.* 1983). Studies on the enzymatic content of cervical mucus indicate significant changes in the concentration of a number of enzymes during this period of vulval wetness (Blackwell 1984, Elstein & Chantler 1991). Two days after ovulation the sensation of vulval wetness disappears as the result of increasing progesterone secretion, which reduces the quantity of mucus produced and alters its characteristics so that it resembles the mucus that preceded the pre-ovulatory surge.

VAGINA

The stratified squamous epithelium of the vagina is exquisitely responsive to the influence of ovarian steroids. Both in childhood and after the menopause, in the absence of oestrogen, the vaginal epithelium is thin and undifferentiated. Oestrogen causes a thickening of the epithelium and its differentiation into the well-recognized basal, intermediate and superficial layers characteristic of the reproductive years. The percentage of superficial cells present in a vaginal smear is an indicator of the amount of oestrogenic activity. Progesterone produces a relative decrease in the number of superficial cells while increasing the number of intermediate cells (Friedrich 1976).

The vaginal epithelium, under the influence of oestrogen, contains a great deal of glycogen. The normal vaginal flora is mixed but lactobacilli and corynebacteria, which predominate, utilize the glycogen to produce lactic acid and a low vaginal pH. This protective environment usually precludes the overgrowth of *Candida* species, which are also present in the vagina. This delicate balance may be disturbed by the use of antibiotics, such as oxytetracycline in the treatment of acne, although other antibiotics are also capable of inhibiting the lactobacilli and corynebacteria and allowing candidal overgrowth. The acidity of the vaginal environment may be reduced by the alkaline secretions of the cervical glands, particularly in the presence of a large eversion of the endocervix, by the alkaline menstrual flow and by frequent acts of coitus, since both the vaginal transudate and the ejaculate are alkaline. A more subtle change takes place in the vagina when the effects of oestrogen are moderated by a relative dominance of progesterone such as occurs during pregnancy and with the use of some oral contraceptives. In these situations glycogen is not so readily available because of a reduction in the numbers of cells in the superficial layer of the vaginal epithelium. The same relative lack of epithelial glycogen occurs in women with diabetes mellitus due to increased glycogenolysis associated with disordered carbohydrate metabolism (Friedrich 1976).

URETHRA AND VULVA

The epithelial lining of the urethra is also influenced by the ovarian hormones and the character of exfoliated urethral epithelial cells changes with the phase of the ovarian cycle. Properly stained smears of epithelial cells in fresh urinary sediment reflects cyclic alterations in oestrogen and progesterone levels in sexually mature women. These cells are more accessible than vaginal epithelial cells in young girls and may be examined for diagnostic purposes when excessive oestrogen production is suspected (Ross & Van de Wiele 1981). Changes corresponding to those in the vaginal epithelium may be observed in the epithelium lining the inner aspects of the labia minora (Tozzini *et al.* 1971).

As already discussed the most obvious physiological vulval change that occurs during a woman's reproductive years is the subjective sensation of wetness, which is present about the time of ovulation. This vulval symptom is a consequence of the changes in the quantity and quality of the cervical mucus secretion during the ovarian cycle. Many of the other vulval signs and symptoms, both physiological and pathological, are the result of changes in the upper reproductive tract, particularly the cervix uteri and vagina. Sexually transmitted diseases are very common and many women are particularly anxious if they have been exposed to the risk of infection. In these circumstances it is important to recognize that a vaginal discharge does not necessarily mean infection and that attempts at self-treatment may worsen the situation and make accurate diagnosis more difficult (Friedrich 1985).

CHANGES RELATED TO COITUS AND PREGNANCY

Many studies have been undertaken to determine any consistent pattern in the female sexual response that could be related to the menstrual cycle. Riley and Trimmer (1991) maintain that in the most reliable studies peaks of sexual interest have been consistently shown to occur in the midfollicular and late luteal phases and that the physiological response is significantly lower during the periovulatory phase than in the immediate postmenstrual and midluteal phases. The difficulties inherent in such studies are evidenced by the fact that vulval and related problems may make sexual intercourse painful, thus influencing the willingness of affected women to engage in sexual activity and that in normal circumstances a substantial minority of women (35–42%) would appear to have very little interest in sexual intercourse (Reader 1991).

During sexual arousal in the female the breasts enlarge and the nipples become erect. This erectile response also occurs in the clitoris, labia minora and the vestibular bulbs on either side of the vaginal opening. The vascular engorgement of the labia minora and vestibular bulbs reduces the size of the introitus by approximately 50% (Burchell & Wabrek 1981, Riley & Trimmer 1991). The upper vagina dilates and the uterus is elevated in the pelvis as a result of pelvic vascular congestion. This vascular congestion, mediated by the parasympathetic nervous system, induces a transudate from the vaginal epithelium that produces the lubrication necessary for coitus. Penetration of the vagina by the penis produces traction on the labia minora and thus an additional stimulus to the clitoris. During orgasm rhythmic contraction of the pelvic floor and perineal musculature occurs. This is followed by decongestion of the pelvic viscera and vasculature during the phase of resolution. The physiological events occurring in the female reproductive tract during coitus facilitate spermatozoal transport, from the site of ejaculation in the upper vagina to the uterine tubes where fertilization normally takes place. Such spermatozoal transport occurs only at or about the time of ovulation, when changes in the cervical mucus allow entry of spermatozoa into the cavity of the uterus.

In the event of fertilization and successful implantation of the embryo the pregnant woman will adapt to a unique hormonal environment created by the steroid and protein hormones produced by the placenta (Casey *et al.* 1992). Blood flow through the pelvic circulation is increased fivefold during the first 2 months of pregnancy and doubles again during the third month (Barrow 1957). Progesterone causes an increase of venous distensibility (Gallagher 1986) and in the progesterone-dominant state of pregnancy predisposes to vulval varicosities. In addition the diminished availability of glycogen from the vaginal epithelium renders the vagina more likely to candidal overgrowth, which is reported to be 10–20 times more common in pregnant than non-pregnant women (Wallenburg & Wladimiroff 1976). The situation is undoubtedly exacerbated by the host's altered immune responsiveness during pregnancy (Toder & Shomer 1990), perhaps to ensure the survival of the fetal allograft, and these alterations appear to make the pregnant woman more susceptible to primary infection, reinfection and reactivated infection (Brabin 1985).

Injury to the genital tract and vulva may occur during delivery of the infant. Rupture of vessels outside the wall of the genital tract may lead to paragenital haematoma formation, in which case a significant distinction must be made between those which lie above and below the levator ani muscle (Beazley 1981). Infralevator haematomas may occur as the result of an inadequate episiotomy repair, which allows a continual ooze into the surrounding tissues. In this way a great quantity of blood can escape into the ischiorectal fossae or paravaginal tissues. Of more direct relevance, in the present context, are injuries to the vaginal wall and vulva that affect the perineum and may occur spontaneously or as a result of episiotomy. These will usually be identified at the time of delivery and appropriately treated; if not they may be associated with serious functional disturbances at a later date.

The menopause and old age

The menopause is defined by the World Health Organization as the permanent cessation of menstruation resulting from the loss of follicular activity. The term perimenopause is used to describe that period beginning with the first symptoms or indications of the approaching menopause and ending 1 year after the final menstrual period (Burger 1996). The term 'menopausal transition' describes that part of the perimenopause ending with the final menstrual period. A prospective study of 2570 women aged 44–55 years, followed for 5 years, showed that menstrual irregularity commenced on average at 47.5 years of age and that the duration of the transition was almost 4 years (McKinlay *et al.* 1992). Despite the WHO's definition of the menopause there is no general agreement as to whether the menopause begins with the last episode of menstruation or after amenorrhoea has persisted for 1 year or longer. However, it would seem from a number of studies that cessation of menstruation occurs at a median age of 50 years in Western industrialized societies but somewhat earlier in non-European women (Ginsberg 1991). Ageing of the ovaries is eventually associated with the inability to secrete sufficient of the hormones necessary to produce endometrial shedding. When menstruation has ceased for at least 1 year the woman is said to be postmenopausal (Davey 1981). Thereafter oestrogen and progesterone levels remain low while gonadotrophin levels increase and may remain elevated for perhaps 20–30 years (Davey 1981).

The postmenopausal changes in the genital and urinary tracts are related to cessation of ovarian hormone secretion but also to the normal ageing process. The body of the uterus is reduced in size, the myometrium is partially replaced by fibrous tissue, the endometrium becomes thin and atrophic and cervical glandular secretion is reduced.

The vagina becomes less rugose, narrower and drier and the vaginal epithelium more easily damaged (Schaffer & Fantl 1996). Microscopically the epithelial layers are reduced in number and the cells lack glycogen, while the stroma is infiltrated with lymphocytes and plasma cells. As a consequence of these changes the vaginal environment becomes alkaline (Davey 1981, Utian 1987). Some time later the vulval skin becomes atrophic and, as a result of the loss of subcutaneous fat, the labia majora and mons pubis are reduced in size and the introitus may gape. Loss of muscle tone encourages the possibility of vaginal and uterine prolapse. Changes comparable to those in the vaginal epithelium also occur in the transitional epithelium of the urethra and bladder with the consequent increased risk of recurrent urethritis and cystitis. These changes may be modified, to an undefined extent, by hormone replacement therapy.

Premature ovarian failure affects approximately 1% of all women under the age of 40 years (Baber *et al.* 1991). Although premature ovarian failure may be caused by some genetic defect, an autoimmune disorder or following treatment for other conditions that may have been life threatening, no definite cause can be established in the majority of affected women. It has also been suggested, on the basis of urinary hormone assays, that oestrogen deficiency may follow tubal ligation in some women (Cattanach 1985).

Incontinence

Incontinence, defined as the inadvertent or uncontrolled passage of faeces or urine or both, is a disability associated with profound social consequences (Swash 1985). In the female it will also have significant clinical effects upon the perineum, which may be difficult to interpret if incontinence is not suspected. Urinary incontinence is present in about 12% of women over 65 years of age and in as many as 9% of younger women (Thomas *et al.* 1980). Faecal incontinence is perhaps less common, although half of the patients investigated for diarrhoea in one study were in fact suffering from faecal incontinence (Leigh & Turnberg 1982).

Neurological causes of incontinence include multiple sclerosis, Parkinson's disease and disorders of the spinal cord or cauda equina. It may also occur in patients with peripheral neuropathy, especially when autonomic nerves are affected, as in diabetes mellitus (Swash 1985). Although local causes of incontinence include urinary or anal fistulae, the commonest local cause is stress incontinence. It now seems evident that, although both urinary and faecal stress incontinence can occur following muscle injury associated with childbirth, the most likely cause of both types of incontinence is nerve injury (Snooks *et al.* 1984). Such nerve injury is associated with repeated straining during defecation (Parks *et al.* 1977) or childbirth (Snooks *et al.* 1984). The nerves involved are those which innervate the levator ani muscle and the external anal sphincter.

Immune responsiveness

The coordinated function of multiple epidermal and dermal cell populations ensures that the skin has a significant role in the immune system, which allows it to respond rapidly and effectively to a wide variety of insults occurring at the interface with the environment. Keratinocytes are the first line of defence in the skin's immune response and the keratinocyte-derived cytokines are pivotal in mobilizing leucocytes from the blood and initiating the involvement of other cutaneous cells. Skin is an important site for antigen presentation and both epidermal Langerhans cells and dermal dendritic cells participate in T-cell-mediated immune responses initiated in the skin (Williams & Kupper 1996). Intact healthy skin in the perineal area is therefore an effective barrier to infection.

The immunological factors which are significant in the physiology and pathophysiology of the lower genital tract have been reviewed recently by Bulmer and Fox (1995). An important component of the genital immune system is the cervical mucus, which contains antibodies, in particular secretory IgA. This locally produced antibody is bactericidal in the presence of lysozyme and complement and can agglutinate bacteria and opsonize them for phagocytosis. In addition, secretory IgA can inactivate antigens by forming non-absorbable complexes with them, can diminish an organism's adhesiveness to mucosa and has the capacity to neutralize viruses.

Large numbers of allogeneic spermatozoa enter the female reproductive tract during coitus and some penetrate the tissues of the female host (Zamboni 1971, Hafez 1976). The invading spermatozoa are destroyed by an immune response that generates cytolytic T lymphocytes specifically effective against the alloantigens expressed by the spermatozoa (McLean *et al.* 1980). This coital immune response is limited, by the immunosuppressive function of seminal fluid, to the immediate post-coital period (Thomas & McLean 1984). Thus, the conceptus, which expresses paternal alloantigens (Heyner 1983), is not subject to immune attack during implantation. Protection against viral infection also requires an effective cytolytic T-lymphocyte response, and any limitation of this response will increase the possibility of an oncogenic virus in the ejaculate escaping destruction. Seminal fluid, by virtue of its physiological role in reproduction, may limit the antiviral response and thereby predispose the female genital tract to viral infection. An additional factor that may render sexually active young women more vulnerable to such infection is the reduced immune responsiveness associated with anovulant contraceptives (Gerretsen *et al.* 1980). It is also generally agreed that a woman is at greater risk of infection when pregnant. This is in part due to a reduced immune responsiveness during pregnancy (Brabin 1985, Toder & Shomer 1990). Therapeutic immunosuppression of renal allograft recipients renders them more susceptible to malignant neoplasia. This was confirmed in a report of squamous cell carcinoma of the vulva in two of 200 such female patients; the two women concerned were both in their early twenties (Caterson *et al.* 1984).

References

Austyn, J.M. (1987) Lymphoid dendritic cells. *Immunology* **62**, 161–170.

Baber, R., Abdalla, H. & Studd, J. (1991) The premature menopause. *Progress in Obstetrics and Gynaecology* **9**, 209–226.

Barmann, J.M., Astore, J. & Pecoraro, V. (1969) The normal trichogram of people over 50 years. In: *Advances in Biology of Skin*, Vol. IX. *Hair Growth* (eds W. Montagna & R.L. Dobson). Pergamon Press, Oxford.

Barrow, D.W. (1957) *The Clinical Management of Varicose Veins*, 2nd edn. Hoebner, New York.

Baruchin, A.M. & Cipollini, T. (1986) Vaginal labioplasty. *British Journal of Sexual Medicine* **13**, 32.

Beazley, J.M. (1981) Maternal injuries and complications. In: *Integrated Obstetrics and Gynaecology for Postgraduates*, 3rd edn (ed. J. Dewhurst), pp. 455–467. Blackwell Scientific Publications, Oxford.

Billewicz, W.Z., Fellowes, H.M. & Hytten, C.A. (1976) Comments on the critical metabolic mass and the age of menarche. *Annals of Human Biology* **3**, 51–59.

Birbeck, M.S., Breathnach, A.S. & Everall, J.D. (1961) An electron microscopic study of basal melanocytes and high-level clear cells (Langerhans cells) in vitiligo. *Journal of Investigative Dermatology* **37**, 51–63.

Bisland, C.A.G. & Milstein, C. (1991) The identification of β2 microglobulin binding antigen encoded by human CD1 gene. *European Journal of Immunology* **21**, 71–78.

Black, J. (1985) Afro-Caribbean and African families. *British Medical Journal* **290**, 984–988.

Blackwell, R.E. (1984) Detection of ovulation. *Fertility and Sterility* **41**, 680–681.

Blaustein, A. (ed.) (1982) *Pathology of the Female Genital Tract*, 2nd edn. Springer-Verlag, New York.

Borgno, G., Micheletti, L., Barbero, M. *et al.* (1990) Topographic distribution of groin lymph nodes. *Journal of Reproductive Medicine* **35**, 1127–1129.

Brabin, B.J. (1985) Epidemiology of infection in pregnancy. *Reviews of Infectious Diseases* **7**, 579–603.

Breathnach, A.S. (1971) Embryology of human skin. *Journal of Investigative Dermatology* **57**, 133–143.

Breathnach, A.S. & Wyllie, L.M. (1965) Electron microscopy of melanocytes and Langerhans cells in human fetal epidermis at 14 weeks. *Journal of Investigative Dermatology* **44**, 51–60.

Brindley, G.S. (1984) New treatment for priapism. *Lancet* **ii**, 220–221.

Bulmer, J.N. & Fox, H. (1995) Immunopathology of the female genital tract. In: *Haines and Taylor Obstetrical and Gynaecological Pathology*, 4th edn (ed. H. Fox), pp. 1299–1332. Churchill Livingstone, London.

Burchell, R.C. & Wabrek, A.J. (1981) Sexual physiology. In: *Scientific Foundations of Obstetrics and Gynaecology*, 2nd edn (eds E.E. Philipp, J. Barnes & M. Newton), pp. 137–143. Heinemann, London.

Burger, H.G. (1996) The menopausal transition. *Clinical Obstetrics and Gynaecology* **10**, 347–359.

Carr, B.R. (1992) Disorders of the ovary and female reproductive tract. In: *Williams' Textbook of Endocrinology*, 8th edn (eds J.D. Wilson & D.W. Foster), pp. 733–798. Saunders, Philadelphia.

Casey, M.L., MacDonald, P.C. & Simpson, E.R. (1992) Endocrinological changes of pregnancy. In: *Williams' Textbook of Endocrinology*, 8th edn (eds J.D. Wilson & D.W. Foster), pp. 977–981. Saunders, Philadelphia.

Caterson, R.J., Furber, J., Murray, J. *et al.* (1984) Carcinoma of the vulva in two young renal allograft recipients. *Transplantation Proceedings* **16**, 559–561.

Cattanach, J. (1985) Oestrogen deficiency after tubal ligation. *Lancet* **i**, 847–849.

Chu, T. & Jaffe, R. (1994) The normal Langerhans cell and the LCH cell. *British Journal of Cancer* **70** (Suppl. XXXIII), S4–S10.

Czernielewski, J.M. & Demarchez, M. (1987) Further evidence for the self reproducing capacity of Langerhans cells in human skin. *Journal of Investigative Dermatology* **88**, 17–20.

Davey, D.A. (1981) The menopause and climacteric. In: *Integrated Obstetrics and Gynaecology for Postgraduates*, 3rd edn (ed. J. Dewhurst), pp. 592–650. Blackwell Scientific Publications, Oxford.

Daw, E. & Riley, S. (1982) Umbilical metastasis from squamous carcinoma of the cervix. Case Report. *British Journal of Obstetrics and Gynaecology* **89**, 1066.

Dewhurst, J. (1980) *Practical Pediatric and Adolescent Gynecology*. Marcel Dekker, New York.

Ebling, F.J.G. (1968) Embryology. In: *Textbook of Dermatology* (eds A. Rook, D.S. Wilkinson & F.J.G. Ebling). Blackwell Scientific Publications, Oxford.

Edwards, J.N.T. & Morris, H.B. (1985) Langerhans cells and lymphocyte subsets in the female genital tract. *British Journal of Obstetrics and Gynaecology* **92**, 974–982.

Elstein, M. & Chantler, E.N. (1991) Functional anatomy of the cervix and uterus. In: *Scientific Foundations of Obstetrics and*

Gynaecology, 4th edn (eds E. Phillip, M. Setchell & J. Ginsberg), pp. 114–135. Butterworth-Heinemann, Oxford.

Etchepareborda, J.J. & Rivero, L.V. & Kesseru, E. (1983) Billings natural family planning method. *Contraception* **28**, 475–480.

Faust, M.S. (1977) Somatic development of adolescent girls. *Monographs of the Society for Research into Child Development* **42**, 1–90.

Fetissof, F., Berger, G., Dubois, M.P. *et al.* (1985) Endocrine cells in the female genital tract. *Histopathology* **9**, 133–145.

Friedrich, E.G. (1976) *Vulvar Disease*. Saunders, Philadelphia.

Friedrich, E.G. (1985) Vaginitis. *American Journal of Obstetrics and Gynecology* **152**, 247–251.

Friedrich, E.G. & Wilkinson, E.J. (1982) The vulva. In: *Pathology of the Female Genital Tract*, 2nd edn (ed. A. Blaustein). Springer-Verlag, New York.

Friedrich, E.G. & Wilkinson, E.J. (1985) Vulvar surgery for neurofibromatosis. *Obstetrics and Gynecology* **65**, 135–138.

Gallagher, P.G. (1986) Varicose veins of the vulva. *British Journal of Sexual Medicine* **13**, 12–14.

Gatter, K.C., Morris, H.B., Roach, B. *et al.* (1984) Langerhans cells and T cells in human skin tumours: an immunohistological study. *Histopathology* **8**, 229–244.

Gerretsen, G., Kremer, J., Bleumink, K.E. *et al.* (1980) Immune reactivity of women on hormonal contraceptives. *Contraception* **22**, 25–29.

Ginsberg, J. (1991) What determines the age at the menopause? *British Medical Journal* **302**, 1288–1289.

Golub, E.S. & Green, D.R. (1991) *Immunology*, 2nd edn. Sinauer, Massachusetts.

Gosling, J.A., Dixon, J.S. & Humpherson, J.R. (1983) *Functional Anatomy of the Urinary Tract*. Churchill Livingstone, Edinburgh.

Gould, V.E., Moll, R., Moll, I., Lee, I. & Franke, W.W. (1985) Biology of disease. *Laboratory Investigation* **52**, 334–352.

Hafez, L.S.E. (1976) *Transport and Survival of Spermatozoa in the Female Reproductive Tract*. Mosby, St Louis.

Hashimoto, K. (1970) The ultrastructure of the skin in human embryos. *Acta Dermatovenereologia* **50**, 241–251.

Herlyn, M. & Shih, I.M. (1994) Interactions of melanocytes and melanoma cells with the microenvironment. *Pigment Cell Research* **7**, 81–88.

Heyner, S. (1983) Alloantigen expression on mouse oocytes and early mouse embryos. In: *Immunology of Reproduction* (eds T.G. Wegmann & T. Gill). Oxford University Press, New York.

Holbrooke, K.A. (1983) Structure and function of the developing human skin. In: *Biochemistry and Physiology of the Skin* (ed. L.A. Goldsmith). Oxford University Press, Oxford.

Hollinshead, W.H. (1971) *Anatomy for Surgeons*, 2nd edn. Harper and Row, New York.

Hu, F. (1981) Melanocyte cytology in normal skin. In: *Masson Monographs in Dermatology I* (ed. A.B. Ackerman). Masson, New York.

Iversen, T. & Aas, M. (1983) Lymph drainage from the vulva. *Gynecologic Oncology* **16**, 169–179.

Jensen, S.T. (1985) Comparison of podophyllin application with simple surgical excision in clearance or recurrence of perianal condylomata acuminata. *Lancet* **ii**, 1146–1148.

Jimbow, K., Fitzpatrick, T.B. & Wick, M.M. (1991) Biochemistry and physiology of melanin pigmentation. In: *Physiology, Biochemistry and Molecular Biology of the Skin* (ed. L.A. Goldsmith). Oxford University Press, New York.

Jimbow, K., Lee, S.K., King, M.G. *et al.* (1993) Melanin pigments and melanosomal proteins as differentiation markers unique to normal and neoplastic melanocytes. *Journal of Investigative Dermatology* **100**, S259–S268.

Kapsenberg, M.L., Teuissen, M.B.M. & Boss, J.D. (1990) Langerhans cells: a unique subpopulation of antigen-presenting dendritic cells. In: *Skin Immune System* (ed. J.D. Boss). CRC Press, Boca Raton.

Kaufman, R.H. (1981) Anatomy of the vulva and vagina. In: *Benign Diseases of the Vulva and Vagina* (eds H.L. Gardner & R.H. Kaufman). Hall, Boston.

Krantz, K.E. (1977) The anatomy and physiology of the vulva and vagina. In: *Scientific Foundation of Obstetrics and Gynaecology*, 2nd edn (eds E.E. Philipp, J. Barnes & M. Newton), pp. 65–78. Heinemann, London.

Leigh, R.J. & Turnberg, L.A. (1982) Faecal incontinence: the unvoiced symptom. *Lancet* **i**, 1349–1351.

Lind, T., Parkin, F.M. & Cheyne, G.A. (1969) Biochemical and cytological changes in liquor amnii with advancing gestation. *Journal of Obstetrics and Gynaecology of the British Commonwealth* **76**, 673–683.

Lozano, G.B.L. & Castenada, P.F. (1981) Priapism of the clitoris. *British Journal of Urology* **53**, 390.

Lunde, O. (1984) A study of body hair density and distribution in normal women. *American Journal of Physical Anthropology* **64**, 179–184.

MacKie, R.M. (1984) *Milne's Dermatopathology*, 2nd edn. Arnold, London.

McKinlay, S.M., Brambilla, D.J. & Posner, J.G. (1992) The normal menopause transition. *Maturitas* **14**, 102–115.

McLean, J.M., Shaya, E.I. & Gibbs, A.C.C. (1980) Immune response to first mating in female rat. *Journal of Reproductive Immunology* **1**, 285–295.

Marshall, W.A. (1978) The relationship of puberty to other maturity indicators and body composition in man. *Journal of Reproduction and Fertility* **52**, 437–443.

Marshall, W.A. & Tanner, J.M. (1969) Variation in the pattern of pubertal changes in girls. *Archives of the Diseases of Children* **44**, 291–303.

Marshall, W.A. & Tanner, J.M. (1981) Puberty. In: *Scientific Foundations of Paediatrics*, 2nd edn (eds J.A. Davis & J. Dobbing). Heinemann, London.

Medawar, P.B. (1953) The microanatomy of the mammalian epidermis. *Quarterly Journal of Microscopical Science* **94**, 481–506.

Melville, H. & Harrison, N. (1985) Persistent priapism in a normal woman. *British Medical Journal* **291**, 516.

Moll, I., Lane, A.T. & Franke, W.W. (1990) Intraepidermal formation of Merkel cells in xenografts of human fetal skin. *Journal of Investigative Dermatology* **94**, 359–364.

Montagna, W. (1960) Cholinesterases in the cutaneous nerves in man. In: *Advances in Biology of Skin*, Vol. 1 (ed. W. Montagna). Pergamon Press, New York.

Montagna, W. & Parakkal, P.F. (eds) (1974) Apocrine glands. In: *The Structure and Function of Skin*, 3rd edn. (eds W. Montagna & P.F. Parakkal). Academic Press, New York.

Morris, H.H.B., Gatter, K.C., Sykes, G., Casemore, V. & Masson, D.Y. (1983) Langerhans cells in the human cervical epithelium: effect of wart virus infection and intraepithelial neoplasia. *British Journal of Obstetrics and Gynaecology* **90**, 412–420.

Niebauer, G. (1968) *Dendritic Cells of the Skin*. Karger, New York.

Odland, G.F. (1983) Structure of the skin. In: *Biochemistry and Physiology of the Skin* (ed. L.A. Goldsmith). Oxford University Press, Oxford.

Omsjo, I.H., Wright, P.B. & Bormer, O.P. (1984) Estrogen and progesterone receptors in normal and malignant vulvar tissue. *Gynecologic and Obstetric Investigation* **17**, 281–283.

O'Rahilly, R. & Muller, F. (1992) *Embryology and Teratology*. Wiley, New York.

Parker, F. (1981) Skin and hormones. In: *Textbook of Endocrinology*, 6th edn (ed. R.H. Williams). Saunders, Philadelphia.

Parks, A.G., Swash, M. & Urich, H. (1977) Sphincter denervation in anorectal incontinence and rectal prolapse. *Gut* **18**, 656–665.

Patterson, J.A.K. & Edelson, R.L. (1982) Interaction of T cells with the epidermis. *British Journal of Dermatology* **107**, 117–122.

Pearse, A.G.E. (1969) The cytochemistry and ultrastructure of polypeptide hormone producing cells of the APUD series and the embryologic, physiologic and pathologic implications of the concept. *Journal of Histochemistry and Cytochemistry* **17**, 303–313.

Pinkus, F. (1910) Development of the integument. In: *Manual of Embryology* (eds F. Keibel & F.P. Mall). Lippincott, Philadelphia.

Pinkus, H. (1958) Embryology of hair. In: *Hair Growth* (eds W. Montagna & R.A. Ellis). Academic Press, New York.

Reader, F. (1991) Disorders of female sexuality. *Progress in Obstetrics and Gynaecology* **9**, 303–318.

Riley, A.J. & Trimmer, E. (1991) Physiology of the human female sexual response. In: *Scientific Foundations of Obstetrics and Gynaecology*, 4th edn (eds E. Phillip, M. Setchell & J. Ginsberg), pp. 179–186. Butterworth-Heinemann, Oxford.

Robboy, S.J., Ross, J.S., Prat, J., Keh, P.C. & Welch, W.R. (1978) Urogenital sinus origin of mucinous and ciliated cysts of the vulva. *Obstetrics and Gynecology* **51**, 347–351.

Ross, G.T. & Van de Wiele, R.L. (1981) The ovaries. In: *Textbook of Endocrinology*, 6th edn (ed. R.H. Williams). Saunders, Philadelphia.

Rowden, G., Lewis, M.G. & Sullivan, A.K. (1977) 1a antigen expression on human epidermal Langerhans cells. *Nature* **268**, 247–248.

Schaffer, J. & Fantl, J.A. (1996) Urogenital effects of the menopause. *Clinical Obstetrics and Gynaecology* **10**, 401–418.

Schmidt, W.A. (1995) Pathology of the vagina. In: *Haines and Taylor's Obstetrical and Gynaecological Pathology*, 4th edn (ed. H. Fox), pp. 135–223. Churchill Livingstone, London.

Serri, F., Montagna, W. & Mescon, H. (1962) Studies of the skin of the fetus and child. *Journal of Investigative Dermatology* **39**, 199–217.

Sinclair, J.D. (1972) Thermal control in premature infants. *Annual Review of Medicine* **23**, 129–148.

Singer, A. (1995) Anatomy of the cervix and physiological changes in cervical epithelium. In: *Haines and Taylor Obstetrical and Gynaecological Pathology*, 4th edn (ed. H. Fox), pp. 225–248. Churchill Livingstone, London.

Slominski, A., Paus, R. & Schadendorf, D. (1993) Melanocytes as sensory and regulatory cells in the epidermis. *Journal of Theoretical Biology* **164**, 103–120.

Smith, W.C.P. & Wilson, P.M. (1991) The vulva, vagina and urethra and the musculature of the pelvic floor. In: *Scientific Foundations of Obstetrics and Gynaecology*, 4th edn (eds E. Phillip, M. Setchell & J. Ginsberg), pp. 84–100. Butterworth-Heinemann, Oxford.

Snooks, S.J., Setchell, M., Swash, M. & Henry, M.M. (1984) Injury to the innervation of pelvic floor sphincter musculature in childbirth. *Lancet* **ii**, 546–550.

Soloman, L.M. & Esterly, N.B. (1970) Neonatal dermatology 1: The newborn skin. *Journal of Paediatrics* **77**, 888–894.

Sparkes, R.A., Purrier, B.G.A., Watt, P.J. & Elstein, M. (1981) Bacteriological colonisation of uterine cavity: role of tailed intrauterine contraceptive device. *British Medical Journal* **282**, 1189.

Swash, M. (1985) New concepts in incontinence. *British Medical Journal* **290**, 4–5.

Swash, M. (1991) Neurology and neurophysiology of the female genital organs. In: *Scientific Foundations of Obstetrics and Gynaecology*, 4th edn (eds E. Phillip, M. Setchell & J. Ginsberg), pp. 110–114. Butterworth-Heinemann, Oxford.

Tanner, J.M. (1962) *Growth at Adolescence*, 2nd edn. Blackwell, Oxford.

Tay, S.K., Jenkins, D., Maddox, P. & Campion, M. (1987a) Subpopulations of Langerhans cells in cervical neoplasia. *British Journal of Obstetrics and Gynaecology* **94**, 10–15.

Tay, S.K., Jenkins, D., Maddox, P. & Singer, A. (1987b) Lymphocyte phenotypes in cervical human papillomavirus infection. *British Journal of Obstetrics and Gynaecology* **94**, 16–21.

Teunissen, M.B. (1992) Dynamic nature and function of epidermal Langerhans cells *in vivo* and *in vitro*: a review with emphasis on human Langerhans cells. *Histochemical Journal* **24**, 697–716.

Thomas, I.K. & McLean, J.M. (1984) Seminal plasma abrogates the post-coital T cell response to spermatozoal histocompatibility antigen. *American Journal of Reproductive Immunology* **6**, 185–189.

Thomas, T.M., Plymar, K.R., Biannan, J. & Meade, T.W. (1980) Prevalence of urinary incontinence. *British Medical Journal* **281**, 1243–1245.

Toder, V. & Shomer, B. (1990) The role of lymphokines in pregnancy. *Immunology and Allergy Clinics of North America* **10**, 65–78.

Tozzini, R., Sobrero, A.J. & Hoovise, E. (1971) Vulvar cytology. *Acta Cytologica* **15**, 57–60.

Tschachler, E., Groh, V. & Popovic, M. (1987) Epidermal Langerhans cells. A target for HTLV III/LAV infection. *Journal of Investigative Dermatology* **88**, 223–237.

Utian, W.H. (1987) The fate of the untreated menopause. *Obstetrics and Gynecology Clinics of North America* **14**, 1–11.

van der Putte, S.C.J. (1991) Anogenital 'sweat' glands. Histology and pathology of a gland that may mimic mammary glands. *American Journal of Dermatopathology* **13**, 557–567.

van der Putte, S.C.J. (1993) Ultrastructure of the human anogenital 'sweat' gland. *The Anatomical Record* **235**, 583–590.

van Roosmalen, J. (1991) Symphyseotomy: a re-appraisal for the developing world. *Progress in Obstetrics and Gynaecology* **9**, 149–162.

Wallenburg, H.C.S. & Wladimiroff, J.W. (1976) Recurrence of vulvovaginal candidosis during pregnancy. *Obstetrics and Gynecology* **48**, 491–494.

Way, J. (1977) The lymphatics of the pelvis. In: *Scientific Foundations of Obstetrics and Gynaecology*, 2nd edn (eds E.E. Phillip, J. Barnes & M. Newton), pp. 118–126. Heinemann, London.

Williams, I.R. & Kupper, T.S. (1996) Immunity at the surface: homeostatic mechanisms of the skin immune system. *Life Sciences* **58**, 1485–1507.

Winkelmann, R.K. (1977) The Merkel cell system and a comparison between it and the neurosecretory or APUD cell system. *Journal of Investigative Dermatology* **69**, 41–46.

Winkelmann, R.K. & Breathnach, A.S. (1973) The Merkel cell. *Journal of Investigative Dermatology* **60**, 2–15.

Woodworth, H., Dockerty, M.B., Wilson, R.B. & Pratt, J.H. (1971) Papillary hidradenoma of the vulva: a clinicopathologic study of 69 cases. *American Journal Obstetrics and Gynecology* **110**, 501–508.

Yu, R.C.H., Morris, J.F., Pritchard, J. & Chu, T.C. (1992) Defective alloantigen-presenting capacity of Langerhans cell histiocytosis cells. *Archives of the Diseases of Childhood* **67**, 1370–1372.

Zamboni, L. (1971) *Fine Morphology of Mammalian Fertilisation*. Harper and Row, New York.

Chapter 3: Historical aspects: principles of examination, investigation and diagnosis

C.M. Ridley & S.M. Neill

Historical and cultural considerations

Vulval lesions are not well described in early medical literature, although references are to be found in the Talmud, the Bible and in Egyptian papyri of the second millenium BC; perhaps the first accurate descriptions were those of Avicenna in the 11th century, and they were followed by those of Renaissance writers such as Severinus Pineus in the 16th century (Fig. 3.1) and Van den Spieghel in the 17th century. In the mid-19th century the histology of the genitalia was described, and gynaecologists and dermatologists began to note and name such conditions as 'leukoplakia' and 'kraurosis'.

Ricci (1943, 1945) is an authority on all historical aspects of gynaecological medicine and surgery; Leonardo (1944), Graham (1950) and Mettler (1947) are also useful; Ploss *et al.* (1935) deal particularly with the anthropological significance of female anatomy and physiology.

The etymological origin of the terms used to describe the anatomical structures is of interest. The vagina (sheath) and mons veneris (hill of Venus) are obvious appellations. Vulva is derived from the Latin for 'covering' and was originally used for the uterus. Isodorus in AD 600 described the labia as being like doors (valvae) and Leonardo (1944) pointed out that in the 4th-century Babylonian Talmud the labia were described as hinges. Clitoris, somewhat more obscurely, is usually thought to come from a Greek word meaning 'door-tender' and, some would say, also 'key'. 'Hymen' obviously suggests a connection with the god of marriage. In ancient Greece, Hymen as a personal divinity was probably called into being to personify a cry 'Hymen' in the wedding song, and was first so recorded in the 5th century BC; the wedding song, itself much older, was known as a *Hymenaios* and the god himself was also entitled Hymenaios. The refrain of the wedding song thus became 'Hymen o Hymenaie'. Although the reference in the wedding song would seem almost certainly to have been to the vaginal membrane, hymen is recorded as a word for any type of membrane, covering skin or patch from the 4th century BC and presumably existed before that time. Moreover, although in 16th-century editions of 4th-century commentaries on Terence and Virgil there are tales of a Hymen who rescued maidens and comments on a vaginal hymen that guarded virginity, the word was not apparently to be found as referring specifically to the vaginal membrane before the 7th century. Its use in this way was firmly established in the 16th century at the time of Vesalius. Conceivably the words for the god and for the membrane were simply homophones, an odd coincidence; alternatively, 'hymen' did originally refer to the vaginal membrane but had lost this connotation by the time it first occurred in the literature as meaning rather a membrane in general, only to acquire it again later (K. Dover, personal communication, 1975).

The subject of female anatomy, especially that of the genital area, is susceptible of very recondite examination. The significance of female nudity, for example, is considered by Warner (1985) in her book on female images in statuary, subtitled 'The allegory of the female form'. Sawday (1995) discusses the development of dissection of the human body in Renaissance culture. He elaborates upon the practices of the anatomy theatres, linking them with concepts of science and religion, particularly as they apply to women and to the female organs of generation (Fig. 3.2).

References to the female genitalia, whether in overt or covert form, are common in art and literature. Weintraub (1972) for example commented on the correspondence between genital landscape and anatomy not only in the obviously erotic *Venus and Tannhaüser* but in the courtly conventions of the medieval *Romaunt of the Rose*; and Bodkin (1963) pointed out that 'psychophysiological echoes' in relation to such archetypal images as caves and water will reinforce and enrich intellectual appreciation of poetry. As regards art, there are the formalized representations on Greek pots, the moulded ceramic 'vulval' plates of Judy Chicago (1996) in her celebration of women down the ages and, indeed, the logo of the International Society for the Study of Vulvovaginal Disease (Fig. 3.3).

General management of vulval problems

Attitudes to vulvovaginal disease will be affected by the

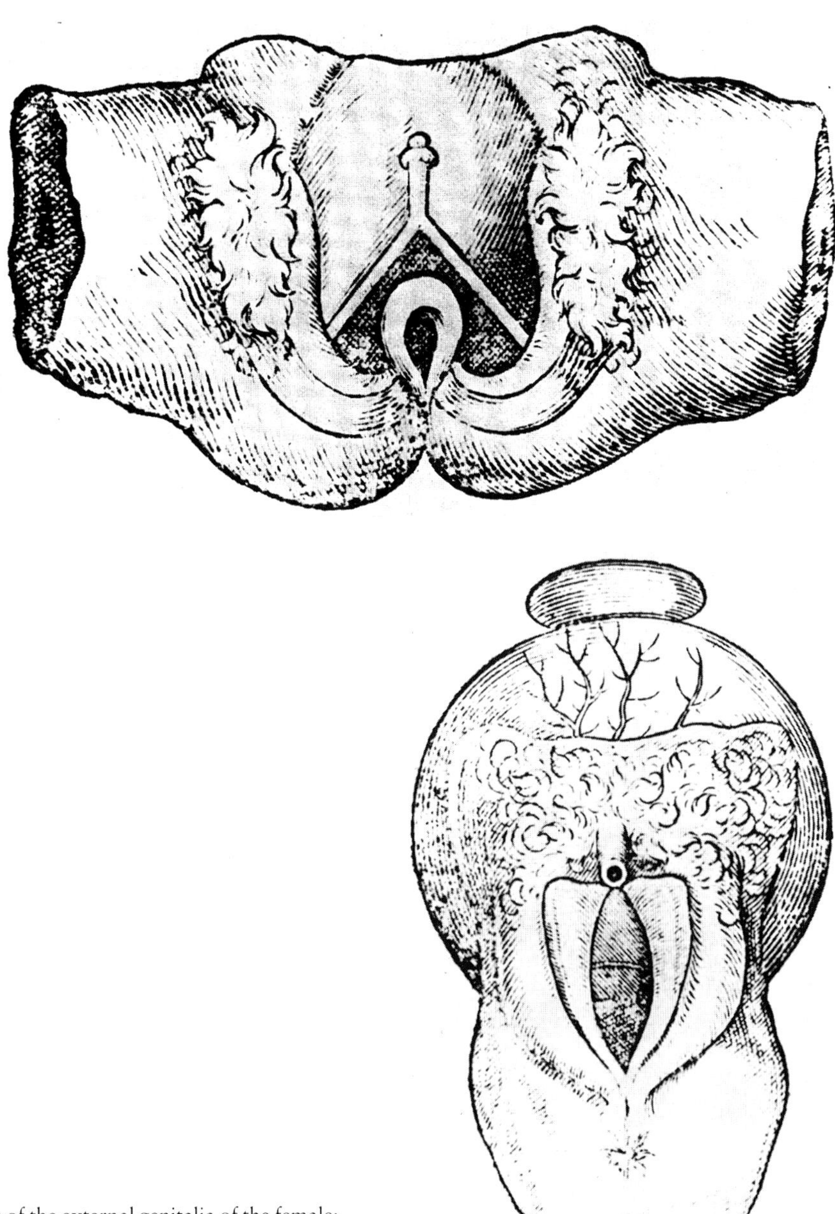

Fig. 3.1 Earliest pictures of the external genitalia of the female: Severinus Pineus (1550–1619).

contemporary social and cultural background. Sociological factors are also of importance in recognition, acceptance and treatment of sexually transmitted disease; the history of that subject and its interaction with society have been intensively considered by Aral and Holmes (1990), Schwartz and Gilmore (1990) and Waugh (1990). The UK is fortunate in its network of clinics for sexually transmitted disease, staffed by specialists in genitourinary medicine and able to deal with the necessary screening and contact tracing; their self-referral system and confidentiality encourage attendance, and are also conducive to the amassing of valid statistics. Trotula in the 11th century (Mason-Hohl 1940) said 'since these organs happen to be in a retired location, women on account of modesty and the fragility and delicacy of the state of these parts dare not reveal the difficulties of their sickness to a male doctor'. There is no doubt that women with vulval problems do still often wish to be seen by a woman doctor, and in the UK there is a substantial proportion of women in dermatology, genitourinary medicine and in general practice (primary care), although the proportion is much lower in gynaecology.

The fact that women with vulval problems may present themselves to any of these doctors offers opportunities of interdisciplinary cooperation, but also of confusion and

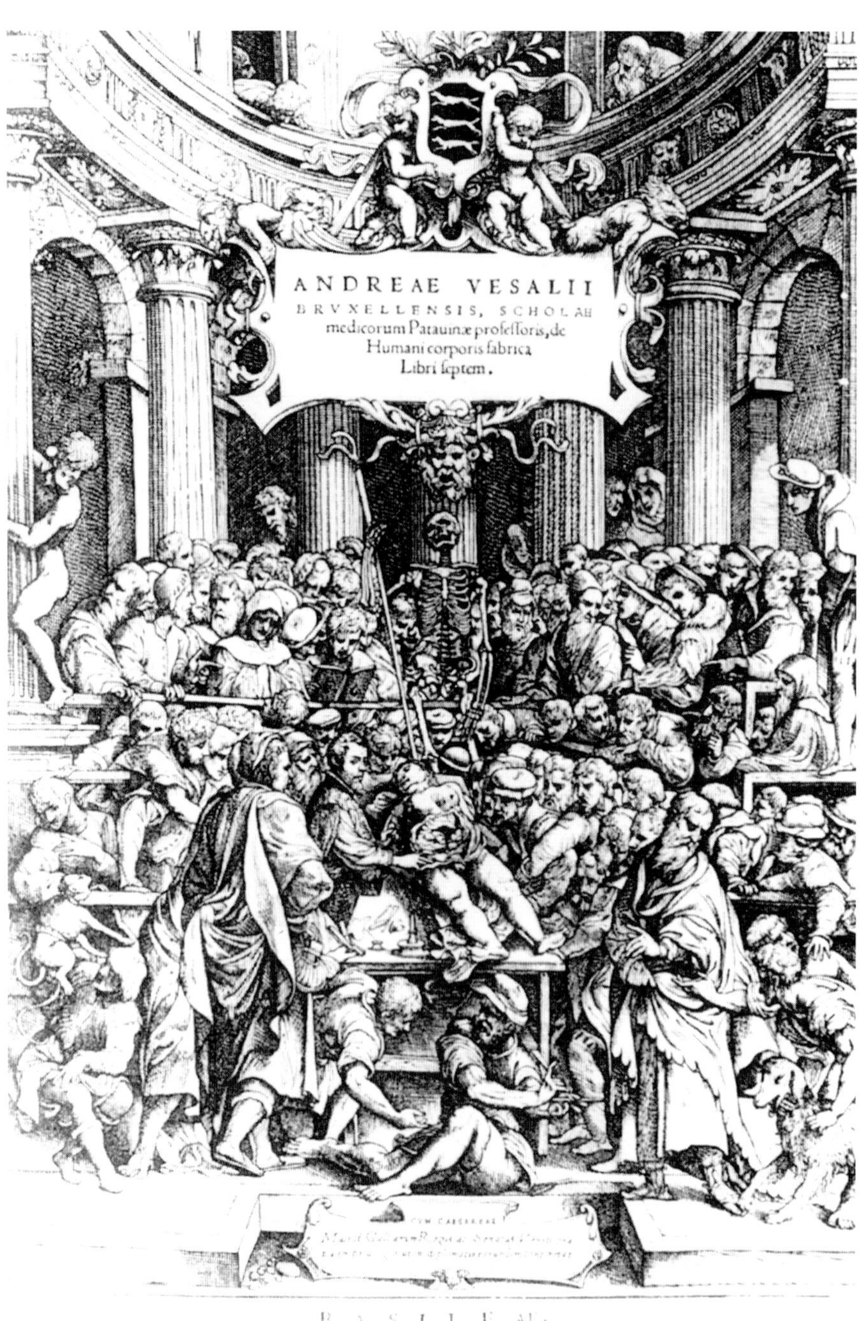

Fig. 3.2 Title page from *De Humani Corporis Fabrica: Vesalius* (1543).

mismanagement. Discussion, and correlation of differing viewpoints on terminology, will often lead to a satisfactory outcome. There are, however, other less easily negotiable difficulties, those inherent in the conditions themselves, and here too cooperation is important.

The role of the pathologist must be stressed. It is the pathologist who will often have the last word in diagnosis and in relation to whom cooperation and understanding are essential. In comparison with the dermatologist, the gynaecologist will tend to lean more heavily on the pathologist and to give him or her greater responsibility. Dermatologists are more likely to have their own ideas on the histology, to want to discuss the sections and to want to refer problems to dermatological pathologists. The pathologist who specializes in gynaecological pathology will be of invaluable help if he or she is interested in vulval, i.e. cutaneous pathology, but not if his or her sphere of interest has been confined to more proximal parts of the lower genital tract. Finally, all pathologists will of course be confused if their own understanding of descriptive terms and of the

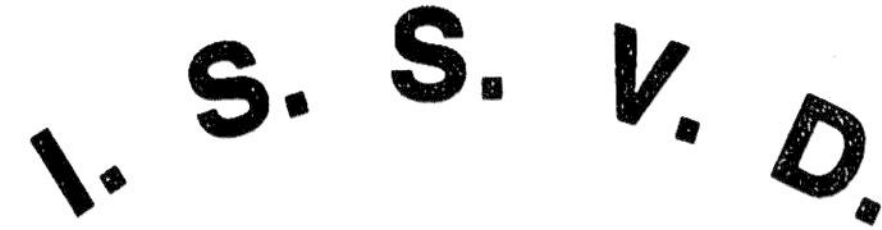

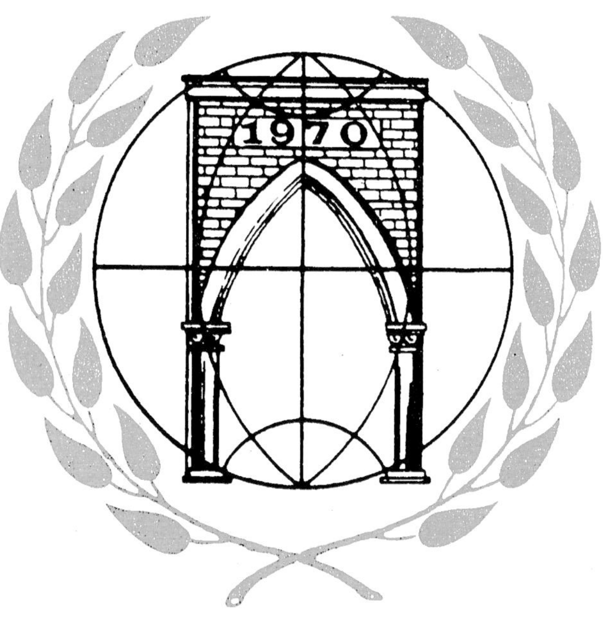

Fig. 3.3 Logo of the International Society for the Study of Vulvovaginal Disease.

current classification (and its shortcomings) is not clear, and if the clinicians cannot agree on the terms they use.

The International Society for the Study of Vulvovaginal Disease was founded in 1970, originally as the International Society for the Study of Vulvar Disease, and its Fellows must demonstrate a particular interest in vulvovaginal conditions; the majority are gynaecologists, dermatologists or pathologists, and they come from many countries. It deals *inter alia* with problems of classification and in so doing has links with the International Federation of Obstetricians and Gynecologists (FIGO), the World Health Organization (WHO) and the International Society of Gynecological Pathologists (ISGP). In addition, several countries now have multidisciplinary groups of varying degrees of formality which are concerned with these conditions; there is, for example, a British Society for the Study of Vulval Disease. Furthermore, a European College for the Study of Vulval Disease has now been inaugurated.

Vulval clinics probably provide the best setting for the doctor to see the patient and the patient to be seen by the doctor. They were first set up in the USA in the 1960s and the published reports on them offer an interesting picture of changing therapies and attitudes (Ridley 1993). Ideally they are multidisciplinary. In practice, at least in the UK, they are mainly organized by a dermatologist, but links with colleagues in gynaecology and genitourinary medicine must be in place. Thus equipped, the clinics offer a valuable repository of experience, which is beneficial in management, teaching and research. It is important, however, that those concerned in looking after the patients should have adequate training and consistency of approach.

The consultation

It is convenient to have a formal protocol as a basis for history taking, and to enlarge upon particular aspects in the light of the individual patient's problem. It is important that the initial interview should take place in a sympathetic atmosphere, and there is no doubt that the function of the clinic as regards teaching may sometimes seem to be at odds with the well-being of the patient. This applies with even more force to the examination. It is essential, therefore, before proceeding, to ensure that the patient is content to have more than one doctor and a nurse present. Most patients readily accede, and they will often also agree to the presence of a male doctor if the importance of discussion and learning is explained. When the doctor carrying out the examination is male, it is essential to have a chaperon present.

The actual examination of the vulva is best performed with the patient in the dorsal and then (for the perianal area) the left lateral position; this arrangement is preferable, as regards both the patient and the doctor, to the lithotomy position. The examination must be thorough and methodical, and include a conscious note of all its parts, as well as of the perineum and perianal area. Depending on the presenting symptoms and signs, the vagina and cervix, the rest of the skin, the nails, mouth and eyes will also be examined. Again, it is helpful to have at hand a list that can be checked, and a diagram to be marked (Fig. 3.4). A good light is essential, as is some form of magnification such as an adjustable magnifying glass on a bracket. The colposcope, giving a magnification of 8–10 times, is not helpful at the vulva; it provides a very small field of examination and shows up little on keratinized skin; moreover, the position that has to be taken up by the patient makes full examination of the whole anogenital area difficult. Colposcopic examination of the vagina and cervix may of course be indicated at some convenient time for certain patients. There is no place for the use of toluidine blue, and little for acetic acid, the only point of which at the vulva might be in delineating areas of vulval intraepithelial neoplasia for biopsy. The confusion caused by misplaced emphasis on acetowhite tissue has been considerable; the light reflection effect produced is essentially non-specific.

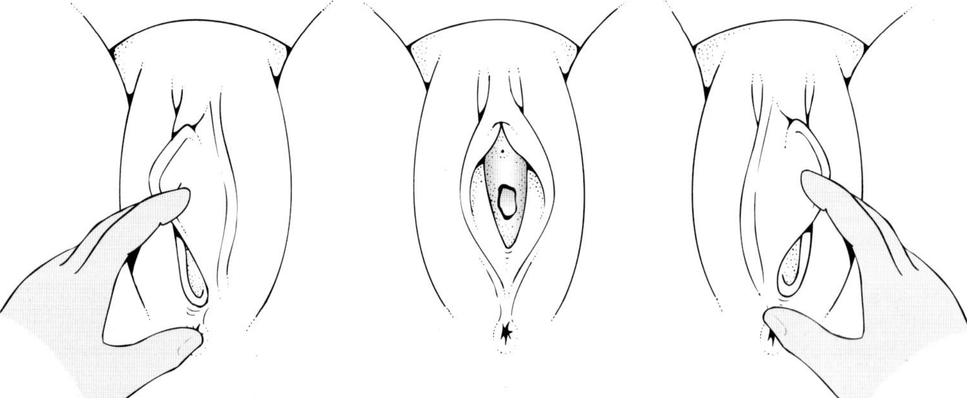

Fig. 3.4 Stylized representation of the vulva.

Most children will permit examination of the vulva and perianal area, either lying on the back or, in the case of very small children and babies, on the knee of the mother or other female attendant. As the labia majora are unformed, visualization is easy, and even the vestibule and hymen are usually readily visible without any need to separate the labia minora.

Factors to be taken into account

With such thoroughness of examination at all ages must go two considerations; appreciation of the influences wrought on the morphology of lesions by local environmental factors, and recognition of variants of normal.

Vulval skin is more easily irritated, is more permeable, and has an increased blood flow compared with skin elsewhere, and it shows age-dependent differences of anatomy and physiology (Oriba *et al.* 1989). In each area—the clitoris, the labia majora, the labia minora, the vestibule, the hymen—the range of normal appearances is wide, and patients must be given firm reassurance where appropriate. One patient (Fig. 3.5) was seen by several specialists and had biopsies before it was recognized that the fimbriated appearance of the edges of the labia minora was normal for her. The same firm reassurance should be given when banal lesions such as small tags, angiokeratomas and seborrhoeic warts can be confidently diagnosed. The vestibule is defined as the area within Hart's line, where there is a clear colour change from keratinized to non-keratinized skin. Routine examination of the vestibule includes the noting of the urethra, the hymen or hymenal ring, and the presence or absence of any minor vestibular gland openings or erythema. Vestibular papillae may be apparent; described under this name by Friedrich (1983) following the earlier description as hirsuties papillaris vulvae by Altmeyer *et al.* (1982), they are now recognized as a variant of normal, and classified as part of the equally normal finding of vestibular papillomatosis (Chapter 6).

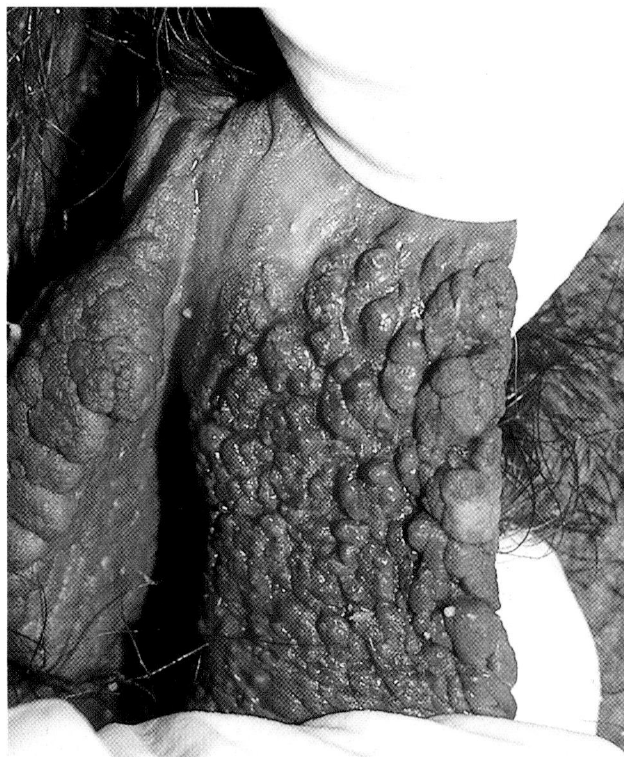

Fig. 3.5 Unusual configuration of the labia minora.

The vulva at birth and for a week or two afterwards is under the influence of maternal oestrogens, and hence oedematous, with some vaginal discharge. The hymen is thickened and the orifice difficult to see. Periurethral cysts, which spontaneously resolve, may be confused with a microperforate hymen.

The prepubertal introital area is brightly erythematous in its normal state, a fact that often gives rise to mistaken suspicion of abnormality. Another important feature in children is the not infrequent presence of labial adhesions (acquired), which can mimic ambiguous genitalia (congenital). With adhesions (Chapter 5) a line of demarcation between the clitoral hood and the labia minora under the clitoris can be seen. The progressive changes encountered between infancy and adolescence have been described by Pokorny (1993).

Although there is a lack of documentation, clinical observation suggests that with increasing age the labia majora diminish in size, presumably because of loss of fat and connective tissue, and that the pubic hair becomes scantier. Minimal evidence of fusion of the clitoral hood is probably acceptable as normal in the elderly. Hormone replacement therapy is now taken by many postmenopausal women; it will tend to restore vaginal and hence introital moistness. Such patients who are not on this treatment may be subject to atrophic vaginitis; this is not relevant to vulval disease except in so far as the discharge may irritate the skin. The vaginitis will be improved by topical or oral oestrogens, but it is important to explain to the patient that this therapy will have no effect on any skin condition.

Investigative techniques

Swabs for bacterial infection, viral transport medium for viral culture and blades for taking scrapings for tinea, *Candida* and erythrasma will be required. Investigations for associated sexually transmitted diseases are best carried out in the genitourinary medicine clinic. With the possible exception of the Tzanck test, to detect acantholytic cells in pemphigus, vulval cytology is now rarely employed; biopsy is more reliable for histological diagnosis.

Investigation in children may pose problems and should be carefully planned, often in consultation with colleagues in gynaecology and genitourinary medicine. This applies with particular force when child sexual abuse (Chapters 5 & 7) is suspected. Pokorny (1992, 1993) has stressed the damage that can be done to the unoestrogenized vaginal mucosa by examination techniques such as a cotton-tipped swab, and discusses alternatives.

BIOPSY

Biopsy excision of lesions follows the general principles governing that of removal of lesions elsewhere. To excise small lesions, or to obtain sample specimens for histology, the disposable biopsy punch is usually satisfactory, in sizes ranging from 2 to 6 mm diameter, and this technique is particularly useful for lesions on the inner aspects of the vulva. Where the specimen is a biopsy only, care must be taken in interpretation (Crawford *et al.* 1995). Clearly where, for example, the depth of a neoplasm is all-important the biopsy specimen can only be accepted where that depth is greater than the critical level; if it is not so, but malignancy is confirmed, then specimens following total excision must be assessed.

Local anaesthesia with lignocaine 1 or 2% is usually preceded by the application of a prilocaine/lignocaine cream (EMLA), absorption being assisted by adduction of the thighs for 10 minutes or so. With this preliminary, and particularly if fine-needle cartridge syringes or 30-gauge needles with conventional syringes are used, discomfort is minimal. The punched-out specimen is removed with sharp scissors. Small biopsies may not require sutures, haemostasis being achieved by pressure or cautery; others may need one or two sutures, for example with 4.0 Vicryl.

Many small lesions such as warts or tags can also be removed in the usual way under local anaesthesia by the hyfrecator, or cautery, or snipping off.

Specimens for immunofluorescence are, after washing in saline, put into liquid nitrogen or into transport medium. Specimens for electron microscopy are put into liquid nitrogen or into glutaraldehyde.

Management

The diagnosis and further management are best discussed with the patient after she has dressed. For many of the conditions, for example vulvodynia or dermatoses, it will be appropriate to give her information leaflets to take away as well as to give information at the time. In some cases further features in the history may need to be checked and indeed are often volunteered by the patient. It is sometimes apparent that psychological or psychosexual advice will be needed; hence it is important for the staff of a vulval clinic to have professional links with an appropriately trained counsellor.

References

Altmeyer, P., Chilf, G.-N. & Holzmann, H. (1982) Hirsuties papillaris vulvae (Pseudokondlyome der vulva). *Der Hautarzt* 33, 281–283.

Aral, S.O. & Holmes, K.K. (1990) Epidemiology of sexual behavior and sexually transmitted disease. In: *Sexually Transmitted Diseases*, 2nd edn (eds K.K. Holmes, P.-A. Märdh, P.F. Starling & P.J. Wiesner), pp. 19–36. McGraw Hill, New York.

Bodkin, M. (1963) The archetype of paradise-hades, or of heaven and hell. In: *Archetypal Patterns in Poetry: Psychological Studies of Imagination*, pp. 112–113. Oxford University Press, London.

Chicago, J. (1996) *The Dinner Party*. Penguin Books, Harmondsworth.

Crawford, R.A.F., Todd, P., Fisher, C., Lowe, D.G. & Shepherd, J.H. (1995) Outpatient vulval biopsy—a note of caution. *British Journal of Obstetrics and Gynaecology* 102, 487–489.

Friedrich, E.G. (1983) The vulvar vestibule. *Journal of Reproductive Medicine* 28, 773–777.

Graham, H. (1950) *Eternal Eve*. Heinemann, London.

Leonardo, R.A. (1944) *History of Gynecology*. Froben Press, New York.
Mason-Hohl, E. (1940) *The Diseases of Women, by Trotula of Salerno*. Ward Ritchie, Los Angeles.
Mettler, C.C. (1947) Venerology, Chap. 9, p. 601. Dermatology, Chap. 10, p. 661. Obstetrics and gynecology, Chap. 13, p. 931. In: *History of Medicine* (ed. F.A. Mettler), Blakiston, Philadelphia.
Oriba, H.A., Elsner, P. & Maibach, H.I. (1989) Vulvar physiology. *Seminars in Dermatology* 8, 2–6.
Ploss, H.H., Bartels, M. & Bartels, P. (1935) The female genitalia: racial and ethnographical characteristics. Anthropological characteristics. In: Woman (ed. E.J. Dingwall) *An Historical Gynaecological and Anthropological Compendium*, pp. 276, 300. Heinemann, London.
Pokorny, S.F. (1992) Prepubertal vulvovaginopathies. *Obstetrics and Gynecology Clinics of North America* 19, 39–68.
Pokorny, S.F. (1993) The genital examination of the infant through adolescence. *Current Opinion in Obstetrics and Gynecology* 5, 753–757.
Ricci, J. (1943) *The Genealogy of Gynaecology 2000 B.C.–1800 A.D.* Blakiston, Philadelphia.
Ricci, J. (1945) *One Hundred Years of Gynaecology*. Blakiston, Philadelphia.
Ridley, C.M. (1993) The 1991 presidential address: International Society for the Study of Vulvovaginal Disease. *Journal of Reproductive Medicine* 38, 1–4.
Sawday, J. (1995) *The Body Emblazoned*. Routledge, London.
Schwartz, P. & Gillmore, M.R. (1990) Sociological perspectives on human sexuality. In: *Sexually Transmitted Diseases*, 2nd edn (eds K.K. Holmes, P.-A. Märdh, P.F. Starling & P.J. Wiesner), pp. 45–53. McGraw Hill, New York.
Warner, M. (1985) *Monuments and Maidens*. George Weidenfeld and Nicolson, London.
Waugh, M.A. (1990) History of clinical developments in sexually transmitted diseases. In: *Sexually Transmitted Diseases*, 2nd edn (eds K.K. Holmes, P.-A. Märdh, P.F. Starling & P.J. Wiesner), pp. 3–16. McGraw-Hill, New York.
Weintraub, S. (1972) The *Savoy* ascendant. In: *Beardsley*, Chap. 8, pp. 165–166. Penguin Books, Harmondsworth.

Chapter 4: Infective conditions of the vulva

J.D. Oriel

Introduction

Normal flora of the adult female genital tract

At puberty, glycogen is formed in the vaginal epithelium in response to oestrogens, and lactobacilli colonize the vulva and vagina. These organisms metabolize glycogen to lactic acid, which helps to maintain a vaginal pH of less than 4.5. This acidic environment restricts the growth of many organisms, with the exception of *Candida* species (Corbishley 1977). Facultative bacteria in low numbers are present in the healthy vagina, including *Staphylococcus epidermidis*, *Gardnerella vaginalis*, coliforms, anaerobic streptococci and *Bacteroides* spp. (Mårdh 1991). Colonization with genital mycoplasmas (*Mycoplasma hominis* and *Ureaplasma urealyticum*) increases with sexual activity (McCormack *et al.* 1972). Neither chlamydiae nor viruses form part of the normal flora.

This complex ecosystem may become destabilized by events such as pregnancy, diabetes mellitus, antimicrobial therapy, or the introduction of a foreign body or pathogen into the lower genital tract. Some organisms may then overgrow at the expense of others, and the patient develop symptoms and signs of vulvovaginal infection.

Sources of infection

In women, infection of the lower genital tract is usually exogenous. Some vulval infections, particularly those caused by fungi or pyogenic cocci, may be transferred to the area by the hands, by fomites or through immersion in contaminated water. The proximity of the vulva to the anus allows colonization of the introitus by coliforms (Fair *et al.* 1970), which may then be inoculated into the urethra and bladder by sexual intercourse and cause urinary tract infection. Organisms such as *Candida* species and threadworms may also reach the vulva and vagina from the anus.

The majority of pathogens reach the vulva and vagina through sexual contact, either genital to genital (with or without intercourse) or mouth to genital. Bacterial infections such as gonorrhoea, syphilis, chancroid and chlamydial infection, viral infections such as genital warts and genital herpes, and protozoal infections such as trichomoniasis are all introduced in this way. Other infections, for example recurrent genital herpes, or candidosis, may be provoked or aggravated by intercourse.

Host defences

ROLE OF NORMAL FLORA

The indigenous flora and incoming vulvovaginal pathogens interact. Both vaginal lactobacilli and *Candida albicans* can inhibit the growth of *Neisseria gonorrhoeae* and other organisms *in vitro* (Hipp *et al.* 1974, Mårdh & Soltesz 1983). Whether this is of any clinical importance is not known.

PHAGOCYTOSIS

Polymorphonuclear leucocytes, monocytes and macrophages play an important part in the defence of epithelia. Phagocytosis involving the attachment of microorganisms to the phagocyte and their subsequent ingestion and death has been studied for *Neisseria gonorrhoeae*, *Chlamydia trachomatis* and *Trichomonas vaginalis* (Dilworth *et al.* 1975, Rein *et al.* 1980, Yong *et al.* 1982). Little is known about the action of phagocytes on other sexually transmitted pathogens.

HUMORAL IMMUNITY

Mucosal antibodies can prevent bacterial attachment, enhance phagocytosis and inactivate viruses. Their action has been reviewed by McNabb and Tomasi (1981). Circulating antibodies to specific microorganisms can be demonstrated in many genital infections but, with the exception of antitreponemal antibodies, there is little evidence that they have any protective effect. Repeated attacks of gonorrhoea, chlamydial infection, genital herpes and trichomoniasis occur despite high titres of circulating antibodies. Little is known about the role of secretory antibodies in the defence against viral infections such as genital herpes and human immunodeficiency virus (HIV).

CELL-MEDIATED IMMUNITY

Patients who have had genital infection caused by *Neisseria gonorrhoeae*, *Treponema pallidum*, *Chlamydia trachomatis*, herpes simplex virus and other pathogens show cellular immune responses to specific antigens, but these are not protective against recurrent infection (Kearns *et al.* 1973, Hanna *et al.* 1979). In acquired immune deficiency syndrome (AIDS), the deficient cellular immunity caused by HIV often results in severe genital infections, for example those of herpes simplex virus and papilloma viruses (Siegal *et al.* 1981). Pregnancy is associated with reduced cellular immunity, which probably accounts for the enlargement of genital warts at this time.

Infection with ectoparasites

Pediculosis

Phthirus pubis, the crab louse, is an insect of the order Anoplura, and occupies a different genus from *Pediculus humanus* with its two forms, the head and body louse. *Phthirus pubis* is a wingless insect 1–2 mm long, grey in colour and dorsoventrally flattened. The last two pairs of its six legs are modified for grasping hairs (Fig. 4.1). After mating, the female lays eggs that are cemented to hairs near their roots, forming nits. Hatching occurs after 7 days, and the louse reaches maturity 2 weeks later. Adult life expectancy is 3–4 weeks. Crab lice feed almost continuously on human blood, and cannot survive for more than 24 hours away from their host (Keh & Poorbaugh 1977).

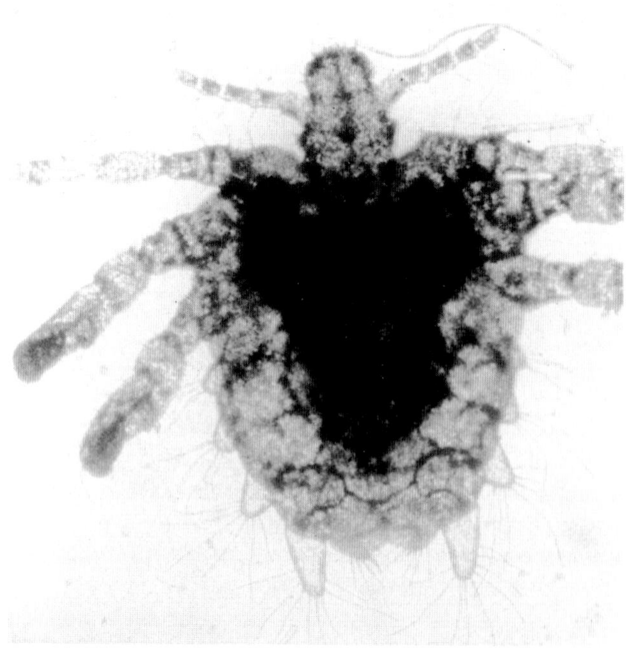

Fig. 4.1 *Phthirus pubis.*

Epidemiology

Infection occurs almost invariably through sexual contact, and the prevalence of pediculosis parallels that of other sexually transmitted diseases (STDs). Below the age of 19 years, women are more often affected than men, but after this age the ratio is reversed (Fisher & Morton 1970). Other STDs are often present in these patients. There has sometimes been speculation that *Phthirus pubis* may act as a vector for other infections, but there is no evidence that this happens.

Clinical features

The incubation period of pediculosis pubis is 1–4 weeks. The commonest symptom is irritation, which is possibly due to sensitization (Orkin & Maibach 1984); some patients present because they have seen the insects moving, and in others the infection is symptomless. The areas most affected are pubic, perianal and perineal, but occasionally the insects are seen on body or axillary hair or on the eyebrows or eyelashes. Nits are commonly present; and their distance from the skin surface indicates the duration of the infection (Fig. 4.2). The scalp is only rarely affected (Elgart & Higdon 1973).

Maculae caeruleae are blue–grey macules on the trunk and thighs, which quickly fade; they may be caused by altered blood pigments, or be a product from the louse's salivary glands. Pediculosis pubis may be complicated by

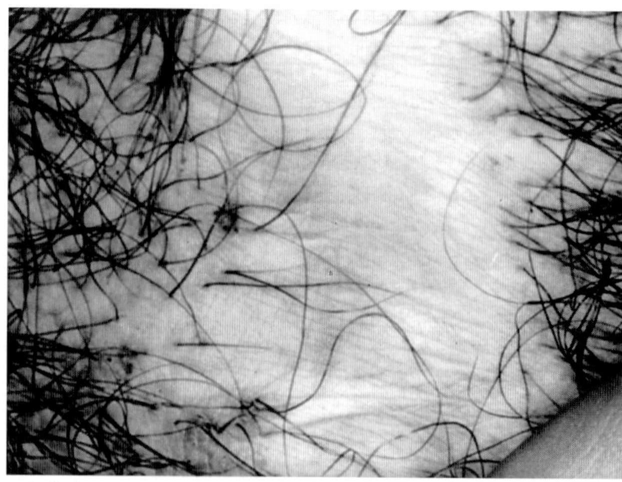

Fig. 4.2 Pediculosis pubis; both pediculi and nits are visible.

impetiginization caused by scratching, particularly in people with poor personal hygiene.

Treatment

Since *Phthirus pubis* is sexually transmitted, a search for associated infections should be made before treatment is started: as a minimum, culture for *Neisseria gonorrhoeae*, an antigen detection test for *Chlamydia trachomatis* and serological tests for syphilis should be performed. Shaving of the pubic or body hair is unnecessary. After a bath or shower, the patient applies 0.5% aqueous malathion or 1% lindane lotion to all hairy areas except the scalp. Alcoholic lotions are not recommended, as they may cause irritation; Vaseline may be used on the eyelashes. The application is washed off after 24 hours, and personal clothing and bed linen are then changed; discarded items are washed at a temperature of at least 50°C. A second application is necessary only for the heaviest infestations. Patients should be warned that egg cases may remain attached to the hairs for a week or two after therapy, but their presence does not mean treatment failure. All sexual contacts of infected women should receive identical treatment as soon as possible.

Scabies

Sarcoptes scabiei is an arachnid of the order Acarina (Johnson & Mellanby 1972). Infection with this parasite causes a widespread and intensely itchy skin eruption. The transmission of scabies requires close and fairly prolonged contact between individuals, and in adults it is regarded as a disease that is predominantly sexually transmitted. Scabies is commonest in the second and third decades of life, and is more often seen in men than in women (Orkin & Maibach 1984). In men with scabies, genital lesions are very common, but in women vulval ones are rare (Fig. 4.3). However, in crusted (Norwegian) scabies the genitalia in both sexes are likely to be affected; this form of scabies is seen in elderly and immunosuppressed patients.

Treatment involves the use of a topical scabicide, and lindane, malathion, benzyl benzoate and crotamiton may be used. Most treatment failures are related to incorrect usage rather than to resistance. It is essential that all members of the household or close contacts of the patient are treated adequately and at the same time.

Infection with nematodes, tapeworms and flukes

Oxyuriasis

Infection with *Enterobius vermicularis* (the threadworm) is common, particularly in children, throughout the world. The worms live in the large bowel, and lay eggs on the perianal and perineal skin during the night. These ova may then be shed and ingested by another person, or the larvae may hatch and re-enter the anal canal. Pruritus ani, sometimes severe, is a common symptom of infection. Vulval irritation and vulvovaginitis may also occur, and the worms are sometimes found in the vagina (Kacker 1973) (Fig. 4.4).

Threadworms are 3–12 mm long, and may be seen around the anus or between the labia. Identification of the ova is made by applying adhesive tape, conveniently mounted on a slide, to the perineum, preferably in the

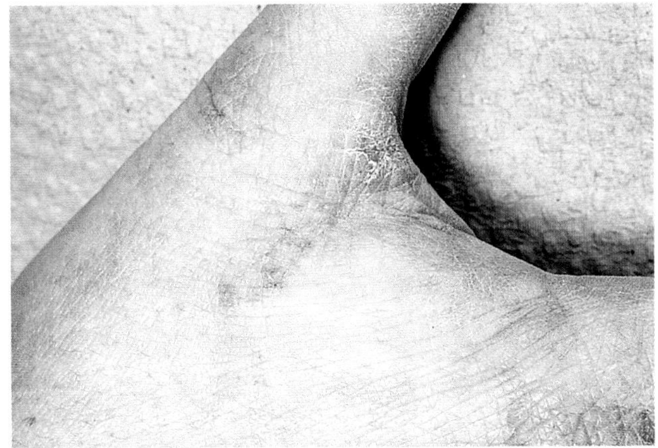

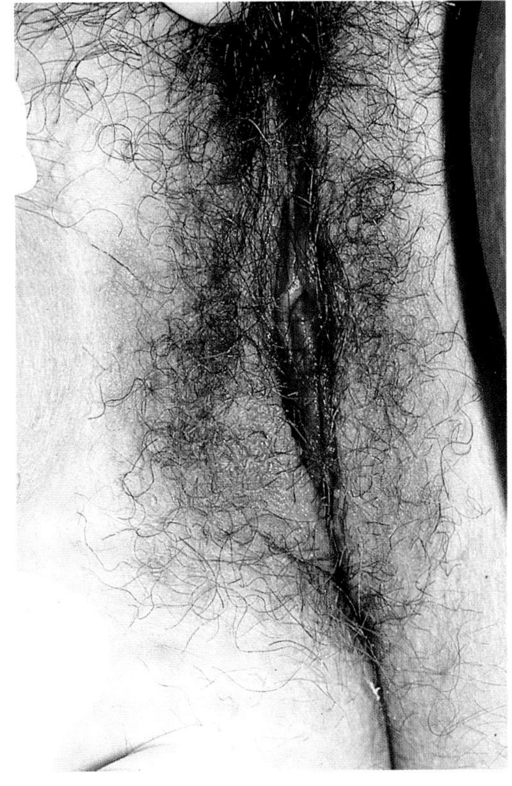

Fig. 4.3 Scabies; lesions of the finger web and vulva.

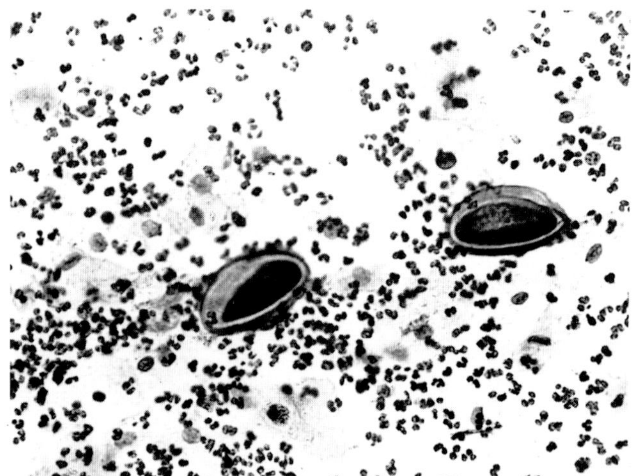

Fig. 4.4 Ova of *Enterobius vermicularis* in cervical smear.

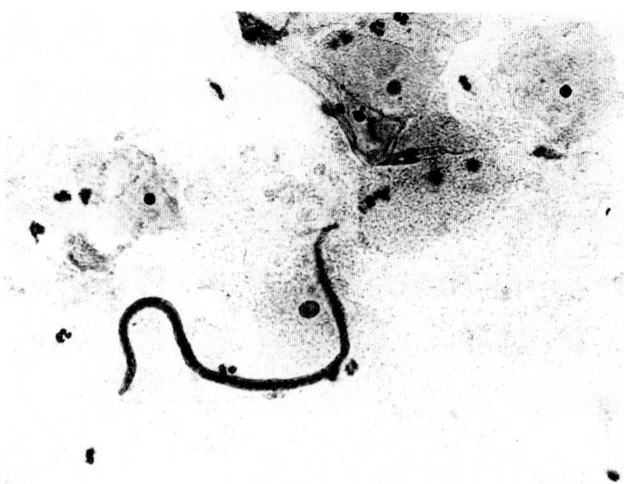

Fig. 4.5 Filarial worm in cytology smear.

morning before washing; the eggs adhere to the tape and can be identified by microscopy. Anthelmintics are relatively ineffective in oxyuriasis, and general measures to prevent self-reinfection are important. The hands should be thoroughly washed and the nails scrubbed before meals and after urination and defecation. If possible, a bath or shower should be taken in the morning to wash off ova deposited during the night. Piperazine salts are widely used. The dosage for piperazine hydrate is: up to 2 years of age, 50–75 mg/kg; 2–4 years, 750 mg; 5–12 years, 1.5 g; children over 12 years and adults, 2 g. These doses are given daily for 7 days. Mebendazole is the drug of choice for all ages over 2 years; 100 mg is given as a single dose. All members of a family should receive treatment.

Other parasitic worms, *Ascaris lumbricoides* (roundworm) and *Trichuris trichiura*, have occasionally been found in the vagina in children (Gardner & Kaufman 1981).

Filariasis

Wuchereria bancrofti and *Brugia malayi* are filarial worms. *Brugia malayi* is confined to Asia, India and the Pacific islands. The infection is transmitted by mosquitoes; microfilariae in human blood are ingested, and the larvae then inoculated into another person. Over a period of years, these develop and reproduce in lymphatic vessels. The subsequent inflammation, if it occurs in inguinal glands, gives rise to genital lymphoedema and elephantiasis.

Filariasis affecting the vulva is usually due to *Wuchereria bancrofti*. By the time lymphoedema appears, there is no evidence of active infection. Both sides of the vulva are affected, although the swelling is often greater on one side. The pathological appearances of affected lymph nodes are usually non-specific, but sometimes histology shows parts of dead worms.

The differential diagnosis is from other forms of lymphatic obstruction with vulval swelling: lymphogranuloma venereum, carcinoma, tuberculosis and following surgery. Diethylcarbamazine is an effective filaricide. Destruction of the microfilariae often induces an allergic response owing to the release of antigen; it is usual to begin treatment with a dose of 1 mg/kg/day, increasing over 3 days to 6 mg/kg/day in divided doses, and this is continued for 3 weeks. Surgical treatment of the elephantiasis may be needed (Lawson 1967).

Onchocerca volvulus is a filarial worm that is endemic in many tropical and subtropical areas. It is transmitted by flies. On the non-genital skin, onchocerciasis causes intensely itchy lichenified eruptions, but the vulva is not affected. The parasite may sometimes be seen in vaginal cytology smears (Fig. 4.5). Treatment is with diethylcarbamazine.

Echinococcosis (hydatid disease)

Echinococcus granularis and *Echinococcus multilocularis* are tapeworms that live in the intestines of dogs and other animals. Ova swallowed by humans develop into larvae, which enter the bloodstream and are carried to distant sites, where hydatid cysts develop. Hydatid cysts of the vulva are rare, but have been described (Anagnostidis 1935, Ricci 1945). They form painless, firm or soft subcutaneous swellings. Treatment is surgical.

Schistosomiasis (bilharzia)

Aetiology

Three main species affect humans: *Schistosoma mansoni* in Africa, the Caribbean and South America, *Schistosoma japonicum* in the Far East, and *Schistosoma haematobium* in Africa and the Middle East. The life cycle is similar for all species, but the intermediate snail host is specific for each. The organisms in the cercarial stage enter the bloodstream via the skin during bathing or wading. The mature stage of male and female parasites is reached in the portal venous system. After copulation, the females migrate to the pelvic venous plexus, *Schistosoma mansoni* and *Schistosoma japonicum* to the mesenteric and *Schistosoma haematobium* to the vesical plexus. Eggs are laid and penetrate the vessels, reaching surrounding tissues and eventually the skin; the clinical and pathological effects are due to immune reactions to these ova. Some ova are excreted via the urine or faeces and hatch miracidia, which are ingested by the snail host, thus completing the cycle.

Clinical features

Involvement of the female genital tract is usually due to *Schistosoma haematobium*, and sometimes to *Schistosoma mansoni*. Vulval lesions occur mainly before puberty, and have been described by Boulle and Notelovitz (1964) and McKee *et al.* (1983). The disease presents as a chronic granulomatous reaction affecting the labia majora first and other parts of the vulva later. The lesions usually resemble condylomata acuminata, and may coalesce or ulcerate; later, scarring and calcification may develop. In some patients the condylomas do not develop for months or even years after the initial infection (Goldsmith *et al.* 1993).

Diagnosis

This depends on identification of the ova. The histology of active lesions shows intense inflammation centred on viable miracidia and degenerating forms, and granulomas and numerous eosinophils are present. Ova may also be found in the urine, faeces and vaginal discharge. Biopsy is probably the best procedure for the diagnosis of vulval schistosomiasis (Fig. 4.6); Berry (1971) has described the use of gynaecological cytology for the diagnosis of ulcerative lesions.

The differential diagnosis is from other chronic infective conditions, including condylomata acuminata, lymphogranuloma venereum, amoebiasis and carcinoma.

Treatment

Praziquantel is effective against all human schistosomes. The dose is 40 mg/kg in two divided doses 4–6 hours apart.

Infection with protozoa

Trichomoniasis

Trichomonas vaginalis is a common human parasite that colonizes the lower genital tract in men and women. In women it is recovered from the vagina, urethra and bladder, and from accessory ducts such as those of Skene's and Bartholin's glands. Trichomoniasis usually causes symptoms, but can be symptomless.

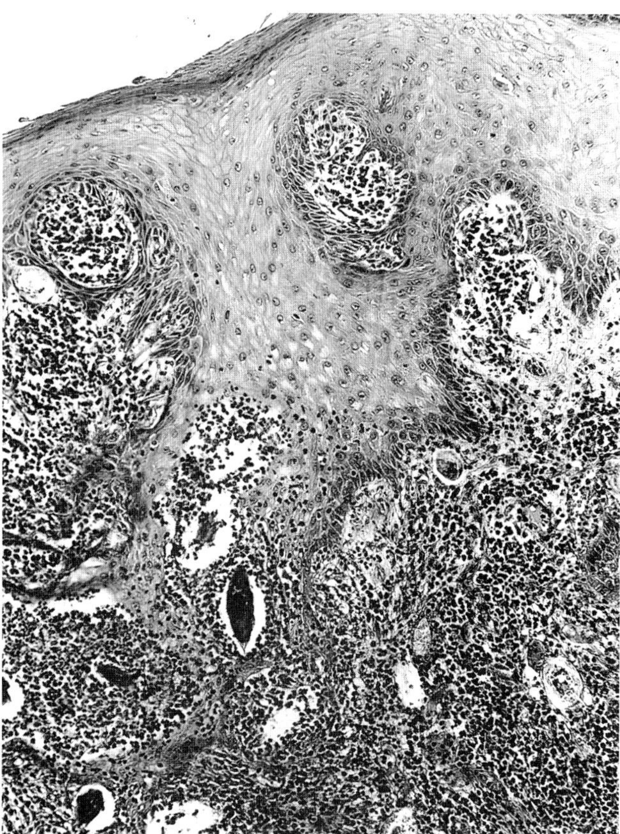

Fig. 4.6 Ova of schistosomiasis.

The organism

Trichomonas vaginalis is a motile, flagellated protozoon (Fig. 4.7). It is 10 μm × 7 μm in size; organisms from patients with acute symptomatic infections may be smaller than from those with chronic or silent infections. They have four anterior flagellae, and a lateral undulating membrane. There is a single oval nucleus near the anterior end of the cell, and an axostyle runs through the centre of the organism and protrudes at its posterior end. *Trichomonas vaginalis* multiplies by binary fission, and does not form cysts (Honigberg 1978). It grows best under moderately anaerobic conditions. It can easily be cultured in nutrient media with added antimicrobials to suppress the growth of bacteria and yeasts, such as Feinberg–Whittington's or Diamond's media.

Trichomonads can ingest small particles by phagocytosis, and their nutrition depends on this property. They can also

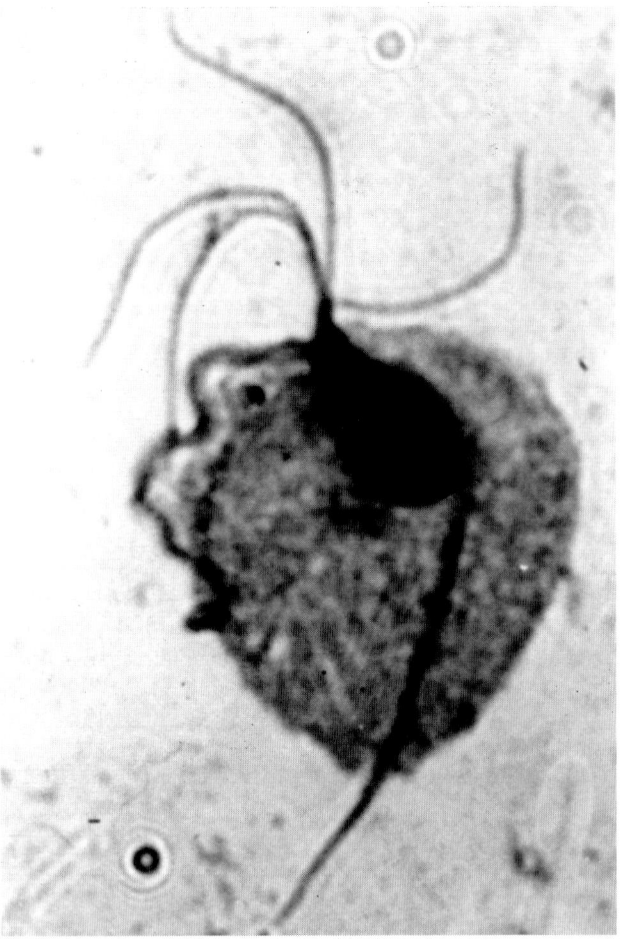

Fig. 4.7 *Trichomonas vaginalis.*

ingest bacteria, which are usually killed within a few hours. It has been claimed that *Neisseria gonorrhoeae* can persist within *Trichomonas vaginalis* for a long period of time, and thereby be protected from the action of gonococcocidal antibodies (Ovcinnikov *et al.* 1975), but this phenomenon, if it exists, does not seem to cause therapeutic problems in clinical practice.

Epidemiology

The prevalence of trichomoniasis is variable. In the USA the reported prevalence varies from 5% or less in healthy women to 33% in women attending STD clinics (Naguib *et al.* 1966, Sparks *et al.* 1975, Fouts & Kraus 1980). It is sexually transmissible; up to 60% of male partners of infected women harbour the parasite (Catterall 1972), and many cases of recurrent trichomoniasis can be cured by the simultaneous treatment of both partners with antitrichomonal drugs (Lyng & Christensen 1981). The inoculation of *Trichomonas vaginalis* into the normal vagina is followed by acute trichomonal vaginitis (Asami & Nakamura 1955). It has been suggested that accidental infection is possible from fomites or in swimming baths, but this has not been reliably documented.

Concurrent infection with other microbes, notably *Neisseria gonorrhoeae*, is common. Gonorrhoea has been reported in 30–46% of women with trichomoniasis (Eriksson & Wanger 1975, Fouts & Kraus 1980), but there is no evidence of any specific association between the two diseases. It has sometimes been reported that trichomoniasis is commoner in black than in white women, but this difference is probably due to socioeconomic rather than racial factors.

Clinical features

The incubation period of trichomoniasis appears to be between 4 and 28 days (Catterall 1972). The clinical picture is variable. The classic description is of an acute vulvovaginitis with a frothy, malodorous, purulent vaginal discharge; in severe infections there may be punctate haemorrhages on the cervix ('strawberry cervix'). The patient complains of vulval soreness and irritation and of vaginal discharge. These symptoms are often worse during or just after menstruation. They are not specifically associated with trichomoniasis (Fouts & Kraus 1980); a diagnosis of the cause of vulvovaginitis based on clinical appearances alone is often wrong, so laboratory investigation is essential (Oriel *et al.* 1972). Between 10 and 50% of women with trichomoniasis are symptomless, and in 15% there is no evidence of vulvovaginitis (Honigberg 1978, Fouts & Kraus 1980). Although the vagina is almost invariably infected, the urethra and Skene's glands are also colonized in 90% of cases (Whittington 1957). In a few women, trichomonads can be recovered from the endocervix. Reinfection of the vagina from these other sites accounted for many treatment failures before the discovery of the nitroimidazoles. There are no local complications of trichomoniasis, and no convincing evidence of any systemic effects. Untreated, the infection may drag on for months or even years.

Diagnosis

The simplest method is microscopy of a drop of vaginal fluid mixed with saline on a slide. Bright-field, phase-contrast and dark-field illumination can all be used. At magnification ×400 the irregular jerky movement of the organisms can be seen; higher power can be used to identify the flagellae and undulating membrane. All glassware used should be warm and clean and the preparation examined as soon as possible, as the organisms rapidly become immobile under adverse conditions. Most workers believe that culture is more sensitive than direct microscopy; Fouts and Kraus (1980) found that wet-mount examination had only half the sensitivity of culture. Others have found much smaller differences (Whittington 1957); no doubt these depend on the culture media used and the skill and experience of the microscopist. Trichomonads can be identified in smears stained by Giemsa, Papanicolaou or acridine orange, but Gram staining is unsatisfactory. During the Papanicolaou process the organisms lose their flagellae and appear as grey-blue, pear-shaped cells with intracytoplasmic granules and small, dark grey nuclei. This technique has a sensitivity of 60–70% in comparison with culture (Thomason *et al.* 1988), and the specificity is also less (Perl 1972).

Treatment

Most strains of *Trichomonas vaginalis* are highly sensitive to the 5-nitroimidazoles. The recommended treatment of trichomoniasis in women is metronidazole 2.0 g given as a single dose (Hager *et al.* 1980). Metronidazole 200 mg three times a day for 7 days was used for many years with good results, but the total dose of the drug is higher and compliance less good than with the single-dose treatment. It is usual to treat sex partners of women with trichomoniasis, and if this is done a cure rate exceeding 95% is achieved. The single-dose metronidazole regimen has not been fully evaluated for men, so the 7-day treatment may be preferable. Metronidazole should not be prescribed during the first 3 months of pregnancy, but may be taken safely after this (Rodin & Hass 1966). In early pregnancy topical treatment is the only choice; a 6-day course of clotrimazole pessaries 100 mg/day can be given, although the cure rate is then only about 50% (Lohmeyer 1974).

Metronidazole has an Antabuse-like action; alcohol during therapy may cause vomiting and is best avoided. Overgrowth of vaginal yeasts after a 7-day course of treatment may occur but this is less likely after single-dose therapy (Hager *et al.* 1980). The possibility of an oncogenic potential of metronidazole arose because prolonged administration in mice increased the frequency of some naturally occurring tumours (Rustia & Shubik 1972), but such effects have never been seen in the 30 years since the drug was first used in humans, and the risk from a short course is now regarded as negligible.

Treatment failure. The re-isolation of *Trichomonas vaginalis* after treatment may be due to poor compliance with a multidose regimen, failure to treat the male partner adequately, inadequate tissue levels and occasionally to trichomonal resistance. When standard courses of treatment have failed and reinfection excluded as far as possible it is usual to treat women with relapsing infections with metronidazole in higher dosage and for a longer period, such as 400 mg orally three times a day for 7–10 days, although this higher dosage may induce vomiting. Although there is little difference in the activity of different 5-imidazoles against *Trichomonas vaginalis in vitro*, if metronidazole is ineffective tinidazole may be tried; it is usually given as a single 2-g dose, and a further 2-g dose may be given if there is no improvement.

Leishmaniasis

Aetiology

Cutaneous leishmaniasis, American mucocutaneous leishmaniasis and visceral leishmaniasis (kala-azar) are all caused by morphologically identical flagellate protozoa; the classification of *Leishmania* associated with different diseases depends on serological, biochemical and cultural features of the organisms, and is not entirely satisfactory (Bray 1974). Genital involvement is commoner in cutaneous leishmaniasis than in the American mucocutaneous variety (Harman 1986). Patients after spontaneous recovery from kala-azar, or after successful treatment with antimony compounds, may develop dermal lesions called leishmanoids; vulval leishmaniasis apparently due to sexual transmission of *Leishmania* from these has been described (Symmers 1960).

Epidemiology

Cutaneous leishmaniasis is endemic in countries bordering the eastern Mediterranean, Asia Minor and India, and American mucocutaneous leishmaniasis in virtually every country in Central and South America. Kala-azar occurs in parts of all continents except Australia. Transmission of all these diseases is by sandflies, and there is a reservoir of infection in alternative mammalian hosts.

Clinical features

The incubation period of cutaneous leishmaniasis is between 2 weeks and several months (Marsden 1979). Dissemination of *Leishmania tropica* after inoculation is followed by the appearance of skin lesions, which can affect the genitals, although the face and extremities are more commonly involved. Nodular, ulcerative and lupoid forms are described (Feinstein 1978).

Diagnosis

The vulval lesions of leishmaniasis must be distinguished from those of syphilis, pyogenic granuloma and donovanosis as well as from malignant tumours. The diagnosis can be confirmed by identifying the parasites as Leishman–Donovan bodies in smears or tissue sections. *Leishmania tropica* can be cultured in special media, and a leishmanin intradermal test, using a *Leishmania tropica* antigen, becomes positive in the majority of patients.

Treatment

Cutaneous leishmaniasis may heal spontaneously, but if the skin lesions are extensive antimony preparations are usually given. The drug of choice is sodium stilbogluconate; a dose equivalent to 600 mg of pentavalent antimony is given daily by intravenous or intramuscular injection for 10 days. There is no agreement as to the efficacy of various other local and systemic treatments; advice on these is often best obtained from experts in tropical medicine.

Amoebiasis

Aetiology

Entamoeba histolytica exists in two forms: the motile trophozoite and the cyst. The trophozoite is the pathogenic form, living in the lumen and/or walls of the colon. When diarrhoea occurs, motile trophozoites can be identified in the faeces. In the absence of diarrhoea *Entamoeba histolytica* usually forms cysts that are highly resistant to environmental changes and can be transmitted either directly through oral–anal contact or via flies, food or water.

Epidemiology

Infection with *Entamoeba histolytica* is worldwide, being particularly common in tropical and subtropical countries, especially where standards of hygiene are low (Krogstad *et al.* 1978). Cases of amoebic dysentery are usually sporadic, but epidemics, usually water-borne, have occurred.

The frequency with which genital lesions occur in patients with amoebiasis is uncertain, but they are regarded as an unusual complication. Cohen (1973) found that only about 100 cases had been described up to 1971, and in most of these the cervix was affected. Majmudar *et al.* (1976) reported a case of clitoral amoebiasis.

Clinical features

Most lesions begin as cutaneous abscesses, which rupture and form painful serpiginous ulcers with slough at the base (Fig. 4.8), or they present as wart-like lesions. The perineum, vulva and cervix may be affected, and local glands are usually also involved (Gogoi 1969). Intestinal amoebiasis is usually present, causing diarrhoea and sometimes liver abscesses (El Zawahry & El Komy 1973). The vulval and perineal lesions are usually due to a direct extension of intestinal disease, but some are believed to arise through sexual inoculation of the organisms.

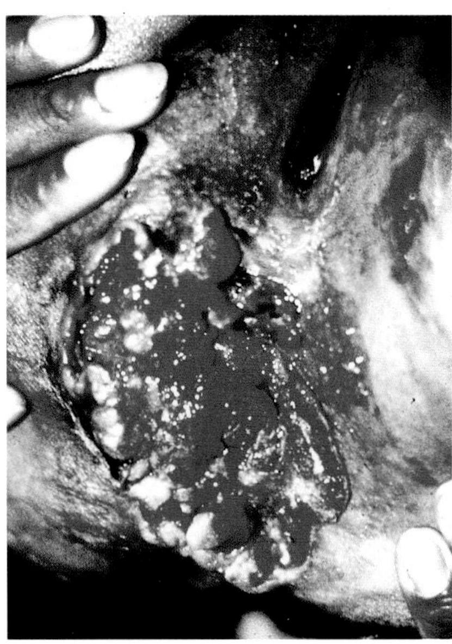

Fig. 4.8 Amoebiasis. Large ulcer with sloughing base.

Diagnosis

Vulval and perineal amoebiasis must be distinguished from donovanosis, lymphogranuloma venereum, deep mycosis and early syphilis. The diagnosis may be established by identifying motile amoebae in scrapings from the ulcers or from the cervix. Histologically there is an inflammatory reaction, and *Entamoeba histolytica* may be seen as a small, round eosinophilic body. Trophozoites or cysts may be found in fresh stool specimens.

Treatment

Metronidazole is very effective in cutaneous amoebiasis, and is given in a dosage of 800 mg three times a day for 5 days. For chronic infections in which cysts rather than trophozoites are present in the faeces, diloxanide furonate 500 mg three times a day for 10 days is the drug of choice.

Mycotic infections

Vulvovaginal yeast infection

Yeasts are oval or spherical cells, which commonly reproduce by budding. In some yeasts the buds elongate into filaments (hyphae) that become linked in chains, resembling a mould mycelium. The genera that usually infect the vulva and vagina are *Candida* (formerly called *Monilia*) and *Torulopsis*; of these, only *Candida* produces hyphae in

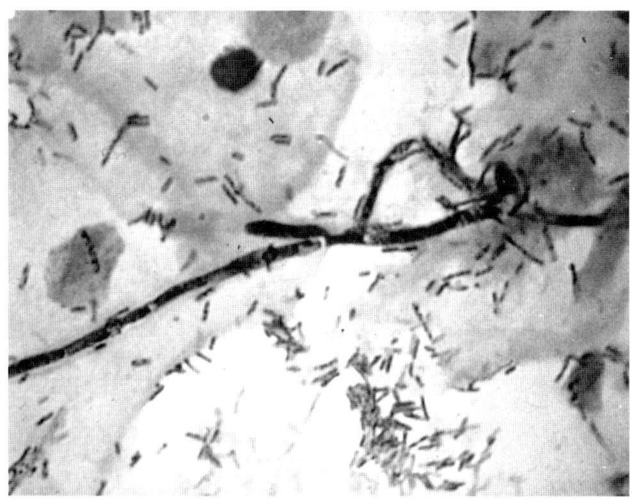

Fig. 4.9 *Candida albicans*. Budding yeasts and hyphae.

culture. The commonest genital yeast is *Candida albicans*; other *Candida* species are uncommon. *Torulopsis glabrata* causes a few infections. Under the microscope *Candida albicans* can appear as ovoid budding yeasts (blastospores), hyphae (Fig. 4.9) and sometimes as refractile chlamydospores; the predominant form in a culture medium depends on the prevailing conditions.

Ecology and epidemiology

The skin, mouth, alimentary tract and vagina all have an endogenous yeast flora. *Candida albicans* can be recovered on rectal culture from up to 20% of unselected women, and this figure may reach 50% in women attending STD clinics (Hilton & Warnock 1975). The isolation rate from the vagina of women who are not pregnant or taking oral contraceptives is about 20% (Odds 1988). Genital yeasts are sexually transmissible. Men whose partners are colonized are four times more likely to yield yeasts from the penis than those with uninfected partners (Davidson 1977). Despite this, sexual transmission is not thought to be of major epidemiological importance to women (Thin *et al.* 1977), and the gastrointestinal tract is more likely to be the initial source of colonization. Neonatal candidosis is much commoner in babies born to women with vaginal candidosis than in babies born to uninfected mothers (Hurley & de Louvois 1979).

Pathogenesis of candidosis

Predisposing factors. Pregnancy, oral contraceptives with a high oestrogen content, diabetes mellitus, antimicrobial therapy and impaired cell-mediated immunity all predispose to vaginal candidosis. In pregnancy, there is not only a higher prevalence of vaginal colonization but a higher rate of symptomatic vulvovaginitis; the margin between simple colonization by yeasts and clinical disease appears to be narrow (Carroll *et al.* 1973). Why pregnancy should predispose to vaginal candidosis is uncertain. It has been suggested that yeasts may overgrow because the high level of reproductive hormones cause an increased vaginal glycogen content. Alternatively, lowered cell-mediated immunity to *Candida albicans* may be responsible (Brunham *et al.* 1983). Vaginal colonization by yeasts is increased by the administration of high-oestrogen oral contraceptives, but this phenomenon does not occur with low-oestrogen oral contraceptives (Davidson & Oates 1985). Both the carriage of yeasts and candidal vulvovaginitis are common in diabetics, and indeed vaginitis may be a presenting symptom of diabetes; its cause may be high vaginal glycogen levels, as in pregnancy. The prevalence of vaginal yeasts is increased by the administration of broad-spectrum antibiotics, and symptomatic vulvovaginitis may follow (Oriel & Waterworth 1975). A similar effect is produced by metronidazole (Beveridge 1962). Although an action on the vaginal flora is postulated as the cause, its exact nature is uncertain.

Host defences. Polymorphonuclear leucocytes can attach themselves to yeast hyphae and subsequently destroy them (Diamond & Krezesicki 1978), and they play an important role in limiting systemic candidosis. These cells are not present in vaginal specimens from women with candidal vulvovaginitis, and they are not thought to play an important part in limiting genital colonization or invasion by *Candida albicans*. Circulating antibodies against and cell-mediated immunity to the organisms have been demonstrated, but their role in limiting infection is uncertain (Odds 1988). The bacterial flora of the vagina may act as a defence against candidosis in some undefined way (Auger & Joly 1980).

The relationship between vaginal colonization by yeasts and the development of symptomatic disease is poorly understood. Previous suggestions that there is an association between mycelium formation and the symptoms and signs of infection are no longer accepted. The concentration of yeasts in the vagina appears to be unrelated to the development of clinical signs of infection (Mursic 1975). It is probable that the transition of *Candida* and *Torulopsis* from commensalism to parasitism is conditioned for the most part by changes in the host that make it easier for the organisms to adhere to and subsequently damage epithelial cells, but an explanation of this phenomenon is not yet forthcoming.

Clinical manifestations

The vulva and vagina are involved together. The cardinal symptom is pruritus, but women also complain of burning, dysuria, vaginal discharge and superficial dyspareunia. On examination, the vulva may show swelling, erythema and scaling, and sometimes excoriation and fissures (Fig. 4.10). The vagina too is erythematous, and a curdy discharge is often present, with plaques of exudate adherent to its walls. The vaginal secretions are not malodorous, and the pH is <4.5. This classical picture is not present in all cases. Some patients show a milder disease, and some women colonized by yeasts show no abnormality. The clinical differentiation between candidosis and other forms of vaginitis such as trichomoniasis is not reliable, and laboratory investigation is always needed.

Laboratory diagnosis

Vaginal yeast infection may be diagnosed by microscopy or culture. A specimen of vaginal fluid may be mixed with a drop of normal saline or 10% potassium hydroxide on a slide and examined as a wet preparation, or stained by Gram's method, which shows blastospores and hyphae as intensely Gram positive. Which of these procedures is used is a matter of choice, but none has more than 50% of the sensitivity of culture. Culture for yeasts is performed on a peptone–glucose–agar medium such as Sabouraud's medium; isolates are confirmed as *Candida albicans* by demonstrating hypha formation by incubation in serum. Other infections may coexist with *Candida*, and should be excluded by appropriate tests.

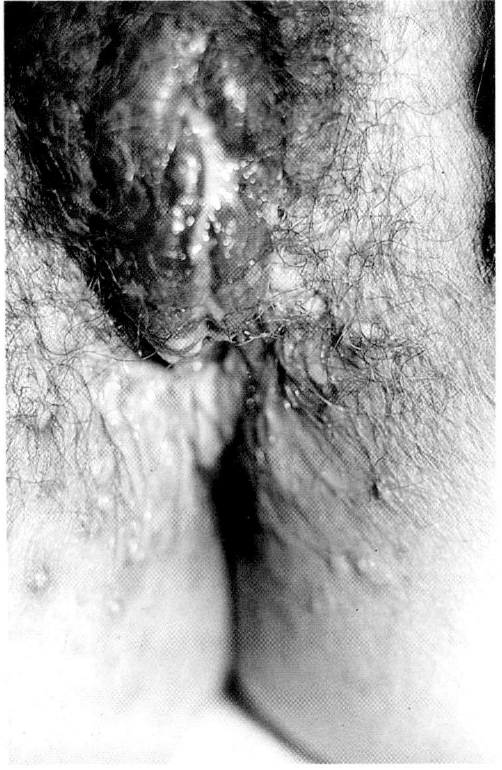

Fig. 4.10 Acute candidal vulvovaginitis.

Treatment

Women with symptomatic candidosis certainly require treatment. Opinion is divided on the management of symptomless yeast carriers, but most physicians are against routine treatment. It is obviously necessary to identify, and treat if possible, any predisposing factors such as diabetes mellitus. It is generally recommended that constrictive underwear and tights should be avoided, and that cotton is preferable to synthetic fabric next to the skin. Potential irritants such as bath oils and vaginal deodorants should not be used.

Most antimycotics fall into one of two groups: the polyenes such as nystatin and amphotericin, and the imidazoles, such as clotrimazole, econazole, isoconazole and miconazole. Imidazoles are usually preferred. Clotrimazole pessaries 100 mg at night for 6 nights, or 200 mg at night for 3 nights, or 500 mg as a single application are equally effective, the single dose being an advantage if compliance is a problem. Intravaginal medication may be supplemented by an antimycotic cream twice daily if there is vulval irritation. Cure rates of 90% or so may be expected with these regimens. The other imidazoles may be used in comparable dosage, and appear to be equally effective. Polyenes are occasionally prescribed if imidazoles give poor results. Nystatin pessaries 100 000 units daily for 14 days, continuing during menstruation, were formerly much used although some patients found their texture and colour disagreeable. Acute vaginal candidosis may also be treated with fluconazole 150 mg orally as a single dose with results similar to those obtained with vaginal imidazoles. Side effects include nausea, abdominal discomfort, diarrhoea and occasionally abnormalities of liver enzymes. Ketoconazole, another imidazole that can be given orally, has been associated with fatal hepatotoxicity.

Recurrent vulvovaginal candidosis. The treatment of this complaint remains difficult. It does not appear to be due to the presence of resistant vaginal yeasts, so switching from one antimycotic to another is of little benefit. The first step is to identify and eliminate any predisposing causes. Abandoning the use of oral contraceptives should certainly be considered, although it may not be helpful to discontinue low-dose oestrogen preparations, particularly when long-term antimycotics are being prescribed (Sobel 1990). Treatment of the male partner with an antimycotic cream has not been shown to be helpful unless he has balanitis. It has been suggested that recurrences may be caused by reinfection from a so-called intestinal reservoir (Miles *et al.* 1977). Supplementary treatment with oral nystatin or amphotericin has been tried, but the results were disappointing (Milne and Warnock 1979). A more usual approach is with intermittent topical therapy (Davidson & Mould 1978). Patients who can identify the onset of a new attack initiate treatment with a short course of treatment, for example with a single 500-mg clotrimazole pessary. Alternatively, antimycotic pessaries may be used regularly, perhaps once a month before or after menstruation, for several months (Miller *et al.* 1984); intermittent oral fluconazole may also be used in this way. Prophylactic antimycotics should be regarded as suppressive rather than curative.

Tinea cruris

Aetiology

Tinea cruris (ringworm of the groin) is a fungal infection that is common in men but uncommon in women (Ingram 1955, Blank & Mann 1975). The usual cause is *Trichophyton rubrum* or *Epidermophyton floccosum*. Heat and humidity are provoking factors, and the condition is most prevalent in people who wear tight, occlusive underwear, particularly during warm weather.

Clinical features

Tinea cruris begins as a small, erythematous, scaly patch, which spreads peripherally and tends to clear in the centre (Fig. 4.11). The groins are chiefly affected, but the disease may encroach on the vulva or spread towards the perineal and perianal area, either as a continuous rash or as inflamed areas separated by normal skin. Where topical corticosteroids have been applied, the typical features may be masked. A focus of infection is often present elsewhere, for example on the feet.

Diagnosis

This may be made by microscopy of scrapings from the edge of the eruption suspended in 10% potassium hydroxide, when the mycelium can be seen, or by culture of the same material; the scrapings can be sent, preferably on black paper so that they can be easily seen, to an experienced laboratory. The main differential diagnoses are flexural psoriasis, which is not usually circinate, erythrasma and cutaneous candidosis. Erythrasma is more uniformly scaly, has a brown colour and gives a coral-red fluorescence in Wood's light. Candidal lesions appear more inflamed than those of tinea cruris, and they have a peripheral sodden fringe; these two diseases may be

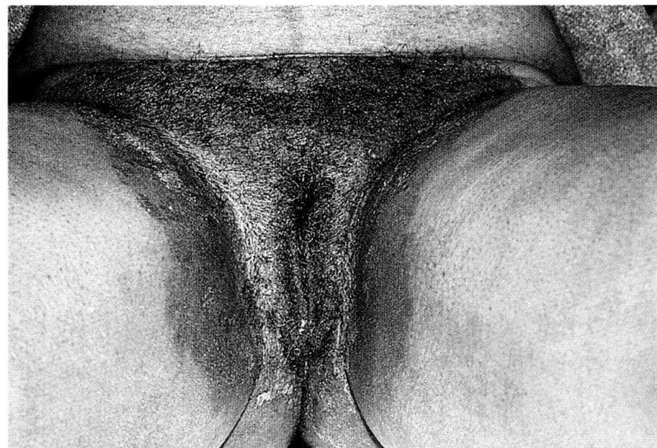

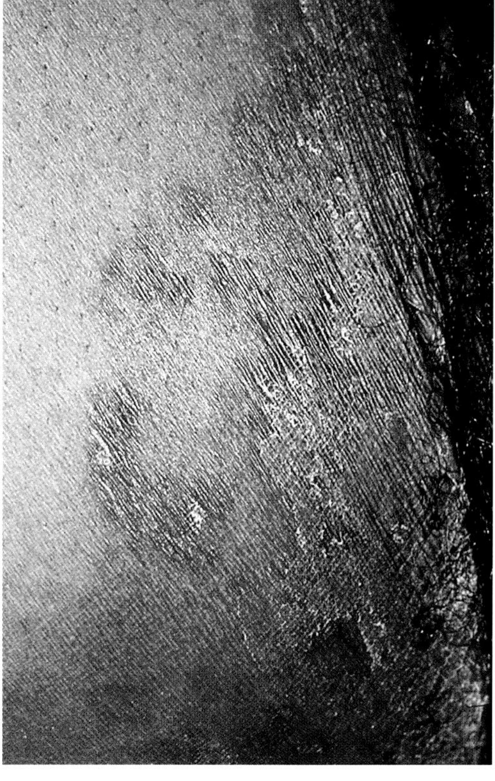

Fig. 4.11 Tinea cruris.

readily differentiated by culture if microscopy is not diagnostic.

Treatment

Imidazole creams have largely replaced benzoic acid preparations, as they are more effective and less messy (Clayton & Connor 1973). Clotrimazole cream 1% may be applied twice daily, and continued for a week or two after clinical clearance. Topical treatment, however, is often not successful in the hair-bearing areas of the vulva. Oral treatment with griseofulvin, or preferably with the newer drug terbinafine, 250 mg/day for 2–4 weeks, is recommended.

Pityriasis versicolor

Aetiology

Pityriasis versicolor (tinea versicolor) is caused by a *Pityrosporum*, usually *Pityrosporon orbiculare* (*Malassezia furfur*). It has maximum prevalence in the hot and humid conditions of the tropics, but is common worldwide.

Clinical features

Brownish, scaly macules appear, principally on the chest, abdomen and back, and may be accompanied by some itching. The genital area usually escapes, but may be involved if the eruption is widespread (Bumgarner & Burke 1949). Strikingly hypopigmented lesions may occur in the napkin area of black infants (Jelliffe & Jacobson 1954).

Diagnosis

Abundant fungal hyphae and spores can easily be seen by microscopy of skin scrapings suspended in 10% potassium hydroxide; culture is unnecessary. Pityriasis versicolor must be distinguished from seborrhoeic dermatitis, pityriasis rosea and secondary syphilis.

Treatment

Clotrimazole cream is usually effective. If it does not cure the eruption itraconazole may be given orally, 200 mg/day for 7 days; it should be avoided if there is a history of liver disease. Selenium sulphide suspension should not be applied to the vulva.

Phycomycosis

The various forms of phycomycosis are caused by fungi of the class *Phycomycetes*. Subcutaneous phycomycosis occurs in children and young adults, and is caused by *Basidiobolus ranarum*. Deep granulomatous masses appear beneath an intact but inflamed epidermis. Infection of the vulva has been described (Lawson 1967, Scott *et al.* 1985). Fluconazole or itraconazole may be effective therapy.

Chromomycosis (chromoblastomycosis)

This chronic fungus infection usually affects the leg or foot in barefooted farm labourers. Kakoti and Dey (1957) described a patient in whom *Hormodendrum compactum* was isolated from a verrucous vulval lesion.

Piedra (trichosporis)

Black and white varieties of this fungal condition are recognized. The causal organisms are *Piedraia hortai* and *Trichosporon beigelii*. Nodules are seen on the hair. The pubic area, as well as other hairy areas, may be affected; this is less frequent in women than in men (Kalter *et al.* 1986). Microscopy and culture on Sabouraud's medium will establish the diagnosis. The differential diagnosis is from trichomycosis nodosa of bacterial origin and pediculosis pubis. Treatment is by cutting off the hair and applying an antifungal compound, but recurrence is common.

Bacterial infections

Gram-positive cocci

STAPHYLOCOCCI

Staphylococcus aureus is present on the skin and in the nose of 30% of healthy people but it can cause many pyogenic infections, which often occur in sites and tissues with lowered host resistance, for example after injury. The organisms produce enzymes, such as coagulase, and toxins, which help to establish them in the host tissues.

On the vulva *Staphylococcus aureus* may cause furuncles and folliculitis. Folliculitis may follow minor trauma such as shaving perigenital hair (Fig. 4.12). Secondary infection by *Staphylococcus aureus*, often in conjunction with other organisms, may complicate pediculosis pubis and indeed almost any variety of vulvitis or vulval dermatosis, the organisms often being introduced by scratching. Furuncles are not uncommon on the vulva, and may recur despite treatment. Multiple furuncles may be associated with diabetes mellitus, immune deficiency or other debilitating diseases. *Staphylococcus aureus* may sometimes cause vulvovaginitis (Lang *et al.* 1958).

Staphylococcus aureus is one of the causes of acute infection of the duct of Bartholin's gland, leading to abscess formation; these abscesses may also be associated with

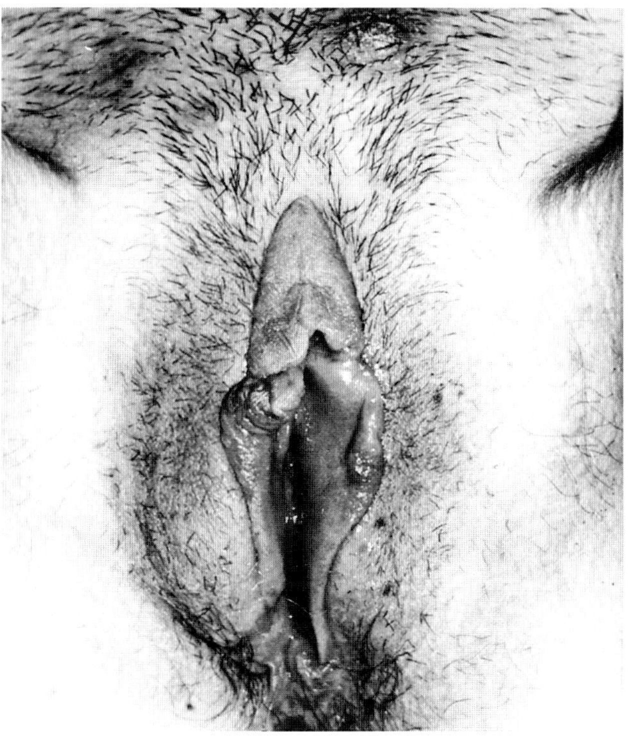

Fig. 4.12 Folliculitis of vulva.

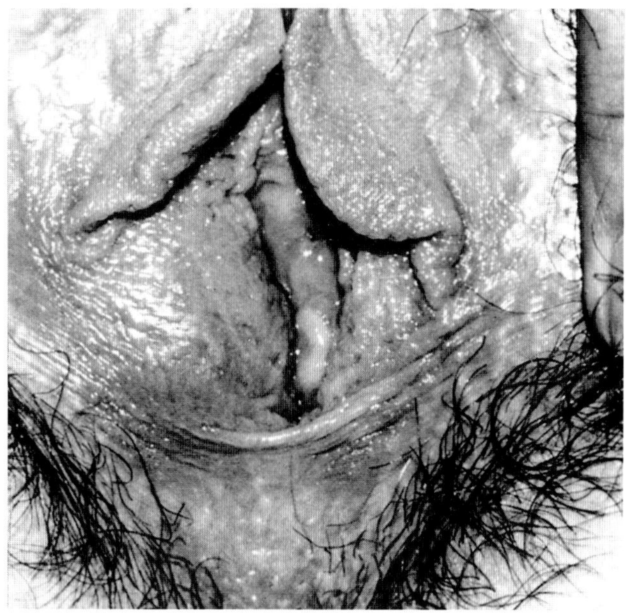

Fig. 4.13 Abscess of Bartholin's gland.

Neisseria gonorrhoeae, *Pseudomonas aeruginosa*, *Escherichia coli* and *Streptococcus faecalis*, and a few are sterile. A tender swelling appears at the affected labium major, and there may be vulval oedema and fever (Fig. 4.13). Some women suffer recurrent attacks; a cyst of Bartholin's gland may precede or follow infection, and is best dealt with surgically.

Coagulase-negative staphylococci have been divided into numerous biotypes. Those of medical importance are *Staphylococcus epidermidis*, which may cause severe infections in immunocompromised patients, and *Staphylococcus saprophyticus*, normally a harmless commensal, but which causes up to 30% of urinary tract infections in young women (Gillespie *et al.* 1978).

STREPTOCOCCI

Most streptococcal infections are caused by the β-haemolytic streptococcus of Lancefield's group A, *Streptococcus pyogenes*. The commonest infection caused by this organism is acute tonsillitis/pharyngitis; at one time it was a common cause of puerperal sepsis, but today other organisms are usually responsible. On the vulva, *Streptococcus pyogenes* causes cellulitis (erysipelas), a spreading inflammation of the dermis, with local redness, heat and swelling; this may extend more deeply into the subcutaneous tissue, and can become chronic. Perianal streptococcal dermatitis has also been described. All these infections may follow fissures and operation wounds and may complicate lymphatic obstruction of all types, and themselves lead to lymphatic obstruction. Cutaneous infection with *Streptococcus pyogenes* is sometimes followed by acute glomerulonephritis. Impetigo, a superficial epidermal infection, may be caused by streptococci, *Staphylococcus aureus* or both organisms (Noble 1981). *Streptococcus milleri* has been associated with anogenital hidradenitis suppurativa (Highet *et al.* 1980).

Group B streptococci are carried asymptomatically in the vagina. Women who do so at term may transmit them to their babies during delivery, causing an early-onset fulminating septicaemia with a high mortality. Infants over the age of 10 days may develop a meningitis syndrome due to group B streptococci, but here infection may be nosocomial.

TREATMENT OF VULVAL INFECTION BY PYOGENIC COCCI

Minor degrees of folliculitis and single furuncles do not usually require systemic antibiotics, but local antiseptics such as chlorhexidine may limit their spread to the surrounding skin. More extensive folliculitis and severe furunculosis merit systemic therapy. Since many staphylococci produce coagulase, erythromycin 250 mg or flucloxacillin 250 mg may be given four times a day for 5–7 days. A similar regimen may be used for the initial treatment of infection of Bartholin's gland pending the results of culture, which may necessitate a modification of treatment. Abscesses of Bartholin's glands require marsupialization or other surgical treatment, with histological examination in middle-aged women to exclude malignancy.

Oral or parenteral penicillin is rapidly effective for cellulitis; erythromycin can be substituted for those allergic to penicillin. Streptococcal lesions also respond well to systemic penicillin or erythromycin, combined with the removal of crusts with 0.05% aqueous chlorhexidine or 10% aqueous povidone iodine. Again, a specimen for microbiology should be taken before treatment is started.

Gram-negative cocci

NEISSERIA GONORRHOEAE

Neisseria gonorrhoeae is a Gram-negative diplococcus with hair-like pili that facilitate attachment to epithelial cells. In women the organism infects the urethra, cervix and anorectum, and from these sites may spread to adjacent structures—the paraurethral glands, Bartholin's glands, the endometrium and Fallopian tubes. The pharynx may also be infected, and from any of these sites gonococci may disseminate and cause systemic disease. Babies may be infected during delivery to mothers with gonorrhoea and develop ophthalmia neonatorum and, rarely, vulvovaginitis.

Epidemiology

Gonorrhoea is one of the commonest infectious diseases in the world. In Europe and North America its incidence markedly increased between the 1960s and 1980s, but has been declining since then. It is commonest in conurbations, and in women who are young, are of low socioeconomic status and belong to ethnic minorities. The risk of a woman acquiring gonorrhoea through a single sexual contact is unknown, but about 90% of sexual partners of men with gonorrhoea become infected (Thin 1970). Condoms give some protection against gonorrhoea (Barlow 1977).

Clinical features

The cervix is infected in 90% of cases of gonorrhoea, the urethra in 75% and the rectum in 50% (Barlow & Phillips 1978); the rectum is the sole infected site in 5% (Thin & Shaw 1979). The adult vagina is not usually infected by *Neisseria gonorrhoeae*, although Judson and Ruder (1979) recorded the recovery of gonococci from the vaginal vault of a woman who had had a hysterectomy. About 50% of women with uncomplicated gonorrhoea are symptomless; the remainder have symptoms of lower genital tract infection—dysuria, vaginal discharge and vulval discomfort—but these symptoms are non-specific and may be due to associated infections such as trichomoniasis. Those who have symptoms apparently due to gonorrhoea give an incubation period of up to 10 days (Wallin 1975). There are no characteristic physical signs. In some women there is evidence of cervicitis, and sometimes purulent material can be expressed from the urethra. The presence of vaginitis indicates trichomonal rather than gonococcal infection.

Local complications. Infection of the paraurethral glands of Skene may cause oedema of the urinary meatus, and sometimes an abscess forms, which can be palpated through the anterior wall of the vagina. Periurethral abscesses are rare (Fig. 4.14). Rees (1967) reported that *Neisseria gonorrhoeae* was isolated from the ducts of Bartholin's glands in 28% of a group of women with gonorrhoea, and one-third of these had enlargement and tenderness of the gland; if untreated, this may progress to abscess formation. The most important complication of gonorrhoea in women is acute salpingitis, which develops in 10–15% of those with lower genital tract infections; it has an adverse effect on both health and fertility, and its prevention by the early treatment of women with uncomplicated infection is of the utmost importance.

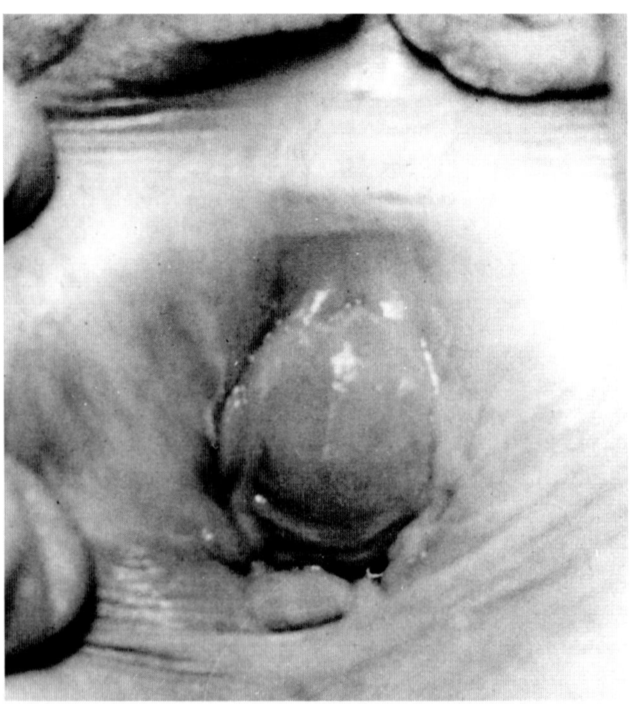

Fig. 4.14 Periurethral abscess, caused by *Neisseria gonorrhoeae*.

Diagnosis

The diagnosis of gonorrhoea in women depends entirely on the results of laboratory tests. Specimens must be taken from all potentially infected sites: the cervix, urethra, anorectum and pharynx. If only one of these is to be sampled, it should be the cervix, but it should be recognized that the urethra, anorectum and pharynx may each be the sole site of infection in 5% of women with gonorrhoea. If indicated, specimens from other sites, such as the ducts of the accessory glands, should be taken. Examination of a high vaginal swab has no place in the laboratory diagnosis of gonorrhoea.

Microscopy of Gram-stained specimens from the genital tract for intracellular Gram-negative diplococci is the first step. Unfortunately, this method is insensitive for specimens from women; it will identify only about 50% of confirmed gonococcal infections in the cervix, urethra and anorectum (Barlow & Phillips 1978), and it is useless for pharyngeal specimens. Culture in the laboratory is essential. Specimens are taken with cotton wool swabs. While direct inoculation of culture plates is preferable, transport media such as Stuart's or Ames' can be used provided they reach the laboratory within 24 hours. Specimens are cultured on selective media, which contain antibiotics to reduce the growth of unwanted organisms, and positive results confirmed by sugar fermentation or immunofluorescence (Stokes & Ridgway 1987). There is at present no serological test of any value for the diagnosis of gonorrhoea.

Treatment

Penicillin was the mainstay of the treatment of gonorrhoea for many years, but there is now evidence of resistance, which has become a serious problem in some parts of the world. In some strains of *Neisseria gonorrhoeae*, chromosomally mediated resistance is so high that penicillin cannot be used for treatment. In 1977 a further problem appeared, because penicillinase-producing strains emerged that were totally resistant to penicillin. These plasmid-mediated strains of *Neisseria gonorrhoeae* (PPNG) have become widely prevalent, particularly in developing countries, where they may comprise >50% of isolates.

In some European countries, including the UK, penicillin derivatives can still be used for the treatment of uncomplicated mucosal gonococcal infections, the recommended schedules being ampicillin or amoxycillin 2.0g with probenecid 1.0g, by mouth as a single dose. In other localities, and for patients unresponsive to penicillin, a single dose of one of the following is advised:

1 ciprofloxacin 500mg by mouth as a single dose;
2 ceftriaxone 250mg i.m. as a single dose;
3 spectinomycin 2.0g i.m. as a single dose.

Associated infections need identification and treatment. Up to one-third of women with gonorrhoea have trichomoniasis, which can be diagnosed and treated without difficulty. Up to 50% of patients have a concomitant cervical infection with *Chlamydia trachomatis*. It is important that this is diagnosed, because it persists after the single-dose treatment of gonorrhoea (Stamm *et al.* 1984) and may cause post-gonococcal salpingitis. Women who are being investigated for possible gonorrhoea should have diagnostic tests for *Chlamydia trachomatis*. If these are not available, it is recommended that after single-dose treatment for gonorrhoea a course of a tetracycline, for example tetracycline 500mg four times a day for 7 days, is given.

After the treatment of gonorrhoea, at least two follow-up examinations, with cultures for *Neisseria gonorrhoeae*, should be performed to confirm cure. The tracing and investigation of sexual contacts is of course mandatory.

Gram-positive bacilli

CORYNEBACTERIA

Erythrasma

This condition is caused by *Corynebacterium minutissimum* or related species (Sarkany *et al.* 1961, Montes & Black 1967). These organisms form part of the normal skin flora, but can cause disease in warm, humid climates or in subjects who are debilitated, for example by diabetes mellitus (Somerville *et al.* 1970).

Erythrasma affects flexural areas such as the axillae, between the toes, the groins and the natal cleft. It is usually symptomless except in the groins, where there may be some itching. Well-defined, brownish, scaly patches appear in the affected areas (Fig. 4.15). The differential diagnosis is from tinea cruris, intertrigo, seborrhoeic dermatitis and flexural psoriasis. Under Wood's light, erythrasma shows a characteristic coral-red fluorescence, caused by the presence of a porphyrin, although this fluorescence is not present in all cases (Mattox *et al.* 1993). It is possible to culture *Corynebacterium minutissimum* in special media from specimens readily obtainable by scraping. The treatment of choice is oral erythromycin 250mg four times a day for 2 weeks. It is effective, but recurrence is common. Clotrimazole cream is useful for long-term local treatment.

Trichomycosis (nodosa)

Trichomycosis is not, despite its name, a fungal disease. It is caused by at least three species of corynebacteria (Freeman

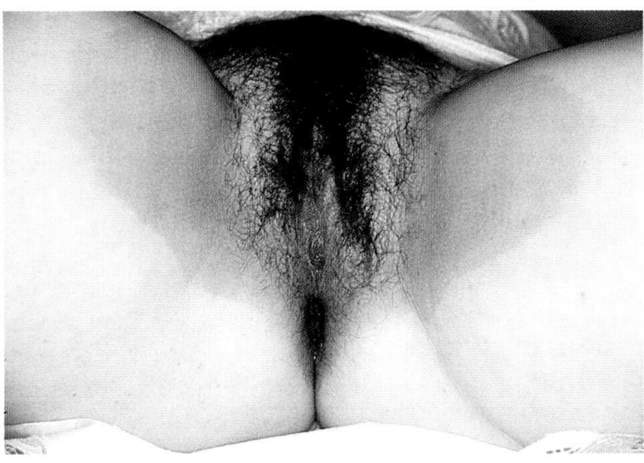

Fig. 4.15 Erythrasma.

et al. 1969). Small nodules of different colours—yellow, red or black (White & Smith 1979)—are firmly attached to the hairs of the axillae or pubic area, and clothing may be stained. The bacteria may inflict some damage to the shafts of the hairs (Orfanos *et al.* 1971), and can elaborate a cement-like substance (Shelley & Miller 1984).

Trichomycosis must be differentiated from piedra, and from the nits of pediculosis pubis. This can be done by microscopy of the affected hairs, or by examination under Wood's light when variably coloured fluorescence may be seen in trichomycosis, or by culture. It is treated by clipping off affected hairs and applying an antibacterial solution.

Cutaneous diphtheria

Diphtheria, caused by *Corynebacterium diphtheriae*, classically presents as a localized inflammation of the throat with a greyish adherent exudate and severe toxaemia. In developed countries it is now a rare disease. Infection of the skin by *Corynebacterium diphtheriae* is common in tropical countries, and can occur elsewhere. It presents with sores and ulcers, often covered by a greyish membrane. These are most common on the legs, but may occur anywhere. Vulval infection has been described, occurring either alone or accompanying respiratory diphtheria. Cases in adults have been reported by Parks (1941) and Machnicki (1953), and in children by Hunt (1954). Toxaemia may be severe. An occasional case of vulvovaginitis in children has been ascribed to *Corynebacterium diphtheriae*, although a true infection must be distinguished from the prodromal vulvovaginitis of many febrile illnesses, including diphtheria.

The rapid diagnosis of diphtheria is all-important, and is made by culture on blood agar and blood tellurite agar. The infection is treated with intramuscular injections of diphtheria antitoxin. *Corynebacterium diphtheriae* is nearly always sensitive to penicillin, so patients should be given a course of the drug, or of erythromycin if they are allergic to it.

Gram-negative bacilli

CHANCROID (*HAEMOPHILUS DUCREYI*)

Chancroid is an acute STD that has become uncommon in the Western world, but in developing countries is a common cause of genital ulceration. The association between genital ulceration and an increased risk of transmission of HIV has made chancroid a particularly important disease.

Aetiology

Haemophilus ducreyi is a small Gram-negative rod, which may show bipolar staining and chain formation—the 'school of fish'. In the past the organism has been difficult to propagate in the laboratory, but much improved media are now available for primary isolation (Hannah & Greenwood 1982, Ronald 1986).

Epidemiology

Chancroid is most common in tropical and subtropical developing countries, but occasional outbreaks occur in Western societies (Hammond *et al.* 1980). It is much commoner in men than in women. This implies that many infected women are not being diagnosed, but whether they have symptomless ulceration or can act as carriers of *Haemophilus ducreyi* is uncertain.

Clinical features

The incubation period is usually 3–10 days. Small, tender papules appear, which soon break down to form ragged, tender, non-indurated ulcers (Fig. 4.16). The lesions may be single, but are more usually multiple. In women, the majority are on the labia, fourchette, perineum and perianal areas, but vaginal and cervical ulcers may occur. Occasionally, secondary infection with fusospirochaetal organisms may lead to a rapidly destructive lesion—phagedena. Inguinal adenitis appears in up to 50% of women with chancroid, which often progresses to form abscesses that rupture spontaneously. Mild constitutional symptoms may occur, but the infection does not disseminate.

Diagnosis

The differential diagnosis is from other causes of the genital ulceration/lymphadenopathy syndrome, in particu-

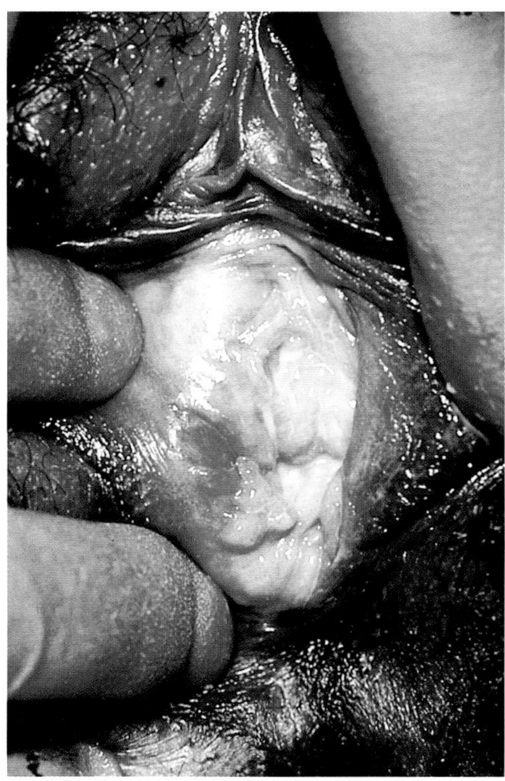

Fig. 4.16 Chancroid.

lar syphilis, genital herpes, lymphogranuloma venereum and donovanosis. The clinical differentiation of these may be difficult, and some patients have genital ulcers of multiple aetiology. Although the appearance of Gram-negative rods in chains may be suggestive of chancroid, the laboratory diagnosis depends on the isolation of *Haemophilus ducreyi* from the ulcers or from bubo pus. No satisfactory serological test is available.

Treatment

The emergence of resistant strains of *Haemophilus ducreyi* has meant that many antimicrobials that were formerly effective for the treatment of chancroid cannot now be used. Trimethoprim/sulphamethoxazole is no longer recommended. At present, the drug of choice is erythromycin; the World Health Organization recommends 500 mg of erythromycin base or stearate three times a day by mouth for 7 days.

DONOVANOSIS (*CALYMMATOBACTERIUM GRANULOMATIS*)

Aetiology

Donovanosis, formerly known as granuloma inguinale, is an STD that causes genital ulceration. The intracellular organisms within the lesions—Donovan bodies—are believed to be its cause. *Calymmatobacterium granulomatis* is a Gram-negative, encapsulated rod, which will not grow on conventional media (Goldberg 1959), although the organisms have been propagated on chick embryo preparations.

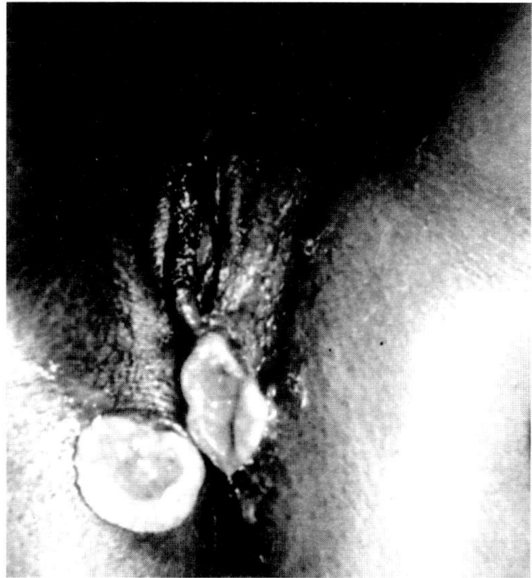

Fig. 4.17 Vulval donovanosis.

Epidemiology

The incidence of donovanosis is now concentrated into only a few tropical regions: New Guinea, India, South Africa and Brazil (Richens 1991). It is associated with poverty, poor hygiene and prostitution, and with other STDs. The disease is only moderately contagious; infection has been detected in 12–52% of regular sexual partners (Hart 1975). It is not known whether a carrier state exists.

Clinical features

The incubation period of donovanosis is uncertain, but may be between 7 and 30 days (Lal & Nicholas 1970). In women, the labia, fourchette and perivulval area are most commonly affected. The initial lesions are papular or nodular, and the overlying skin breaks down to form deep, red, soft ulcers with granulation tissue at their base. These progressively spread to involve a large area, including the perineum and anus (Fig. 4.17). They are relatively painless unless secondarily infected. Regional lymphadenitis does not occur, although granulomatous lesions may develop in the inguinal area. Vulval granulation tissue may extend into the vagina and affect the cervix, and primary infection of the cervix may also occur. Haematogenous spread of the infection is unusual but may happen, particularly in women (Brigden & Guard 1980). The manifestations of donovanosis may progress rapidly during pregnancy. In long-standing infections lymphoedema and vulval or anal stenosis may develop.

Diagnosis

The differential diagnosis is from other causes of vulval ulceration, notably syphilis and chancroid. Other infections, including HIV, are not uncommon in women with donovanosis, and screening for these is important. The laboratory diagnosis depends on the demonstration of Donovan bodies in tissue smears; the best specimens are biopsy or curettings of the ulcer base, stained with Leishman or Giemsa stain (Plummer *et al.* 1984). Histological examination is valuable for both diagnosis and the exclusion of malignancy (Sowmini 1983); haematoxylin and eosin do not stain Donovan bodies well.

Treatment

The treatment of choice is tetracycline 500 mg orally four times a day, or erythromycin base or stearate 500 mg orally four times a day, for 2–3 weeks. Sexual partners should be examined, and treated if necessary.

Mycobacteria

TUBERCULOSIS (*MYCOBACTERIUM TUBERCULOSIS*)

Epidemiology

Although the lung is the most common site of tuberculosis, other sites may be infected, either directly or by spread from distant areas. Tuberculosis of the female genital tract is not uncommon, particularly in developing countries. In comparison with infection of the upper genital tract, vulval tuberculosis is rare (Moore 1954). It may occur:

1 as a primary exogenous infection through contact with sputum or secretions from a sex partner with pulmonary or urogenital tuberculosis (Bjornstad 1947);
2 by distal spread from the upper genital tract; or
3 by haematogenous spread from tuberculosis elsewhere.

An association between tuberculosis and HIV infection is well known, and genitourinary tuberculosis is more common in HIV-positive patients.

Clinical features

In a true primary tuberculosis complex the initial lesion is an inconspicuous brown-red papule, but this may be missed so that the clinical picture is dominated by inguinal or femoral adenitis. The primary tuberculous lesion usually heals after a few months, but the enlarged glands may persist and break down.

In other forms of vulval tuberculosis, cutaneous and/or mucosal lesions appear either as nodules which break down to form ulcers with soft, ragged edges, or as indurated fungating masses. In the chronic stage, fibrosis leads to scarring and sinus formation. Involvement of regional lymph nodes may lead to caseation and scarring, or to vulval lymphoedema (Ashworth 1974). Infection of Bartholin's glands, usually unilateral, presents as a painless, hard vulval swelling, or as a cold abscess (Schaefer 1959).

Diagnosis

Tuberculous lesions of the vulva must be distinguished from lymphogranuloma venereum, donovanosis, hydradenitis and carcinoma. Histology of biopsy material may show tubercles and caseation, and tubercle bacilli may be demonstrated by microscopy of pus or tissue sections stained by a Ziehl–Nielsen technique. Suspected tuberculous material may be cultured for *Mycobacterium tuberculosis*, with care to differentiate the organism from opportunist mycobacteria.

Treatment

This follows the general principles of antituberculous chemotherapy.

LEPROSY (*MYCOBACTERIUM LEPRAE*)

Various forms are described, the spectrum depending on the host's ability to develop specific cell-mediated immunity. Cutaneous lesions range between lepromatous and tuberculoid types (Jopling & Harman 1986). The female genital tract may be infected by *Mycobacterium leprae* by haematogenous spread; the ovaries, cervix, uterus and Fallopian tubes may be affected (Bonar & Rabson 1957). Direct infection of the vulva can also occur (Grabstold & Swan 1952).

Actinomycosis

Actinomycosis is an uncommon granulomatous disease. *Actinomyces israelii* and *Actinomyces gerencseriae* are the most frequent causal agents. The organisms are Gram-positive branching bacilli with a tendency to form fungus-like colonies in tissue; they are anaerobic or microaerophilic. They are regularly found in the mouths of healthy adults, and sporadically in the gastrointestinal and genital tracts. Colonization of intrauterine contraceptive devices within the cervical canal is not uncommon, but is usually symptomless. The factors that determine the onset of active disease are largely unknown. In the tissues the organisms cause a chronic granulomatous infection characterized by the formation of abscesses, which drain to the surface through sinuses.

Genital tract infection is rare. It usually arises from the extension of bowel disease (Wagman 1975). Cases of an invasive actinomycotic infection associated with intrauterine contraceptive devices have been described, involving the cervix, uterus and adnexa (Lomax *et al.* 1976, Purdie *et al.* 1977); many years ago three cases of actinomycosis affecting the vulva alone were described by Daniel and Mavrodin (1954). Penicillin is the agent of choice for the treatment of actinomycosis, but prolonged high dosage may be required.

Spirochaetes

SYPHILIS (*TREPONEMA PALLIDUM*)

The introduction of antibiotics 50 years ago had a profound effect on this old disease. Early infections were readily curable, and late syphilis became rare. The incidence of syphilis, at least in Western societies, declined steeply. Within the last few years this picture has changed. In the USA, for example, the number of new cases is rising in both men and women, fuelled by socioeconomic deprivation and drug addiction, and congenital syphilis has reappeared (Drusin 1996). In developing countries syphilis has always been a problem, but in some parts of the world, particularly Africa and the Far East, it is escalating. In all areas, the association between syphilis and HIV infection is causing serious problems.

Aetiology

The pathogenic species are *Treponema pallidum* (which causes venereal and endemic syphilis), *Treponema pertenue* (causing yaws) and *Treponema carateum* (causing pinta). These organisms are morphologically and serologically indistinguishable, and have not yet been propagated *in vitro*. There are many non-pathogenic treponemes.

Treponema pallidum is 6–15 μm long and less than 0.25 μm wide. It is too narrow and has too little protoplasm to be easily visible by light microscopy (although Schaudinn and Hoffmann, its discoverers, did so). Dark-field microscopy reveals it as a slender, spiral organism, which undergoes characteristic movements: rotation, angulations, and coil compression and expansion. The organism multiplies by binary fission (Turner & Hollander 1957).

Epidemiology

Syphilis is an STD, and as such is inexorably linked to human behaviour. In Western industrialized countries its incidence reached a peak during and after the Second World War, and subsequently showed a marked fall; this was probably due partly to more settled conditions, but mostly to the use of antibiotics. During the 1970s and 1980s the number of cases of early syphilis in men increased, largely because of more widespread homosexual practices. In Europe, the incidence in women remained low. In the USA, however, although the number of cases in homosexual men declined, it rose in heterosexual men and in women. This was related to promiscuous sexual intercourse among underprivileged subjects living in major conurbations, many of whom were drug abusers (Drusin 1996). In developing countries, prostitution also made a major contribution to the spread of syphilis.

Pathology

Treponema pallidum probably gains entry to the tissues through small abrasions produced during intercourse. The organisms multiply locally, and at the same time some reach the regional lymph nodes. Polymorphonuclear leucocytes are attracted to the area, and these are followed by lymphocytes and macrophages (Lukehart *et al.* 1980). Proliferation of blood vessels and endarteritis occur, and the whole complex now forms a primary chancre. Ulceration of its surface is due to perivascular infiltration and endarteritis. Similar changes cause enlargement of the regional lymph nodes.

Circulating antibodies appear early. Lipoidal antigens (reagin) are present in syphilis and some other diseases and can be measured by flocculation tests such as Venereal Disease Research Laboratory (VDRL) and rapid plasma reagin (RPR) tests. These tests are negative during the incubation period of syphilis, but usually become positive with, or shortly after, the appearance of the chancre. Specific treponemal antibodies can be detected by the fluorescent treponemal antibody (absorbed) (FTA-ABS) test and by the *Treponema pallidum* haemagglutination assay (TPHA) test. The FTA-ABS test is the first to become reactive, and is positive in most cases of primary syphilis. The TPHA test is slower to respond, but is positive by the end of the primary stage in most patients.

In primary syphilis, the operation of cell-mediated and humoral immunity leads to the slow resolution of the primary chancre and the enlarged regional glands. The immune response is incomplete because, although the local disease is contained, treponemes have reached the bloodstream and are disseminated to other organs and tissues. Between 4 and 6 weeks after the primary chancre has appeared, this treponemal septicaemia is expressed clinically as secondary syphilis, during which all serological tests are strongly positive. This persists, with exacerbations and remissions, for up to 9–12 months, after which all clinical signs of the infection have disappeared. But again, although the infection has been contained, it has not been eradicated, and true immunity has not developed. A period of latency now follows, of variable duration. Incomplete suppression of the infection may lead to a partial return of the lesions of secondary, or even primary, syphilis but eventually all physical signs die away, although the serology remains positive.

Less than a third of patients with untreated early syphilis progress to late syphilis; in the remainder, latency is prolonged for life. Tertiary syphilis presents 3–20 years after the original infection, as gummas, cardiovascular syphilis and neurosyphilis. A gumma is a granuloma showing infiltration with lymphocytes and mononuclear cells and endarteritis. They are very rare today. Patients with late syphilis usually have reactive lipoidal antigen tests, and the specific tests are invariably positive (King *et al.* 1980).

If a woman suffering from primary, secondary or early latent syphilis becomes pregnant, the fetus is almost sure to become infected unless the mother receives adequate treatment. The later in pregnancy the mother becomes infected, the more severe will be the neonatal disease. Because of a decline in adult syphilis, and routine serological tests during pregnancy, congenital syphilis in the Western world had almost disappeared by the 1970s. Recently, the incidence of congenital syphilis has begun to rise again in some localities, and it has always been a serious problem in developing countries.

Vulval lesions in early syphilis. The incubation period of syphilis is 10–90 days, commonly about 2 weeks, and the untreated primary stage lasts for 3–8 weeks. The first lesion is a macule, which soon becomes papular, then ulcerates to form a primary chancre. A classical (Hunterian) chancre is an indurated, painless ulcer with a dull red base. In the majority of cases the regional lymph nodes enlarge within a week of the appearance of the chancre; they are usually painless, firm and smooth.

The clinical signs of syphilis have always been variable, and there is some evidence that these are becoming milder. It has been suggested that the 'classical' chancre may now be unusual (Chapel 1978). Multiple chancres are common, they may be tender because of secondary infection, and in some series only a minority of women with primary syphilis show regional lymph node enlargement (Duncan *et al.* 1984). In developing countries the difficulty of diagnosing primary syphilis is compounded by multiple infections, particularly of syphilis and chancroid.

In a classical study Fournier (1906) reported that 46% of chancres were on the labia majora, 22% on the labia minora and 5% on the cervix. Davies (1931) believed that most chancres were on the cervix, but recent experience is that the vulva is much more commonly affected (King *et al.* 1980, Duncan *et al.* 1984) (Figs 4.18 & 4.19). Vulval lesions can cause marked labial oedema. Enlargement of the inguinal or femoral lymph nodes may be unilateral or bilateral; overlying erythema occurs only if the glands are secondarily infected.

The commonest effects of secondary syphilis are constitutional symptoms such as malaise and fever, lesions of skin and mucous membranes, and generalized lymphadenopathy. The vulva is affected by skin eruptions and mucous patches. The skin rashes of secondary syphilis may be macular, papular, papulosquamous or pustular, and any of these may occur on the vulva. At times, they can resemble many dermatoses, but itching is minimal. Condylomata lata are a variant of papular syphilides. They develop at the periphery of the vulva and around the anus, and are confluent, soft, spongy masses with flat tops and broad bases; they may become eroded, and exude highly infectious serum (Fig. 4.20). Mucous patches usually appear at the same time as maculopapular skin lesions; they are painless, round, greyish-white eroded areas, affecting the labia minora.

Vulval lesions in late syphilis. These are now very rare. Gummas affecting the skin of the vulva appear as squamous lesions or subcutaneous nodules, which sometimes ulcerate.

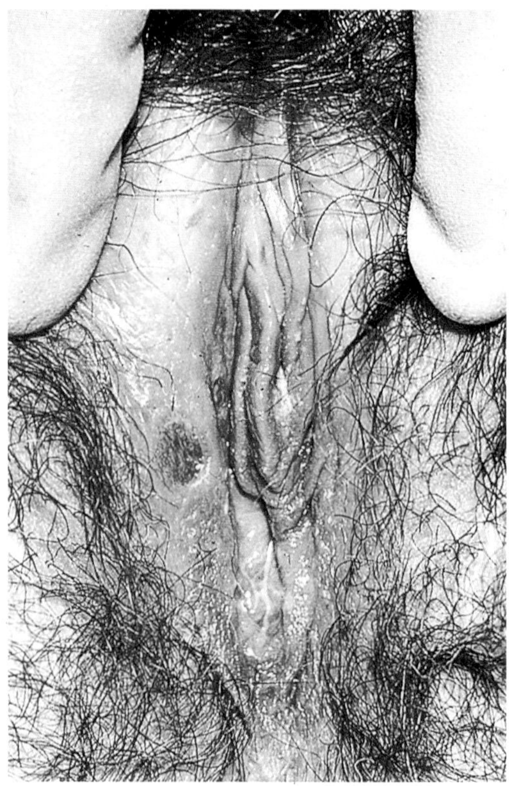

Fig. 4.18 Primary chancre of labium majus.

Cases were described by Matras (1935) and Konrad (1936).

Diagnosis

Primary chancres in women need to be differentiated from other types of vulval ulceration, including genital herpes, pyogenic lesions, infected injuries and, in developing countries, chancroid, lymphogranuloma venereum and donovanosis. Rarer causes of genital ulcers include fixed drug eruptions, Behçet's disease and squamous-cell carcinoma. Clinical impressions of the cause of vulval ulcers are often inaccurate, and laboratory investigation is always necessary. Herpetic lesions are initially vesicular and are painful but not indurated. The ulcers of chancroid are painful, vascular and not indurated; if the regional lymph nodes are infected there is overlying erythema, and suppuration is common. Ulcers in lymphogranuloma venereum are small and inconspicuous, while adenopathy is marked. It must be remembered that vulval ulcers may have multiple causation, particularly in developing countries.

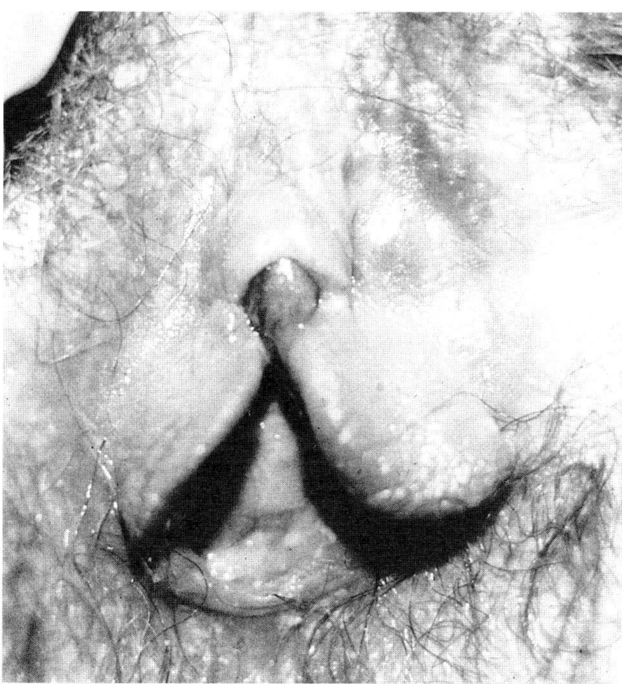

Fig. 4.19 Primary chancre of clitoris.

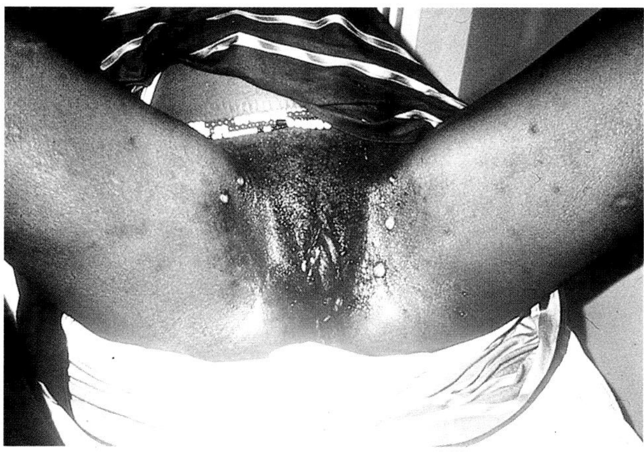

Fig. 4.20 Secondary syphilis: condylomata lata.

The vulval lesions of secondary syphilis may resemble many dermatoses, although other signs of syphilis are likely to be present. The macular rash may be mistaken for seborrhoeic dermatitis, drug eruptions and exanthemata, and the papular rash may resemble papular urticaria, pityriasis rosea or lichen planus. Condylomata lata may be confused with condylomata acuminata, and mucous patches with genital herpes, fixed drug eruptions and Behçet's syndrome.

The laboratory diagnosis of early syphilis depends on dark-field examination for *Treponema pallidum* and serological tests. Dark-field microscopy is a valuable, highly specific technique, which can be used when there are ulcers or papular lesions of the skin or mucous membranes. The area to be examined is first cleaned with normal saline. If the lesion is moist, enough serum for examination may be obtained by squeezing. If it is dry, it must be scarified at its edge so that it bleeds; after the clot has retracted, a specimen of serum is obtained. Specimens are examined at a magnification of ×400 or ×900 to detect motile treponemes. If no organisms are seen on examination of a suspicious lesion, the examination should be repeated daily for 3 days. If the suspect chancre is healing, or has been treated with local antiseptics, it may be possible to aspirate fluid from enlarged regional lymph nodes for dark-field microscopy.

Serological tests for syphilis should always be performed. The VDRL and RPR tests are positive in 50–70% of patients with primary syphilis (Wende *et al.* 1971), and is invariably positive at high titre in secondary syphilis. After this the titre slowly declines, but is unlikely to become negative for many years. A fall in titre occurs after the successful treatment of early syphilis; most patients have negative cardiolipin tests 1 year after treatment of primary syphilis, and 2 years after treatment of secondary syphilis (Fiumara 1980). The FTA-ABS is reactive in 70–90% of patients with primary syphilis (Fiumara 1980). The FTA-ABS is reactive in 70–90% of patients with primary syphilis (Duncan *et al.* 1974), and the TPHA test in 64–87% (Lesinski *et al.* 1974). Both these tests are positive in virtually all cases of secondary syphilis, and thereafter remain positive indefinitely.

Treatment

Penicillin has been the treatment of choice for syphilis for half a century, and there is no evidence that *Treponema pallidum* has become resistant to it. There are several recommended treatment schedules. For early syphilis (primary, secondary and latency present for less than 1 year) the following are recommended (World Health Organization 1993):

1 procaine penicillin 1200 units i.m. daily for 10 days;
2 benzathine penicillin G 2.4 million units as a single intramuscular injection.

Patients who are allergic to penicillin should receive tetracycline 500 mg by mouth four times a day for 15 days; if pregnant, they should receive erythromycin 500 mg by mouth four times a day for 15 days.

The prognosis for patients treated for early syphilis with adequate penicillin dosage is very good (Goldmeier & Hay 1993). Experience of treatment with non-penicillin regimens is limited, and post-treatment surveillance of patients treated in this way must be careful. All patients treated for early syphilis should be assessed clinically and serologically at the end of treatment, then monthly for 3 months, then 3-monthly for at least a year. Early syphilis rapidly becomes non-infectious with antimicrobial therapy, and intercourse may safely be resumed on the completion of treatment. It is clearly important to locate, examine and if necessary treat the sexual partners of women with early syphilis.

Syphilis and human immunodeficiency virus infection

Syphilis and HIV infection are closely linked by sexual behaviour, and indeed may be acquired together (Minkoff *et al.* 1990). Furthermore, it is now established that diseases such as syphilis that cause genital ulceration increase the liability to HIV infection.

Genital mycoplasmas

Three *Mycoplasma* species are thought to cause disease of the human genital tract: *Mycoplasma hominis*, *Ureaplasma urealyticum* and *Mycoplasma genitalium*. Although the first isolation of *Mycoplasma hominis* was from an abscess of Bartholin's gland (Dienes & Edsall 1937), subsequent studies have produced no evidence that the organism is a major cause of this disease (Lee *et al.* 1977). Women with bacterial vaginosis (see p. 95) often have positive cultures for *Mycoplasma hominis*, but its role in the disease is uncertain. The organism and probably *Mycoplasma genitalium* appear to be implicated in pelvic inflammatory disease and in post-partum and post-abortion fever (Glatt *et al.* 1990, Taylor-Robinson 1995).

Ureaplasma urealyticum causes some cases of non-gonococcal urethritis in men, but is not known to cause any disease of the lower urogenital tract in women. Like *Mycoplasma hominis*, it is recovered from the normal vagina, this colonization being related to sexual activity. *Ureaplasma urealyticum* is present in 75%, and *Mycoplasma hominis* in 20% of women who have had several sex partners (McCormack *et al.* 1972).

Chlamydia trachomatis

Chlamydia trachomatis is a Gram-negative intracellular bacterium with a unique life cycle. The infecting particle is the elementary body (EB), which after entry into a susceptible cell undergoes a series of replicative changes culminating in the formation of a cytoplasmic inclusion. This ruptures and releases further EBs, which infect other cells. The following serovars of *Chlamydia trachomatis* have been identified (Grayston & Wang 1975), associated with different diseases: A–C cause trachoma, D–K a group of oculogenital infections, including non-gonococcal urethritis and related disorders in both sexes, and L1–3 cause lymphogranuloma venereum (LGV).

OCULOGENITAL INFECTIONS

Epidemiology

Serovars D–K are sexually transmissible. In up to 50% of cases of non-gonococcal urethritis, chlamydiae can be detected, and about two-thirds of female sex partners of men with chlamydial infection become infected themselves. The risk of infection from a single sexual contact is unknown. In many countries, particularly in the West, chlamydial infection is the commonest STD.

Clinical features

In women, the major target for infection is the columnar epithelium of the endocervix. Infection of the urethra is not uncommon (Paavonen 1979); it can occur alone, but usually there is a concomitant infection of the cervix. Chlamydiae do not infect the vagina. Canalicular spread from the cervix leads to endometritis, salpingitis and perihepatitis; and exposure of infants during delivery may lead to neonatal conjunctivitis and respiratory infection (Taylor-Robinson 1991).

Chlamydial infection of the lower genital tract in women is often symptomless, although mucopurulent cervicitis may cause vaginal discharge. The impact of *Chlamydia trachomatis* on the vulva is slight. Infection may cause urethritis, but this is almost always asymptomatic, and the dysuria and frequency of micturition of the urethral syndrome is not usually associated with chlamydial infection (Feldman *et al.* 1986). Although the organisms have been recovered from the ducts of Bartholin's glands, most of the reported cases also had gonococcal infections (Davies *et al.* 1978), and it is not thought that chlamydiae alone cause infection of Bartholin's glands.

Diagnosis

Specimens are collected from the urethra and cervix with cotton wool-tipped swabs. Cell culture is the standard diagnostic procedure. The specimens are centrifuged on to a cell monolayer, and after incubation chlamydial inclusions are identified by staining with iodine or Giemsa (Fig. 4.21). This method is technically demanding, and in most laboratories antigen detection based on either immunofluorescence or enzyme-linked immunosorbent assay (ELISA) are preferred; recently DNA amplification tests such as polymerase chain reaction (PCR) and ligase chain reaction have appeared to be both sensitive and specific (Thomas *et al.* 1993). Neither serological tests nor Papanicolaou-stained cervical smears are of value in clinical diagnosis.

Treatment

The tetracyclines are widely used for the treatment of genital infection by *Chlamydia trachomatis*. With a course of tetracycline hydrochloride 500 mg four times a day for 7 days, or doxycycline 100 mg twice daily for 7 days, a cure rate of over 90% may be expected. Women who cannot take tetracyclines because of pregnancy, lactation or intolerance to the drugs may be treated with erythromycin base or stearate 500 mg four times a day for 7 days. Recently the azalide macrolide, azithromycin, which shows good *in vitro* activity against *Chlamydia trachomatis*, has been shown to be successful against genital infection by the organism. A single dose of azithromycin 1 g eradicates chlamydiae from virtually 100% of cases of chlamydial urethritis and cervicitis (Ridgway 1996). Its single dosage is a major advantage. The tracing and treatment of contacts of patients with chlamydial genital infection is of particular importance, because they are often symptomless.

LYMPHOGRANULOMA VENEREUM

The serovars 1–3 of *Chlamydia trachomatis* are more invasive than the oculogenital strains and, unlike them, cause disease in lymphatic tissue. The highest prevalence of LGV is in tropical and subtropical regions such as sub-Saharan Africa, South-East Asia and South America, but it has also occurred in small outbreaks in temperate regions. LGV is reported more often in men than in women, who are less likely to be diagnosed before the onset of late complications (Schachter & Dawson 1978).

Clinical features

The incubation period of LGV is between 3 days and 3 weeks. The primary lesion is a small, painless papule, vesicle or ulcer, which rapidly heals. In women, this lesion is

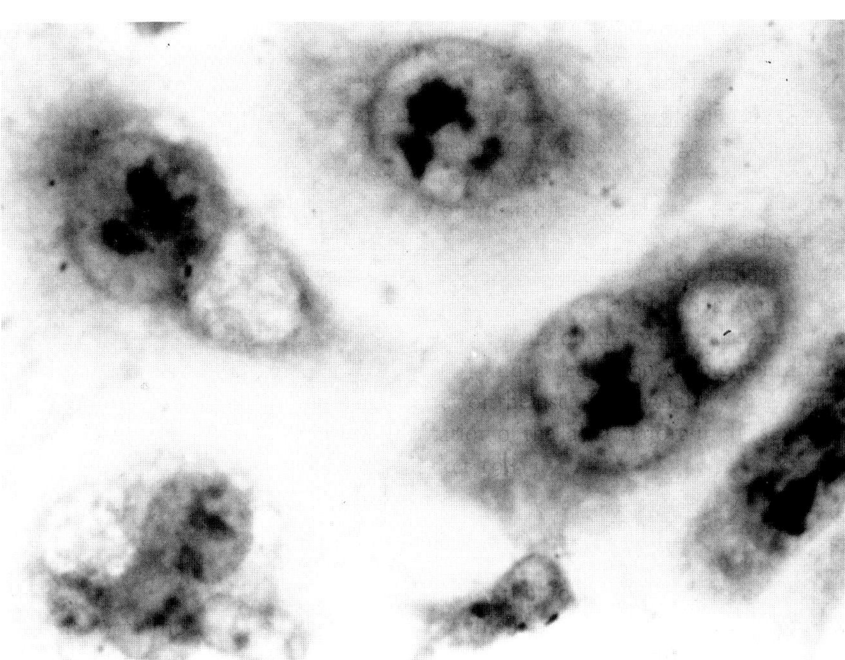

Fig. 4.21 Cell monolayer, showing *Chlamydia trachomatis* inclusions.

commonest on the fourchette (Greenblatt *et al.* 1959), but it may also occur on the labia or cervix, or escape notice altogether. The secondary stage of LGV comprises an 'inguinal' and 'anorectal' syndrome. Lymphadenopathy, a characteristic feature of LGV, develops several weeks later. In women with primary vulval lesions the inguinal glands are affected (Fig. 4.22); they enlarge to form a painful mass, which in most cases suppurates and forms sinuses. Healing is slow, with extensive scarring, and in some patients this persists for months or years. The external and internal iliac lymph nodes may become affected if the primary lesion is on the cervix. In these cases there may be fever and malaise, and a tender adnexal mass palpable on bimanual examination (Perine *et al.* 1980).

The anorectal syndrome is due to extension of the infection to rectal and perirectal lymphatics. It begins with acute proctocolitis, with the passage of blood, mucus and pus. The rectal mucosa is friable and eroded, and perirectal abscesses and anal fissures or fistulae may form (Fig. 4.23). Later, perirectal fibrosis may lead to the formation of a rectal stricture. The late stages of LGV are rarely seen nowadays. Vulval elephantiasis is attributed to chronic active infection combined with lymphatic obstruction. Esthiomene is due to persistent oedema combined with sclerosis and ulceration; there may be much tissue loss (Fig. 4.24).

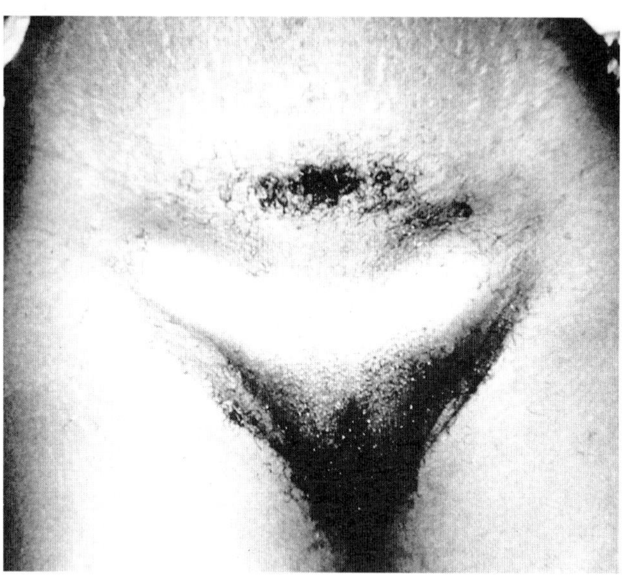

Fig. 4.22 Lymphogranuloma venereum: inguinal adenitis.

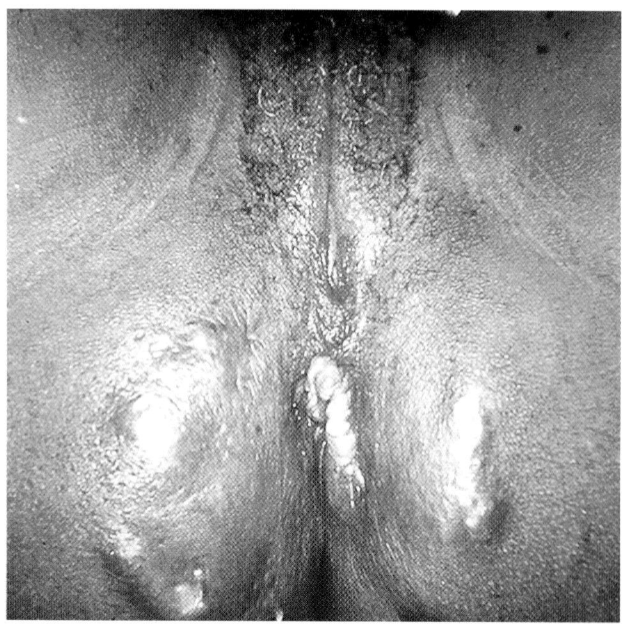

Fig. 4.23 Lymphogranuloma venereum: perianal sinuses.

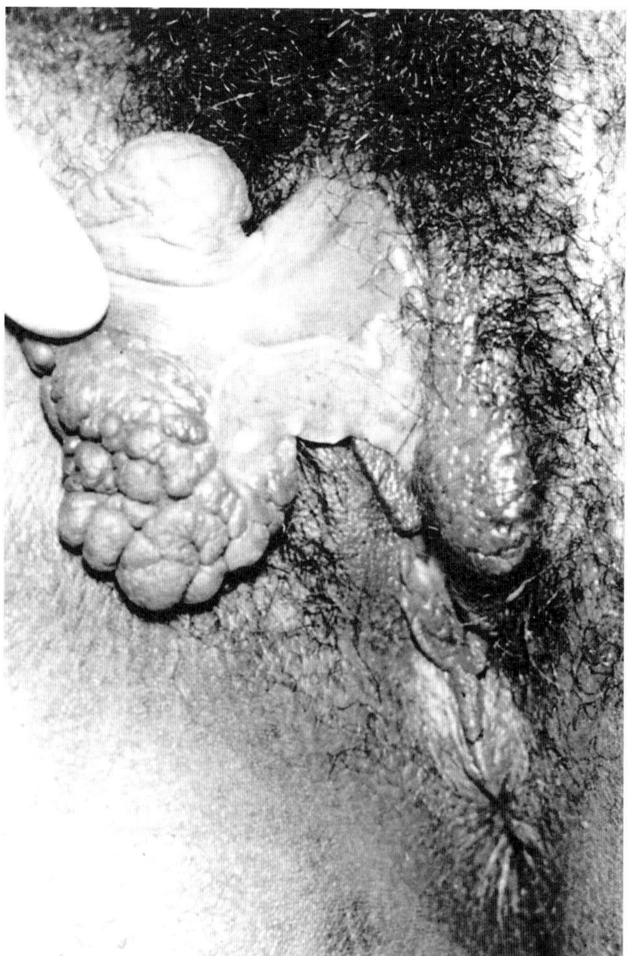

Fig. 4.24 Lymphogranuloma venereum: vulval elephantiasis with esthiomene.

Diagnosis

LGV must be differentiated from other causes of genital ulceration and lymphadenopathy, particularly syphilis, and from cat-scratch disease, filariasis and lymphoma. The best diagnostic laboratory test is cell culture for *Chlamydia trachomatis*; specimens from any site may be examined, but aspirated pus is the best material. The LGV complement fixation test is widely used. It is usually impracticable to wait for rising titres of antibodies and if the clinical signs of LGV are present a titre of > 64 is regarded as confirmatory (Schachter & Dawson 1978). The Frei skin test is now obsolete.

Treatment

Early LGV responds well to tetracyclines, although prolonged treatment may be necessary. Tetracycline hydrochloride 2 g daily in divided doses for 2–3 weeks is a common regimen; it may need to be prolonged if the response is slow. Erythromycin 2 g daily or a sulphonamide such as sulphadiazine 4 g daily are possible alternatives. Surgical treatment should not be undertaken before adequate antimicrobial therapy. Aspiration of a fluctuant bubo may prevent sinus formation; elephantiasis, esthiomene and rectal stricture may require surgical treatment.

Mixed infections

Bacterial vaginosis

Aetiology

Bacterial vaginosis (formerly called non-specific vaginitis) is one of the commonest causes of abnormal vaginal discharge (Blackwell *et al.* 1983). It is due not to a single organism but to a complex disturbance of the entire vaginal flora, with loss of the normal lactobacilli and an overgrowth of *Mycoplasma hominis*, *Gardnerella vaginalis* and various anaerobes. These anaerobes include *Bacteroides* and *Peptococcus* species and a curved, motile rod now named *Mobiluncus* (Hillier *et al.* 1991). The discharge contains some polymorphonuclear leucocytes, but the characteristic cells are squamous epithelial, plastered with adherent bacteria (clue cells). The cause of bacterial vaginosis is unknown. It is most often seen in sexually active women, but there is no evidence that it is sexually transmitted.

Clinical features and diagnosis

Women usually complain of a vaginal discharge that smells unpleasant, and sometimes of mild vulval and vaginal irritation, but some are symptomless (Amsel *et al.* 1983). Vulvitis is absent, but there is a homogeneous vaginal discharge. The vaginal pH is >4.5. A fishy amine odour can be smelt when the secretions are mixed with a drop of 10% potassium hydroxide on a slide. A wet mount shows numerous bacteria and clue cells, and motile *Mobiluncus* species may also be seen. Culture of vaginal specimens is not necessary for the diagnosis (Easmon 1986).

There has been some evidence of pelvic complications of bacterial vaginosis—post-abortion and post-partum endometritis, infection of the vaginal cuff following hysterectomy and pelvic inflammatory disease (Soper *et al.* 1990, Larson *et al.* 1992). This appears to justify prophylactic treatment of women found to have bacterial vaginosis before gynaecological surgery. There is some evidence linking bacterial vaginosis with complications of pregnancy such as amniotic fluid infection. Metronidazole treatment is safe after the first trimester, but high dosage should be avoided.

Treatment

The nitroimidazoles are effective for the treatment of bacterial vaginosis (Pheifer *et al.* 1978). Metronidazole 200 mg three times a day for 7 days is usually curative. Clindamycin is also effective, and can be used topically; a course of 2% clindamycin cream applied daily for 3 days has been shown to give good results (Ahmed-Jushuf *et al.* 1995). Recurrences after treatment are common.

Erosive vulvitis

This is loosely related to acute ulcerative tonsillitis (Vincent's angina) and erosive balanitis. All are inflammatory conditions, associated with a coarse spirochaete (*Borrelia vincenti*) and a fusiform organism now classified as *Leptotrichia*, both of which are strict anaerobes.

Erosive balanitis is quite common; multiple irregular erosions occur as a complication of other infections or as a result of poor subpreputial hygiene. Erosive vulvitis is rarer, but has comparable predisposing causes. It is treated by frequent bathing with normal saline, combined with a course of metronidazole 200 mg three times a day for 7 days. Predisposing causes should be corrected. Non-infective erosive vulvitis may be seen in various dermatological conditions.

Synergistic (synergic) gangrene

This is a rapidly spreading gangrene of the abdominal wall with widespread destruction of skin and subcutaneous tissue, first described by Meleny *et al.* (1945). 'Necrotizing fasciitis' is probably a synonym for the same condition

(Stone & Martin 1972). The initiating lesion may be an operation or trivial injury. The causal organisms are various combinations of strict anaerobes, including *Bacteroides* species (Rea & Wyrick 1970); the source of these is usually the gastrointestinal tract. Factors that predispose to the disease, or worsen the prognosis, are diabetes mellitus, corticosteroid therapy, debilitating diseases and irradiation for malignancy.

The earliest sign is an erythematous or violaceous discoloration of the skin, with subcutaneous induration and oedema, and marked tenderness. Later, bullae and subcutaneous necrosis develop, and gas formation may be detected clinically or radiologically (Fisher *et al.* 1979). Toxaemia is profound, and the prognosis is poor, particularly if treatment is delayed. The vulva is a site of election. Cases have been described by Borkawf (1973), Hammar and Wanger (1977), Shy and Eschenbach (1981), Meltzer (1983) and Addison *et al.* (1984). The cases described by Ewing *et al.* (1979), where three of four patients who developed oedema post-partum died, may fall into this group. Roberts and Hester (1972) described four patients with synergistic bacterial gangrene that originated in abscesses of the vulva or Bartholin's glands; all were diabetic, and three of them died.

Successful treatment requires early diagnosis and wide debridement of infected tissue combined with antianaerobic chemotherapy. It is important to distinguish these conditions from pyoderma gangrenosum (Hutchinson *et al.* 1976), the treatment of which is radically different from that of synergistic bacterial gangrene.

Hidradenitis

See Chapter 5.

Infection with viruses

Genital papillomavirus infection

Virology

Papillomaviruses are unenveloped, icosahedral particles 50–55 nm in diameter (Fig. 4.25). The structural proteins are arranged as 72 subunits, and the capsid contains a double-stranded genome. It has not been possible to replicate papillomaviruses in tissue culture, so they could not be classified by conventional methods, but during the 1970s DNA hybridization techniques enabled the comparison of strains of virus extracted from different lesions. It was decided empirically that if a human papillomavirus (HPV) showed less than 50% homology with any virus already isolated it would be assigned to a new type. So far, more than 70 types of HPV have been identified (Cossart *et al.* 1995).

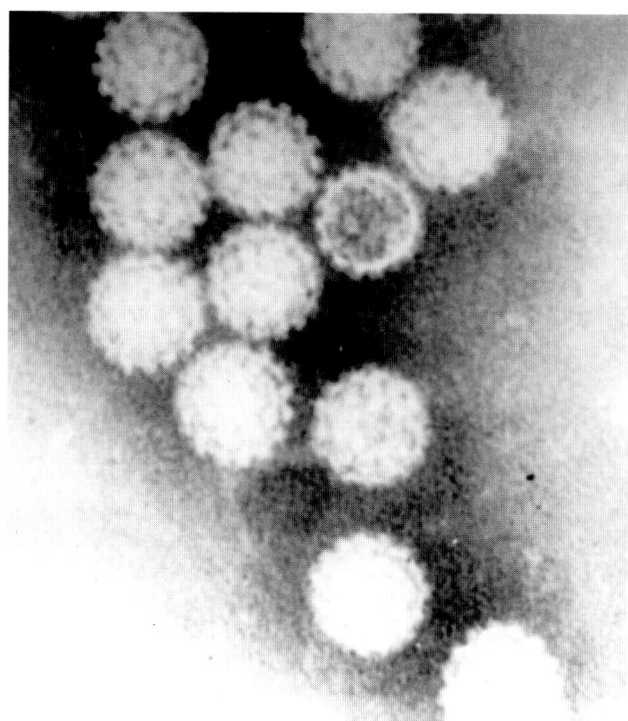

Fig. 4.25 Human papillomavirus particles.

About one-third of these are associated with lesions of the genital tract, falling into two broad groups. HPV types 6 and 11 are associated with lesions of low malignant potential: genital and perianal warts, laryngeal papillomas of children and some cases of the lower grades of cervical intraepithelial neoplasia (CIN). On the other hand, HPV types 16 and 18 are characteristically associated with carcinoma-*in-situ*, the higher grades of CIN and squamous cell cancer of the cervix, vulva, penis and anus. Types 31, 33 and 35 are classed as 'intermediate'. Sequences of HPV DNA can quite often be found in normal epithelia.

Factors in transformation. The progression of benign viral papillomas to malignancy depends not only on the HPV type present but on the operation of cofactors. There are many examples of this process in animal and human tumours. In cattle, bovine papillomavirus type 4 causes benign oesophageal and intestinal papillomas, which become malignant if the animal is fed on bracken rather than grass (Jarrett *et al.* 1978). In humans, epidermodysplasia verruciformis is characterized by widespread benign plane warts. One-third of the patients develop skin cancers, notably those whose lesions contained sequences of HPV 5 and have been exposed to sunlight (Jablonska & Orth 1983). In the case of human genital cancers, the cofactors may include the presence of other STDs such as herpes simplex infections, smoking and oral contraception (zur

Hausen 1992). Double infections with HPV types of low and high malignant potential are not uncommon, but their significance is not clear; whether it is possible for a single cell to be infected by two viruses at the same time is unknown.

Pathology

Histology. The cell most characteristic of HPV infection is the koilocyte. This is a vacuolated squamous epithelial cell, whose nucleus is basophilic and pyknotic; binucleate cells are common. Electron microscopy shows that these nuclei are the site of mature virus formation. Koilocytes were first defined on Papanicolaou-stained cervical smears by Meisels *et al.* (1977), but are present in HPV-associated lesions in all parts of the genital tract. Dyskeratosis, characterized by sheets of cells with orangophilic cytoplasm due to abnormal keratin formation, is often present in HPV infection, although it is not pathognomonic.

There are two kinds of lesion caused by HPV infection. The first is the wart. Its histological features are well known (Lever & Schaumberg-Lever 1975). The dermal papillae are elongated. The basal cell layer is intact, and the prickle-cell layer hyperplastic (acanthosis). The granular cell layer is often well developed, and contains koilocytes. The stratum corneum is of variable thickness, depending on the site of the wart (Fig. 4.26). Four clinical types of wart are described: common warts (verrucae vulgaris), plane warts, plantar warts and condylomata acuminata. In the last, acanthosis is marked, constituting most of the lesion, and the stratum corneum is poorly developed, often consisting of a few layers of parakeratotic cells. There is a correlation between the type of wart and the infecting virus. Thus, common warts contain HPV 1, 2 or 4, plane warts contain HPV 1, and genital warts usually contain HPV 6 or 11.

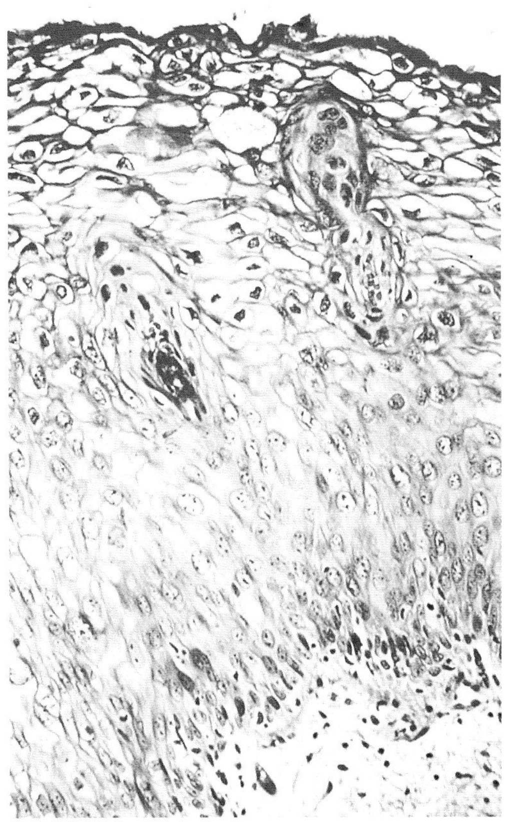

Fig. 4.26 Vulval wart histology, showing acanthosis and superficial vacuolated cells.

The second histological reaction to HPV infection is a lesion designated flat condyloma, or subclinical HPV infection. It is best defined on the cervix (Fig. 4.27), where it can be seen by colposcopy as a variable-sized area of flat, shiny-white epithelium, often with a raised and roughened surface (Reid *et al.* 1980). These lesions can be identified in other genital areas, including the vulva, after pretreatment with dilute acetic acid; however, an 'acetowhite' epithelium is not diagnostic of HPV infection, as it occurs in other conditions.

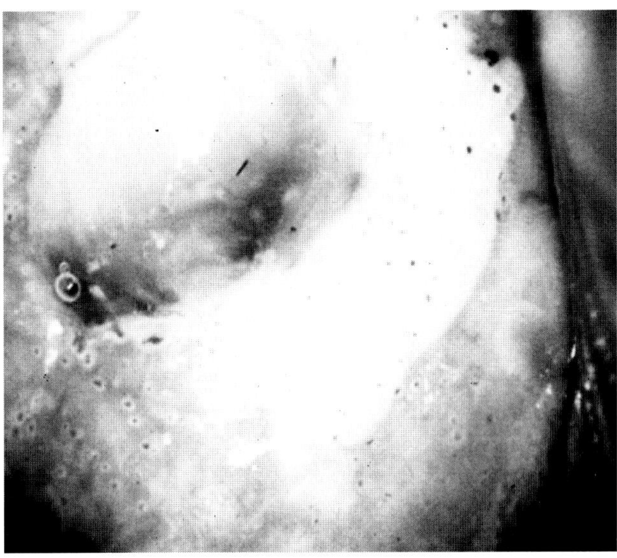

Fig. 4.27 Subclinical papillomavirus infection of cervix.

It is possible to demonstrate HPV in the cells of condylomas. In about 50% of cases virus particles can be seen with an electron microscope, and immunochemical methods have been used to show capsid antigen in the nuclei of infected cells. These techniques will give positive results only in the superficial cell layers, where virion assembly is taking place.

DNA detection. Various hybridization techniques are now available for the detection and typing of HPV genomes in exfoliated cells and tissue specimens, such as Southern blot, dot blot and *in situ* hybridization (Tenover 1988). Recently PCR has been favoured for its simplicity and sensitivity (Guerrero & Shah 1991). The value of these procedures in clinical practice is undecided. It was suggested that low-grade squamous intraepithelial lesions at genital sites, if associated with a 'high-risk' HPV such as HPV 16, might require more aggressive treatment and intensive follow-up than similar lesions associated with 'low-risk' viral types. Unfortunately, the significance of the presence of a 'high-risk' virus in these circumstances was weakened by studies showing that HPV 16 is often present in normal genital epithelia (de Villiers *et al.* 1986).

Epidemiology

Genital HPV infections are common among sexually active young people. The first manifestation to be studied were genital warts. After the resolution of an early misconception that these lesions were related to cutaneous warts, it became clear that they constituted an STD (Oriel 1971). About 60% of subjects sexually exposed to the disease develop warts themselves, the incubation period being between 3 weeks and 8 months. The peak age of onset in women is between 19 and 22 years; women with genital warts admit to an earlier age of first intercourse and more lifetime sex partners than those without the disease (Syrjänen *et al.* 1984). Women with vulval warts, whether they are seen in STD clinics or in dermatological practice, often have other STDs (Fairris *et al.* 1984). Genital warts are a common disease, the incidence of which is increasing (Aral & Holmes 1990). There are no reliable data on the epidemiology of subclinical HPV infection.

HPV may be present in clinically normal genital epithelia. There have been many studies of the prevalence of genotypes in cellular specimens from women with normal cervical cytology. The estimates vary with the sensitivity of the technique used; with PCR it appears to lie between 4 and 40% (Critchlow & Kousky 1995). Risk factors for the presence of HPV in the normal cervix include an early age of first intercourse, the number of sexual partners, suppression or alteration of immune status, young age and current oral contraceptive use (Schneider 1993). Because of the difficulty of obtaining satisfactory specimens, data on the prevalence of HPV in the normal vulva are not available. HPV was detected in 8% of cells scraped from the normal penis in a group of 365 men aged 16–35 years (Grussendorf-Conen *et al.* 1986); it is not unreasonable to suppose that HPV DNA is present in some women with normal vulval epithelia, but the natural history of these colonizations is at present unknown.

Immune responses

Immune responses are important in limiting disease caused by HPV. It has been difficult to study humoral response because of the problem of obtaining adequate amounts of viral antigen. Genital warts contain too few virions to be of value, and *in vitro* systems for the production of virions are rudimentary. Such information as there is (Lutzner 1985) indicates that antibodies do not have a significant role in preventing or limiting HPV infection.

The importance of cell-mediated immunity is shown by the behaviour of HPV infections in immunosuppressed individuals. The proliferation of cutaneous and genital warts in renal allograft recipients was noted many years ago (Spencer & Andersen 1970). Women with lymphoma, who often have defective cell-mediated immunity, are liable to recalcitrant vulval condylomas (Shokri-Tabibzadeh *et al.* 1981) (Fig. 4.28), and these lesions are a common complication of HIV infection (Kiviat *et al.* 1990). In immunosuppressed people, warts not only increase in size and number but also respond poorly to treatment and may be subject to pre-malignant or malignant change (Schneider *et al.* 1983).

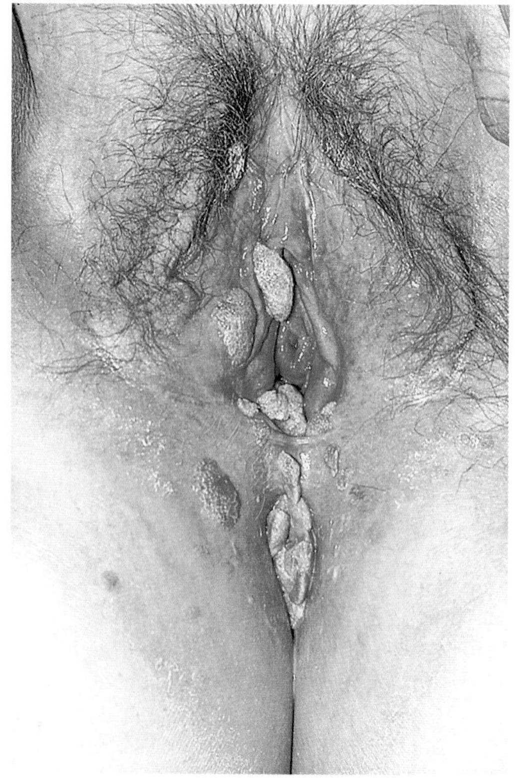

Fig. 4.28 Vulval warts in an immunosuppressed patient.

Clinical features

Genital warts. HPV can infect any part of the vulva, and may be expressed in several ways. Of these, genital warts are the commonest and best recognized. Condylomata acuminata are irregular, fleshy, vascular tumours, which can affect any part of the vulva. The earliest lesions appear most often on areas traumatized during coitus such as the fourchette and adjacent labia. They may be seen around the urethra and above the clitoris; they often extend into the lower part of the vagina, and sometimes the whole vagina is involved. The disease can extend backwards to affect the perineum and perianal area, and lesions may appear in the genitocrural folds (Fig. 4.29). During pregnancy, physiological immunosuppression causes condylomas to enlarge. They may reach a large size (Fig. 4.30), and even compromise delivery because of obstruction of the birth canal and haemorrhage (Wilson 1973); after delivery they regress, and may disappear altogether. Very large condylomas may affect women with severe immunosuppression following organ transplantation or HIV infection. Papular warts also affect the vulva (Fig. 4.31). These are small, raised, rounded lesions, commonly multiple; they often appear alone, but may accompany condylomata acuminata. Dürst *et al.* (1983) have shown that the predominant viral types present in vulval warts are HPV 6 and 11; HPV 16 is rarely present.

Genital HPV infection is multicentric; it is believed that the area infected is considerably greater than clinical examination would suggest. Anal warts are present in about 20% of women with vulval warts (Oriel 1971), and the cervix is also commonly involved. Cervical condylomas have been reported in 8% of women with vulval warts (Chuang *et al.* 1984). Subclinical cervical epithelial abnormalities, detected by cytology and/or colposcopy, are much commoner. Rowen *et al.* (1991) reported these in 44% of a group of 97 women with a history of genital warts, and histological evidence of CIN 1–2 in 13%; Walkinshaw *et al.* (1988) found histologically proved CIN in 29% of 59 women with vulval warts. It has been concluded that women attending for the first time with vulval warts require screening for CIN.

Subclinical HPV infection. The concept of subclinical infection originated with studies of the cervix. 'Flat condylomas' were identified by colposcopy after acetic acid staining; previously these had often been misdiagnosed as mild dysplasia, but there is no doubt that they are viral (Meisels *et al.* 1982). Subsequently, the idea arose of studying external genital epithelia in a similar way, and after the applica-

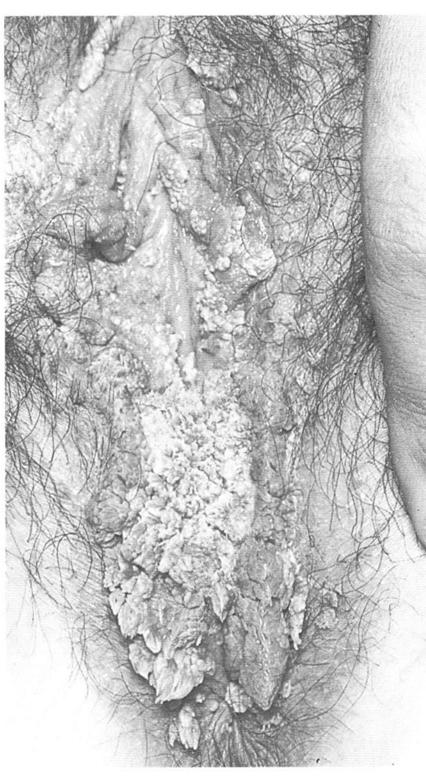

Fig. 4.29 Extensive condylomata acuminata.

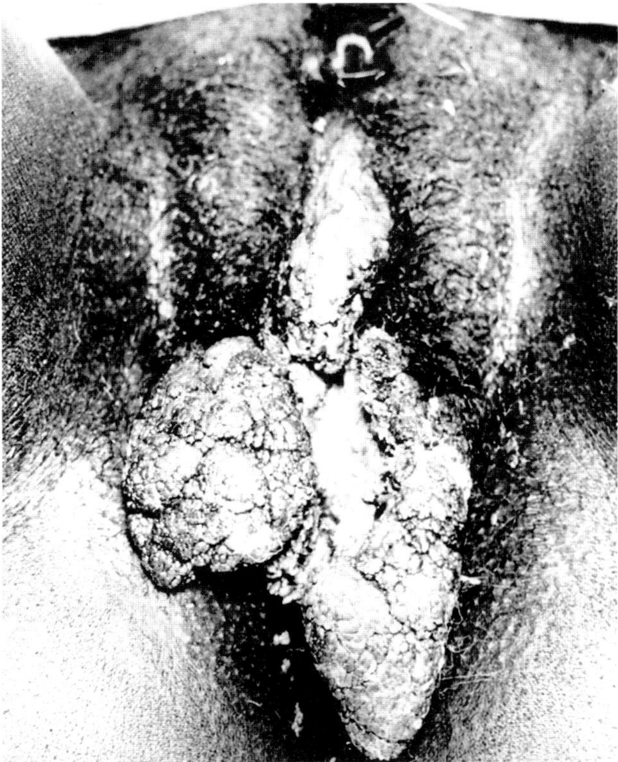

Fig. 4.30 Large condylomata acuminata in a pregnant woman: these lesions regressed completely after delivery.

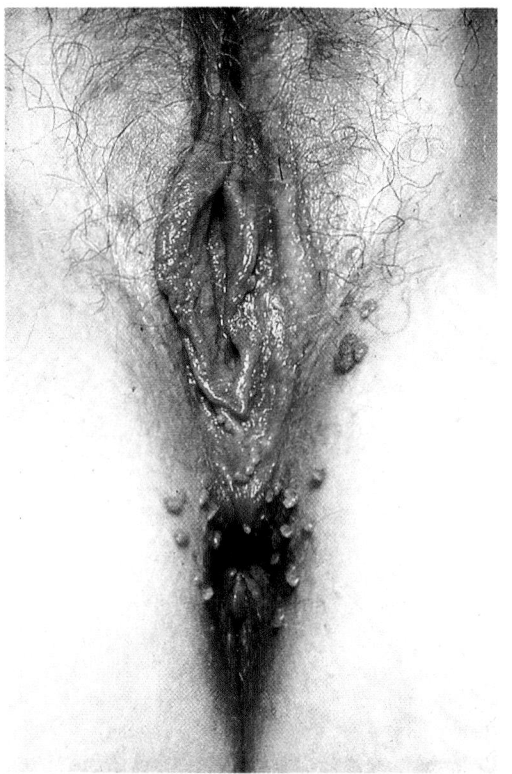

Fig. 4.31 Vulval and perianal papular warts.

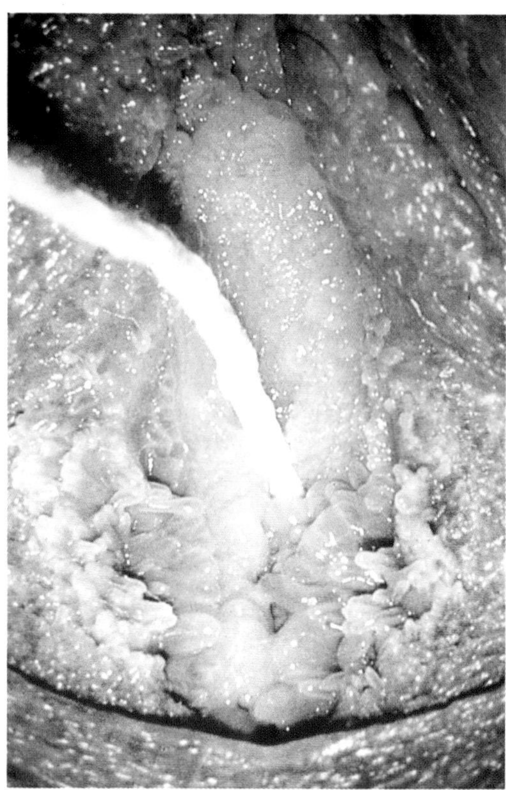

Fig. 4.32 Vestibular papillae.

tion of 5% aqueous acetic acid areas of white epithelial discontinuity, often with a punctate vascular pattern, were identified on the penis, anus and vulva. These subclinical lesions may be associated with warts, or they may be the sole evidence of HPV infection. In women, if present at the fourchette they may be associated with fissuring and cause dyspareunia (McKay 1989). On the vulva, areas of acetowhite epithelium are commonly due to HPV infection, but not exclusively so. Vulval intraepithelial neoplasia or some dermatoses, for example lichen sclerosus, may show a similar appearance. For this reason, unless the changes are obvious and typical, biopsy for histology is advisable.

Recently it has been suggested that some cases of vulvodynia, pruritus and superficial dyspareunia may be due to subclinical HPV infection. Dennerstein *et al.* (1994) investigated 13 such patients in whom the diagnosis had been made on clinical, colposcopic or histological grounds, but were unable to detect HPV in any of them.

Vulval and vestibular papillae. In many women, small filiform papillae are present around the introitus, described as 'vestibular papillae' by Friedrich in 1983. They are usually symptomless, but are sometimes associated with soreness or dyspareunia (Fig. 4.32). Their nature is controversial. For a long time they were regarded as an anatomical variant, but there have been reports of histological evidence of HPV infection (Growdon *et al.* 1985). However, this has been disputed (Moyal-Barraco *et al.* 1990). Virology is inconclusive (Costa *et al.* 1991), and the lesions do not appear to enlarge or progress. The weight of evidence at present is that vestibular papillae are not caused by HPV infection. This condition is also discussed elsewhere (Chapter 6).

Vulval intraepithelial neoplasia (see also Chapter 10). The acronym VIN covers a group of dysplastic lesions previously termed Bowen's disease and Bowenoid papulosis (Fig. 4.33). The clinical presentation of VIN is variable. The lesions are usually multifocal, they may be dark or red, papular or erosive, and smooth or keratinized (Reid & Greenberg 1991). Histologically, VIN is graded 1–3 according to its severity. VIN 3 is both multifocal and multicentric, being often associated with neoplasms in other parts of the genital tract, particularly the cervix (Friedrich *et al.* 1980, Bornstein *et al.* 1988).

HPV DNA is present in 50–100% of VIN lesions (Gross *et al.* 1985), and is more commonly present in lesions of young women. In low-grade VIN, sequences of HPV 6 and 11 are likely to be present, while VIN 3 strongly associated

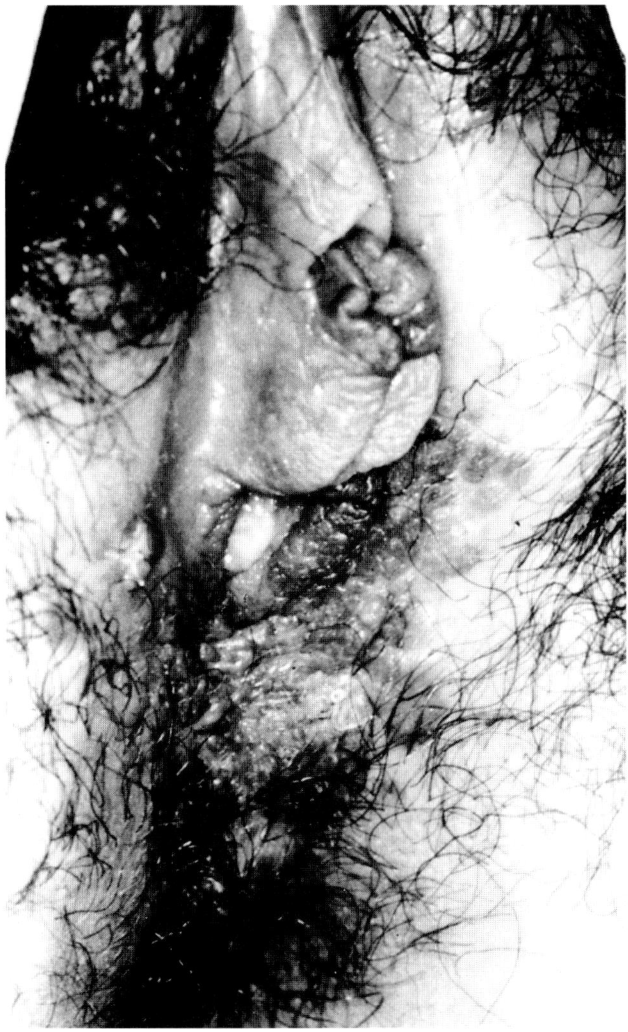

Fig. 4.33 Bowenoid papulosis (VIN): it is important to distinguish these pre-malignant lesions from condylomata acuminata.

with HPV 16 (Ikenberg *et al.* 1983). A hypothesis can be made that women infected by HPV 6 or 11 develop vulval, vaginal and cervical lesions that do not progress to malignancy, and indeed may regress spontaneously; on the other hand, women infected by HPV 16 may be at greater risk for VIN or CIN and cancer. It seems highly probable that cofactors are also involved, because the number of individuals infected by HPV 16 far exceeds the number developing overt malignant disease. There is no doubt that VIN and HPV infection are associated, or that some cases of VIN in young women progress via carcinoma-*in-situ* to invasive cancer. Hording *et al.* (1993) found that 19 (31%) of 62 squamous-cell vulval cancers contained DNA of HPV 16, 18 or 33, but none contained HPV 6 or 11. The aetiology of vulval carcinoma in elderly women is uncertain, but it does not seem that HPV infection is a factor.

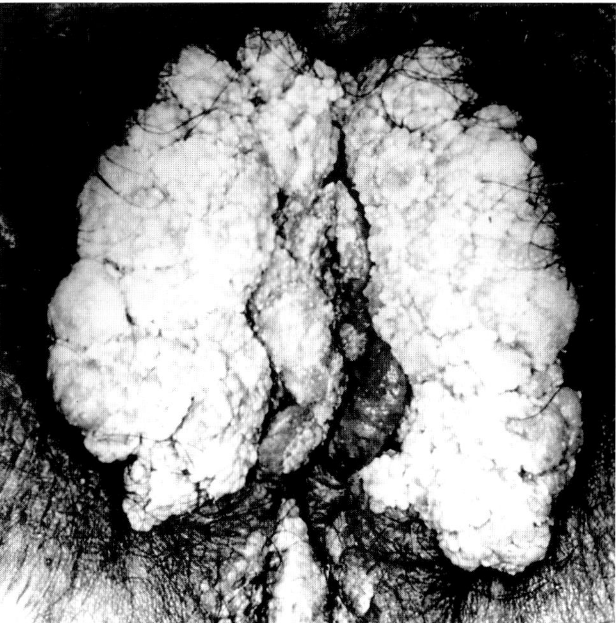

Fig. 4.34 Giant condyloma of vulva.

Giant condyloma. This is a rare tumour, first described by Buschke and Loewenstein (1925). In most reported cases the penis has been affected, but cases with lesions of the vulva and anal canal have been described (Baird *et al.* 1979). The disease starts as a small warty tumour, and this relentlessly enlarges, bulging inwards into the connective tissue and causing much destruction (Fig. 4.34). Clinically it appears to be malignant, but histologically it is benign, resembling condyloma acuminatum. It has been suggested that giant condyloma is a slow-growing malignant tumour from the outset, and that it closely resembles, or is identical to, verrucous carcinoma (Bogomoletz *et al.* 1985). Both tumours have been reported to contain HPV 6 DNA (Gissmann 1982, Rando *et al.* 1986).

Diagnosis

These various manifestations of vulval HPV infection must be distinguished from each other and from other papular conditions of the area. Among infective conditions are molluscum contagiosum, the papules and condylomata lata of secondary syphilis, and donovanosis. Rarely, warts are mimicked by lymphangiectasia (Chapter 5) and neurofibromatosis (Chapter 9). Fibroepithelial polyps are common benign lesions. Others, such as fibroma, lipoma, hidradenoma, adenoma and endometrioma are usually diagnosed histologically after biopsy. The distinction of vulval warts from VIN and invasive carcinoma is very important but may be difficult, particularly since the diseases may occur together. Biopsy of all vulval lesions of uncertain nature, or which are responding poorly to treatment, is essential.

Treatment

Before treatment of HPV-induced lesions of the vulva is undertaken it is necessary:

1 to confirm that they are benign (see above);

2 to determine the extent of the disease, using vulval/cervical colposcopy, cervical cytology with biopsy if indicated; and

3 to exclude associated infections.

It is important that sexual partners of these patients are examined, as they often have genital HPV lesions (Levine *et al.* 1984). In view of the frequent concurrence of other infections and the need for contact tracing, there is a good case for the initial management of vulval warts, particularly in young women, being in the hands of a genitourinary physician.

Spontaneous remission of some genital warts does occur, but is very unusual. There are many treatment modalities; all will cure some patients, but none will cure all. The following are in current use.

Cytotoxic agents.

Podophyllin has been used for half a century. It is a resin extracted from the roots of the podophyllum plant; the most active component being podophyllotoxin. Podophyllin is applied as a 15–25% solution in ethanol or compound benzoin tincture once or twice a week, and washed off after 4 hours. It has several disadvantages, and in some countries it is not used at all. Its composition is not standardized, and it is irritating to the normal skin, which means that it must be applied by medical or paramedical personnel rather than by the patient. Furthermore, it is potentially toxic. While small quantities are well tolerated, a liberal application to extensive warts has been followed by absorption and systemic effects, which include blood dyscrasias, peripheral neuritis, coma and death (Montaldi *et al.* 1974). This toxicity is particularly disastrous in pregnancy (Chamberlain *et al.* 1972). For these reasons, not more than 0.5 ml of 25% solution should be applied during one treatment session, prolonged treatment should be avoided, and the agent not used at all during pregnancy or, because it has teratogenic properties, to cervical lesions. Podophyllin preparations are effective for the treatment of condylomata acuminata, particularly of short duration; they are less active against papular or keratinized lesions. Treatment should not be prolonged beyond 4–6 weeks if progress is not being made.

Podophyllotoxin has recently become available for the treatment of genital warts. It is a pure standardized preparation, more reliable and less irritating than podophyllin. It is usually used as a buffered alcoholic 0.5% solution, which is painted on the warts twice a day for 3 days, followed by a 4-day interval, and the regimen is continued for 3 or 4 weeks. A 0.15% podophyllotoxin cream is also available. The efficacy of these preparations is about the same as that of podophyllin (Handley *et al.* 1991), but they are less irritating and can be applied by the patient at home.

Trichloracetic acid is applied as a 50–75% solution at weekly intervals. It is difficult to apply it precisely, and it is painful. It is sometimes used for the treatment of genital warts in pregnancy, but there are better alternatives (see below).

5-Fluorouracil is a cytotoxic agent that has been used as a 5% cream for the treatment of vulvovaginal warts (Ferenczy 1984a). Again, it is difficult to confine its action to the warts, and side effects, which include severe skin irritation, are not uncommon. It has never found a secure place in the treatment of warts.

Surgery. There are many destructive procedures, and which is used is largely a matter of availability and personal choice. Cryotherapy with a liquid nitrogen spray or nitrous oxide cryoprobe are useful for the treatment of vulval warts unless these are numerous; the procedure is painful, and local anaesthesia may be necessary. Electrocautery or coagulation under local anaesthesia is an effective out-patient treatment, but unsuitable for large or extensive lesions. For these, and for warts that have been recalcitrant to other modalities, destruction under general anaesthesia is necessary.

For this purpose, the carbon dioxide laser is now widely used (Landthaler *et al.* 1990). Its advantages over other techniques are its precision both in the area treated and the depth of destruction. If it is performed under colposcopic control; any associated cervical disease can be treated at the same time. Ferenczy *et al.* (1985) have detected papillomavirus sequences in histologically normal skin adjacent to genital warts, and noted that recurrences after laser therapy of the warts occurred in some of these patients. This raises the possibility that extension of the field of therapy may reduce the risk of recurrence (Reid 1985).

For the treatment of warts confined to the anus and anal canal, the scissor excision procedure developed by Thomson and Grace (1978) is very satisfactory. Postoperative discomfort is small and scarring is radial, so there is no risk of anal stenosis.

Immunomodulating therapy. Recurrence is a major problem after the treatment of genital warts, and is probably due to the persistence of HPV or HPV DNA in apparently normal tissue. It has been suggested that interferons (IFN), which have antiviral, antitumour and immune-modulating properties, might be of value in dealing with this problem. IFN are now classified as α, β and γ according to their biological properties, and they have been used topically, by intralesional injection, parenterally and in combination with other therapies. A considerable literature has developed, which has been reviewed by Gross (1990). The subject will not be discussed in detail here, but some general conclusions have emerged from recent studies.

IFN undoubtedly have an effect on genital warts. Topical treatment is the least effective. Intralesional treatment, involving repeated injections into individual warts, is obviously of limited practical value. Parenteral therapy has had some success, but its value is reduced by side effects such as fever and leucopenia. The most promising approach seems to lie in ablative treatment, such as laser, followed by either topical or systemic low-dose IFN, although this is not always successful (Armstrong *et al.* 1996). Whether α, β or γ IFN, or some combination of these, is preferable has not been decided.

Imiquimod, an immune response modifier, is a new topical agent of promise (Barrasso 1998).

Treatment of vulval warts during pregnancy. Recent advances in the epidemiology of HPV infections have raised some problems concerning the management of genital warts in pregnancy. On the one hand, vulval warts usually regress after delivery, so that although they may become large it may be best to leave them untreated, or with minimal treatment; this is the traditional view. On the other hand, there is a possibility of transmission of the infection to the infant, resulting in anogenital warts or, much more seriously, laryngeal papillomatosis (Mounts & Shah 1984). The risk of these diseases has not been quantified, but is believed to be low (Watts *et al.* 1998), and has to be weighed against the risks of caesarean section. If treatment is considered necessary, podophyllin should not be used because of its toxicity. Cryotherapy for small lesions and carbon dioxide laser for large lesions are both safe (Ferenczy 1984b).

Management of subclinical human papillomavirus vulval infections. There is no unanimity about this. Some clinicians recommend biopsy if the lesions persist for more than 6 weeks. If histology then shows intraepithelial neoplasia, ablation must be considered. There is no satisfactory treatment for uncomplicated subclinical HPV infection. Many workers think that attempts to eradicate them may do more harm than good, and that they are best left alone.

Genital herpesvirus infection

The first description of genital herpes was given by the French physician Jean Astruc in 1736. By the end of the 19th century it had become quite common; Unna said in 1883 that he had seen 200 cases in 4 years in prostitutes attending an STD clinic in Hamburg. Herpes simplex virus (HSV) was first grown in the laboratory in the mid-1920s. Lipschütz pointed out in 1921 the clinical and epidemiological differences between oral and genital herpes, and 40 years later it was shown that there were two antigenic types of virus, designated HSV 1 and HSV 2, and that the viral type recovered was related to the site of the lesions. During the last three decades genital herpes has become important. It is common, and recurrences and the possibility of passing it to a sexual partner cause much anxiety and distress. It can cause major illness or death to neonates, and herpetic ulceration may lead the way to HIV infection.

Virology

The core of the virion is composed of double-stranded linear DNA, and this is surrounded by an icosahedral protein capsid composed of 162 subunits. Outside this is an impermeable envelope composed of glycoproteins (Nahmias & Roizman 1973) (Fig. 4.35). The subtypes HSV 1 and HSV 2 can be differentiated by cultural and serological methods, and their nucleic acids show approximately 50% homology.

Life cycle of herpes simplex virus. The virus is introduced directly into epithelial cells; for genital herpes this occurs

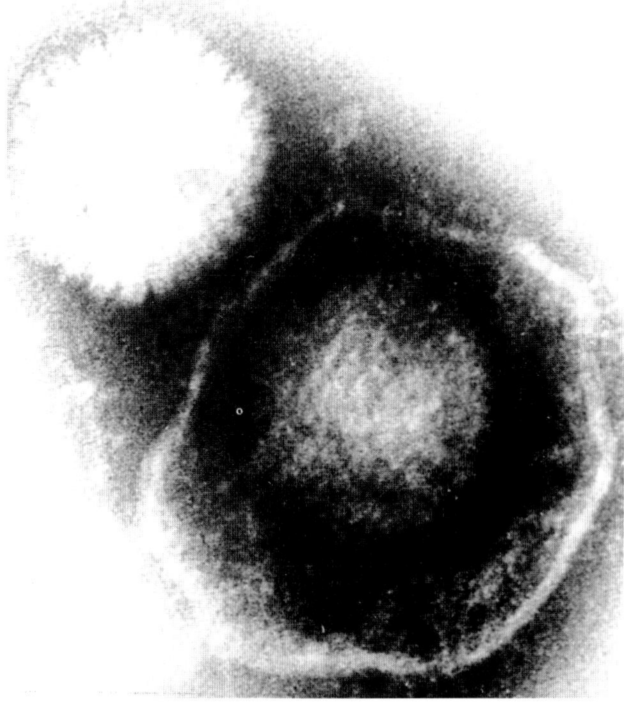

Fig. 4.35 Herpes simplex virus particles.

during intercourse or orogenital contact. A productive phase of infection ensues, which lasts for 5–6 hours and culminates with the assembly of new virus particles and their release with the death and lysis of the host cell (Raab & Lorincz 1981).

Animal experiments have shown that about 24 hours after inoculation the virus begins to spread from the infected epithelium along sensory nerves to regional sensory ganglia. In the case of human genital herpes, HSV 2 and less often HSV 1 can be recovered from the nerve root ganglia of S3 and S4 (Barringer 1974). After a brief productive infection, the stage of latency begins; no viral antigen can be demonstrated, but, if the ganglia are excised and cultured, infectious virus can be isolated. Latency persists indefinitely and reactivation, leading to repeated attacks of disease, can occur at any time. Recurrences may be provoked by intercourse, menstruation and psychological stress, but are often inexplicable. HSV 2 infections are more liable to recur than those due to HSV 1.

Pathology

The lesions of primary and recurrent herpes are histologically identical. Initial dermal congestion, with intracellular and extracellular oedema, culminates in the formation of an epidermal vesicle, which ruptures to form a shallow ulcer. The intraepidermal vesicles do not extend below the basement membrane, so do not result in permanent scarring. The nuclei of infected cells contain inclusions that are initially basophilic but later eosinophilic. Both vesicles and ulcerated areas contain multinucleated giant cells, some of whose nuclei also contain inclusions. The inflammatory infiltrate around the herpetic lesion is initially composed of mononuclear cells, but later polymorphonuclear leucocytes predominate.

Immunology

Antibodies to HSV can be detected by several methods, of which complement fixation (CF) and neutralization are the best known (Eberle & Courtney 1981). They can be detected in convalescent sera from 95% of patients with first attacks of genital herpes, and persist after the attack has resolved. Their presence does not appear to have any influence on the development of recurrent infections. It is, however, likely that circulating antibodies have a protective effect. The presence of antibodies to HSV 1 appears to mitigate the severity of first episodes of genital infections from HSV 2, and indeed may prevent them (Corey & Holmes 1983). Cowan *et al.* (1994) have used a new type-specific antibody test for HSV 2, and found that it may be a useful tool for studying the epidemiology of sexually transmitted herpetic infections.

An intact cell-mediated immune (CMI) system appears to be essential in preventing or moderating genital herpes (Corey *et al.* 1978). Immunocompromised individuals, such as those with AIDS or those receiving immunosuppressive drugs, are subject to severe or atypical genital herpes infections (Whitley *et al.* 1994). The role of CMI in recurrent infections is uncertain, and it is impossible to say why some people exposed to the infection never develop it, or why some individuals have so many more recurrences than others.

Epidemiology

In the UK the number of women attending STD clinics because of genital herpes doubled between 1981 and 1990. Some of this increase may be due to increased public awareness of the disease, but it is likely that there has been a true increase in incidence. Although exact data are not available, there is little doubt that genital herpes is becoming commoner in other countries. Serological surveys in North America have shown that up to one-third of city dwellers have antibodies to HSV 2; only a minority of those with antibodies give a history of genital herpes, which suggests that most of these infections have been silent (Mertz 1990).

Genital herpes in women is acquired through vaginal intercourse or orogenital contact with an individual shedding the virus. The source contact may have obvious genital or oral lesions, but in many situations this is not the case and the partner has either minimal or no signs of infection. Asymptomatic shedding of virus is an important source of infection; it has been demonstrated in saliva (Spruance 1984) and seminal secretion (Centifanto *et al.* 1972). Such viral shedding in men may also be from penile lesions too small to be identifiable by examination, perhaps in a subject with recurrent genital herpes. The majority of genital herpes is caused by HSV 2, but about 25% of episodes of first attacks are due to HSV 1 (Corey & Holmes 1983), most of them attributable to oral sex.

Clinical features

The incubation period of a first attack of genital herpes is 2–10 days. Genital or perigenital burning or itching may precede the appearance of lesions by 2 or 3 days. The lesions themselves are at first erythematous, but soon become vesicular, then rupture to form single, multiple or grouped shallow ulcers, 1–2 mm in diameter (Fig. 4.36). These may coalesce to form larger ulcerated areas. The ulcers are not indurated, and are very painful and tender. In women they are commonest on the labia majora and minora, clitoris, perineum and perianal areas. Oedema of the labia is not unusual, and the pain of a severe attack may make it almost impossible to examine the genital area

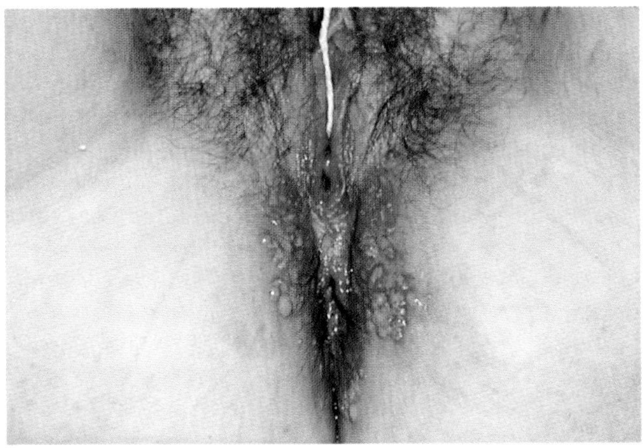

Fig. 4.36 Genital herpes, showing vesicular and ulcerative lesions.

thoroughly. In 80% of cases of primary vulval herpes the cervix is involved (Corey & Holmes 1983); it appears congested, and multiple shallow ulcers, or even areas of necrosis, can be seen. Dysuria is a common symptom, due either to the contact of urine with periurethral lesions or to herpetic ulceration of the urethra itself. Moderate enlargement of inguinal and/or femoral lymph nodes occurs in the second week of the illness. The nodes are tender, but do not suppurate. These varied symptoms are usually accompanied by general malaise, and often by fever.

The symptoms of primary genital herpes reach a maximum after 7–10 days, and thereafter gradually subside. The ulcers on the labia majora and perineum begin to crust (mucosal ulcers do not crust) and after 14–21 days healing may be virtually complete. However, the formation of new lesions occurs in 75% of patients, and these will slow recovery. When all lesions have healed, the patient may be regarded as non-infective.

Complications. Pharyngeal infection, usually symptomatic, may be associated with primary genital infection by HSV 1 or HSV 2 (Embil *et al.* 1981). Severe and prolonged headache may indicate the onset of aseptic meningitis, which occurs in about one-third of women with first attacks of genital herpes (Corey & Holmes 1983). The meningitis is usually mild and self limiting. Lumbosacral herpetic radiculitis is not uncommon, indicated by the development of perineal and sacral anaesthesia, constipation and retention of urine (Caplan *et al.* 1977); retention of urine may also be due to severe dysuria.

Extragenital skin lesions develop in at least one-quarter of women with primary infections. They occur during the second week of the disease, and mostly affect the thighs and buttocks; disseminated blood-borne infection is rare (Nahmias 1970). Secondary bacterial infection of herpetic lesions is uncommon except in immunosuppressed patients. Superinfection by yeasts is common, developing in the second week of the attack.

Recurrent infections. About 50% of women with primary genital herpes caused by HSV 1 and 80% with primary infections with HSV 2 develop recurrences within the year following infection (Reeves *et al.* 1981). The pattern of recurrence is variable. Some women have only one or two a year, but in one study in the USA two-thirds of patients were having more than five attacks a year (Knox *et al.* 1982). Women with HSV 1 infections have fewer recurrences than those with HSV 2. Recurrences are usually shorter and less severe than first attacks; their duration is on average 7 days. Cervical involvement is much reduced; only 15–30% of women shed virus from the cervix, and there are usually no clinical abnormalities (Guinan *et al.* 1981). Dissemination to other sites does not occur.

Genital herpes and vulval neoplasia. Early suspicions that HSV might be involved in the pathogenesis of genital neoplasia were largely based on seroepidemiological studies that indicated that women with CIN were up to 10 times more likely to have antibodies against HSV 2 than controls (Nahmias & Roizman 1973). When the cases and controls were carefully matched for possible confounding factors, these results were not confirmed (Vonka *et al.* 1984). There is no evidence that HSV induces the proliferation of latently infected cells, and HSV DNA, unlike HPV DNA, cannot regularly be detected in cervical carcinoma. It is not now thought that herpes viruses have a major role in neoplasia of the cervix.

Although it has been less intensively studied, much the same arguments apply to vulval neoplasia. HSV 2-induced protein antigens in carcinoma have been reported, but their significance is uncertain (Schwartz & Naftolin 1981). While it is unlikely that HSV is an important aetiological agent in vulval neoplasia, it is conceivable that HPV and HSV may cooperate in some way in oncogenesis (zur Hausen 1982).

Diagnosis

The clinical diagnosis of genital herpes in its vesicular stage is straightforward, but once ulcerated it must be differentiated from other causes of genital ulceration. Among infective causes, primary and secondary syphilis must always be excluded, even in confirmed cases of herpes, because the two diseases may occur together. In women who live in, or have recently travelled to, the tropics, chancroid, lymphogranuloma venereum and donovanosis may be differentiated by appropriate laboratory tests. Non-infective causes of genital ulceration include aphthous ulcers, Lipschütz ulcer, Behçet's and Crohn's disease; in these diseases the duration of ulceration is more prolonged, and the ulcers larger and deeper than in genital herpes.

Laboratory diagnosis. Viral culture is the most sensitive procedure (Levin 1991). Specimens of vesicle fluid or from the base of ulcers are placed in virus transport medium; it is important, in a first attack, to sample the cervix as well. In the laboratory, specimens are inoculated on to a suitable cell line, incubated at 37°C and examined regularly for a cytopathic effect. If the inoculum is large, this will be apparent in 1–7 days. The viral isolates can be typed by various procedures, of which immunofluorescence is the one favoured by most laboratories.

Cytology can also be used for diagnosis. Scrapings of vulval lesions or cervical smears are stained by Papanicolaou or Wright–Giemsa methods and examined microscopically for intranuclear inclusions and giant cells. These methods are specific but insensitive. Immunological tests include a direct immunofluorescence test; provided enough cells have been collected, its sensitivity is 75–90% that of culture. Serological tests are of no value for diagnosis.

Treatment

General measures. Associated infections should be excluded by appropriate tests. Women with primary herpes often feel unwell because of viraemia and anxiety about the condition. Rest is important, and analgesia given as required. If there is evidence of incipient complications such as meningitis or difficulty with urination, admission to hospital is indicated. Frequent bathing with 0.9% saline is soothing. Bacterial secondary infection is unusual, but if it should occur cotrimoxazole (which has no antitreponemal action) is the drug of choice. Superinfection with *Candida* species is common, and needs treatment with antimycotics. Retention of urine can usually be avoided if a high fluid intake is maintained and the patient encouraged to urinate, perhaps in a warm bath. If it should occur, an indwelling catheter will be needed for a few days. Suprapubic drainage is unnecessary.

Counselling is important. Patients are often concerned about the likelihood of recurrence, pregnancy and the possibility of infecting their sexual partners. This risk is low once genital lesions have healed, and women should be encouraged to lead a normal sex life, avoiding intercourse during attacks. Nevertheless, there is a small risk of infecting others in between attacks. The advisability of the patient telling her partner that she has recurrent herpes is a delicate and emotive problem, which she may like to discuss. Some people derive benefit from self-help groups.

Antiviral agents. Aciclovir is the best drug for the treatment of genital herpes (Wagstaff *et al.* 1994). For a first attack, oral aciclovir, 200 mg five times a day, has a marked effect on the duration and severity of symptoms and the duration of viral shedding. It should be started as soon as the diagnosis has been made, and may have an effect even if this has been delayed for a week after the onset of symptoms. The application of aciclovir cream 5% every 4 hours also reduces pain and viral shedding (Fiddian *et al.* 1983), but topical therapy has no effect on systemic manifestations. Intravenous aciclovir, 5 mg/kg body weight given 8-hourly for 5 days is highly effective (Mindel 1991), and should be considered for complicated and neonatal infections, and for genital herpes in immunosuppressed patients. Aciclovir therapy for primary herpes, however administered, has no influence on the rate of recurrence.

Patients with mild and infrequent recurrences need only symptomatic treatment. If recurrences are more severe, antiviral therapy may be considered. Aciclovir cream slightly reduces the duration of viral shedding, but has little effect on the time taken for the lesions to heal. Oral therapy is a little more effective, particularly if it is started during the prodromal period of an attack (Reichman *et al.* 1984). Patients with frequent recurrences undoubtedly benefit from suppressive therapy. This should begin with aciclovir 200 mg four times a day and continued for 6–8 weeks. If there have been no recurrences the dose is then progressively reduced. After a year, treatment is discontinued for a few weeks to assess the frequency of recurrences, then resumed if necessary. Continuous aciclovir therapy makes a lot of difference to the lives of many women, and side effects are very uncommon.

Prevention

Health education is important; for example, it is surprising how many people do not realize that genital herpes can be contracted through oral sex. The use of condoms during foreplay and intercourse may reduce the transmission of HSV, although this has not been established in clinical trials. Attempts are currently being made to develop a vaccine against genital herpes, but hitherto without success.

Varicella–zoster

Varicella–zoster virus is another member of the herpesviridae. It causes disease of two clinical types, varicella (chickenpox) mostly in children, and herpes zoster (shingles), mostly in adults. After the primary infection with varicella the virus becomes latent in the sensory root ganglia, and later in life may be reactivated and causes herpes zoster. The reasons for this reactivation are not known, but it is much more likely to occur in patients with neoplasms (such as lymphoma) affecting cell-mediated immunity, patients on immunosuppressive therapy and people with HIV infection. The histology of the lesions of varicella and zoster are identical. There are intraepidermal vesicles, with ballooning of adjacent prickle cells. Acidophil intranuclear inclusions and multinucleate giant cells are present, and there is some dermal inflammation.

Varicella. This is a highly contagious disease, with an incubation period of 14–21 days. The eruption starts with faint macules, which rapidly become vesicular; successive crops appear over the next few days. Eventually the lesions scab and normally disappear without scarring. Vulval lesions occur as part of the exanthem, but there is no specific association. Patients receiving corticosteroids or immunosuppressive drugs for organ transplants, or who have AIDS, are likely to have a more severe varicella infection of longer duration, and sometimes a widespread systemic illness.

Zoster. This is a disease of the nerves of the skin and of the tissues they supply; although cervical and thoracic nerves are the most commonly affected, lumbosacral nerves are involved in 15% of cases. The rash of zoster is usually preceded and accompanied by local itching or pain, and is essentially unilateral. Vulval lesions appear if the dermatome of S3 is affected (Fig. 4.37). The eruption is vesicular; after a few days crusts form, which eventually separate, leaving no scarring. Vaginal lesions have been recorded (Janson 1959), and transient enlargement of the inguinal lymph glands often occurs. Zoster of S2 and below may lead to acute retention of urine (Waugh 1974). About 10% of patients with zoster experience some degree of post-herpetic neuralgia, and this becomes commoner and more distressing in the elderly.

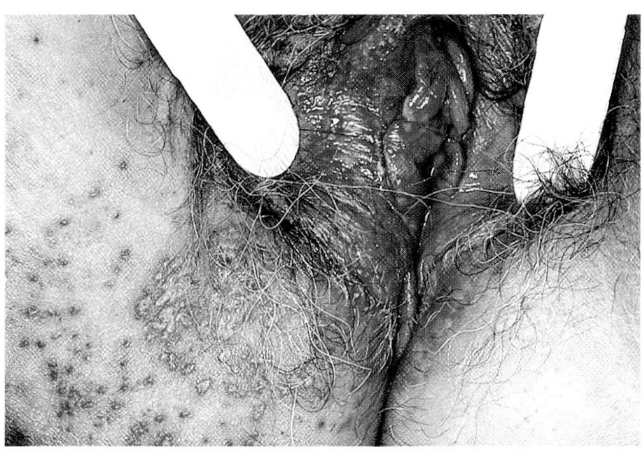

Fig. 4.37 Vulval herpes zoster: the third sacral nerve root is involved.

Zoster is not only more likely to occur in people who are immunocompromised, but if it does so it will probably be more severe; in these cases dissemination of the virus may occur and lead to a life-threatening illness.

Diagnosis and treatment

The diagnosis of vulval zoster is usually easy, but if the lesions are scanty genital herpes will need to be excluded by culture of vesicle fluid. Varicella is usually a mild disease requiring only symptomatic treatment, but in adults with severe infections, and in the immunocompromised, antiviral therapy may be needed. Vulval zoster is so uncomfortable and distressing that this is widely used. Aciclovir is the drug of choice, but higher dosage is required than for herpes simplex infections. The oral dose is 800 mg five times a day, and this is continued until no new lesions have appeared for 48 hours. The effect of aciclovir on post-herpetic neuralgia is controversial, but there is some evidence of its efficacy (Huff *et al.* 1993). Severe infections with the varicella–zoster virus, particularly in immunocompromised patients, may require intravenous aciclovir 10 mg/kg 8 hourly.

Epstein–Barr virus

Epstein–Barr virus (EBV) is another human herpesvirus. It causes infectious mononucleosis, and is also associated with several lymphomas, nasopharyngeal carcinoma and oral hairy leukoplakia. Although some cutaneous manifestations of infectious mononucleosis are recognized, genital ulceration is rare (Brown & Stenchever 1977). Portnoy *et al.* (1984) described a young woman with virologically and serologically confirmed infectious mononucleosis who developed painful vulval ulceration; EBV was recovered from the ulcers (see also Chapter 5). No association between EBV and vulval neoplasia has been demonstrated (Cheung *et al.* 1993).

Genital poxvirus infections

MOLLUSCUM CONTAGIOSUM

Virology

The virus of molluscum contagiosum is a brick-shaped particle, 200 × 100 μm; the outer tubular structures are arranged spirally, giving a 'ball of wool' appearance (Fig. 4.38). The genome is double-stranded DNA. It has not been possible to propagate the virus in the laboratory, and, although circulating antibodies have been detected by various techniques (Brown *et al.* 1981), their significance is uncertain.

Pathology

The molluscum lesion is an umbilicated papule. Its base is composed of acanthotic prickle cells; as these move towards the surface, cytoplasmic virus particles appear, which replicate to form a large inclusion, which pushes the nucleus to the periphery of the cell. Eventually the nucleus disappears, and the cell is now occupied by a 'molluscum body', which has been described as a 'sack of virus' (Blank & Rake 1955). The central core of the lesion is composed of these bodies together with cell debris (Fig. 4.39).

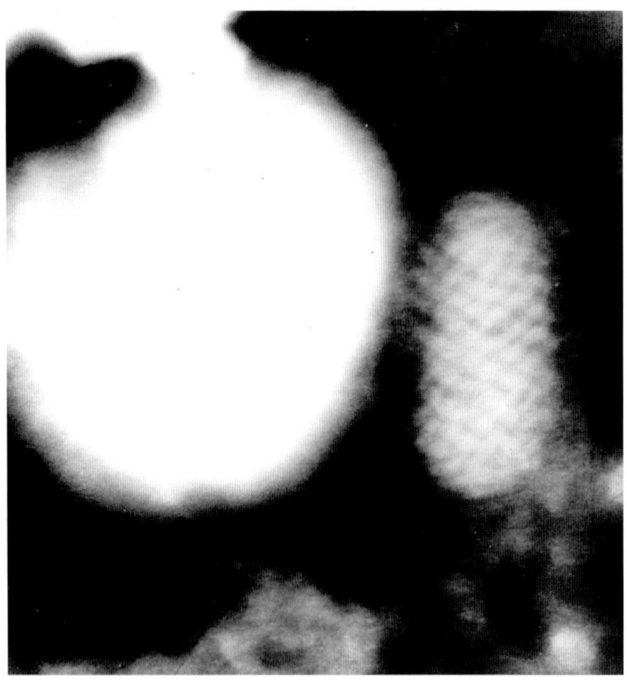

Fig. 4.38 Molluscum contagiosum: virus particle.

Epidemiology

The incidence of molluscum is biphasic, with peaks in childhood and in young adult life. In children the papules usually appear on the face, trunk and limbs, but in adults they are predominantly on the genitals; in this case they may be sexually transmitted (Cobbold & MacDonald 1970).

Clinical features

The incubation period is 2–6 weeks (Felman & Nikitas 1980). The lesions are firm hemispheric papules, usually 2–5 mm in diameter, with a dimpled centre from which cheesy material may be squeezed. In women they appear on the lower abdomen, pubis, labia majora and adjacent skin (Fig. 4.40); they do not affect the vagina or cervix. The number of lesions present is usually between one and 20; they are very numerous in patients with impaired immunity (Pauly *et al.* 1978), and multiple mollusca on the face may be a feature of AIDS (Katzman *et al.* 1987).

Diagnosis

Molluscum lesions may be mistaken for genital warts, and if solitary they may sometimes resemble other vulval conditions such as basal cell carcinoma. If secondarily infected, they may mimic furuncles, and if they ulcerate they

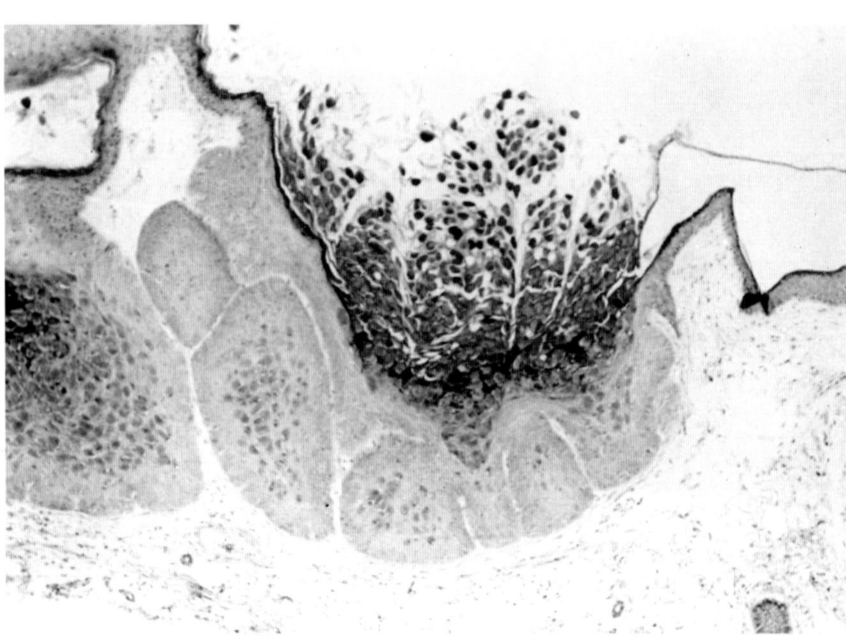

Fig. 4.39 Molluscum contagiosum: histology, showing acanthosis and amorphous molluscum bodies.

will have to be distinguished from other types of genital ulcer. For laboratory diagnosis, biopsy may be performed. Alternatively, the core of the lesion may be scraped out with a small curette and mixed with a drop of 10% potassium hydroxide on a slide. At magnification ×400 molluscum bodies appear as irregular masses about 35 μm in diameter.

Treatment

The tumours may be curetted under local anaesthesia or treated by cryotherapy. Small mollusca can be ablated by introducing liquid phenol with a sharpened stick. In patients with AIDS the lesions are unresponsive to treatment, and liable to recur.

ORF

This disease of sheep and lambs is caused by a pox virus. It causes large pustules with a central depression, which may be haemorrhagic. Human meat handlers may be infected with orf, and a case of vulval orf in a child who lived on a farm has been described (James 1968).

Human immunodeficiency virus infection

HIV infection is a major worldwide health problem. Like syphilis in bygone years, it has an impact on all organs and tissues; here, only its effect on the vulva and its diseases will be discussed. The first cases of AIDS were described in homosexual and bisexual men, and in northern Europe and the USA most HIV infections still occur in this group. A smaller epidemic exists among intravenous drug abusers. In Africa and the Far East AIDS predominantly affects heterosexuals, and it is in these localities that most infections of women are seen.

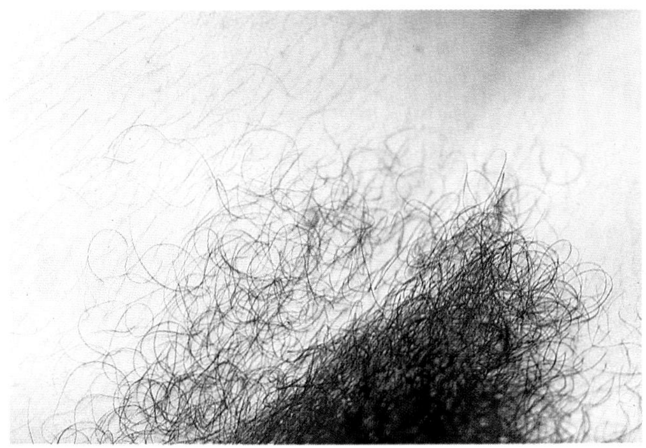

Fig. 4.40 Molluscum contagiosum: vulval lesions.

EFFECTS OF HUMAN IMMUNODEFICIENCY VIRUS INFECTION ON OTHER VULVAL INFECTIONS

Immunosuppression has a major impact on the natural history of many of these conditions. Among bacterial infections, *chancroid* is of particular importance in Africa. In women with HIV, there is a more extensive local disease and because of altered host responses the regional adenitis is less. The response to antimicrobial therapy may be unsatisfactory. In early *syphilis* there may be a delay in treponemal seropositivity (Hicks *et al.* 1987); persistent seronegativity does not occur. *Folliculitis*, *impetigo contagiosum* and *furunculosis* are all worsened by immunosuppression. Long *et al.* (1996) have reported bacillary angiomatosis of the cervix and vulva in a patient with AIDS. *Candidosis* is one of the commonest opportunist infections in HIV-positive patients and recurrent vulvovaginal candidosis often occurs, its severity increasing with advancing immunosuppression.

Viral disorders often affect women with chronic HIV infection. Severe *genital herpes* is among the commonest of these, and recurrent attacks become more frequent and more prolonged. *Herpes zoster* develops at some time in 20% of adults infected by HIV, and may be severe. *Molluscum contagiosum* is also common; multiple facial lesions are a notorious sign of infection (Katzman *et al.* 1987), and multiple vulval mollusca also occur. *HPV infection* with low-risk and high-risk genotypes is common at all stages of HIV infection (Ho *et al.* 1994). In some patients this may be the only hint of impaired immunity. The prevalence of these warts in HIV-seropositive patients may be as high as 20% (Rudlinger *et al.* 1990). They are multiple and widespread, and bleed easily. Their response to treatment is poor, and recurrences are common. A cytomegalovirus (CMV) napkin rash in an infant with systemic CMV lesions and congenital HIV infection has been reported (Thiboutot *et al.* 1991).

HUMAN IMMUNODEFICIENCY VIRUS AND VULVAL NEOPLASIA

Anorectal dysplasia in homosexual men has been linked with HPV and HIV infection (Frazer *et al.* 1986). There has also been speculation that carcinoma of the cervix may also be associated with these viruses (Maiman *et al.* 1990); in HIV-seropositive women, this disease has recently been designated an AIDS-defining condition. Other epithelial malignancies have been reported in HIV-infected patients, and multicentric primary squamous neoplasia of the female genital tract may occasionally occur (Rose & Fraire 1993). VIN appears to be more common than expected in women with HIV infections, but there is no evidence that invasive tumours develop more often in these patients. Kaposi's sarcoma is a neoplastic proliferative disorder that is the commonest tumour in HIV-infected individuals, constituting a diagnostic criterion for AIDS. It mostly affects homosexual men, and is uncommon in other risk groups. Kaposi's sarcoma of the vulva associated with HIV infection is rare in women, but has been described (Rajah *et al.* 1990, Macasaet *et al.* 1995).

VULVAL LESIONS PREDISPOSING TO HUMAN IMMUNODEFICIENCY VIRUS INFECTION

Co-infection with HIV and other STDs is common. In New York, co-infection with syphilis is often seen, and has been attributed to prostitution fuelled by the need for 'crack' cocaine (Drusin 1996). Patients with syphilis are more likely to be seropositive for HIV than others attending an STD clinic (Quinn *et al.* 1990). Elsewhere in the USA, a previous HSV 2 infection has been reported as a risk factor for HIV (Holmberg *et al.* 1988). Among Nairobi prostitutes, a simultaneous infection with HIV and chancroid is common.

In some cases multiple infections may simply have been contracted together from one sexual contact. There is no doubt, however, that the presence of some infections predisposes patients to contract HIV (Greenblatt *et al.* 1988). This applies particularly to genital ulcer diseases such as chancroid, herpes and syphilis. The most convincing data come from Africa where genital ulceration, particularly due to chancroid, is very common. Women with chancroid who are exposed to HIV are up to eight times more likely to contract this infection than women without chancroid. Conversely, the presence of genital ulcers in an HIV-infected woman heightens the risk of infection to the male partner (Kreiss *et al.* 1980). It is likely that the same phenomena occur in association with other types of genital ulceration (Plourde *et al.* 1994). It has been noted that gonorrhoea is an independent cofactor facilitating the acquisition and transmission of HIV, presumably because of disruption of epithelial protection. It is clear that the control of STD, and in particular genital ulceration, would have a significant effect on the epidemiology of HIV in both sexes; this aim is currently being actively pursued.

Vulval infection in children

(see also Chapter 5 and 7)

After the menarche, vulval infections are the same as in adults. In young children, the presentations are different. The vaginal epithelium is columnar rather than squamous, there is no glycogen, and the pH is 6.5–7.5. Because of this the flora is not dominated by lactobacilli, as it is in adults; there is an assortment of organisms, with a high prevalence of diphtheroids and *Staphylococcus epidermidis* (Heller *et al.* 1969). Vaginitis rather than cervicitis is the clinical feature of infections such as gonorrhoea. The ways in which the vulva may become infected in children are:

1 transplacental, as in congenital syphilis;
2 perinatal, as in herpes simplex infections and some cases of anogenital warts;
3 accidental, as in threadworm infestation, poor hygiene and via fomites like towels and flannels;
4 sexual abuse.

Vulvovaginitis

The clinical features are similar whatever its cause, with itching, discharge, crusting and erythema of the labia and introitus (Fig. 4.41). Its cause has to be identified by laboratory tests. Possible pathogens include *Streptococcus pyogenes*, *Neisseria gonorrhoeae*, *Trichomonas vaginalis*, *Candida* species and threadworms. In prepubertal children, vaginal infection with *Neisseria gonorrhoeae* is likely to be due to sexual contact. In the past, epidemic non-venereal gonococcal vulvovaginitis due to defective hygiene in children in institutions was common (Holt 1905), but gonorrhoea from this cause is now rare (Farrell *et al.* 1981). *Trichomonas vaginalis* vulvovaginitis may occur in children

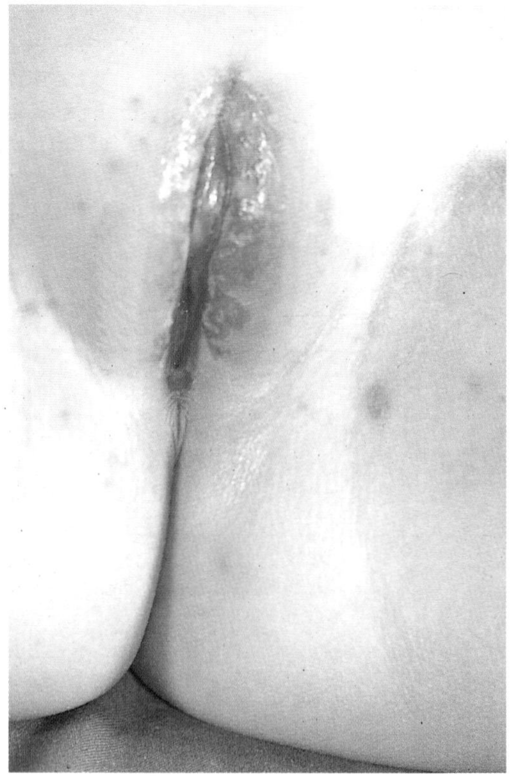

Fig. 4.41 Streptococcal vulvovaginitis in a child.

through sexual contact, but female infants born to women with trichomoniasis can acquire the infection during delivery, although the risk is low (Bramley 1976). The organisms disappear from the vagina in about 6 weeks, when the influence of maternal oestrogens has waned. McLaren *et al.* (1983) suggested that trichomonads may be a rare cause of neonatal pneumonia.

Ulcerative conditions

In early congenital syphilis, bullous, papular and papulosquamous lesions appear on the vulva as part of the characteristic dermatosis. Mucous patches and moist erosions also occur. Other signs of congenital syphilis will probably be present. Vulval condylomata lata develop later, typically towards the end of the first year of life (Nabarro 1954). The incidence of congenital syphilis can be reduced to vanishing point by the use of serological tests during pregnancy.

Infection by either HSV 1 or 2 can occur in children. Perinatal infection occurs 24–72 hours after birth (Stagno & Whitley 1990). Infection of the neonate by HSV during delivery is much more likely to occur if the mother has a first attack of herpes at the time than if she has a recurrence (Nahmias *et al.* 1971). In one study, about 25% of neonatal infections were with HSV 1 (Whitley *et al.* 1980), which suggests that some neonatal herpetic infections may be nosocomial. Neonatal herpes is a serious disease. The lesions may be localized to the skin or mouth, but in 50–65% of cases viral dissemination occurs and rapidly progresses to convulsions, cranial nerve palsies and visceral infection. The mortality rate is 65%, and most of the survivors have neurological sequelae.

Neonatal herpes should be preventable, and several strategies have been proposed. One is that women with a history of genital herpes should have repeated viral cultures near to term, but this has failed to predict the infant's risk at delivery (Arvin *et al.* 1986). It has been recommended that if suspect lesions are present at or near the time of delivery, caesarean section should be performed, preferably before the membranes rupture (Committee on Foetus and Newborn 1980). If a woman is having her first attack of herpes, where the risk of neonatal infection may be as high as 50% (Corey & Holmes 1983), this is undoubtedly an indication for caesarean section. The risk to a baby born to a woman with recurrent herpes, even if she is shedding virus at the time of delivery, is low (Prober *et al.* 1987), and the argument for surgical intervention is much less strong. Recently, the use of antivirals, notably aciclovir, during late pregnancy has been seriously considered (Mercey & Mindel 1991).

Genital herpes in older children has the same clinical features as in adults (Fig. 4.42), except that cervical infection does not occur. Children can transmit HSV to the vulva from infection in their own mouths (Nahmias *et al.* 1968), and occasionally a mother's herpetic whitlow may be responsible. Sexual transmission of HSV to abused children is well known (Gardner & Jones 1984).

Papular and condylomatous lesions

Genital warts in children are not uncommon, and both condylomata acuminata and papular lesions may be seen (Figs 4.43 & 4.44). The number of prepubertal children with vulval warts is increasing (Bender 1986). Since the disease is not difficult to diagnose, this probably reflects a true increase in incidence. Transmission of HPV to children may occur:

1 vertically, from a mother with HPV infection;
2 by autoinoculation from cutaneous warts;
3 as a result of sexual abuse.

Transmission of HPV from an infected mother can result in anogenital condylomata acuminata in her infant (Cohen *et al.* 1990). It is uncertain whether infection occurs through the intact amnion or during delivery. Exceptionally, condylomas may be present at birth (Tang *et al.* 1978), but most reports allude to an incubation period of up to 11 months (Oriel & Robinson 1995). Laryngeal papillomatosis in infants born to women with genital warts is rare but well authenticated (Mounts & Shah 1984). The majority of anogenital warts in children contain sequences of HPV 6 or 11, but other genotypes, even HPV 16, ma y be present. Some workers have reported a frequent association with HPVs that are responsible for cutaneous warts (Obalek *et al.* 1990). The explanation of this is not altogether clear, but one case of undoubted autoinoculation with HPV 2 from a finger wart has been described (Fleming *et al.* 1987).

Pre-menarchal girls with vulval warts are often infected with HPV at internal mucosal sites such as the vagina and

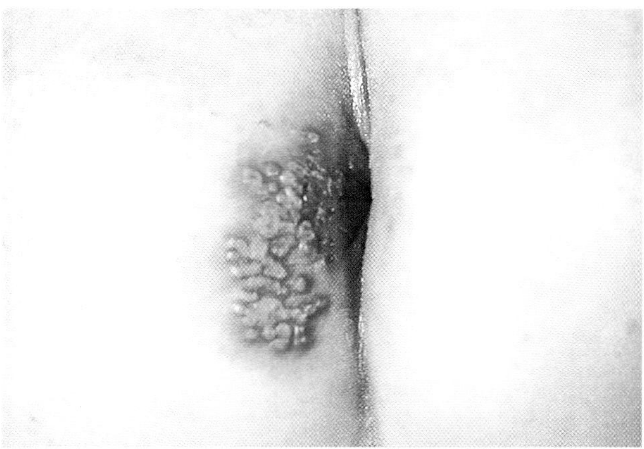

Fig. 4.42 Genital herpes in a child.

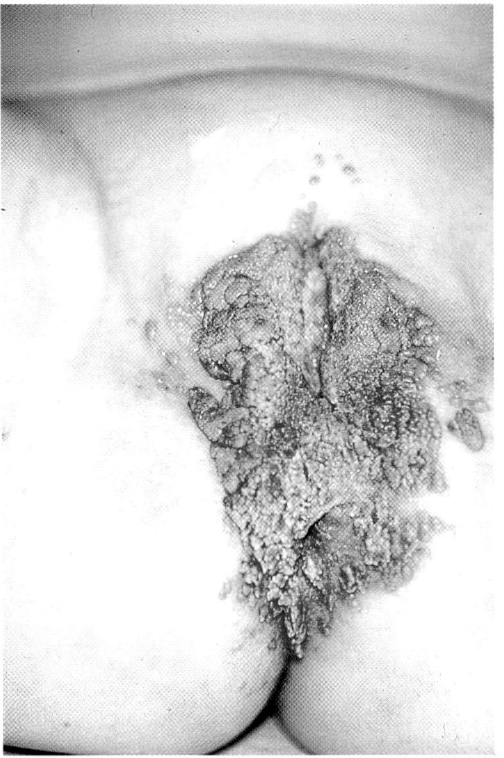

Fig. 4.43 Condylomata acuminata in a child.

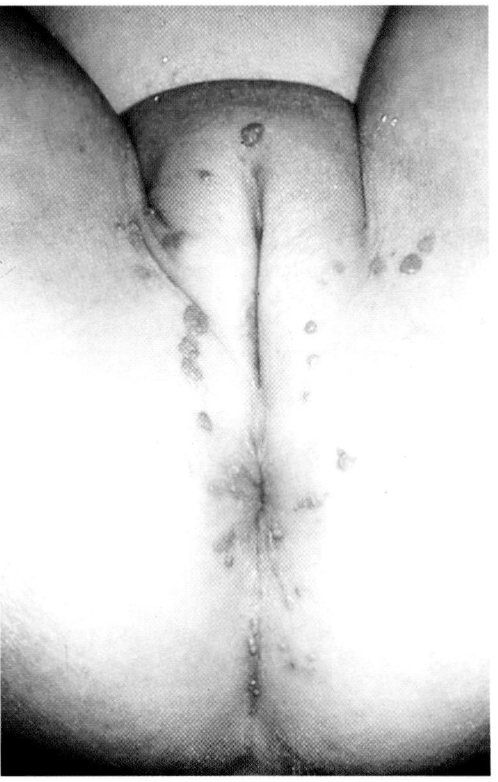

Fig. 4.44 Papular warts in a child.

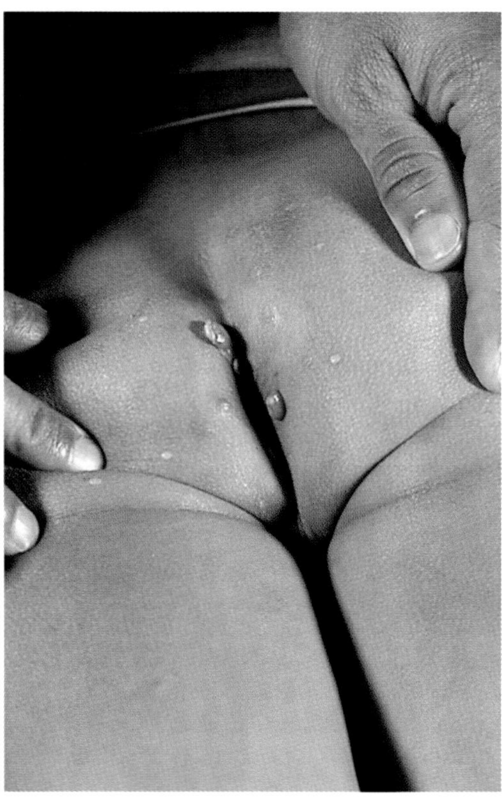

Fig. 4.45 Large perianal mollusca contagiosa lesions in a child.

anal canal (Gutman *et al.* 1994). During the last decade the need to consider sexual abuse in children with genital warts has been repeatedly stressed (American Academy of Dermatology Task Force on Pediatric Dermatology 1984). While there is no doubt about this connection, there has been disagreement over the proportion of affected children who have been abused (Oriel & Robinson 1995). There are difficult medical and social problems involved in female children with the disease (Bender 1986). It is obvious that doctors and other health workers must detect sexual abuse if it is occurring. On the other hand, the desire to protect a child should not lead to an innocent adult being accused of sexual assault. Schachner and Hankin (1985) have listed criteria that may be helpful in assessing the possibility of sexual assault in these cases. HPV identification and typing may prove helpful in determining the site of origin of an infection, but not necessarily its mode of transmission (Padel *et al.* 1990, Handley *et al.* 1993).

Molluscum contagiosum is sexually transmissible between adults. In children, the infection is more likely to reach the vulva through casual contact, but may follow child abuse (Bargman 1986). The appearance of the papules is similar to that in adults (Fig. 4.45). Sometimes lesions elsewhere on the body antedate vulval mollusca.

References

Addison, W.A., Livengood, C.H., Hill, G.B. *et al.* (1984) Necrotising fasciitis in diabetes. *Obstetrics and Gynecology* **63**, 473–478.

Ahmed-Jushuf, I.H., Shahmanesh, M., Arya, O.P. *et al.* (1995) The treatment of bacterial vaginosis with a 3-day course of 2% clindamycin cream. *Genitourinary Medicine* **71**, 254–256.

American Academy of Dermatology Task Force on Pediatric Dermatology (1984) Genital warts and sexual abuse in children. *Journal of the American Academy of Dermatology* **1**, 529–530.

Amsel, R., Totten, P.A., Speigel, C.A. *et al.* (1983) Nonspecific vaginitis. Diagnostic criteria and microbial and epidemiologic associations. *American Journal of Medicine* **74**, 14–22.

Anagnostidis, N. (1935) Kyste hydatique de la grande lèvre de la vulve et mécanisme de sa production. *Gynécologie et Obstétrique* **32**, 356–358.

Aral, S.O. & Holmes, K.K. (1990) Epidemiology of sexual behaviour and sexually transmitted diseases. In: *Sexually Transmitted Diseases*, 2nd edn (eds K.K. Holmes, P.-A. Mardh, P.F. Sparling & P.J. Wiesner), pp. 19–36. McGraw-Hill, New York.

Armstrong, D.K.B., Maw, R.D., Dinsmore, W.W. *et al.* (1996) Combined therapy trial with interferon alpha-2a and ablation therapy in the treatment of anogenital warts. *Genitourinary Medicine* **72**, 103–107.

Arvin, A.M., Hensleigh, P.A., Prober, C.G. *et al.* (1986) Failure of antepartum maternal cultures to predict the infant's risk of exposure to herpes simplex virus at delivery. *New England Journal of Medicine* **315**, 796–800.

Asami, K. & Nakamura, A.M. (1955) Experimental inoculation of bacteria-free *Trichomonas vaginalis* into human vaginae and its effect on the glycogen content of vaginal epithelia. *American Journal of Tropical Medicine and Hygiene* **4**, 254–258.

Ashworth, F.L. (1974) Tuberculous lymphoedema. *British Medical Journal* **iv**, 167–169.

Auger, P. & Joly, J. (1980) Microbial flora associated with *Candida albicans*. *Obstetrics and Gynecology* **55**, 397–401.

Baird, P.J., Elliott, P., Stening, M. *et al.* (1979) Giant condyloma acuminatum of the vulva and anal canal. *Australian and New Zealand Journal of Obstetrics and Gynaecology* **19**, 119–122.

Bargman, H. (1986) Is genital molluscum contagiosm a cutaneous manifestation of sexual abuse? *Journal of the American Academy of Dermatology* **14**, 847–849.

Barlow, D. (1977) The condom and gonorrhoea. *Lancet* **i**, 811–812.

Barlow, D. & Phillips, I. (1978) Gonorrhoea in women: diagnostic, clinical and laboratory aspects. *Lancet* **i**, 761–763.

Barrasso, R. (1998) Genital warts: treatment with the immune response modifier 'Imiquimod'. Report from the XVth FIGO World Congress of Gynaecology and Obstetrics. *Journal of Obstetrics and Gynaecology* **18**, (Suppl. 2) 5.69–5.83.

Barringer, J.R. (1974) Recovery of herpes simplex virus from human sacral ganglia. *New England Journal of Medicine* **291**, 828–834.

Bender, M.E. (1986) New concepts of condylomata acuminata in children. *Archives of Dermatology* **122**, 1121–1124.

Berry, A. (1971) Evidence of gynaecological bilharziasis in cytologic material. A morphological study for cytologists in particular. *Acta Cytologica* **15**, 482–486.

Beveridge, M.M. (1962) Vaginal moniliasis after treatment of trichomonal infection with 'Flagyl'. *British Journal of Venereal Diseases* **38**, 220–222.

Bjornstad, R. (1947) Tuberculous primary infection of genitalia—two cases of venereal genital tuberculosis. *Acta Dermato-venereologica (Stockholm)* **27**, 106–109.

Blackwell, A.L., Fox, A.R., Phillips, I. *et al.* (1983) Anaerobic vaginosis (non-specific vaginitis): clinical, microbiological and therapeutic findings. *Lancet* **ii**, 1379–1382.

Blank, F. & Mann, S.J. (1975) *Trichophyton rubrum* infections according to age, anatomical distribution and sex. *British Journal of Dermatology* **92**, 171–174.

Blank, H. & Rake, H. (1955) *Viral and Rickettsial Infections of the Skin, Eye and Mucous Membranes*, pp. 182–192. Churchill Livingstone, London.

Bogomoletz, SW.V., Potet, F. & Molas, G. (1985) Condylomata acuminata, giant condyloma (Buschke–Loewestein tumour) and verrucous carcinoma of the perianal and anorectal regions: a continuous precancerous spectrum? *Histopathology* **9**, 1155–1169.

Bonar, B.E. & Rabson, A.S. (1957) Gynaecological aspects of leprosy. *Obstetrics and Gynecology* **9**, 33–38.

Borkawf, H.I. (1973) Bacterial gangrene associated with pelvic surgery. *Clinical Obstetrics and Gynecology* **16**, 40–45.

Bornstein, J., Kaufman, R.H., Adam, E. *et al.* (1988) Multicentric intraepithelial neoplasia involving the vulva. *Cancer* **62**, 1601–1604.

Boulle A. & Notelovitz, M. (1964) Bilharzia of the female genital tract. *South African Journal of Obstetrics and Gynaecology* **18**, 48–50.

Bramley, M. (1976) Study of female babies of women entering confinement with vaginal trichomoniasis. *British Journal of Venereal Diseases* **52**, 58–62.

Bray, R.S. (1974) Leishmania. *Annual Review of Microbiology* **28**, 189–199.

Brigden, M.B. & Guard, R. (1980) Extragenital granuloma inguinale in North Queensland. *Medical Journal of Australia* **2**, 565–567.

Brown, S.T., Nalley, J.F. & Kraus, S.J. (1981) Molluscum contagiosum. *Sexually Transmitted Diseases* **6**, 10–13.

Brown, Z.A. & Stenchever, M.A. (1977) Genital ulceration and infectious mononucleosis: report of a case. *American Journal of Obstetrics and Gynecology* **127**, 673–674.

Brunham, R.L., Martin, D.H., Hubbard, T.W. *et al.* (1983) Depression of the lymphocyte transformation response to microbial antigens and to phytohaemagglutinin during pregnancy. *Journal of Clinical Investigation* **72**, 1629–1638.

Bumgarner, F.E. & Burke, R.C. (1949) Pityriasis versicolor. Atypical clinical and mycological variants. *Archives of Dermatology* **59**, 192–194.

Buschke, A. & Loewenstein, L. (1925) Uber carcinomahnliche Condylomata Acuminata. *Klinische Wochenschrift* **4**, 1726–1728.

Caplan, L.R., Kleeman, F.J. & Berg, S. (1977) Urinary retention probably secondary to herpes genitalis. *New England Journal of Medicine* **297**, 920–921.

Carroll, C.J., Hurley, R. & Stanley, V.C. (1973) Criteria for diagnosis of *Candida* vulvovaginitis in pregnant women. *Journal of Obstetrics and Gynaecology of the British Commonwealth* **80**, 258–263.

Catterall, R.D. (1972) Trichomonal infection of the genital tract. *Medical Clinics of North America* **56**, 1203–1209.

Centifanto, Y.M., Drylie, D.M., Deardourff, S.L. *et al.* (1972) Herpesvirus type 2 in the male genitourinary tract. *Science* **178**, 318–319.

Chamberlain, M.J., Reynolds, A.L. & Yeoman, W.B. (1972) Toxic effect of podophyllum in pregnancy. *British Medical Journal* iii, 391–392.

Chapel, T.A. (1978) The variability of syphilitic chancres. *Sexually Transmitted Diseases* **5**, 68–70.

Cheung, A.N.Y., Khoo, V.S., Kwong, K.Y. *et al.* (1993) Epstein–Barr virus in carcinoma of the vulva. *Journal of Clinical Pathology* **46**, 849–851.

Chuang, T.Y., Perry, H.O., Kurland, L.T. *et al.* (1984) Condylomata acuminata in Rochester, Minnesota, 1950–1978. Epidemiology and clinical features. *Archives of Dermatology* **120**, 469–475.

Clayton, Y.M. & Connor, B.L. (1973) Comparison of clotrimazole cream, Whitfield's ointment and nystatin ointment for the topical treatment of ringworm infections, pityriasis versicolor, erythrasma and candidosis. *British Journal of Dermatology* **89**, 197–199.

Cobbold, R.J.C. & MacDonald, A. (1970) Molluscum contagiosum as a sexually transmitted disease. *Practitioner* **204**, 416–420.

Cohen, B.A., Honig, P. & Androphy, A. (1990) Anogenital warts in children. *Archives of Dematology* **126**, 1575–1580.

Cohen, C. (1973) Three cases of amoebiasis of the cervix uteri. *Journal of Obstetrics and Gynaecology of the British Commonwealth* **80**, 476–480.

Committee on Foetus and Newborn (1980) Committee on infectious disease, perinatal herpes simplex infections. *Pediatrics* **66**, 147–148.

Corbishly, C.M. (1977) Microbial flora of the vagina and cervix. *Journal of Clinical Pathology* **30**, 745–748.

Corey, L. & Holmes, K.K. (1983) Clinical course of genital herpes simplex virus infection in men and women. *Annals of Internal Medicine* **48**, 973–983.

Corey, L., Reeves, W.C. & Holmes, K.K. (1978) Cellular immune responses in genital herpes simplex virus infections. *New England Journal of Medicine* **299**, 286–291.

Cossart Y.E., Thomspson, C. & Rose, B. (1995) Virology. In: *Genital Warts: Human Papillomavirus Infection* (ed. A. Mindel), pp. 1–34. Edward Arnold, London.

Costa, S., Rotola, A., Terzano, P. *et al.* (1991) Is vestibular papillomatosis associated with human papillomaviruses? *Journal of Medical Virology* **35**, 7–13.

Cowan, F.M., Johnson, A.M., Ashley, R., Corey, L. & Mindel, A. (1994) Antibody to herpes simplex virus type 2 as serological marker of sexual lifestyle in populations. *British Medical Journal* **309**, 1325–1329.

Critchlow, C.W. & Kousky, L.A. (1995) In: *Genital Warts: Human Papillomavirus Infection* (ed. A. Mindel), pp. 53–81. Edward Arnold, London.

Daniel, C. & Mavrodin, A. (1954) L'actinomycose génitale de la femme. *Revue Française de Gynécologie et d'Obstétrique* **29**, 1–11.

Davidson, F. (1977) Yeasts and circumcision in the male. *British Journal of Venereal Diseases* **53**, 121–122.

Davidson, F & Mould, R. (1978) Recurrent genital candidosis in women and the effect of intermittent prophylactic treatment. *British Journal of Venereal Diseases* **54**, 176–183.

Davidson, F. & Oates, J.K. (1985) The pill does not cause 'thrush'. *British Journal of Obstetrics and Gynaecology* **92**, 1265–1266.

Davies, J.A., Rees, E., Hobson, D. *et al.* (1978) Isolation of *Chlamydia trachomatis* from Bartholin's duct. *British Journal of Venereal Diseases* **54**, 409–413.

Davies, T.A. (1931) *Primary Syphilis in the Female.* Oxford University Press, Oxford.

Dennerstein, G.J., Scurry, J.P. & Garland, S.M. (1994) Human papillomavirus vulvitis: a new disease or an unfortunate mistake? *British Journal of Obstetrics and Gynaecology* **101**, 992–998.

de Villiers, E.M., Schneider, A., Gross, G. & zur Hausen, H. (1986) Analysis of benign and malignant urogenital tumours for human papillomavirus infection by labelling cellular DNA. *Medical Microbiology and Immunology* **174**, 281–286.

Diamond, R.D. & Krezesicki, R. (1978) Mechanisms of attachment of neutrophils to *Candida albicans* pseudohyphae in the absence of serum, and of subsequent damage to pseudohyphae by microbicidal processes of neutrophils *in vitro*. *Journal of Clinical Investigation* **61**, 360–365.

Dienes, L. & Edsall, G. (1937) Observations on the L-organisms of Kleinberger. *Proceedings of the Society for Experimental Biology and Medicine* **36**, 740–745.

Dilworth, J.A., Hendley, J.O. & Mandell, G.L. (1975) Attachment and ingestion of gonococci by human neutrophils. *Infection and Immunity* **11**, 512–516.

Drusin, L.M. (1996) Syphilis makes a comeback. *International Journal of STD and AIDS* **7**, 7–9.

Duncan, M.O., Ballard, R.C., Bilgeri, Y.R. *et al.* (1984) Sexually acquired genital ulceration in urban black women. *Southern Africa Journal of Sexually Transmitted Diseases* **4**, 23–27.

Duncan, W.C., Knox, J.M. & Wende, R.D. (1974) The FTA-ABS test in darkfield positive primary syphilis. *Journal of the American Medical Association* **228**, 859–860.

Dürst, M., Gissmann, L., Ikenberg, H., zur Hausen, H. (1983) A papilloma-virus DNA from a cervical carcinoma and its prevalence in cancer biopsies from different geographical regions. *Proceedings of National Academy of Science USA* **80**, 3812–3815.

Easmon, C.S.F. (1986) Bacterial vaginosis. In: *Recent Advances in Sexually Transmitted Diseases 3* (eds J.D. Oriel & J.W.R. Harris) 185–193. Churchill Livingstone, Edinburgh.

Eberle, R. & Courtney, R.J. (1981) Assay of type-specific and type-common antibodies to herpes simplex virus types 1 and 2 in human sera. *Infection and Immunity* **31**, 1062–1072.

Elgart, M.L. & Higdon, R.S. (1973) *Pediculosis pubis* of the scalp. *Archives of Dermatology* **107**, 916.

El Zawahry, M. & El Komy, M. (1973) Amoebiasis cutis. *International Journal of Dermatology* **12**, 305–310.

Embil, J.A., Manuel, F.R. & McFarlane, E.S. (1981) Concurrent oral and genital infection with an identical strain of herpes virus type 1. *Sexually Transmitted Diseases* **8**, 70–72.

Eriksson, G. & Wanger, L. (1975) Frequency of *N. gonorrhoeae*, *Trichomonas vaginalis* and *Candida albicans* in female venereological patients. A one-year study. *British Journal of Venereal Diseases* **51**, 192–197.

Ewing, T.L., Smale, L.E. & Elliott, F.A. (1979) National deaths associated with post-partum vulval oedema. *American Journal of Obstetrics and Gynaecology* **134**, 173–179.

Fair, W.R., Timothy, M.M., Miller, M.A. *et al.* (1970) Bacteriologic and hormonal observations of the urethra and vaginal vestibule in normal premenopausal women. *Journal of Urology* **104**, 426–431.

Fairris, G.M., Stratham, B.N. & Waugh, M.A. (1984) The investigation of patients with genital warts. *British Journal of Dermatology* **111**, 736–738.

Farrell, M.K., Billmire, M.E., Sharroy, J.A. *et al.* (1981) Prepubertal gonorrhoea: a multidisciplinary approach. *Pediatrics* **67**, 151–153.

Feinstein, R.J. (1978) Cutaneous leishmaniasis. *Dermatology* **1**, 45–50.

Feldman, R.G., Johnson, A.L., Schober, P.C. *et al.* (1986) Aetiology of urinary symptoms in sexually active women. *Genitourinary Medicine* **62**, 333–341.

Felman, Y.M. & Nikitas, J.A. (1980) Genital molluscum contagiosum. *Cutis* **26**, 28–35.

Ferenczy, A. (1984a) Comparison of 5-fluorouracil and carbon dioxide laser treatment of vaginal condylomata. *Obstetrics and Gynaecology* **64**, 773–778.

Ferenczy, A. (1984b) Treating genital condylomas during pregnancy with the carbon dioxide laser. *American Journal of Obstetrics and Gynaecology* **148**, 9–12.

Ferenczy, A., Mitao, M., Nasai, N. *et al.* (1985) Latent papillomavirus and recurring genital warts. *New England Journal of Medicine* **313**, 784–788.

Fiddian, A.P., Kinghorn, G.R., Goldmeier, D. *et al.* (1983) Topical acyclovir in the treatment of genital herpes: a comparison with systemic therapy. *Journal of Antimicrobial Chemotherapy* **12** (Suppl. B), 67–77.

Fisher, I. & Morton, R.S. (1970) *Phthirus pubis* infestation. *British Journal of Venereal Diseases* **46**, 326–329.

Fisher, J.R., Conway, M.J. & Takeshita, R.T. (1979) Necrotising fasciitis. Importance of roentgenographic studies for soft-tissue gas. *Journal of the American Medical Association* **241**, 803–807.

Fiumara, N.J. (1980) Treatment of primary and secondary syphilis: serological response. *Journal of the American Medical Association* **243**, 2500–2503.

Fleming, K.A., Venning, V. & Evans, M. (1987) DNA typing of genital warts and a diagnosis of sexual abuse in children. *Lancet* **ii**, 454.

Fournier, J.A. (1906) Quoted by Stokes, J.H. (1944) *Modern Clinical Syphilology*, p. 492. Saunders, Philadelphia.

Fouts, A.C. & Kraus, S.J. (1980) *Trichomonas vaginalis*: re-evaluation of its clinical presentation and laboratory diagnosis. *Journal of Infectious Diseases* 141, 137–143.

Frazer, I.H., Medley, G. & Crapper, R.M. (1986) Association between anorectal dysplasia, human papillomavirus and human immunodeficiency virus in homosexual men. *Lancet* **ii**, 657–660.

Freeman, R.G., McBride, M.E. & Knox, J.M. (1969) Pathogenesis of trichomycosis axillaris. *Archives of Dermatology* **100**, 90–93.

Friedrich, E.G. (1983) The vulval vestibule. *Journal of Reproductive Medicine* **28**, 773–777.

Friedrich, E.G., Wilkinson, E.J. & Fu, Y.S. (1980) Carcinoma *in situ* of the vulva: a continuing challenge. *American Journal of Obstetrics and Gynaecology* 136, 830–843.

Gardner, H.L. & Kaufman, R.H. (1981) Pediatric vulvovaginitis. In: *Benign Diseases of the Vulva and Vagina*, 2nd edn, p. 415. Hall, Boston.

Gardner, M. & Jones, J.G. (1984) Genital herpes acquired from the sexual abuse of children. *Journal of Pediatrics* **104**, 243–244.

Gillespie, W.A., Sellin, M.A., Gill, P. *et al.* (1978) Urinary tract infections in young women, with special reference to *Staphylococcus saprophyticus*. *Journal of Clinical Pathology* **31**, 348–350.

Gissmann, L., de Villiers, E.M. & zur Hausen, H. (1982) Analysis of human genital warts (condylomata acuminata) and other genital tumours for human papillomavirus type 6 DNA. *British Journal of Cancer* **29**, 143–147.

Glatt, A.E., McCormack W.M. & Taylor-Robinson, D. (1990) Genital mycoplasmas. In: *Sexually Transmitted Diseases*, 2nd edn (eds K.K. Holmes, P.-A. Mardh, P.F. Sparling & P.J. Wiesner), pp. 279–293. New York, McGraw-Hill.

Gogoi, M.P. (1969) Amoebiasis of the female genital tract. *American Journal of Obstetrics and Gynaecology* **105**, 1281–1286.

Goldberg, J. (1959) Studies on granuloma inguinale. iv. Growth requirements of *Donovania granulomatis*. *American Journal of Syphilis* 37, 60–70.

Goldmeier D. & Hay, P. (1993) A review and update on adult syphilis. *International Journal of STD and AIDS* **4**, 70–78.

Goldsmith, P.C., Leslie, T.A., Sams, V. *et al.* (1993) Lesions of schistosomiasis mimicking warts on the vulva. *British Medical Journal* **307**, 556–557.

Grabstold, H. & Swan, L. (1952) Genitourinary lesions in leprosy, with special reference to atrophy of the testis. *Journal of the American Medical Association* **149**, 1287–1291.

Grayston, J.T. & Wang, S.-P. (1975) New knowledge of chlamydiae and the diseases thay cause. *Journal of Infectious Diseases* **132**, 87–105.

Greenblatt, R.B., Dienst, R.B. & Baldwin, K.R. (1959) Lymphogranuloma venereum and granuloma inguinale. *Medical Clinics of North America* **43**, 1493–1506.

Greenblatt, R.M., Lukehart, S.A., Plummer, F.A. *et al.* (1988) Genital ulceration as a risk factor for human immunodeficiency infections. *AIDS* **2**, 47–50.

Gross, G. (1990) Interferons in genital HPV disease. In: *Genital Papillomavirus Infections* (eds G. Gross, S. Jablonska, H. Pfister & H.E. Stegner), pp. 393–430. Springer-Verlag, Berlin.

Gross, G., Hagedorn, M., Ikenberg, H. *et al.* (1985) Bowenoid papulosis: presence of human papillomavirus structural antigens and of HPV-related DNA sequences. *Archives of Dermatology* **121**, 858–863.

Growdon, W.A., Fu, Y.S., Lebherz, T.B. *et al.* (1985) Pruritic vulval squamous papillomatosis evidence for human papillomavirus aetiology. *Obstetrics and Gynaecology* **66**, 564–568.

Grussendorf-Conen, E.I., de Villiers, E.M. & Gissmann, L. (1986) Human papillomavirus genomes in penile smears of healthy men. *Lancet* **ii**, 1092.

Guerrero, E. & Shah, K.V. (1991) Polymerase chain reaction in HPV diagnosis. *Papillomavirus Reports* **2**, 115–118.

Guinan, M.E., MacCallum, J., Kern, E. *et al.* (1981) Course of an untreated episode of recurrent genital herpes infection in 27 women. *New England Journal of Medicine* **304**, 759–763.

Gutman, L.T., St Claire, K.K. & Everett, V.D. (1994) Cervicovaginal and intra-anal HPV infection of young girls with external genital warts. *Journal of Infectious Diseases* **1170**, 339–343.

Hager, W.D., Brown, S.T., Kraus, S.J. *et al.* (1980) Metronidazole for vaginal trichomoniasis: seven day vs single dose regimens. *Journal of the American Medical Association* **244**, 1219–1220.

Hammar, H. & Wanger, L. (1977) Erysipelas and necrotising fasciitis. *British Journal of Dermatology* **96**, 409–419.

Hammond, G.W., Slutchuk, M., Scatliff, J. *et al.* (1980) Epidemiologic, clinical, laboratory and therapeutic features of an urban outbreak of chancroid in North America. *Review of Infectious Diseases* **2**, 867–879.

Handley, J.M., Maw, R.D., Horner, T. *et al.* (1991) Self-treatment of primary anogenital warts in males with podophyllin 0.5% in ethanol vs podophyllotoxin 0.5%: a randomised double blind comparative study. *Venereology* **4**, 84–87.

Handley, J.M., Maw, R.D., Bingham, E.A. *et al.* (1993) Anogenital warts in children. *Clinical and Experimental Dermatology* **18**, 241–247.

Hanna, L., Schmidt, L., Sharp, M. *et al.* (1979) Human cell-mediated immune responses to chlamydial antigens. *Infection and Immunity* **23**, 412–417.

Hannah, P. & Greenwood, J.R. (1982) Isolation and rapid identification of *Haemophilus ducreyi*. *Journal of Clinical Microbiology* **16**, 861–864.

Harman, R.R.M. (1986) Parasitic worms and protozoa. In: *Textbook of Dermatology*, 4th edn (eds A. Rook, D.S. Wilkinson & F.J.G. Ebling) Chap. 26. Blackwell Scientific Publications, Oxford.

Hart, G. (1975) *Chancroid, Donovanosis, Lymphogranuloma Venereum*. US Department of Health, Education & Welfare Publication No. CDC 75-8302.

Heller, R.H., Joseph, J.M. & Davis, H.J. (1969) Vulvovaginitis in the premenarcheal child. *Journal of Pediatrics* **74**, 370–377.

Hicks, C.B., Benson, P.M. & Lupton, G.P. (1987) Seronegative secondary syphilis in a patient infected with the human immunodeficiency virus with Kaposi's sarcoma: a diagnostic dilemma. *Annals of Internal Medicine* **107**, 492–495.

Highet, A.S., Warren, R.E., Staughton, R.C.D. *et al.* (1980) *Streptococcus milleri* causing treatable infection in perineal hidradenitis suppurativa. *British Journal of Dermatology* **103**, 375–382.

Hillier, S.L., Critchlow, C.W., Stevens, C.E. *et al.* (1991) Microbiological, epidemiological and clinical correlates of vaginal infection by *Mobiluncus* spp. *Genitourinary Medicine* **67**, 26–31.

Hilton, A.L. & Warnock, D.W. (1975) Vaginal candidosis and the role of the digestive tract as a source of infectoion. *British Journal of Obstetrics and Gynaecology* **82**, 922–926.

Hipp, S.S., Lawton, W.D., Chen, N.C. *et al.* (1974) Inhibition of *Neisseria gonorrhoeae* by a factor produced by *Candida albicans*. *Applied Microbiology* **27**, 192–196.

Ho, G.Y.F., Burk, R.D., Fleming, I. *et al.* (1994) Risk of genital human papillomavirus infection in women with HIV-induced immunosuppression. *International Journal of Cancer* **56**, 788–792.

Holmberg, S.D., Stewart, J.A., Gerber, A.R. *et al.* (1988) Prior HSV type 2 infection as a risk factor for HIV infections. *Journal of the American Medical Association* **259**, 1048–1050.

Holt, L.E. (1905) Gonococcus infections in children, with especial reference to their prevalence in institutions and means of prevention. *New York Medical Journal* **81**, 521–526, 589–592.

Honigberg, B.M. (1978) Trichomonads of importance in human medicine. In: *Parasitic Protozoa*, Vol. 2 (ed. J.P. Kreiser), p. 275. New York, Academic Press.

Hording, U., Kringsholm, B., Andreasson, B. *et al.* (1993) Human papillomavirus in vulval squamous cell carcinoma and in normal vulval tissues: a search for a possible impact of HPV on vulval cancer progression. *International Journal of Cancer* **55**, 394–396.

Huff, J.C., Drucker, J.L., Clemmer, A. *et al.* (1993) Effect of oral acyclovir on pain resolution in herpes zoster: a reanalysis. *Journal of Medical Virology* (Suppl. 1), 93–96.

Hunt, E. (1954) Ulcers of the vulva. In: *Diseases Affecting the Vulva*, 4th edn, p. 122. Henry Kimpton, London.

Hurley, R. & de Louvois, J. (1979) Candida vaginitis. *Postgraduate Medical Journal* **55**, 645–649.

Hutchinson, P.E., Summerly, R. & Lawson, R.S. (1976) Progressive postoperative gangrene: a reminder. *British Journal of Dermatology* **194**, 89–95.

Ikenberg, H., Gissmann, L., Gross, G. *et al.* (1983) Haman papillomavirus type 16-related DNA in genital Bowen's disease and Bowenoid papulosis. *International Journal of Cancer* **32**, 563–565.

Ingram, J.T. (1955) Tinea of the vulva. *British Medical Journal* **ii**, 1500.

Jablonska, S. & Orth, G. (1983) Human papillomavirus. In: *Recent Advances in Dermatology 6* (eds A.J. Rook & H.I. Maibach), p. 1. Churchill Livingstone, Edinburgh.

James, J.R.E. (1968) Orf in man. *British Medical Journal* **iii**, 804–806.

Janson, P. (1959) Seltere Zoster verlaufeformen. *Zeitschrift für Haut und Geschlechtskrankheiten* **26**, 292.

Jarrett, W.F.H., McNeil, P.E., Grimshaw, W.T.R. *et al.* (1978) High incidence area of cattle cancer with a possible interaction between an environmental carcinogen and a papillomavirus. *Nature* **274**, 215–217.

Jelliffe, D.B. & Jacobson, F.W. (1954) The clinical picture of tinea versicolor in negro infants. *Journal of Tropical Medicine and Hygiene* **57**, 290–292.

Johnson, C.G. & Mellanby, K. (1972) The parasitology of human scabies. *Parasitology* **39**, 285–290.

Jopling, W.H. & Harman, R.R.M. (1986) Leprosy. In: *Textbook of Dermatology*, 4th edn (eds A. Rook, D.S. Wilkinson & F.J.G. Ebling), p. 823. Blackwell Scientific Publications, Oxford.

Judson, F.N. & Ruder, M.A. (1979) Effect of hysterectomy on genital infections. *British Journal of Venereal Diseases* **55**, 434–438.

Kacker, T.P. (1973) Vulvovaginitis in an adult with threadworms in the vagina. *British Journal of Venereal Diseases* **49**, 314–315.

Kakoti, L.M. & Dey, N.C. (1957) Chronic blastomycosis in India. *Journal of the Indian Medical Association* **28**, 351.

Kalter, D.C., Tschen, J.A., Cernoch, P.K. *et al.* (1986) Genital white piedra: epidemiology, microbiology and therapy. *Journal of the American Academy of Dermatology* **14**, 982–993.

Katzman, M., Carey, J.T., Elmets, C.A. *et al.* (1987) Molluscum contagiosum and the acquired immunodeficiency syndrome: clinical and immunological details of two cases. *British Journal of Dermatology* **116**, 131–138.

Kearns, D.H., Seibert, G.B., O'Reilly, R. *et al.* (1973) Paradox of the immune response to uncomplicated gonococcal urethritis. *New England Journal of Medicine* **289**, 1170–1174.

Keh, B. & Poorbaugh, J.H. (1977) Understanding and treating infestations of lice on humans. *California Vector Views* **47**, 349–356.

King, A., Nicol, C.S. & Rodin, P. (1980) *Venereal Diseases*, 4th edn, pp. 53, 215. Baillière Tindall, London.

Kiviat, N., Rompalo, A., Bowden, R. *et al.* (1990) Anal human papillomavirus infection among human immunodeficiency virus seropositive and seronegative men. *Journal of Infectious Diseases* **162**, 358–361.

Knox, S.R., Corey, L., Blough, H.A. *et al.* (1982) Historical findings in subjects from a high socioeconomic group who have genital infections with herpes simplex virus. *Sexually Transmitted Diseases* **9**, 15–20.

Konrad, K. (1936) Ulceroses Syphilid zwei Jahre nach durchgefuhrer Malariakur. *Zentralblatt fur Hant- und Geschlechtskrankheiten* **53**, 150.

Kreiss, J.K., Coombs, R., Plummer, F. *et al.* (1980) Isolation of human immunodeficiency virus from genital ulcers in Nairobi prostitutes. *Journal of Infectious Diseases* **160**, 380–384.

Krogstad, D.J., Spencer, H.C. & Healy, G.R. (1978) Current concepts in parasitology: amoebiasis. *New England Journal of Medicine* **298**, 262–265.

Lal, S. & Nicholas, C. (1970) Epidemiological and clinical features in 165 cases of granuloma inguinale. *British Journal of Venereal Diseases* **46**, 461–463.

Landthaler, M., Hohenleutner, U., Haina, D. *et al.* (1990) Laser therapy of anogenital papillomavirus infections—the view of the dermatologist. In: *Genital Papillomavirus Infections* (eds G. Gross, S. Jablonska, H. Pfister & H.E. Spegner), pp. 341–348. Springer-Verlag, Berlin.

Lang, W.R., Israel, S.L. & Fritx, M.A. (1958) Staphylococcal vulvovaginitis: a report of two cases following antibiotic therapy. *Obstetrics and Gynecology* **11**, 352–354.

Larson, P., Platz-Christenseri, J., Thejis, H. *et al.* (1992) Incidence of pelvic inflammatory disease after first-trimester legal abortion in women with bacterial vaginosis. *American Journal of Obstetrics and Gynecology* **166**, 100–103.

Lawson, J.B. (1967) Chronic lymphoedema and elephantiasis of the vulva. In: *Obstetrics and Gynaecology in the Tropics and Developing Countries* (eds J.B. Lawson & D.B. Stewart), p. 466. Arnold, London.

Lee, Y.-H., Rankin, J.S., Albert, S. *et al.* (1977) Microbiological investigation of Bartholin's gland abscesses and cysts. *American Journal of Obstetrics and Gynecology* **129**, 150–153.

Lesinski, J., Krach, J. & Kadziewicz, E. (1974) Specificity, sensitivity and diagnostic value of the TPHA test. *British Journal of Venereal Diseases* **50**, 334–340.

Lever, W.F. & Schaumberg-Lever, G. (1975) *Histology of the Skin*, 5th edn, pp. 337–360. Lippincott, Philadelphia.

Levin, M.J. (1991) Genital herpes simplex. In: *Laboratory Methods for the Diagnosis of Sexually Transmitted Diseases*, 2nd edn (eds B.B. Wentworth, F.N. Judson & M.J.R. Gilchrist), pp. 128–164. American Public Health Association, Washington.

Levine, R.U., Crum, C.P., Herman, E. *et al.* (1984) Cervical papillomavirus infection and intra-epithelial neoplasia: a study of male sex partners. *Obstetrics and Gynecology* **64**, 16–20.

Lohmeyer, H. (1974) Treatment of candidosis and trichomoniasis of the female genital tract. *Postgraduate Medical Journal* **50**, S81.

Lomax, C.W., Harbert, G.M. & Thornton, W.N. (1976) Actinomycosis of the female genital tract. *Obstetrics and Gynecology* **48**, 341–346.

Long, S.R., Whitfield, M.J., Eades, C., Korn, A.P. & Zaloudek, C.J. (1996) Bacillary angiomatosis of the cervix and vulva in a patient with AIDS. *Obstetrics and Gynecology* **88**, 709–711.

Lukehart, S.A., Baker-Zander, S.A., Lloyd, R.M. *et al.* (1980) Characterisation of lymphocyte responsiveness in early experimental syphilis. II Nature of cellular infiltration and *Treponema pallidum* distribution in testicular lesions. *Journal of Immunology* **124**, 461–467.

Lutzner, M. (1985) Papillomavirus lesions in immunodepression and immunosuppression. *Clinical Dermatology* **3**, 165–169.

Lyng, J. & Christensen, J.A. (1981) A double-blind study of the value of treatment with a single-dose timidazole of partners to females with trichomoniasis. *Acta Obstetrica Gynecologica Scandinavica* **60**, 199–204.

Macasaet, M.A., Duerr, A., Thelmo, W. *et al.* (1995) Kaposi sarcoma presenting as a vulval mass. *Obstetrics and Gynecology* **86**, 695–697.

McCormack, W.M., Almeida, P.C., Bailey, P.E. *et al.* (1972) Sexual activity and vaginal colonisation with genital mycoplasmas. *Journal of the American Medical Association* **221**, 1375–1377.

Machnicki, S. (1953) Diphtheria of the vulva and vagina. *Zeitschrift für Haut- und Geschlechtskrankheiten* **86**, 386.

McKay, M (1989) Vulvodynia. *Archives of Dermatology* **125**, 256–262.

McKee, P.H., Wright, E. & Hutt, M.S.R. (1983) Vulval schistosomiasis. *Clinical and Experimental Dermatology* **8**, 189–194.

McLaren, L.C., Davis, L.E., Healy, G.R. *et al.* (1983) Isolation of *Trichomonas vaginalis* from the respiratory tract of infants with respiratory disease. *Pediatrics* **71**, 888–890.

McNabb, P.C. & Tomasi, T.B. (1981) Host defence mechanisms at mucosal surfaces. *Annual Review of Microbiology* **35**, 477–496.

Maiman, M., Fruchter, R.G., Serur, E. *et al.* (1990) Human immunodeficiency virus infection and cervical neoplasia. *Gynecologic Oncology* **38**, 377–382.

Majmudar, B., Chaiken, M.C. & Lee, K.U. (1976) Amoebiasis of clitoris mimicking carcinoma. *Journal of the American Medical Association* **236**, 1145–1146.

Mårdh, P.-A. (1991) The vaginal ecosystem. *American Journal of Obstetrics and Gynecology* **165**, 1163–1168.

Mårdh, P.-A. & Soltesz, L. (1983) *In vitro* interactions between lactobacilli and other micro-organisms occurring in the vaginal flora. *Scandinavian Journal of Infectious Diseases* (Suppl. 40), 47–51.

Marsden, P.D. (1979) Current concepts in parasitology: leishmaniasis. *New England Journal of Medicine* **300**, 350–355.

Matras, G. (1935) Lues III. Ulcer gummosa. *Zentralbum für Haut und Geshlechtskrankheiten* **51**, 89.

Mattox, T.F., Rutgers, J., Yoshimori, R.N. *et al.* (1993) Non-fluorescent erythrasma of the vulva. *Obstetrics and Gynecology* **81**, 862–864.

Meisels, A., Fortin, R. & Roy, M. (1977) Condylomatous lesions of the cervix and vagina II. Cytologic, colposcopic and histopathologic study. *Acta Cytologica* **21**, 379–390.

Meisels, A., Morin, C. & Casas-Cordero, M. (1982) Human papillomavirus infection of the cervix. *International Journal of Gynecologic Pathology* **1**, 75–94.

Meleney, F.L., Friedman, S.T. & Harvey, H.D. (1945) The treatment of progressive bacterial synergistic gangrene with penicillin. *Surgery* **18**, 423–435.

Meltzer, R.M. (1983) Necrotising fasciitis and progressive synergistic bacterial gangrene. *Obstetrics and Gynecology* **61**, 757–760.

Mercey, D.E. & Mindel, A. (1991) Preventing neonatal herpes? *Genitourinary Medicine* **67**, 1–2.

Mertz, G.J. (1990) Genital herpes simplex virus infection. *Medical Clinics of North America* **74**, 1433–1454.

Miles, M.R., Olsen, L. & Rogers, A. (1977) Recurrent vaginal candidiasis. Importance of an intestinal reservoir. *Journal of the American Medical Association* **238**, 1836–1837.

Miller, P.I., Humphries, M. & Grassick, K. (1984) A single-blind comparison of oral and intravaginal treatments in acute and recurrent vaginal candidosis in general practice. *Pharmatherapeutica* **3**, 582–587.

Milne, J.D. & Warnock, D.W. (1979) Effect of simultaneous oral and vaginal treatment on the rate of cure and relapse in vaginal candidosis. *British Journal of Venereal Diseases* **55**, 362–365.

Mindel, A. (1991) Antiviral chemotherapy for genital herpes. *Reviews in Medical Virology* **1**, 111–118.

Minkoff, H.L., McCalla, S., Delke, I. *et al.* (1990) The relationship of cocaine use to syphilis and human immunodeficiency virus infections among inner city parturient women. *American Journal of Obstetrics and Gynecology* **163**, 521–526.

Montaldi, D.H., Giambrone, J.P., Courey, N.G. *et al.* (1974) Podophyllin poisoning associated with the treatment of condylomata acuminata: a case report. *American Journal of Obstetrics and Gynecology* **119**, 1130–1131.

Montes, L.F. & Black, S.H. (1967) Fine structure of diphtheroids of erythrasma. *Journal of Investigative Dermatology* **48**, 342–346.

Moore, D. (1954) Genito-peritoneal tuberculosis—a review of 26 cases. *South African Medical Journal* **28**, 666–673.

Mounts, P. & Shah, K.V. (1984) Respiratory papillomatosis: etiology related to genital tract papillomaviruses. *Progress in Medical Virology* **29**, 90–114.

Moyal-Barraco, M., Leibowitch, M. & Orth, G. (1990) Vestibular papillae of the vulva. *Archives of Dermatology* **126**, 1594–1598.

Mursic, V.P. (1975) Diagnosis, pathogenicity and therapy of candidosis. *Munchen Medische Wochenschrift* **117**, 893–896.

Nabarro, D. (1954) *Congenital Syphilis*. Edward Arnold, London.

Naguib, S.M., Cornstock, G.W. & Davis, H.J. (1966) Epidemiologic study of trichomoniasis in normal women. *Obstetrics and Gynecology* **27**, 607–616.

Nahmias, A.J. (1970) Disseminated herpes simplex virus infection. *New England Journal of Medicine* **282**, 684–686.

Nahmias, A.J. & Roizman, B. (1973) Infection with herpes simplex viruses 1 and 2. *New England Journal of Medicine* **289**, 666–673, 719–725, 781–789.

Nahmias, A.J., Dowdle, W.R., Naib, Z.M. *et al.* (1968) Genital infection with herpesvirus hominis types 1 and 2 in children. *Pediatrics* **42**, 659–666.

Nahmias, A.J., Josey, W.E., Naib, Z.M. *et al.* (1971) Perinatal risk associated with maternal genital herpes simplex virus infection. *American Journal of Obstetrics and Gynecology* **110**, 825–834.

Noble, W.C. (1981) *Microbiology of Human Skin*, 2nd edn. Lloyd Luke, London.

Obalek, S., Jablonska, S., Favre, M. *et al.* (1990) Condylomata acuminata in children: frequent association with human papillomaviruses responsible for cutaneous warts. *Journal of the American Academy of Dermatology* **23**, 205–213.

Odds, F.C. (1988) *Candida and Candidosis*, 2nd edn. Baillière Tindall, London.

Orfanos, C.E., Schloesser, E. & Mahrie, G. (1971) Hair destroying growth of *Corynebacterium tenuis* in the so-called trichomycosis axillaris. *Archives of Dermatology* **103**, 632–636.

Oriel, J.D. (1971) Natural history of genital warts. *British Journal of Venereal Diseases* **47**, 1–13.

Oriel, J.D. & Robinson, A. (1995) Human papillomavirus in children. In: *Genital Warts: Human Papillomavirus Infection* (ed. A. Mindel), pp. 237–251. Edward Arnold, London.

Oriel, J.D. & Waterworth, P.M. (1975) Effect of minocycline and tetracycline on the vaginal yeast flora. *Journal of Clinical Pathology* **28**, 403–406.

Oriel, J.D., Partridge, B.M., Denny, M.J. *et al.* (1972) Genital yeast infections. *British Medical Journal* **iv**, 761–764.

Orkin, M. & Maibach, H.I. (1984) Current views of scabies and pediculosis pubis. *Cutis* **33**, 85–97.

Ovcinnikov, N.M., Delektorskii, V.V., Turanova, E.N. *et al.* (1975) Further studies of *Trichomonas vaginalis* with transmission and scanning electron microscopy. *British Journal of Venereal Diseases* **51**, 357–375.

Paavonen, J. (1979) *Chlamydia trachomatis* induced urethritis in female partners of men with non-gonococcal urethritis. *Sexually Transmitted Diseases* **10**, 271–275.

Padel, A.F., Venning, V.A., Evans, M.F., Quantrill, A.M. & Fleming, K.A. (1990) Human papillomaviruses in anogenital warts in children: typing by *in situ* hybridisation. *British Medical Journal* **300**, 1491–1494.

Parks, J. (1941) Diphtheritic vaginitis in the adult. *American Journal of Obstetrics and Gynecology* **41**, 714–718.

Pauly, C.R., Artis, W.M. & Jones, H.E. (1978) Atopic dermatitis, impaired cellular immunity and molluscum contagiosum. *Archives of Dermatology* **114**, 391–396.

Perine, P.L., Andersen, A.J., Krause, D.W. *et al.* (1980) Diagnosis and treatment of lymphogranuloma venereum in Ethiopia. In: *Current Chemotherapy and Infectious Diseases* (ed. K.K. Holmes), pp. 1280–1282. American Society for Microbiology, Washington DC.

Perl, G. (1972) Errors in the diagnosis of *Trichomonas vaginalis* infection as observed among 1199 patients. *Obstetrics and Gynecology* **39**, 7–12.

Pheifer, T.A., Forsyth, P.S., Durfee, M.A. *et al.* (1978) Non-specific vaginitis: role of *Haemophilus vaginalis* and treatment with metronidazole. *New England Journal of Medicine* **298**, 1429–1434.

Plourde, P.J., Pepin, J., Agoki, E. *et al.* (1994) HIV Type 1 seroconversion in women with genital ulcers. *Journal of the American Academy of Dermatology* **5**, 249–263.

Plummer, F.A., Kraus, S.J., Sottnek, F.O. *et al.* (1984) Chancroid and granuloma inguinale. In: *Laboratory Methods for the Diagnosis of Sexually Transmitted Diseases*, 2nd edn (eds B.B. Wentworth, F.N. Judson & M.J.R. Gilchrist), pp. 237–257. American Public Health Association, Washington DC.

Portnoy, J., Ahronheim, G.A., Ghibu, F. *et al.* (1984) Recovery of Epstein–Barr virus from genital ulcers. *New England Journal of Medicine* **311**, 966–968.

Prober, O.G., Sullender, W.M., Yasukawa, L.L. *et al.* (1987) Low risk of herpes simplex infections in neonates exposed to the virus at the time of delivery to mothers with recurrent genital herpes simplex virus infection. *New England Journal of Medicine* **316**, 240–244.

Purdie, D.W., Carty, M.J. & McLeod. (1977) Tubo-ovarian actinomycosis and the intrauterine contraceptive device. *British Medical Journal* **ii**, 1392.

Quinn, T.C., Cannon, R.O., Glasser, D. *et al.* (1990) The association of syphilis with risk of human immunodeficiency virus infection in patients attending sexually transmitted diseases clinics. *Archives of Internal Medicine* **150**, 1297–1302.

Raab, B. & Lorincz, A.L. (1981) Genital herpes simplex—concepts and treatment. *Journal of the American Academy of Dermatology* **5**, 249–263.

Rajah, Moodley, J., Pudifin, D. *et al.* (1990) Kaposi's sarcoma associated with acquired immunodeficiency syndrome presenting as vulval papilloma. *South African Medical Journal* **77**, 585–586.

Rando, R.F., Sedlacek, T.V., Hunt, J. *et al.* (1986) Verrucous carcinoma of the vulva associated with an unusual type 6 human papillomavirus. *Obstetrics and Gynecology* **67**, 70S–75S.

Rea, W.J. & Wyrick, W.J. (1970) Necrotising fasciitis. *Annals of Surgery* **172**, 957–963.

Rees, E. (1967) Gonococcal bartholinitis. *British Journal of Venereal Diseases* **43**, 150–156.

Reeves, W.C., Corey, L., Adams, H.G. *et al.* (1981) Risk of recurrence after first episode of genital herpes: relation to HSV type and antibody response. *New England Journal of Medicine* **305**, 315–319.

Reichman, R.C., Badger, G.J., Mertz, G.J. *et al.* (1984) Treatment of recurrent herpes simplex infection with oral acyclovir. *Journal of the American Medical Association* **251**, 2103–2107.

Reid, R. (1985) Superficial laser vulvectomy 1. The efficiency of extended superficial ablation for refractory and very extensive condylomas. *American Journal of Obstetrics and Gynecology* **151**, 1047–1052.

Reid, R. & Greenberg, M.D. (1991) Human papillomavirus-related diseases of the vulva. *Clinical Obstetrics and Gynecology* **34**, 630–650.

Reid, R., Laverty, C.R., Coppleson, M. *et al.* (1980) Noncondylomatous cervical wart virus infection. *Obstetrics and Gynecology* **151**, 1047–1052.

Rein, M.F., Sullivan, J.A. & Mandell, G.L. (1980) Trichomonacidal activity of human polymorphonuclear leucocytes: killing by disruption and fragmentation. *Journal of Infectious Diseases* **142**, 575–585.

Ricci, J. (1945) *One Hundred Years of Gynecology, 1800–1900*, p. 470. Blakiston, Philadelphia.

Richens, J. (1991) The diagnosis and management of donovanosis (granuloma inguinale). *British Journal of Venereal Diseases* **67**, 441–452.

Ridgway, G.L. (1996) Azithromycin in the management of *Chlamydia trachomatis* infections. *International Journal of STD and AIDS* **7**, (Suppl. 1), 5–8.

Ridley, C.M. (1984) Vulval dysplasia. *British Journal of Hospital Medicine* **159**, 223.

Roberts, D.B. & Hester, L.L. (1972) Progressive synergistic bacterial gangrene arising from abscesses of the vulva and Bartholin's gland. *American Journal of Obstetrics and Gynecology* **114**, 285–290.

Rodin, P. & Hass, G. (1966) Metronidazole and pregnancy. *British Journal of Venereal Diseases* **42**, 210–212.

Ronald, A.R. (1986) Laboratory diagnosis of *Haemophilus ducreyi* infection. In: *Recent Advances in Sexually Transmitted Diseases 3* (eds J.D. Oriel & J.R.W. Harris), pp. 59–69. Churchill Livingstone, Edinburgh.

Rose, P.G. & Fraire, A.E. (1993) Multiple gynaecological neoplasms in a young HIV-positive patient. *Journal of Surgical Oncology* **53**, 269–272.

Rowen, D., Carne, C.A., Sonnex, C. *et al.* (1991) Increased incidence of cervical cytological abnormalities in women with genital warts or contact with genital warts: a need for increased vigilance? *Genitourinary Medicine* **67**, 460–463.

Rudlinger, R., Buchmann, P., Grob, F. *et al.* (1990) Genitoanal HPV infections in immunodeficient individuals. In: *Genital Papillomavirus Infections* (eds G. Gross, S. Jablonska, H. Pfister & H.E. Stegner), pp. 249–260. Springer-Verlag, Berlin.

Rustia, M. & Shubik, P. (1972) Induction of lung tumours and malignant melanomas in mice by metronidazole. *Journal of the National Cancer Institute* **48**, 421–428.

Sarkany, I., Taplin, D. & Blank, H. (1961) Erythrasma. *Journal of the American Medical Association* **177**, 130–133.

Schachner, L. & Hankin, D.E. (1985) Assessing child abuse in childhood condylomata acuminata. *Journal of the American Academy of Dermatology* **12**, 157–160.

Schachter, J. & Dawson, C.R. (1978) *Human Chlamydial Infection*, pp. 45–62. PSG Publishing Company, Littleton, MA.

Schaefer, G. (1959) Diagnosis and treatment of female genital tuberculosis. *Clinical Obstetrics and Gynecology* **2**, 530–535.

Schneider, A. (1993) Pathogenesis of genital HPV infection. *Genitourinary Medicine* **69**, 165–173.

Schneider, V., Kay, S. & Lee, H.M. (1983) Immunosuppression as a high-risk factor in the development of condyloma acuminatum and squamous neoplasia of the cervix. *Acta Cytologica* **27**, 220–224.

Schwartz, P.E. & Naftolin, F. (1981) Type 2 herpes simplex virus and vulval carcinoma in situ. *New England Journal of Medicine* **305**, 517–518.

Scott, R.A., Gallis, H.A. & Livengood, C.H. (1985) Phycomycosis of the vulva. *American Journal of Obstetrics and Gynecology* **153**, 675–676.

Shelley, W.B. & Miller, M.A. (1984) Electron microscopy, histochemistry and microbiology of bacterial adhesion in trichomycosis axillaris. *Journal of the American Academy of Dermatology* **10**, 1005–1014.

Shokri-Tabibzadeh, S., Koss, L., Molnar, J. *et al.* (1981) Association of human papillomavirus and neoplastic processes in the genital tract of four women with impaired immunity. *Gynecologic Oncology* **12**, S129–S140.

Shy, K.K. & Eschenbach, D.A. (1981) Fatal perineal cellulitis from an episiotomy site. *Obstetrics and Gynecology* **54**, 292–298.

Siegal, F.P., Lopez, C., Hammer, G.S. *et al.* (1981) Severe acquired immunodeficiency in male homosexuals manifested by chronic perianal ulcerative herpes simplex lesions. *New England Journal of Medicine* **305**, 1439–1444.

Sobel, J.D. (1990) Vulvovaginal candidiasis. In: *Sexually Transmitted Diseases*, 2nd edn (eds K.K. Holmes, P.-A. Mardh, P.F. Sparling & P.J. Wiesner), pp. 521–522. McGraw-Hill, New York.

Somerville, D.A., Seville, R.H., Cunningham, R.C. *et al.* (1970) Erythrasma in a hospital for the mentally subnormal. *British Journal of Dermatology* **82**, 355–358.

Soper, D.E., Bump, R.C. & Hurt, W.G. (1990) Bacterial vaginosis and trichomonal vaginitis are risk factors for cuff cellulitis after abdominal hysterectomy. *American Journal of Obstetrics and Gynecology* **163**, 1016–1023.

Sowmini, C.N. (1983) In: *International Perspectives on Neglected Sexually Transmitted Diseases* (eds K.K. Holmes & P.-A. Mardh), p. 205. Hemisphere, Washington DC.

Sparks, R.A., Williams, G.C., Boyce, J.M.H. *et al.* (1975) Antenatal screening for candidiasis, trichomoniasis and gonorrhoea. *British Journal of Venereal Diseases* **51**, 110–115.

Spencer, E.S. & Andersen, H.K. (1970) Viral infections in renal allograft recipients treated with long term immunosuppression. *British Medical Journal* **ii**, 829–830.

Spruance, S.L. (1984) Pathogenesis of herpes simplex labialis: excretion of virus into the oral cavity. *Journal of Clinical Microbiology* **19**, 675–679.

Stagno, S. & Whitley, R.J. (1990) Herpes virus infections in the neonate and children. In: *Sexually Transmitted Diseases*, 2nd edn (eds K.K. Holmes, P.-A. Mardh, P.F. Sparling & P.J. Wiesner), pp. 863–887. McGraw-Hill, New York.

Stamm, W.E., Guinan, M.E., Johnson, C. *et al.* (1984) Effect of treatment regimens for *Neisseria gonorrhoeae* on simultaneous infections with *Chlamydia trachomatis*. *New England Journal of Medicine* **310**, 545–549.

Stokes, E.J. & Ridgway, G.L. (1987) *Clinical Microbiology*, 6th edn, pp. 103–106. Edward Arnold, London.

Stone, H.H. & Martin, J.D. (1972) Synergistic necrotising cellulitis. *Annal of Surgery* **175**, 702–711.

Symmers, W. StC. (1960) Leishmaniasis acquired by contagion. A case of marital infection in Britain. *Lancet* **i**, 1276.

Syrjänen, K., Vayrynen, M., Castren, O. *et al.* (1984) Sexual behaviour of women with human papillomavirus lesions of the uterine cervix. *British Journal of Venereal Diseases* **60**, 243–248.

Tang, C.K., Shermeta, D.W. & Wood, C. (1978) Congenital condylomata acuminata. *American Journal of Obstetrics and Gynecology* **131**, 912–913.

Taylor-Robinson, D. (1991) Genital chlamydial infections: clinical aspects, diagnosis, treatment and prevention. In: *Recent Advances in Sexually Transmitted Diseases and AIDS* (eds J.R.W. Harris & S.M. Forster), pp. 219–262. Churchill Livingstone, Edinburgh.

Taylor-Robinson, D. (1995) The history and role of *Mycoplasma genitalium* in sexually transmitted diseases. *Genitourinary Medicine* **71**, 1–8.

Tenover, F.C. (1988) Diagnostic deoxyribonucleic acid probes for infectious diseases. *Clinical Microbiology Reviews* **1**, 82–101.

Thiboutot, D.M., Beckford, A., Mart, C.A., Sexton, M. & Maloney, M.E. (1991) Cytomegalovirus diaper dermatitis. *Archives of Dermatology* **127**, 396–398.

Thin, R.N.T. (1970) Direct and delayed methods of immunofluorescent diagnosis of gonorrhoea in woman. *British Journal of Venereal Diseases* **47**, 27–30.

Thin, R.N.T. & Shaw, E.J. (1979) Diagnosis of gonorrhoea in women. *British Journal of Venereal Diseases* **55**, 10–13.

Thin, R.N.T., Leighton, M. & Dixon, M.J. (1977) How often is genital yeast infection sexually transmitted? *British Medical Journal* **ii**, 93–94.

Thomas, B.J., MacLeod, E.J. & Taylor-Robinson, D. (1993) Evaluation of the sensitivity of 10 diagnostic assays for *Chlamydia trachomatis* by use of a simple laboratory procedure. *Journal of Clinical Pathology* **46**, 408–411.

Thomason, J.L., Gelbart, S.M., Sobun, J.F. *et al.* (1988) Comparison of four methods to detect *Trichomonas vaginalis*. *Journal of Clinical Microbiology* **26**, 1869–1870.

Thomson, J.F.S. & Grace, R.H. (1978) Treatment of perianal and anal condylomata acuminata. A new operative technique. *Journal of the Royal Society of Medicine* **71**, 181–185.

Turner, T.B. & Hollander, D.H. (1957) *Biology of the Treponematoses*, p. 42. WHO Monograph Series 35. WHO, Geneva.

Vonka, V., Kanka, J., Jelinek, K. *et al.* (1984) Prospective study on the relationship between cervical neoplasia and herpes simplex type 2 virus. 1. Epidemiological characteristics. *International Journal of Cancer* **33**, 49–60.

Wagman, H. (1975) Genital actinomycosis. *Proceedings of the Royal Society of Medicine* **68**, 228–230.

Wagstaff, A.J., Faulds, D. & Goa, K.L. (1994) Acyclovir. A reappraisal of its antiviral activity, pharmacokinetic properties and therapeautic efficacy. *Drugs* **47**, 153–205.

Walkinshaw, S.A., Dodgson, J., McCance, D.J. *et al.* (1988) Risk factors in the development of cervical intraepithelial neoplasia in women with vulval warts. *Genitourinary Medicine* **64**, 316–320.

Wallin, J. (1975) Gonorrhoea in 1972. A one year study of patients attending the VD unit in Uppsala. *British Journal of Venereal Diseases* **51**, 41–47.

Watts, H., Kontsky, L.A., Holmes, K.K., Goldman, D., Kuypers, J., Kiviat, N.B. & Galloway, D.A. (1998) Low risk of perinatal transmission of human papillomavirus: Results from a prospective cohort study. *American Journal of Obstetrics and Gynecology* **178**, 365–373.

Waugh, M.A. (1974) Herpes zoster of the anogenital area affecting urination and defaecation. *British Journal of Dermatology* **90**, 235–238.

Wende, R.D., Mudd, R.L., Knox, J.M. & Holder, W.R. (1971) The VDRL slide test in 322 cases of dark-field positive primary syphilis. *Southern Medical Journal* **64**, 633–634.

White, S.W. & Smith, J. (1979) Trichomycosis pubis. *Archives of Dermatology* **115**, 444–445.

Whitley, R.J., Nahmias, A.J., Visintine, A.M. *et al.* (1980) The natural history of herpes simplex virus infection of mother and new-born. *Pediatrics* **66**, 489–494.

Whitley, R.J., Levin, M., Barton, N. *et al.* (1984) Infections caused by herpes simplex virus in the immunocompromised host: natural history and topical acyclovir therapy. *Journal of Infectious Diseases* **150**, 323–329.

Whittington, M.J. (1957) Epidemiology of infections with *Trichomonas vaginalis* in the light of improved diagnostic methods. *British Journal of Venereal Diseases* **33**, 80–91.

Wilson, J. (1973) Extensive vulval condylomata acuminata necessitating Caesarian section. *Australian and New Zealand Journal of Obstetrics and Gynaecology* **13**, 121–124.

World Health Organization (1993) *Draft Recommendations for the Treatment of Sexually Transmitted Diseases*, pp. 24–31. WHO Advisory Group Meeting 1993 WHO/GPA/STD/93.1. WHO, Geneva.

Yong, E.C., Klabanoff, S.J., Kuo, C-C. *et al.* (1982) Toxic effect of human polymorphonuclear leucocytes on *Chlamydia trachomatis*. *Infection and Immunity* **37**, 422.

zur Hausen, H. (1982) Human genital cancer; synergism between two virus infections or synergism between a virus infection and initiating events? *Lancet* **ii**, 1370–1372.

zur Hausen, H. (1992) Viruses in human tumours. In: *Gynaecological Oncology* (ed. M. Coppleson), pp. 55–69. Churchill Livingstone, Edinburgh.

Chapter 5: Non-infective cutaneous conditions of the vulva

C.M. Ridley & S.M. Neill

Introduction

In this chapter the cutaneous conditions affecting the vulva will be discussed, grouped for convenience under appropriate headings; an entirely logical arrangement is impossible to achieve. As regards the dermatological entities, or dermatoses, those to be considered comprise those conditions which have a predilection for the vulva, those which are common there and elsewhere, and those which, while rare, have some particular academic or clinical importance.

It is recognized that some conditions tend to be clinically and histologically less distinct when they occur in the vulval area. They are influenced by the particularities of physiology mentioned in Chapter 3. Lesions on the non-keratinized surfaces are especially difficult to categorize. Secondary infection and, occasionally, contact dermatitis from remedies applied can complicate the picture. Furthermore, they are modified by warmth and moisture, which lead to maceration and to scaling that is less apparent or pale and soggy rather than crisp or white.

Finally, it should be remembered that intraepithelial neoplastic conditions tend to mimic benign dermatoses (Figs 5.1 & 5.2). For this reason biopsy of any lesion not clearly categorized or not responding to simple treatment is essential.

Classification of non-infective, non-neoplastic lesions

With successive accounts of vulval disease, this section becomes more straightforward. In short, all that is required is a simple listing of the conditions found at this site in appropriate groupings, such as the authors hope they have here supplied. Such a scheme is at present being discussed by the International Society for the Study of Vulvovaginal Disease (ISSVD). For historical reasons, however, and also as an aid to interpreting the literature, it is necessary to summarize briefly previous classifications.

These schemes were directed primarily at the epithelial dermatological disorders; and they were imposed because such disorders were not clearly categorized, a state of confusion dating back to the first descriptions of vulval disease towards the end of the 19th century. Dermatological and gynaecological literature developed separately and many different names were given to identical conditions. Jeffcoate and Woodcock (1961) preferred to sweep away the former plethora of terms and to substitute the all-embracing concept of a 'dystrophy'. This in turn led to the classification adopted by the fledgeling ISSVD in 1976 (Friedrich 1976), featuring lichen sclerosus and dystrophy, the latter of mixed and hypertrophic types, with and without atypia. Later, atypia was taken up into the new concept of intraepithelial neoplasia, which was given its own classification. Non-malignant conditions were classified as lichen sclerosus, other dermatoses and squamous cell hyperplasia in 1987, a listing still in force at the time of writing (Table 5.1). Although an improvement on the earlier schemes, the concept of squamous cell hyperplasia appeared out of place in the otherwise essentially clinically determined terminology. In the current discussions it is planned that the term will be dropped. An orderly system, will embrace, as appropriate, all dermatological conditions.

Symptoms

As with any cutaneous lesion, all these disorders often lead to varying degrees of itching and soreness, although occasionally they come to attention solely because of their appearance. The inflammatory element in many of them and the presence of erosion often give rise to soreness, but symptoms consisting predominantly of pain, burning and soreness, occurring with few visible signs, or persisting after adequate treatment of some particular lesion, are likely to be in the category of vulval vestibulitis or dysaesthetic vulvodynia and are discussed in Chapter 6.

Itching, or pruritus, is the commonest complaint. It is best defined as a sensation that leads to a wish to scratch. Lesions tend to be more pruritic at this site than those elsewhere. This may be attributable in part to the local environment, and in part to psychological and psychosexual factors. The mechanism of itch is not well understood, but

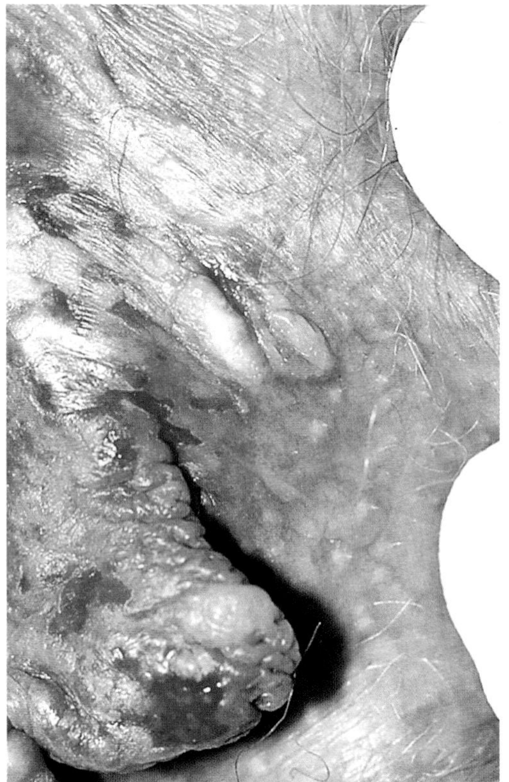

Fig. 5.1 Vulval intraepithelial squamous neoplasia (VIN).

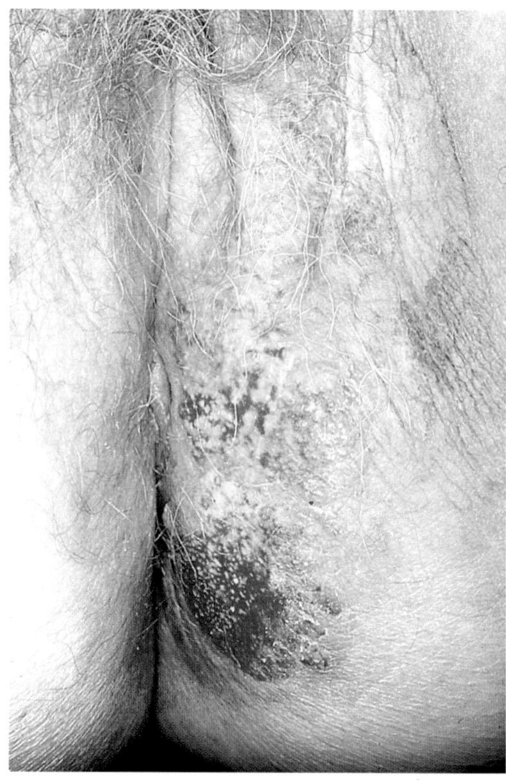

Fig. 5.2 Extramammary Paget's disease: 'eczematoid' appearance.

Table 5.1 Classification of non-neoplastic disorders of the vulva: International Society for the Study of Vulvovaginal Disease and International Society of Gynecological Pathologists, 1987. (Adapted from Ridley *et al.* 1989.)

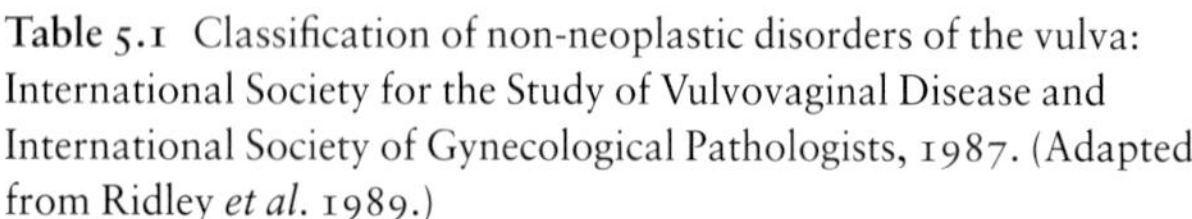

1 Lichen sclerosus
2 Squamous cell hyperplasia (formerly hyperplastic dystrophy)
3 Other dermatoses

Mixed epithelial disorders may occur. In such cases it is recommended that both conditions be reported. For example: lichen sclerosus with associated squamous cell hyperplasia (formerly classified as mixed dystrophy) should be reported as lichen sclerosus and squamous cell hyperplasia. Squamous cell hyperplasia with associated vulval intraepithelial neoplasia (formerly hyperplastic dystrophy with atypia) should be diagnosed as vulval intraepithelial neoplasia.

Squamous cell hyperplasia is used for those instances in which the hyperplasia is not attributable to another cause.

Specific lesions or dermatoses involving the vulva (e.g. psoriasis, lichen planus, lichen simplex chronicus, *Candida* infection, condyloma acuminatum) may include squamous cell hyperplasia, but should be diagnosed specifically and excluded from this category.

it is probably mediated by free unmyelinated nerve endings, distinct from those serving pain sensation, near the dermal–epidermal junction. Encephalins (opioids), in conjunction with histamine released from mast cells, and perhaps prostaglandin E and neuropeptides, are also likely to be involved (Greaves 1992). The sensation is greatly influenced by psychological factors and by warmth. It is obliterated by pain, patients will stop scratching when the itch has been replaced by pain, which many find preferable. Rarely, intense pruritus arises on normal skin. Itching and rubbing are frequently followed by the thickening of lichenification, to which the genital area appears to be especially susceptible. This change was at one time termed neurodermatitis, referring to the role of the nerve fibres, rather than to a psychological origin (Whitlock 1976), and the term may have influenced the practice of such undesirable treatments as alcohol injections (Ward & Sutherst 1975) and denervation procedures (Mering 1952). The word is now best avoided.

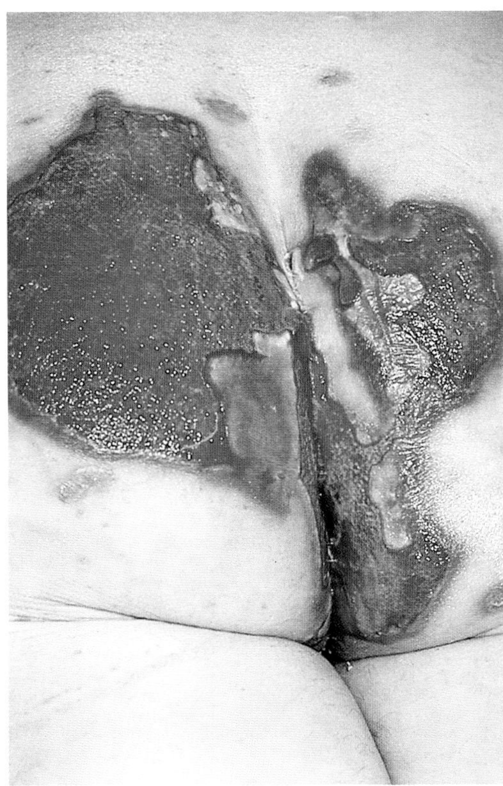

Fig. 5.3 Epidermolysis bullosa, junctional type: anogenital ulceration.

Genetic disorders

Epidermolysis bullosa

Aetiology

This title is applied to a genetically determined group of conditions, inherited by way of either dominant or recessive genes. They are characterized by increased fragility of the skin and mucosae, with a tendency to form bullae, which may arise spontaneously or in response to mild trauma. The appearances and pathogenesis are heterogeneous; electron microscopy, together with immunohistological and immunogenetic techniques, is used to define the different types (Tidman & Eady 1990).

The forms that involve the genital area are the junctional type, where the splitting occurs in the lamina lucida of the basement membrane, and the dystrophic type, where the splitting takes place below the lamina densa. An example of the latter was described by Petersen *et al.* (1996).

Clinical features

Extensive scarring in the anogenital area may follow healing (Fig. 5.3). The patient of Shackleford *et al.* (1982) had anal scarring leading to constipation and bladder compression, narrowing of the vestibule and partial fusion of the labia, while that of Steinkampf *et al.* (1987) had vaginal adhesions.

Differential diagnosis

The early onset, often with a family history, together with the presence of lesions elsewhere, will usually make the diagnosis of epidermolysis bullosa straightforward.

Management

Genetic counselling and pre-natal diagnosis may be offered where appropriate. Many patients have been helped by the support group, the Dystrophic Epidermolysis Bullosa Research Association. Dedicated attention to detail in avoiding friction and pressure is required. Drug therapy, for example with phenytoin, has had variable results.

Benign familial chronic pemphigus (Hailey–Hailey disease)

Aetiology

This rare dermatosis is inherited through an autosomal dominant gene. Not all patients will give a positive family history; lack of recognition of mild lesions, and the relatively late onset, may be the reason rather than a mutation. The pathogenesis is thought to be a defect in keratinocyte adhesion, with a breakdown in desmosome–keratin filaments possibly associated with the activation of a protease (Burge 1992).

Clinical features

Lesions usually begin to appear between the second and fourth decades, and affect the genital area as well as flexures elsewhere. In general they fluctuate and tend to improve with time. Cases have been reported where the lesions were apparently confined to the vulva (Thiers *et al.* 1968, Hazelrigg & Stoller 1977) and in a similar case (Lyles *et al.* 1958) the lesions appeared in pregnancy and remitted post-partum. The appearance is typically of moist, red plaques with fissuring and erosions (Fig. 5.4). Pustules and vesicles are also common. The lesions are sore and itching. Fresh lesions can be triggered off by heat, friction, infection, for example herpes simplex, bacterial and *Candida* infections, and by contact allergy. Vaginal lesions have been reported (Václavínková & Neumann 1982, Brandrup *et al.* 1990).

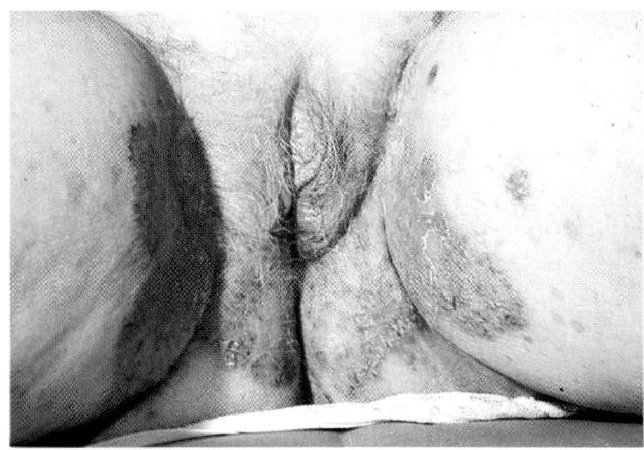

Fig. 5.4 Benign familial chronic pemphigus: moist, scaly, fissured erythema.

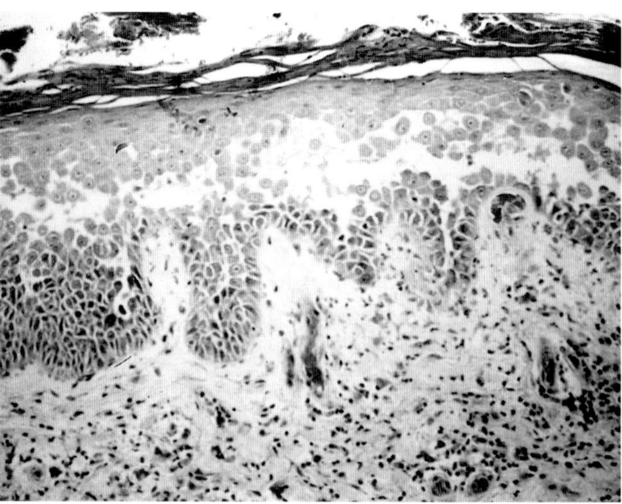

Fig. 5.5 Benign familial chronic pemphigus: extensive acantholysis.

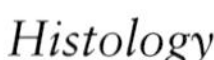

Histology

Histology shows suprabasal splitting and extensive intraepidermal acantholysis, the latter giving rise to the description of a 'dilapidated brick wall' (Fig. 5.5). Occasionally there are a few *corps ronds* or *grains* high up in the epidermis. Immunofluorescence is negative.

Differential diagnosis

The differential diagnosis is mainly from Darier's disease. The different balance of the histological features and several clinical features, for example white bands but no notches on the nails, absence of horny papules and palmar pits, later onset and precipitation of lesions by trauma in benign familial chronic pemphigus, will usually suffice to distinguish between the two. Sometimes the appearance is mistaken for that of a banal inflammation; resistance to treatment under these circumstances should always alert the clinician to the need for biopsy. Lesions confined to the anogenital area may appear as papules and be mistaken for warts (Langenberg *et al.* 1992), and they may be suggestive of other infective processes, since as well as being precipitated by infective agents they also mimic them.

Management

The mainstays of treatment, apart from general measures to avoid friction, the use of bland emollients and antibacterial washes such as potassium permanganate, are topical corticosteroids combined with antibacterial and antifungal agents such as tetracycline, fusidic acid and clotrimazole. The potency of the corticosteroid required for control varies with the severity of the lesions. Long-term antibiotics by mouth, and occasionally courses of oral steroids, can be useful. Recently, good results have been reported with oral cyclosporin (Berth-Jones *et al.* 1995). Grenz rays have been shown to help (Sarkany 1959) and a variety of drugs and surgical procedures have yielded variable success (Burge 1992); of these, grafting appears to be the most satisfactory.

Other acantholytic lesions

Unilateral linear acantholytic lesions with features suggestive of Darier's disease or of benign familial chronic pemphigus have been described. They are probably best regarded as special forms of epidermal naevi. One in the latter category and involving the anogenital area was that of Vakilzadeh and Kolde (1985) occurring in a girl of 5 with its onset at the age of 3 months, although the mother and maternal grandmother had a history of anogenital vesicular lesions so the possibility of benign familial chronic pemphigus arises.

Ackerman (1972) classified focal acantholytic dyskeratoses as multiple, whether permanent (Darier's disease) or transient (Grover's disease), and as single, whether clinically inapparent, papular or nodular. Duray *et al.* (1983) described three examples of the nodular form at the vulva; the lesions did not recur after excision. Chorzelski *et al.* (1984) reported a patient whose papular vulval lesions were suggestive of Darier's disease, and essentially similar cases were reported by Cooper (1989), Barrett *et al.* (1989), van Joost *et al.* (1991) and Salopek *et al.* (1993). Langenberg *et al.* (1992) believe that many if not all of these cases represent mild examples of benign familial chronic pemphigus, and this view is supported by the observation of Burge (1992) that diagnosis of that condition is often delayed.

Darier's disease (keratosis follicularis)

Aetiology

This rare condition (Burge & Wilkinson 1992, Burge 1994) is inherited by way of an autosomal dominant gene. Not all patients will give a family history, however, and reasons for this include non-recognition of mild early disease, non-paternity of putative fathers (Munro 1992) and new mutations. As well as the cutaneous lesions, association with disorders of other systems, particularly neurological, have been noted; however, these authors found that most of the affected patients did not have other medical problems. The pathogenesis is complex (Burge 1994). The characteristic acantholysis is probably caused by a mutation in a structural protein, which leads to an instability of adhesion junctions between the desmosomes and the keratin filaments and hence to a breakdown of the complexes between them.

Clinical features

The lesions tend to develop in childhood or adolescence and to worsen gradually, with fluctuations but no remissions. The primary lesions consist of horny papules. All aspects of the vulva, as well as skin and mucosal surfaces elsewhere, are often involved. Oral lesions are well recognized but vaginal lesions do not appear to have been recorded. Maceration and secondary bacterial infection is common, leading in severely affected patients to malodorous masses, which are common in the genital area. The lesions are also susceptible to viral infection, of which the herpes simplex virus is the commonest. Lesions are aggravated by heat and warmth, and also by oral lithium carbonate.

Histology

Histologically there is dyskeratosis with the formation of *corps ronds* and *grains*, clefts within the epidermis and focal areas of acantholysis in the suprabasal layer.

Differential diagnosis

The differential diagnosis is mainly from benign familial chronic pemphigus (Hailey–Hailey disease), which can show considerable overlap with Darier's disease both clinically and histologically. The morphology of extragenital lesions will usually be helpful, particularly those of nail changes, since, although both may show white bands, only in Darier's disease does one see red and white bands with a split or notch, and horny papules and palmar pits are typical of Darier's disease.

Management

Bland emollients, corticosteroids and antibacterial agents are of limited value. The apparent resemblance to the lesions of vitamin A deficiency (of which there is no evidence) led to the trial of retinoids. Topical retinoic acid may help a little, but is irritant. Systemic administration of etretinate and now of acitretin is of great benefit, although less so in flexural lesions; but unfortunately this therapy is limited by its teratogenicity and its side effects, including potential danger to bones. Many patients decide not to continue, or to take the drug intermittently. Recently, cyclosporin has been favourably reported on (Martini *et al.* 1995). Radiation therapy, dermabrasion and the laser have been employed, with varying success.

Neurofibromatosis

The neurofibromatoses occur in various forms; of these, type 2 rarely manifests cutaneous signs. The others, of which type 1 (von Recklinghausen's disease) is the commonest, are characterized by tumours, discussed in Chapter 9, and by so-called freckling which, while usually in the axillae, has been reported in the vulval area (Crowe 1964).

Cowden's disease (multiple hamartoma syndrome)

This rare condition, reviewed by Starink and Hausman (1984), is determined by an autosomal dominant gene; hamartomatous lesions involve ectodermal, mesodermal and endodermal tissues. The skin may show acral, facial and oral mucosal lesions. The vulva may be affected by the acral type, namely keratotic papillomas, sometimes showing a follicular origin (Burnett *et al.* 1975, Brownstein *et al.* 1979), or by other lesions, for example an apocrine cystadenoma in the case of Salem and Steck (1983). Excision of any troublesome lesion is indicated. Many other gynaecological lesions have been reported, perhaps representing chance associations (Buckley 1995).

Pseudoxanthoma elasticum

This condition may be inherited by way of autosomal recessive or dominant genes. The elastic tissue, ground substance and collagen are abnormal and the main hazard is the serious risk of systemic vascular lesions and lesions of the eye. Although there are potential risks in pregnancy, Viljoen *et al.* (1987) found only a possibly increased rate of spontaneous abortion and a marked incidence of striae. The skin is a site of election. Cases where the vagina or vulva were involved were reported by Kissmeyer and With (1922), Szymanski and Caro (1955) and Goodman *et al.* (1963).

Clinical features

The lesions are yellowish papules, confluent in larger plaques, often with purpura and telangiectasia. Lesions elsewhere on the body are likely and the 'plucked-chicken' appearance is easily recognizable.

Histology

Histologically the main feature is the presence of dystrophic elastic fibres showing deposition of calcium.

Management

No treatment is possible apart from limited surgical removal if requested.

Ehlers–Danlos syndrome

Ehlers–Danlos syndrome (EDS) is now known to comprise at least 10 types, all characterized by different abnormalities of the connective tissue. In type IV, inherited as an autosomal dominant condition, the skin is transparent and fragile but hyperelasticity is slight. Arterial and bowel rupture may be fatal. The fault lies in the production of type III collagen. Rudd *et al.* (1983) studied 20 women in four families with EDS type IV. Ten had been pregnant with a total of 20 pregnancies and five patients had died as a result. Complications and fatalities had arisen from rupture of bowel, large vessels or uterus, lacerations of the vagina and post-partum haemorrhage. Twelve of the live-born babies had EDS IV and two died during delivery; two were aborted. Lurie *et al.* (1998) have reviewed further cases of EDS IV and discussed management. This appears to be the main type of EDS in which there are risks in pregnancy. The need for counselling and supervision is obvious.

Netherton's syndrome (ichthyosis linearis circumflexa)

This rare condition is determined by an autosomal recessive gene. Ichthyosis linearis circumflexa is associated with trichorrhexis invaginata or other abnormalities of the hair shaft. The skin is red and scaly and the changes are marked in the flexures. Kübler *et al.* (1987) have reported a patient with a vulval carcinoma superimposed on the warty tissue.

White sponge naevus

White hyperkeratotic lesions of the oral mucosa, often inherited as an autosomal dominant condition, have been described. In some cases, for example those of Dégos and Ebrard (1958), genital lesions have also been present (Figs 5.6 & 5.7). Jorgenson and Levin (1981) reviewed the subject. Later examples with vulval involvement were described by Buchholz *et al.* (1985) and Nichols *et al.* (1990).

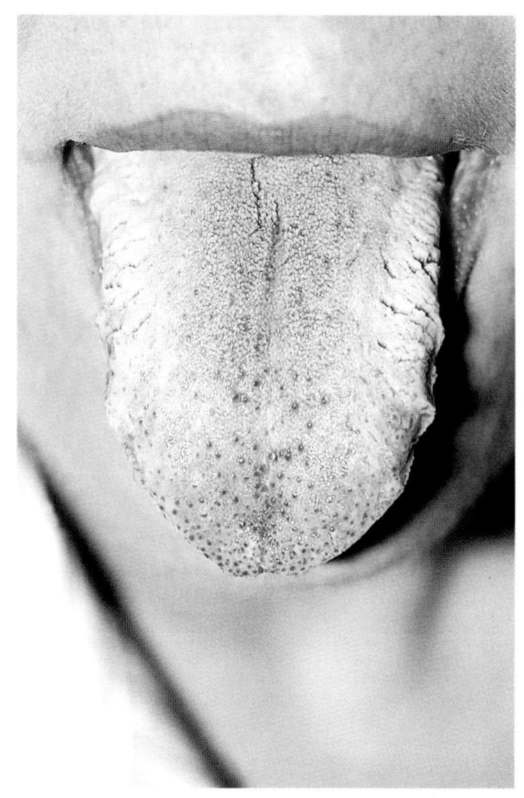

Fig. 5.6 White sponge naevus: white plaques on the tongue.

Histology

Histology of the white plaques shows acanthosis, individual cell keratinization and large vacuolated cells.

Differential diagnosis

The differential diagnosis includes lichen planus, human papillomavirus and *Candida* infection, and vulval intraepithelial neoplasia.

Management

If symptoms are present, treatment with topical tetracycline has been helpful in oral lesions, and so is worth trying for the genital area (McDonagh *et al.* 1990, Lim and Ng, 1992).

Dyskeratosis congenita

This rare condition, commoner in males and usually inherited through an X-linked recessive gene, is characterized by

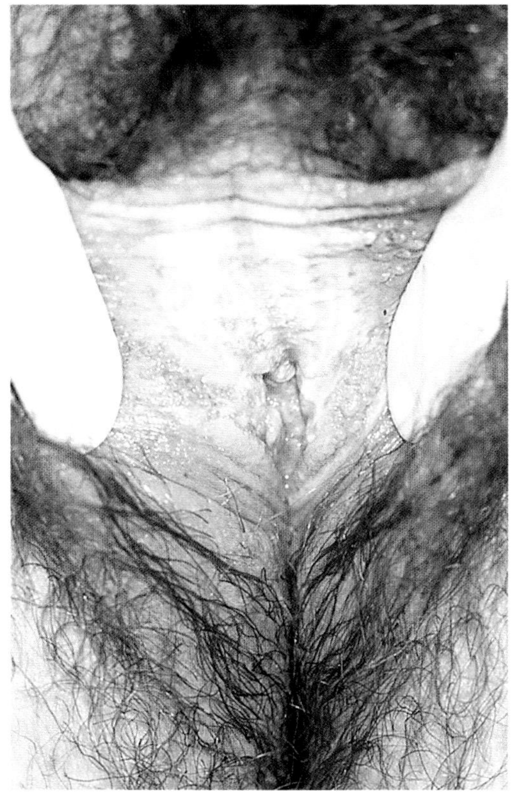

Fig. 5.7 White sponge naevus: white plaque at the vulva.

cutaneous atrophy and pigmentation with a nail dystrophy. Leukoplakia of the oral cavity may be accompanied by similar changes in the eye and urogenital mucosa. Carcinomas are frequent, affecting the skin, mucosae and other organs, and one female patient described by Sorrow and Hitch (1963) had a carcinoma of the cervix and vagina.

ACQUIRED DYSKERATOTIC LEUKOPLAKIA

Under this title, James and Lupton (1988) described a woman of 38 who developed white plaques of the palate, lips and gums, followed by similar lesions on the labia minora. There was no family history and the status of the condition remains uncertain.

Histology

The histology showed clusters of dyskeratotic cells in the epidermis but sparing the basal layer, and did not appear to fit in with that of any known entity.

Management

Treatment with oral steroids and retinoids, and with the laser, was ineffective.

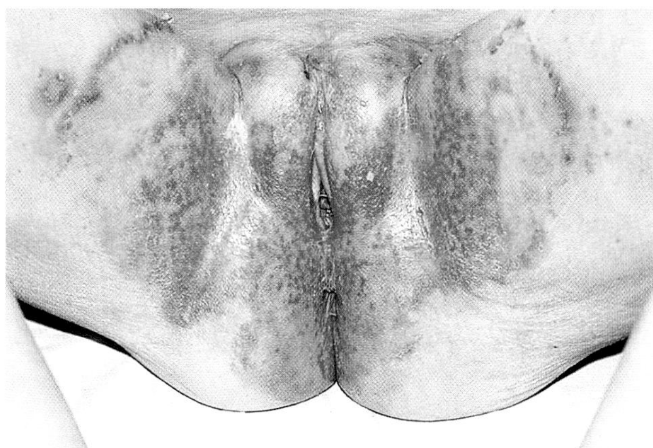

Fig. 5.8 Glucagonoma syndrome: scaly and moist serpiginous rash.

Conditions associated with systemic disease

Necrolytic migratory erythema (glucagonoma syndrome)

This distinctive eruption affects many areas of the body, but mainly the genital area. The first cases were associated with the rare pancreatic islet-cell glucagonoma, as have been almost all since. Exceptions, however, with cirrhosis and diabetes but without a glucagonoma or glucagonaemia, were reported by Kasper and McMurry (1991) and by Masri-Fridling and Turner (1992), who speculate as to a hepatic pathogenesis for the rash. Other theories include amino-acid deficiency, essential fatty acid deficiency and elevation of epidermal arachidonic acid caused by a raised plasma glucagon.

Clinical features

The subject is usually a middle-aged woman who is ill, with weight loss, stomatitis, glossitis and often diabetes. The lesions are erythematous and bullous, extending and then healing at the edges to form a serpiginous pattern (Fig. 5.8).

Histology

The histology shows epidermal necrolysis and a mild lymphocytic dermal infiltrate.

Differential diagnosis

In the differential diagnosis, pustular psoriasis, bullous dermatoses, acrodermatitis enteropathica and toxic epidermal necrolysis have to be considered, although the latter is more acute. The clinical picture is, however, fairly typical.

Management

Where a glucagonoma, usually but not invariably of the pancreas, is found, surgical removal leads to rapid improvement. Secondary deposits may be present at the time of diagnosis and require treatment. Hepatic artery embolization and therapy with octreotide acetate, a synthetic octapeptide analogue of somatostatin, have been shown to be helpful (Altimari *et al.* 1986, Wermers *et al.* 1996).

Acrodermatitis enteropathica

Aetiology

This condition is related to zinc deficiency, whether genetically determined because of a defect in absorption inherited as a recessive characteristic, or acquired through such causes as total parenteral nutrition, Crohn's disease, jejunoileal bypass surgery, alcoholism, prematurity, penicillamine given for cystinuria or Wilson's disease, or chelating agents given for iron overload in thalassaemia (Leigh *et al.* 1979, Ridley 1982). The genetically determined examples, and some of the others, are seen in infancy. Adults may suffer from the acquired type, and from relapses of the genetic type, as in the patient of Verburg *et al.* (1974) who developed lesions in pregnancy having been previously well controlled on zinc therapy.

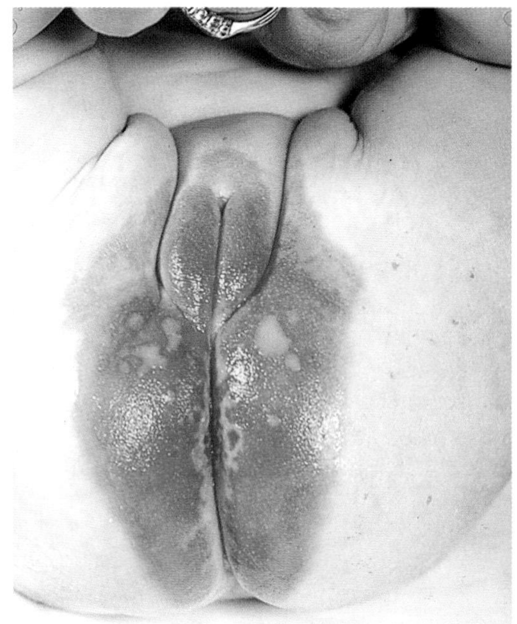

Fig. 5.9 Acrodermatitis enteropathica: fiery erythema of the anogenital area.

Clinical features

The lesions are red, eroded and vesicopustular; they affect not only the genital area but other parts, particularly the face, and there is loss of hair (Figs 5.9 & 5.10). The course is chronic in the absence of treatment.

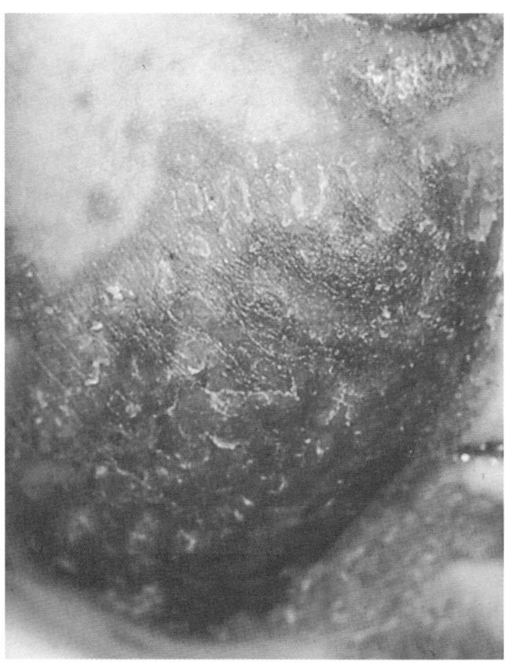

Fig. 5.10 Acrodermatitis enteropathica: fiery erythema of the face.

Histology and differential diagnosis

The histology is non-specific so the differential diagnosis is on clinical and microbiological grounds from candidosis, seborrhoeic dermatitis and other banal eruptions; a rare differential diagnosis is Netherton's syndrome where, in association with ichthyosis, atopy and hair abnormalities, chronic anogenital lesions are somewhat similar (Greene & Muller 1985). Serum zinc determinations are useful in cases of doubt, although they are not entirely reliable; falsely low values are found in hypoalbuminaemia.

Management

Oral zinc is now the accepted treatment, although before its lack was incriminated di-iodoquine was given with limited success.

Inflammatory bowel disease

For convenience, ulcerative colitis and Crohn's disease may be considered separately. Clinically, however, the distinction is not always easy to make.

Ulcerative colitis

Anogenital lesions are much rarer than in Crohn's disease. Verbov (1973) found only one definite example out of 40 patients. Forman (1966) described a pustular vegetative eruption in the groins in some patients. Although it was clinically suggestive of pemphigus vegetans the histology showed only rare acantholysis, and immunofluorescence was negative; it was named pemphigus vegetans, Hallopeau type or pyodermite végétante.

Crohn's disease

Anogenital lesions are not unusual; in the series of McCallum and Kinmont (1968), Mountain (1970) and Verbov (1973) up to 30% of patients were so affected. The lesions may be a direct continuation of bowel involvement. If they are well clear of the anogenital area, particularly if normal skin intervenes, they are referred to as metastatic (Fig. 5.11). Such metastatic lesions, often at flexural sites, were described by Parks *et al.* (1965) and later accounts include those of Mountain (1970), McCallum and Gray (1976), Reyman *et al.* (1986) and the review by Shum and Guenther (1990).

Clinical features

Lesions of Crohn's disease, whether contiguous with affected bowel or metastatic, may precede or follow the recognition of bowel disease, often by many years, and even after resolution or removal of the affected intestine. Children and adolescents as well as adults may be affected (Lally *et al.* 1988, Kim *et al.* 1992, Werlin *et al.* 1992).

The patients present with oedema, often very marked and sometimes with lymphangiectases, firm swelling, oedematous perianal tags and ulcers, fissures, sinuses and fistulae (Fig. 5.12). The oedema and swelling may occur alone and may be unilateral (Martin & Holdstock 1997) (Fig. 5.13). Symptoms are often severe and may include dyspareunia (Hamilton *et al.* 1977). The course is chronic. Bowen's disease was reported in one case (Prezyna and Kalyanaraman 1977) and anal carcinoma is a recognized, although rare, hazard; the mechanism is unclear but may result from the long-standing inflammatory process, from a defect in immune status, or from the effect of immunosuppressive drugs used in treatment (Ball *et al.* 1988).

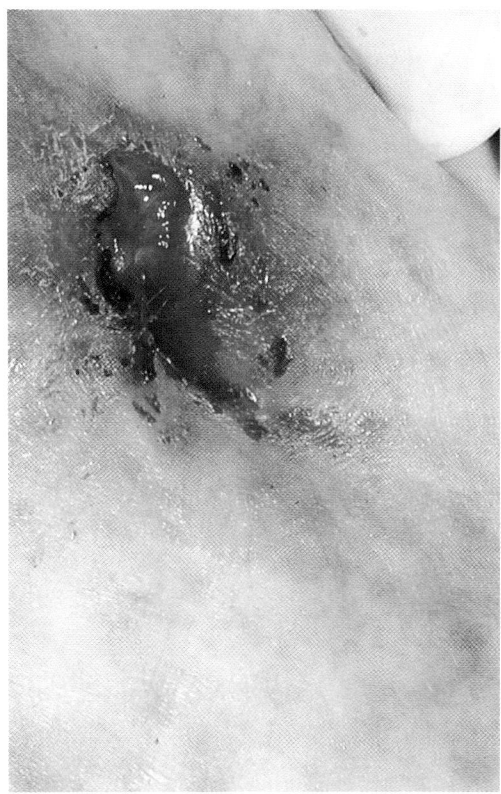

Fig. 5.11 Crohn's disease: metastatic umbilical lesion.

Histology

Histology may show non-caseating granulomas or only oedema.

Differential diagnosis

The pleomorphic physical signs and variable, often nonspecific histology can render diagnosis difficult, particularly in association with the fact that the diagnosis is not excluded by the absence of demonstrable bowel disease. One common difficulty is to distinguish it from hidradenitis suppurativa; the presence of bridged scars and comedones in the latter condition is helpful. However, the two conditions have been known to coexist (Ostlere *et al.* 1991, Burrows and Russell Jones 1992). Other diagnoses to consider include chronic infections and, in children, sexual abuse.

Management

The lesions respond to some extent to medical treatment of the bowel condition, measures reviewed by Scully (1989) and including oral steroids, antibiotics, especially metronidazole (Duhra & Paul 1988, Kingsland and Alderman 1991), and immunosuppressive drugs such as azathioprine

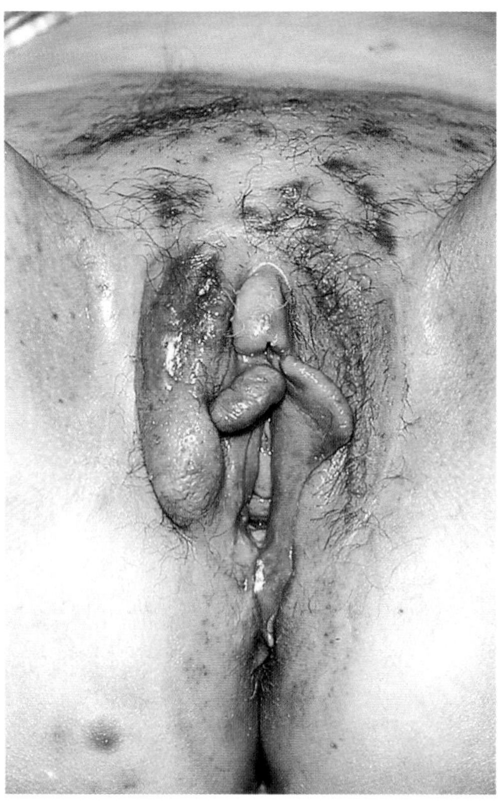

Fig. 5.12 Crohn's disease: indurated oedema, tags, fissures and sinuses.

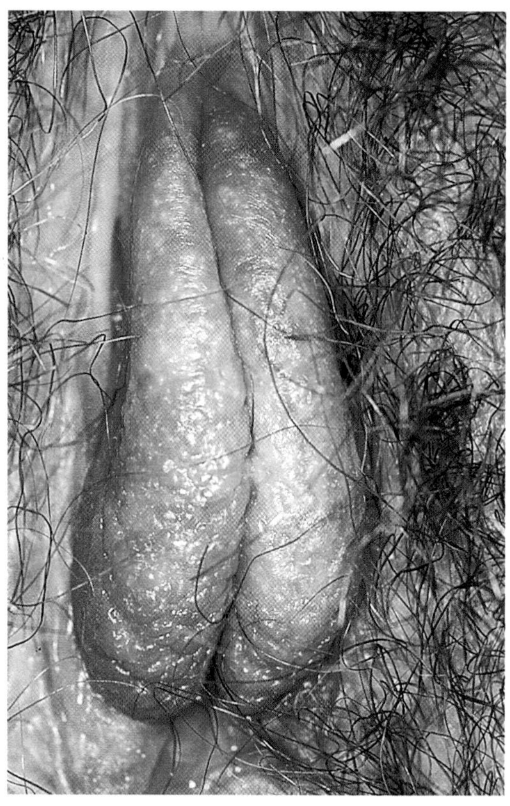

Fig. 5.13 Crohn's disease: gross oedema of labia.

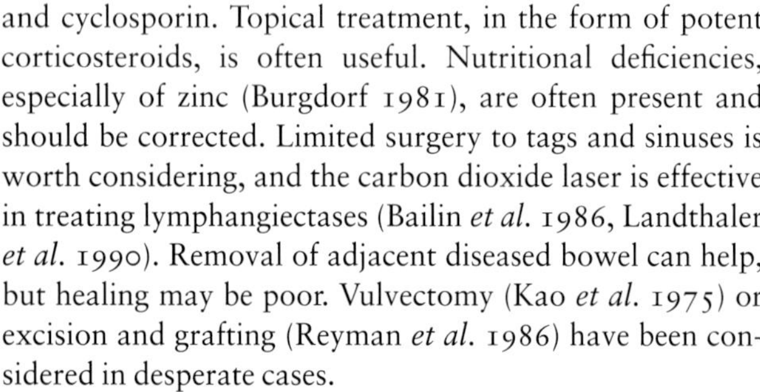

and cyclosporin. Topical treatment, in the form of potent corticosteroids, is often useful. Nutritional deficiencies, especially of zinc (Burgdorf 1981), are often present and should be corrected. Limited surgery to tags and sinuses is worth considering, and the carbon dioxide laser is effective in treating lymphangiectases (Bailin *et al.* 1986, Landthaler *et al.* 1990). Removal of adjacent diseased bowel can help, but healing may be poor. Vulvectomy (Kao *et al.* 1975) or excision and grafting (Reyman *et al.* 1986) have been considered in desperate cases.

Acute febrile neutrophilic dermatosis (Sweet's syndrome)

Sweet (1979) reviewed a group of patients whom he had earlier reported as having this condition of unknown aetiology. They had fever, painful, erythematous, raised plaques on the skin, and neutrophilia; the condition occurred mainly in middle-aged women. Vulval involvement has been reported (Delke *et al.* 1981, Lindskov 1984, Keefe *et al.* 1988). There have also been reports of its association with Behçet's syndrome (Mizoguchi *et al.* 1987, Cho *et al.* 1989) and myeloproliferative disorders.

Histology

Histologically, there is leucocytoclasis and a severe inflammatory process, which, although predominantly neutrophilic, may in some instances be lymphocytic or mixed (Jordaan 1989).

Management

The response to oral prednisolone is usually good.

Pyoderma gangrenosum

The aetiology of this rare condition is undetermined, but there is a strong association with rheumatoid arthritis and ulcerative colitis, and sometimes Crohn's disease (Burgdorf 1981, Gellert *et al.* 1983) as well as with blood and myeloproliferative disorders. Its indolent ulcerative lesions have been reported at the vulva (Work 1980, Davidson *et al.* 1989, McCalmont *et al.* 1991, Lebbe *et al.* 1992), although the diagnosis is often difficult to make with certainty. For example, a patient of Work (1980), who responded to extensive surgery, had had lesions over many years and suffered from Crohn's disease, which could perhaps account for them directly.

Clinical features

There are multiple punched-out, pepperpot-like, small ulcers, or a single large ulcer, set in an area of induration. The edges tend to be dusky, overhanging and oedematous.

Histology

The histology is usually inflammatory but non-specific, although there may be evidence of a vasculitis.

Differential diagnosis and management

The differential diagnosis is from infective ulcerations and in particular from synergistic bacterial gangrene (post-operative progressive gangrene) (Chapter 4). The correct diagnosis is vital since treatment is not surgical, but medical, with systemic steroids, often with the addition of dapsone, azathioprine and minocycline; cyclosporin was also effective (Buckley & Rogers 1995, in a patient whose hidradenitis suppurativa also improved; Nisar *et al.* 1995).

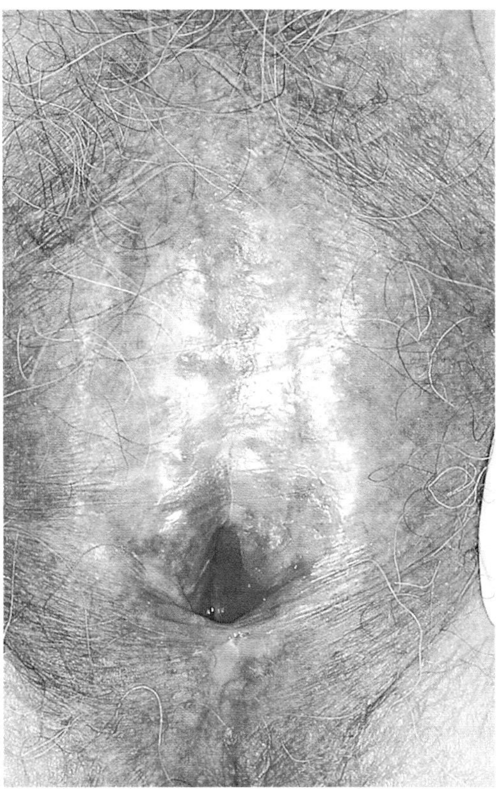

Fig. 5.14 Vulval amyloidosis: atrophy and loss of architecture.

ASSOCIATION BETWEEN ACUTE FEBRILE NEUTROPHILIC DERMATOSIS AND PYODERMA GANGRENOSUM

The case of Lebbe *et al.* (1992) was unusual in having a scleral ulcer and extensive pulmonary neutrophilic non-infective infiltrates. These authors, whilst believing that pyoderma gangrenosum was the most likely diagnosis, discuss the overlap found between that condition, other lesions associated with inflammatory bowel disease, and Sweet's syndrome. Sweet's syndrome and pyoderma gangrenosum have been found together also in myeloproliferative disorders such as myeloid leukaemia, and it was been suggested that they are then part of a continuum of non-infective and non-metastatic inflammatory neutrophilic dermatoses associated with these states (Caughman *et al.* 1983, Kuroda *et al.* 1995).

Amyloidosis (see also Chapter 8)

Lesions are typically glassy or waxy, showing purpura and telangiectasia, but clinical appearances are nevertheless variable. Vulval examples are rare (Goltz 1952). Northcutt and Vanover (1985) reported an example, which appeared to be the third case, in a woman of 53 with nodular lesions that were reddish, ulcerated and simulated malignancy. They recurred 6 years after excision but the patient remained well with no evidence of systemic disease. Histology showed dermal amyloid material of immunoglobulin light chain origin. The previous two cases had also shown no evidence of systemic disease. The case of Gorodeski *et al.* (1988) appeared to be of lichen amyloidosis affecting the vulva. Taylor *et al.* (1991), however, reported an example in a woman of 74 with typical waxy nodules at the vulva and elsewhere and with evidence of a monoclonal serum abnormality and Bence-Jones protein in the urine, and Buezo *et al.* (1996) described a patient with multiple myeloma whose presentation was that of perianal, warty, amyloid-containing lesions. A personal case with a paraproteinaemia showed confluent changes clinically suggestive of lichen sclerosus, without nodulation (Fig. 5.14).

Histology

Histology shows immunoglobulin light chain amyloid with typical straight filaments on electron microscopy. It surrounds vessel walls, accounting for the purpura noted clinically.

Management

The patient should be evaluated and followed up from the point of view of systemic disease. Treatment will be dictated mainly by the presence or absence of lesions elsewhere or of systemic disease. Localized deposits can be treated by surgical excision or the laser.

Sarcoidosis

A patient with vulval nodular sarcoidosis was reported by de Oliveira Neto (1972). Neill *et al.* (1984) reported an example of vulval ulcerated sarcoidosis. The patient had proven sarcoidosis elsewhere, and there was no evidence of Crohn's disease or infection that might mimic sarcoidosis. The lesions were extensive, painless, shallow ulcers affecting the submammary and perianal area and the labia majora; histology was compatible with sarcoidosis. Tatnall *et al.* (1985) reported on a patient with papular lesions of the vulva and perianal areas. The patient had a raised serum angiotensin-converting enzyme, a positive Kveim test and pulmonary lesions; the histology was that of sarcoidosis.

Histology

Histology shows epithelioid cells aggregated into discrete non-caseating granulomas with a variably developed surround of lymphoid cells and, sometimes, multinucleate giant cells.

Management

This will be as for the lesions of sarcoidosis elsewhere.

OTHER GRANULOMATOUS CONDITIONS

Some of the reported cases with such histology may have had Crohn's disease, inadequately investigated, or before the onset of bowel lesions. However, several cases have been categorized as variants of the Melkersson–Rosenthal syndrome (Westermark & Henriksson 1979, Wagenberg and Downham 1981); the evidence for this has been reviewed, with the addition of a further example, a woman with lesions of the anal and perineal areas, by Hackel *et al.* (1991). These authors conclude that whether or not these lesions are part of the classical Melkersson–Rosenthal syndrome remains open for discussion. Samaratunga *et al.* (1991) described a patient in this category who in addition to the granulomatous vulval lesions had a squamous cell carcinoma of the vulva at the age of 31; she had, in addition, evidence of a human papillomavirus (types 6 and 11) and systemic lupus erythematosus.

Langerhans cell histiocytosis (see also Chapter 8)

Langerhans cell histiocytosis (LCH), previously known as histiocytosis X, may affect the vulva as a solitary manifestation or as part of a widely disseminated disease process (Blaauwgeers *et al.* 1993). It is probably best regarded as a disorder of immune regulation (Axiotis *et al.* 1991) and occurs in forms which are benign and localized (eosinophilic granuloma), chronic and progressive (Hand–Schuller–Christian) and acute with systemic illness (Letterer–Siwe).

Clinical features

The age range of patients with vulval lesions ranged from 8 months to 85 years in the review of Axiotis *et al.* (1991). In infants a typical presentation is of yellowish, often purpuric papules in the napkin area and elsewhere. In adults, the lesions are papular or nodular, sometimes ulcerated.

Differential diagnosis

The differential diagnosis is wide, including neoplasia and dermatoses; definitive diagnosis depends on the specific histology.

Management

Treatment is that of the underlying disease process, and will include excision where feasible, radiotherapy, steroids, vinblastine, vincristine and other chemotherapeutic drugs (Dupree & Lee 1973, Issa *et al.* 1980, Axiotis *et al.* 1991).

Malacoplakia (see also Chapter 8)

This condition probably results from an inadequate or atypical inflammatory response to *Escherichia coli.* Genital tract involvement is well recognized, and was reviewed by Chen and Hendricks (1985). Nodules or ulcers may be found.

The clinical differential diagnosis includes Crohn's disease and other granulomatous conditions, and malignancy. The histological appearance is typical.

Management

Chen and Hendriks (1985) found treatment with cholinergic agonists, which raise the level of cyclic guanosine monophosphate in mononuclear cells, helpful. Van Furth *et al.* (1992) reported good results with ciprofloxacin, which penetrates well into macrophages, in a patient with malacoplakia of the bladder.

Ligneous disease

This rare condition (*Lancet* 1990) is usually manifested as a membranous or pseudomembranous conjunctivitis but can affect other tissues including the lower genital tract. Ocular involvement may precede or follow such lesions. It is not clear whether it is triggered off by local factors or is a multisystem disease with multifocal manifestations. Its aetiology is unknown. Rubin *et al.* (1989) reported a woman with extensive cervical and gingival lesions that defied diagnosis until the history of eye problems in childhood was elucidated; subsequently she was found to have similar lesions around the Fallopian tubes (Ridley & Morgan 1993). Scurry *et al.* (1993b) have reported the cases of two women, who so far are without ocular involvement. One had lesions of the cervix, endometrium and a Fallopian tube, the other of the cervix, vagina and possibly of the endometrium.

The clinical appearance is of firm and sometimes necrotic plaques and nodules, which recur and spread after local biopsy or destructive procedures.

Histology

There is a subepidermal hyaline deposit, which is amorphous and eosinophilic and contains albumin, fibrin and immunoglobulin, together with a variable mixed cellular component and sometimes areas of granulation tissue. The epidermis may be ulcerated or hyperplastic. Stains for amyloid are negative.

Management

There is no effective treatment, whether surgical, topical or systemic, with the possible exception of azathioprine.

Lupus erythematosus

Burge *et al.* (1989) found that in a series of 121 patients, male and female, with lupus erythematosus 21% of those with systemic disease and 24% of those with chronic cutaneous disease had mucosal involvement (nose, eyes, mouth). No specific genital lesions were found in 48 female patients with systemic lupus erythematosus, although one had vaginal lesions possibly referable to Sjögren's syndrome. Vulval lesions were, however, found in two out of 42 women with chronic cutaneous lupus erythematosus. Of these two, one had erythema and ulceration and later scarring near the introitus; the other had erythema and white reticulate vulval lesions, with lichen planus-like lesions in the mouth, but histology was diagnostic at neither site.

Sjögren's syndrome

Sjögren's syndrome, characterized by dryness of mucous membranes related to abnormality of exocrine secretion, is rare. Most cases are associated with other mainly autoimmune diseases, especially rheumatoid arthritis, systemic sclerosis and lupus erythematosus.

Although anogenital symptoms are not uncommon in affected patients, the true incidence of vulval or vaginal involvement is unknown. Bloch *et al.* (1965) described 62 cases and commented that vaginal dryness was present in 20 of the 59 women (11 of them premenopausal) in the series; patients complained of burning and dyspareunia and the mucosa was noted to be red; a biopsy in one patient was non-specific. Capriello *et al.* (1988) noted complaints of dryness, burning and dyspareunia in a high proportion of their patients and descibed an 'erythematous vulvitis' in 12 out of 26 women, again not confined to the postmenopausal.

Which glands can be inculpated in these changes is unclear, since vaginal moisture is largely a matter of transudation, the vagina containing no glandular structures; cervical and vulval tissue may be at fault, although the changes described are essentially somewhat non-specific and commonly encountered in patients with no evidence of the syndrome. However, vaginal atresia has been attributed to the condition on one occasion (Ricard-Rothiot *et al.* 1979).

Management

No specific treatment is available and drugs given for associated disease appear to be of little help. Symptomatic treatment with lubricating agents is indicated.

Dermatomyositis

Lavery *et al.* (1985) have described vulval involvement in one case; otherwise it appears not to have been reported.

Behçet's syndrome

Definition and aetiology

This syndrome was originally defined in 1937 as a triad of oral and genital ulceration and ocular lesions (uveitis). It is now recognized as a multisystem disease that may sometimes be diagnosed only after a period of observation of an evolving clinical picture. In 1990 diagnostic criteria were outlined by an International Study Group for Behçet's syndrome (1990), (Wechsler & Piette 1992). Recurrent oral ulceration is obligatory and must be accompanied by two of the following: recurrent genital ulceration, eye lesions, cutaneous lesions and a positive pathergy test. The causative agent may be viral, and the pathogenesis of the lesions is probably vascular. An association with HLA B5 has been described but immunogenetic factors may vary in different parts of the world.

Clinical features

The onset is usually in adult life before the age of 50 years. The oral ulcers are indistinguishable from recurrent aphthous ulcers. The vulval ulcers are recurrent, painful and often on the labia minora (Fig. 5.15). They eventually heal, often with scarring. Vaginal ulcers have been reported (Morgan *et al.* 1988) in an atypical case. Cutaneous lesions include pyodermatous plaques, erythema nodosum and sterile pustules following trauma such as a needle prick (pathergy).

Histology

Histologically the appearances may be non-specific or show thrombosed arterioles or other manifestations of arteriolar or venous disease.

Differential diagnosis

The important differential diagnosis is from recurrent aphthous disease, where in general scarring is less evident, there is more likely to be a family history, and lesions elsewhere will be lacking.

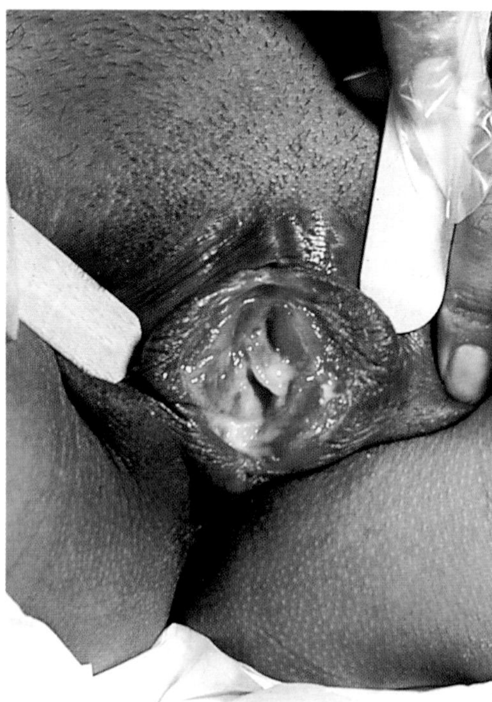

Fig. 5.15 Behçet's disease: deep vulval ulcers.

Management

The condition is not as a rule life threatening but blindness and neurological complications can lead to severe disability, and management is difficult. Many drugs are employed, with varying success, for example colchicine, steroids, dapsone, levamisole, thalidomide and immunosuppressive drugs. Those with most experience (Wechsler & Piette 1992) recommend colchicine and aspirin to prevent acute exacerbations, corticosteroids for ocular and neurological involvement and anticoagulants for thrombotic disease. Thalidomide is effective for mucosal ulcers although difficult to obtain (in the UK, only on a named-patient basis (Powell 1996)), teratogenic and with side effects such as neuropathy. Alli *et al.* (1997) report good results from intralesional recombinant human granulocyte/macrophage colony-stimulating factor (rhGM-CSF) for a large genital ulcer. Fortunately, where the ulcers are mild topical tetracycline and corticosteroids are helpful.

Recurrent aphthous ulceration

The fairly common condition of mild recurrent aphthous ulceration affects the mouth primarily but some patients have the major form, with more severe, scarring lesions (Fig. 5.16), and it may then be associated with recurrent vulval ulceration. It is unaccompanied by any manifestations of systemic disease, and has an onset usually in childhood or adolescence. There may be a family history. Oral aphthous ulcers are classified as major, minor or herpeti-

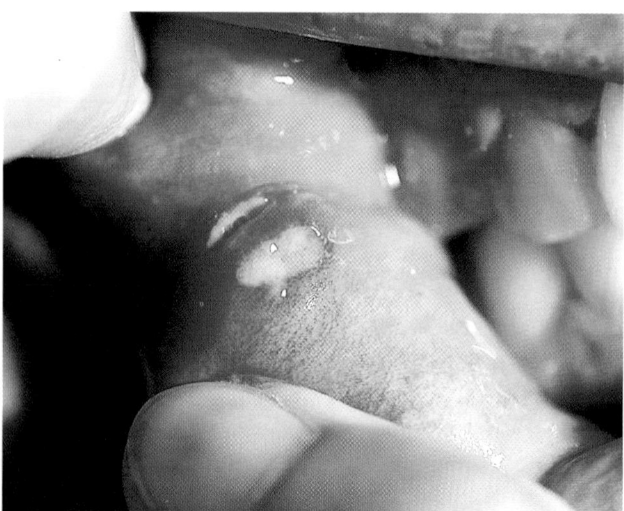

Fig. 5.16 Major aphthous ulcer of the mouth.

form, but these distinctions are not readily made at the vulva.

Aetiology

The aetiology is uncertain. Possibly there are cross-reactions between bacterial antigens and the mucosa; some significant HLA links have been reported (Scully 1992).

Clinical and histological features

The vulval ulcers are sharply defined, of varying sizes, with a yellowish base and a red halo (Fig. 5.17). The histology is non-specific.

Differential diagnosis

The important differential diagnoses for the vulval ulcers are herpes simplex, Stevens–Johnson syndrome and, above all, Behçet's sydrome, for which condition other manifestations are required.

Management

Topical corticosteroids and tetracycline are useful in treatment. The corticosteroids can be used as a proprietary preparation in an adhesive base. A readily prepared empirical remedy (5 ml of triamcinolone acetonide (10 mg per ml) mixed with 95 ml of tetracycline syrup) is helpful, as is 5% lignocaine ointment.

OTHER NON-INFECTIVE ULCERS

Other ulcers, particularly those described in the older literature, are difficult to categorize and may not be distinct entities.

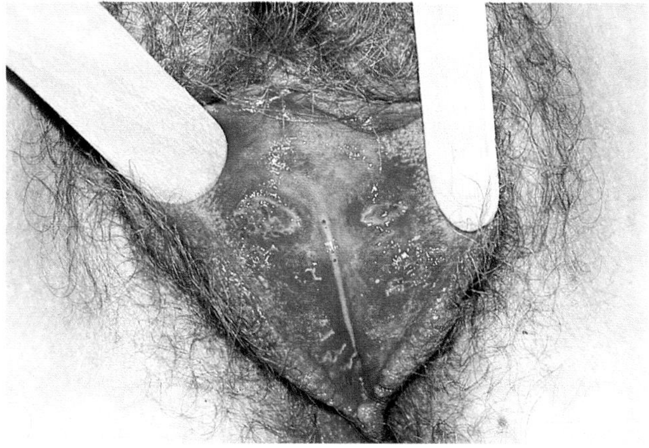

Fig. 5.17 Major aphthous ulcers of the vulva.

Sutton's ulcers (Sutton 1935) were described, originally in 1913, as recurrent, solitary or few, deep and painful, more often occurring in the mouth than at the vulva; they may well have been identical to major aphthous ulcers.

Lipschutz (1913) described ulcers of sudden onset with fever and pain in young girls; they affected the inner labia minora, were multiple and healed over a few days to leave faint scars; another variety lasted for weeks, and could affect other areas of the vulva. The latter may well have been of the aphthous type. The former, however, seem rather to resemble those now sometimes seen in young girls, of uncertain origin but often associated with fever. They have also been reported in patients with pityriasis lichenoides (Joulia & le Coulant 1954, Burke *et al.* 1969). They have been found in association with infectious mononucleosis, caused by the Epstein–Barr virus (McKenna *et al.* 1994); the female cases in the literature were reviewed, with an additional example, by Lampert *et al.* (1996). In one example (Portnoy *et al.* 1984) the virus was recovered from an ulcer. The Epstein–Barr virus is known to be subclinically harboured, in both sexes, in the genital tract, which may provide a reservoir of infection and permit sexual transmission (Näher *et al.* 1992).

Ulceration was reported in association with syphilis and with diphtheria (Parks 1941, Machnicki 1953). Boyce and Valpey (1971) reported an outbreak of painful ulcers in the wives of servicemen returning from Asia who were themselves symptom free. Muram and Gold (1993) have reported vulval ulcers, not caused by infection or by leukaemic infiltration, in girls with myelocytic leukaemia, and the authors postulated a multifactorial aetiology.

Histology

In all these ulcers the histology is non-specific.

Differential diagnosis

The differential diagnosis will include infections, particularly, in the acute forms, herpes simplex and varicella–zoster.

Management

Treatment is symptomatic, as for aphthous ulcers.

Pigmentary disorders

Pigmentation related to haemosiderin

This pigmentation tends to have a reddish-brown tinge, rather than the brownish- or bluish-black colour found with melanin.

It occurs as a result of extravasation of blood and is a feature of lichen sclerosus, Zoon's vulvitis, caruncles and prolapsed tissue of cervical, vaginal, rectal or urethral origin (Fig. 5.18).

Pigmentation related to melanin

There is considerable variation in the normal pigmentation of the keratinized vulval skin in relation to ethnicity, age and hormonal status. These appearances are usually even and diffuse and offer no diagnostic difficulty.

HYPERPIGMENTATION

Post-inflammatory pigmentation

This is usually the sequel of lichen planus, less often of lichen sclerosus. The pattern of the discoloration and the association of the disease are helpful in diagnosis (Fig. 5.19) but if there is any doubt a biopsy should be carried out.

Histologically there is pigmentary incontinence, with pigmented macrophages in the upper dermis.

Fixed drug eruption is a cause of localized post-inflammatory pigmentation.

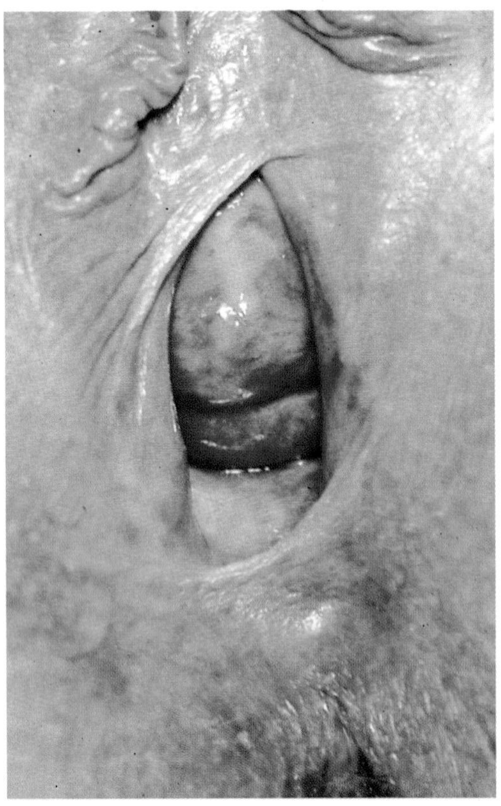

Fig. 5.18 Haemosiderin deposition on the prolapsed vaginal wall, in a patient with lichen planus.

Melanosis

Pigmentation that is patchy and intense, extensive or sparse, symmetrical or asymmetrical, affecting either keratinized or non-keratinized areas or both, often presents diagnostic problems. Such lesions should always be subjected to biopsy. Histology may reveal evidence of flat seborrhoeic warts, lentigines, melanocytic naevi or vulval intraepithelial neoplasia.

In some cases, however, the histology will reveal only basal hypermelanosis with, usually, an increased number of melanocytes and some pigmentary incontinence but no melanocytic proliferation (Fig. 5.20). Some choose to call such lesions, particularly if there is any associated oral pigmentation, examples of Laugier–Hunziker disease (Laugier *et al.* 1977). Others use the term vulval melanosis (Jackson 1984, Sison-Torre & Ackerman 1985, Dupré and Viraben 1990, Kanj *et al.* 1992, Estrada & Kaufman 1993). Gerbig

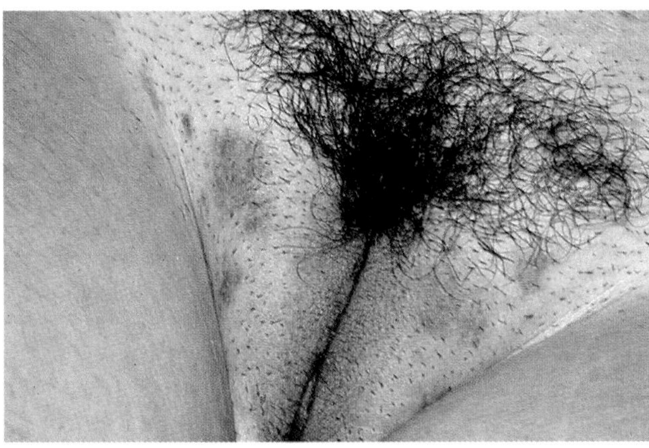

Fig. 5.19 Post-inflammatory pigmentation on the pubic area, in a patient with lichen planus.

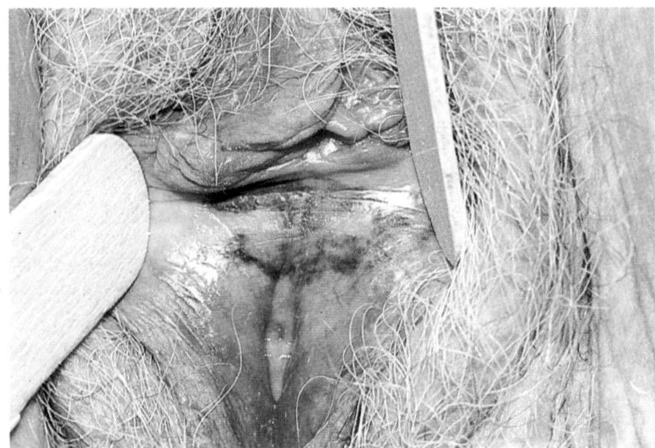

Fig. 5.20 Melanosis: extensive patchy pigmentation.

and Hunziker (1996) have now suggested the term idiopathic lenticular mucocutaneous pigmentation. Barnhill *et al.* (1990) however, in a detailed review of 10 reported cases in men and seven current and reported examples in women, prefer the term genital lentiginosis whenever there is, as is often the case in these lesions, evidence of melanocytic hyperplasia (to demonstrate which special stains may be required), reserving the term melanosis for those where it is absent. These authors prefer to keep an open mind as to the potential of such lesions for malignancy. Although a commoner view is that, on the analogy with apparently similar (though solitary) oral lesions (Ho *et al.* 1993), these lesions are unlikely to become malignant, follow-up is certainly recommended since long-term observation has not been reported. Photographs or diagrams are important aids where change is being looked for. Lesions that have changed in some way should be biopsied.

Lentigines (see also Chapter 10). Lentigines may be sporadic, or part of a syndrome. The LAMB syndrome (lentigines, atrial myxoma, mucocutaneous myxomas, blue naevi) has been described by Rhodes *et al.* (1986) in a girl of 13, who as well as an atrial myxoma and other lesions had lentigines of the face and vulva, confirmed by histology. Lentigines were not found on the vaginal or oral mucosa. A further case, with a review of the literature, was added by Reed *et al.* (1986).

Vaginal pigmentation. Melanocytes are to be found in only about 3% of vaginas (Schmidt 1995) but pigmented macules, melanosis and malignant melanoma are all recognized. Any pigmented vaginal lesion should be biopsied.

Acanthosis nigricans

This rare disease in all its forms is now thought to be related to insulin resistance (Rendon *et al.* 1989). In children it is benign and may be hereditary. In adults it may be benign or linked with malignancy, usually an adenocarcinoma but occasionally a lymphoma or epithelial carcinoma (Brown & Winkelmann 1968, Mikhail *et al.* 1979). Very rarely, the condition is drug induced; nicotinic acid (Tromovitch *et al.* 1964) and triazinate (Greenspan *et al.* 1985) have been incriminated.

Clinical features. The lesions chiefly affect the face, the mucosae and the flexures, and the genital area is a site of predilection. They are dark, at first velvety and then warty, and all aspects of the vulva may be involved.

Histology. The histology shows hyperkeratosis and papillomatosis, some acanthosis, and pigmentation. Horny inclusions are sometimes present.

Management. Only symptomatic measures, and treatment where feasible of the underlying condition, are possible.

Pseudoacanthosis nigricans

This name is given to the banal darkening and thickening of flexural skin, often accompanied by skin tags, in obese patients, particularly if they have a somewhat dark skin (Fig. 5.21). Again, the effect may be mediated by insulin resistance induced by the obesity; the changes remit if weight is lost.

Differential diagnosis. The main differential diagnosis for acanthosis nigricans and pseudoacanthosis nigricans is from one another, and will depend on associated features and investigations; the histology is different only in degree from true acanthosis nigricans.

Miscellaneous causes of pigmentation

Staining of vulval skin. Trichomycosis and chromidrosis may lead to some discoloration of the skin. A proprietary laxative, Dorbanex, was reduced in the bowel to dithranol and was responsible for staining of skin in contact with faeces as well as reddish-brown discoloration of urine and vaginal secretions (Barth *et al.* 1984, Greer 1984); and related compounds may cause similar effects.

HYPOPIGMENTATION AND DEPIGMENTATION

Post-inflammatory hypopigmentation

Patchy hypopigmentation is a common sequela of inflammation, especially obvious in a dark skin (Fig. 5.22).

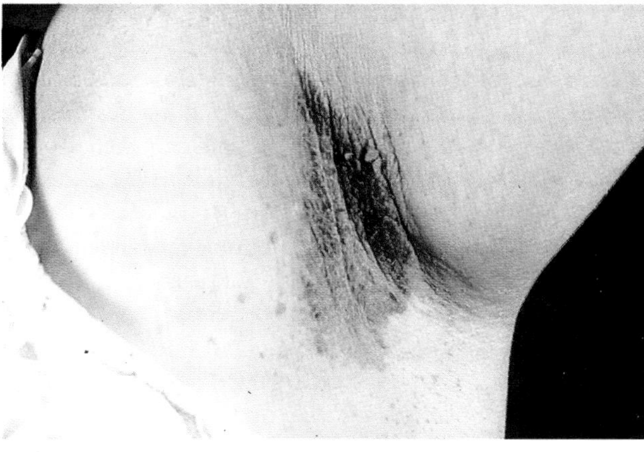

Fig. 5.21 Pseudoacanthosis nigricans: darkening and tags in a flexure.

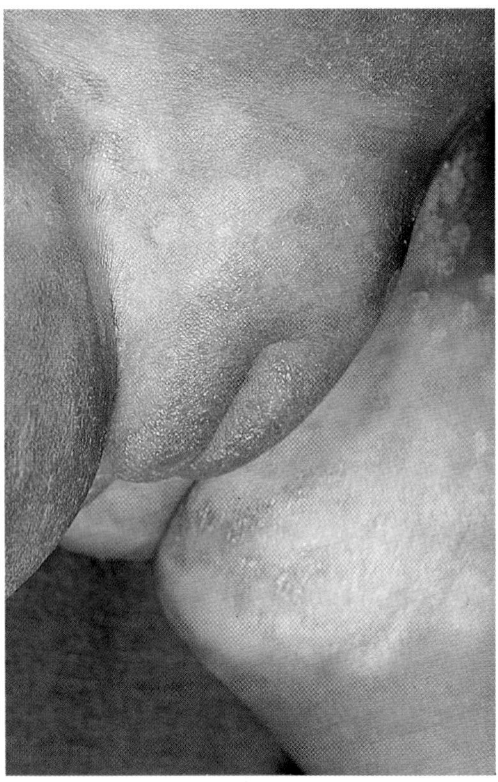

Fig. 5.22 Post-inflammatory hypopigmentation in a child with a psoriasiform napkin rash.

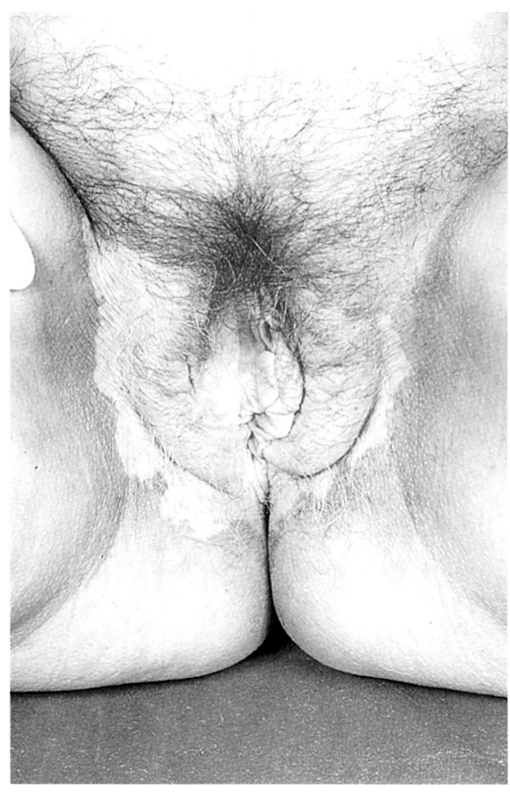

Fig. 5.23 Vitiligo: total loss of pigment in a symmetrical pattern.

Vitiligo

Aetiology. Vitiligo is of uncertain aetiology but autoimmune and neurohumoral mechanisms have been suggested.

Clinical features. There is complete depigmentation of an area of skin that is in all other respects normal. The patch is well defined and the condition is usually symmetrical (Fig. 5.23). In hairy areas, the hair may or may not retain its colour.

Histology. The histology shows that melanocytes are reduced in number, apparently normal but non-functional, or absent, a loss demonstrable by electron microscopy. There is a mild lymphocytic infiltrate.

Differential diagnosis. The differential diagnosis from the pale thickening of lichenification is usually easy, but to distinguish it from a mild lichen sclerosus (with which it is not infrequently associated) can be almost impossible. Post-inflammatory hypopigmentation is usually incomplete and ill defined. Occupational depigmentation from paratertiary butyl phenol, reported in the genital area in men (Moss & Stevenson 1981), is unlikely in women.

Management. There is no effective treatment; measures that might be tried elsewhere would be inappropriate at this site.

Disorders of skin appendages

Disorders of sebaceous glands

Clinical features

Sebaceous glands may be clinically apparent on the labia majora and minora, either as yellowish specks known as Fordyce spots and analogous to the oral lesions, or as aggregated sheets (Fig. 5.24). On the labia minora, they end where Hart's line marks the boundary of the vestibule. Secretion from the glands may accumulate between the labia, and patients who complain of soreness or a subjective sensation of swelling in this area often have unusually profuse glands. Blockage of sebaceous gland ducts leads to the temporary or permanent formation of yellow papules, nodules and cysts, which may give rise to symptoms.

Rocamora *et al.* (1986) have described a case where sebaceous lobules surrounding a duct formed soft polypoid lesions. They were thought to represent sebaceous gland hyperplasia.

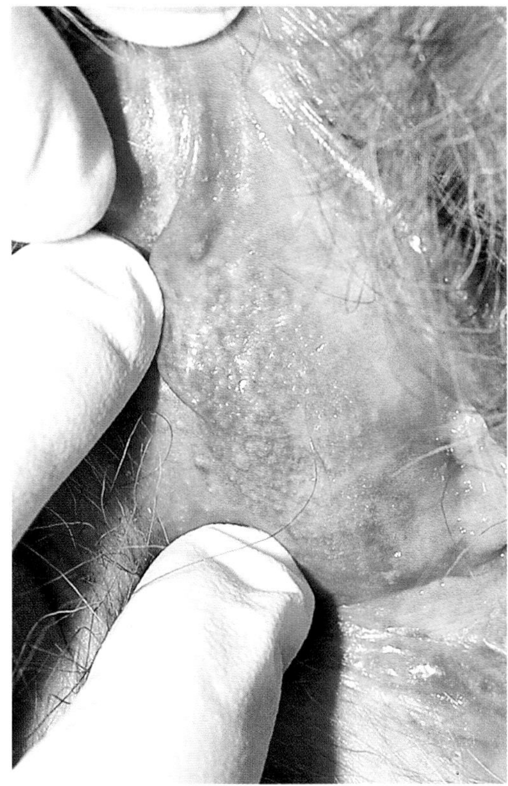

Fig. 5.24 Fordyce spots: aggregated yellow specks on the inner labium minus.

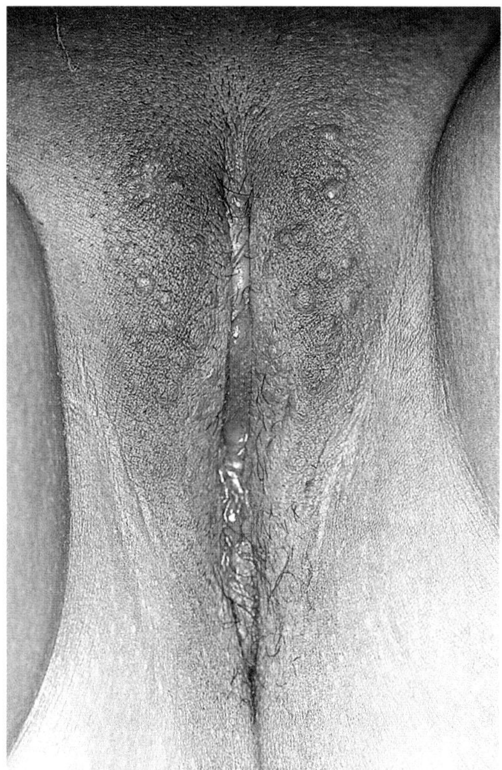

Fig. 5.25 Syringomas: multiple skin-coloured papules.

Management

Treatment is not usually indicated, but if the lesions give rise to symptoms cautery or the hyfrector is effective.

Disorders of sweat glands

ECCRINE MILIARIA

Occlusion of the sweat-gland orifices, under conditions of heat and humidity, leads to the appearance of papulovesicles. They are encountered mainly in infants. The obstruction may result in a subcorneal vesicle or in vesiculation proximal to a deeper obstruction at the dermal–epidermal junction. The problem is self limiting.

SYRINGOMAS (see also Chapter 10)

These benign adenomas of the eccrine sweat ducts appear as skin-coloured papules at the vulva, with or without lesions elsewhere (Fig. 5.25).

APOCRINE MILIARIA

These are poorly documented, but probably not uncommon, appearing as transient painful papules often with a cyclical (menstrual) pattern. Grimmer (1968) reported them in an elderly woman.

CHROMHIDROSIS

This refers to the secretion of coloured sweat, usually arising in apocrine glands. The colour varies from black or brown to yellow or green. The vulva is not a common site, but Joosse *et al.* (1964) reported lesions there. Areas of pigmentation under the skin were found to be a lipofuscin, probably a normal tissue constituent; however, the granules were larger than normal and more numerous. Surgical treatment, sometimes considered elsewhere, is unlikely to be feasible in the genital area.

FOX–FORDYCE DISEASE

This rare eruption of unknown aetiology is characterized by closely set, skin-coloured papules, which are very itchy and which affect the axillae, breasts and anogenital area (Fig. 5.26). They develop after puberty and become more itchy at menstruation, improving in pregnancy and after the menopause.

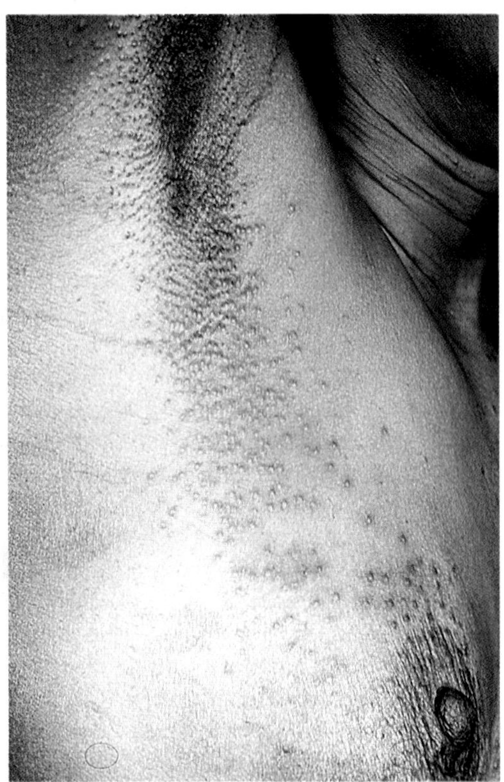

Fig. 5.26 Fox–Fordyce disease: skin-coloured papules in and around a flexure.

Histology

The ducts of the apocrine glands are obstructed by keratin plugs, leading to retention of sweat. There may be surrounding inflammation. Complete obstruction of a duct can result in rupture of a retention vesicle.

Differential diagnosis

The differential diagnosis histologically is from apocrine miliaria, and clinically from syringomas (which, however, rarely itch).

Management

The contraceptive pill may improve the symptoms. Topical corticosteroids are of limited value. Ultraviolet irradiation or topical retinoic acid to exfoliate the surface have been advocated. Surgical measures may be used as a last resort.

Disorders of hair

PILONIDAL SINUSES

Vulval examples are less common than are sacrococcygeal ones, but do occur. Most if not all arise as a reaction to penetration of the skin by a hair. Cases have been reported by Betson *et al.* (1962) and by Radman and Bhagavan (1972). The lesion is painful and may present as an abscess requiring incision; definitive treatment is by excision.

Histology

There is a tract lined by granulation tissue and fragments of hair can often be seen.

FOLLICULITIS

This is not uncommon, particularly on the mons pubis. Chemical irritants such as sugar, used as a depilatory, or physical factors such as trauma from shaving, with or without infection, may be responsible. The lesions are follicular papulopustules.

Histology

There are inflammatory changes, mainly at the follicular ostium.

Differential diagnosis

It is important not to miss an infection with pediculosis pubis or scabies as an underlying cause.

Management

Treatment is by removing any underlying irritant, attention to local hygiene, application of antiseptics such as povidone iodine and topical or systemic antibacterial agents if necessary. Should there be problems of recurrence or of poor response, the possibility of unsuspected underlying factors and of perineal carriage of organisms may have to be explored.

PSEUDOFOLLICULITIS PUBIS

A reaction to ingrowing hairs, analogous to that seen in the beard area, may occur after preoperative shaving, following regular shaving of the pubic area as practised in some cultures, or after shaving or waxing of the 'bikini line'.

Management

Avoidance of shaving, or instruction in improved techniques, will lead to improvement.

HIDRADENITIS SUPPURATIVA

Aetiology

This inflammatory condition has in the past been considered to involve mainly the apocrine glands. Yu and Cook (1990), however, considered that the basic pathogenesis is in the follicular epithelium rather than in the apocrine gland, a view supported by Boer and Weltevreden (1996), who found that the earliest event is a spongiform infundibular folliculitis.

The aetiology is uncertain. Although occlusion of the axillary skin can lead to bacterial proliferation in the glands and to a clinical lesion it is not thought that antiperspirants or deodorants are culpable. While *Streptococcus milleri* is frequently found in the lesions (Highet *et al.* 1980), it is not held to be responsible for their causation. Mortimer *et al.* (1986a) suggested that androgen metabolism is involved; in 42 women patients a significant incidence of clinical and biochemical endocrine abnormalities was found, in that the patients more often had irregular periods, premenstrual exacerbation of disease, acne and hirsutes, a higher concentration of free testosterone and a higher free androgen index than did normal control subjects. These findings were in accord with the incidence in the reproductive years and with the impression that acne is a frequent accompanying condition. However, Barth *et al.* (1996) have found that these findings are no longer significant when the results are controlled for body weight, and conclude that there is no evidence of hyperandrogenism.

Clinical features

It is rare before puberty and tends to involute after the menopause, although cases occasionally present at or even after that time (Barth *et al.* 1996). Anogenital lesions are common, being found in the genitocrural folds and on the mons pubis and buttocks; the axillae and breasts may also be affected. Black subjects are said to be affected more often than are white.

Tender nodules form, soften and may lead to abscesses; spontaneous discharge is uncommon. Widespread sinuses, induration and scarring develop and there may be fistulae that open into the anus. When the condition is quiescent an important diagnostic feature is the presence of bridged scars and comedonal plugs (Fig. 5.27).

Histology

Histologically there is often distension of apocrine glands and accumulations of polymorphs, which tend to migrate to adjacent tissue. The gland may become necrotic, with an infiltrate of lymphocytes, plasma cells and macrophages.

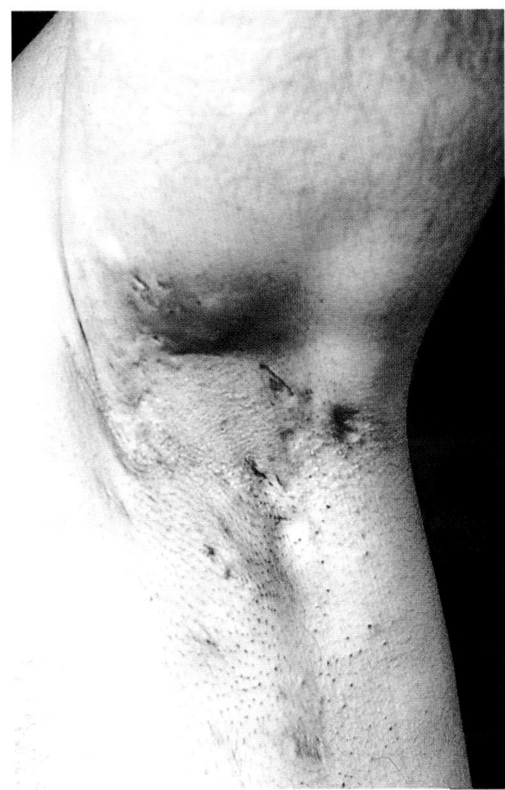

Fig. 5.27 Hidradenitis suppurativa: comedones and bridged scars in a flexure.

Ultimately the changes include sinuses lined by keratinized epithelium, fibrosis, foreign body reactions and sometimes pseudoepitheliomatous hyperplasia. At least nine cases of squamous cell carcinoma have been reported (Sparks *et al.* 1985), two of these being in women with buttock lesions.

Differential diagnosis

The differential diagnosis is in the early stages from a simple folliculitis, and later from deep infections and, in particular, from Crohn's disease, which it may closely resemble and with which it may sometimes coexist (Ostlere *et al.* 1991, Burrows & Russell Jones 1992).

Management

The first approach in treatment is long-term antibiotics. Mortimer *et al.* (1986b) found antiandrogen therapy helpful in a double-blind cross-over study. Etretinate, now prescribed as acitretin, and isotretinoin have been used with variable results (Dicken *et al.* 1984, Stewart & Light 1984, Norris & Cunliffe 1986, Hogan & Light 1988), acitretin being preferred; however, side effects and teratogenicity limit the application of these drugs. Cyclosporin may prove useful (Buckley & Rogers 1995). Severe cases often result in extreme destruction and debility, and here the best approach is surgical (Banerjee 1992). The carbon dioxide laser is helpful for small areas (Finley & Ratz 1996). Small areas may be excised with primary closure, but sometimes grafting or healing by secondary intention is required. There may, however, be recurrence in spite of these surgical measures.

ALOPECIA AREATA

Aetiology

Alopecia areata is a common condition in the aetiology of which genetic, autoimmune and other immune factors are probably involved.

Clinical features

Genital hair is lost in alopecia totalis. Patchy loss may be seen in milder examples of the disease. The patches are round, non-inflamed and symptom free. Lesions are usually to be found elsewhere.

Histology

This shows follicles that are smaller and higher in the dermis than usual; in the early stages there is a lymphocytic infiltrate round the hair bulb.

Management

Treatment is unsatisfactory and would be rarely advised at this site. A topical corticosteroid would be safer than sensitizing agents, as are sometimes used elsewhere, but may have no more than placebo value.

Other causes of alopecia

The pubic hair becomes thinner with age, but does not disappear entirely.

Bullous (blistering) diseases

Those conditions which rarely if ever affect the vulva (porphyria, dermatitis herpetiformis, pemphigoid gestationis, pemphigus foliaceus) will not be considered here.

Epidermolysis bullosa, benign familial chronic pemphigus (Hailey–Hailey disease) and Darier's disease are discussed above.

Stevens–Johnson syndrome

Mucosal involvement (oral, ocular, genital) is the essential feature of this variant of erythema multiforme, lesions on the skin not being necessary for the diagnosis.

Aetiology

The condition may arise spontaneously, but attacks are often precipitated by infection, particularly herpes simplex, or by drugs.

Clinical features

The onset is acute and often accompanied by systemic symptoms. As regards the genital area, there are painful, shallow ulcers and flaccid bullae of all aspects of the labia, often involving also the surrounding skin (Fig. 5.28). Vaginal stenosis (Graham-Brown *et al.* 1981) and vulvovaginal adenosis (Marquette *et al.* 1985, Wilson & Malinak 1988, Bonafe *et al.* 1990) have been described as sequelae (see below).

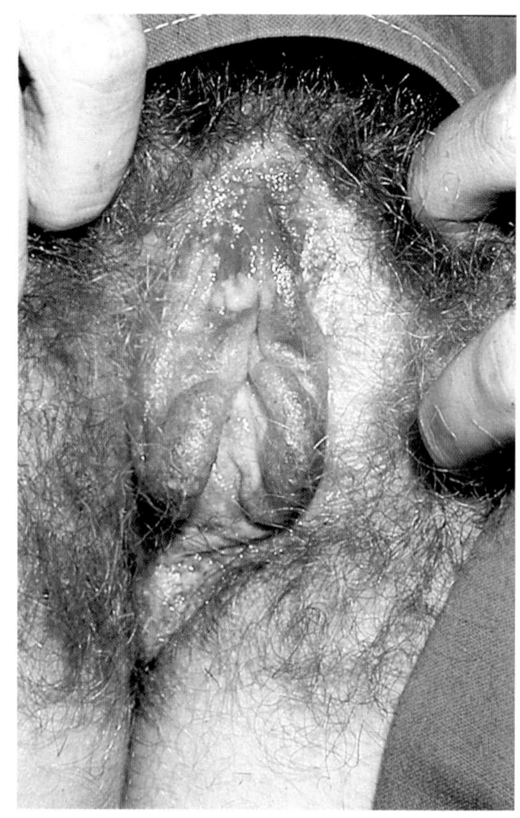

Fig. 5.28 Stevens–Johnson syndrome: multiple vulval ulcers and erosions.

Histology

The histology shows a perivascular infiltrate and extravasation of red cells, oedema and varying degrees of epidermal necrosis, particularly of the basal layer; a subepidermal bulla may form.

Differential diagnosis

The diagnosis is usually easily made except in respect of toxic epidermal necrolysis (TEN); typical cutaneous lesions of erythema multiforme, if present, will be helpful. It is sometimes difficult, however, to tell if a focus of genital or oral herpes is, or has been, present to account for the eruption, or to incriminate a specific drug as the cause.

Management

When the syndrome is precipitated by recurrent herpesvirus attacks, long-term aciclovir is beneficial as a preventive measure. Good nursing is essential and in severe cases the patient should be under the care of a burns unit. Controversy remains as to the role of systemic steroids; some advocate pulsed doses, others think that they are best avoided. Cyclosporin may be used in difficult cases. Antibiotics should not be given without guidance from swab results, since resistant strains may become a problem. Bonafe *et al.* (1990) found treatment with the laser helpful in dealing with adhesions; surgical procedures may also be employed (Chapter 11).

Staphylococcal scalded skin syndrome and toxic epidermal necrolysis

Aetiology

These conditions are histologically but not clinically distinct. In children the cause is a staphylococcal exotoxin, usually of phage type 2, which results in the staphylococcal scalded skin syndrome (SSSS). Although this has been reported in adults (O'Keefe *et al.* 1987) they are more likely to have TEN. In TEN, although idiopathic cases may occur, there is often a drug that is responsible, commonly a phenazone or a sulphonamide.

Clinical features

The onset is acute with systemic illness and exquisitely painful lesions rapidly causing denudation of the epidermis. The vulval area is often involved in both types, sometimes with vulvovaginal scarring, especially in TEN (Meneux *et al.* 1997). The soreness and redness may indeed begin in the genital area. The outcome, especially in TEN, may be fatal.

Histology

SSSS has an intraepidermal split below the granular layer. In TEN, the whole epidermis is necrotic with a subepidermal bulla and much basal cell destruction. Frozen sections are advised in case of doubt.

Differential diagnosis

The differential diagnosis between the two is vital since the treatment will be different. That from Stevens–Johnson syndrome can be difficult or impossible clinically and, in TEN, also histologically; typical iris lesions of erythema multiforme on the skin are helpful if present.

Management

In both conditions, good nursing is essential and admission to a burns unit is often indicated. In SSSS the treatment is with antibiotics, usually flucloxacillin; in TEN any suspected drug must be withdrawn. In TEN, the use of systemic steroids is controversial, the balance of opinion being in favour of their avoidance. As in the Stevens–Johnson syndrome, cyclosporin may be helpful in severe cases, while antibiotics given blindly will tend to lead to resistant strains. Further practical details of management have been well discussed by Creamer *et al.* (1996).

Fixed drug eruption

Aetiology

In this condition lesions appear at the same site or sites when a particular drug is ingested. Its mechanism remains essentially unexplained (Ackroyd 1985). It is well recognized on the penis but reports of vulval examples are sparse. Klostermann (1972) had an illustration of such a lesion. Sinha (1982) reported a vulval example caused by dapsone, Sehgal and Gangwan (1986) found two examples (one vaginal and one vulval) in women out of a total of 29 cases in the genital area, and Hughes *et al.* (1987) reported two cases at the vulva related to trimethoprim. The drugs responsible vary with prescribing patterns. In the past, barbiturates, phenazones and phenolphthalein were often involved whereas now sulphonamides are probably the commonest group. Seminal fluid as a cause of a fixed drug eruption, affecting areas elsewhere as well as the vulva and vagina, was reported by Best *et al.* (1988); mefenamic acid was helpful as a preventive agent.

Clinical features

The lesion is a pigmented plaque, which flares up to produce an oedematous, often frankly bullous, area when the drug is ingested, and then subsides to leave pigmentation, which tends to persist.

Histology

There is epidermal necrosis with dermal inflammatory changes and later deposition of melanin in the epidermis and in dermal melanophages.

Differential diagnosis

The clinical differential diagnosis is from herpes simplex and from other causes of an acute bulla or plaque, and in the quiescent stage from melanocytic lesions and pigmented intraepithelial neoplasia.

Management

Much depends on persistence in exploring the history. A challenge test can be diagnostic and discontinuation of the offending drug is curative.

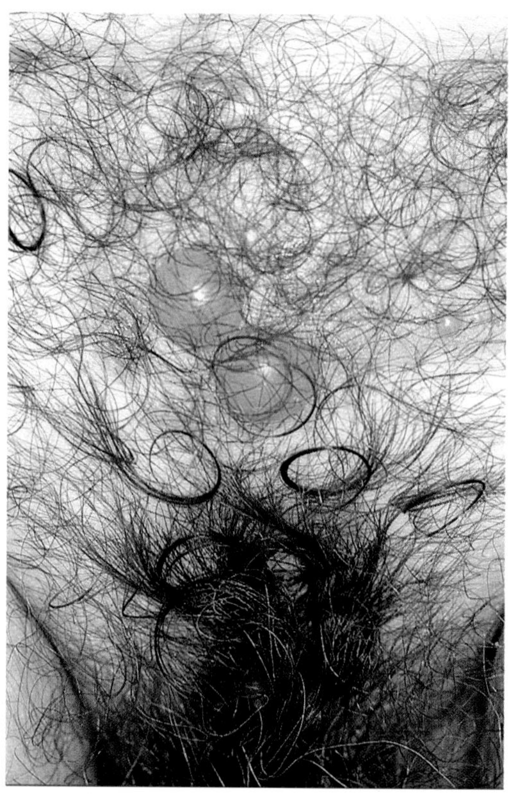

Fig. 5.29 Bullous pemphigoid: tense bullae and erythema of the pubic area.

Immunobullous disorders

These disorders affect skin and mucosae. In those to be discussed, anogenital involvement is common and important in management. Marren *et al.* (1993), for example, in a large series of female patients with immunobullous disease found that such lesions occurred in over 50% of their adult patients with bullous or cicatricial pemphigoid; in the patients with linear IgA disease they were found in 80% of the children and almost 50% of the adults.

Aetiology and classification

The pathogenesis of the immunobullous disorders lies in the development of antibodies that react against normal epidermal and basement membrane zone tissue. The target antigens are those molecules promoting adhesion between the cells and of the cells to the underlying dermis, hence the development of a blister. Immunofluorescence (IMF) of non-lesional skin and sometimes of other sites is an all-important technique in investigation. Indirect IMF, using the patient's serum, can also be useful.

Their classification was originally under clinically determined titles, but is likely now to give way to names that are a more precise characterization in terms of the target antigens, as in the case of linear IgA disease. Techniques of increasing sophistication and specificity used in recently reported work mean that the true nature of some cases reported earlier may sometimes be doubtful, and that the headings employed here may be subject to modification in the future.

The differential diagnosis and management of these conditions will be considered together.

BULLOUS PEMPHIGOID

Bullous pemphigoid (BP) mainly affects the elderly, but cases have been described in children, where in both sexes there may be mucosal involvement, which is sometimes genital (deCastro *et al.* 1985, Guenther & Shum 1990, Levine *et al.* 1992, Saad *et al.* 1992, Marren *et al.* 1993, Nagano *et al.* 1994, Wakelin *et al.* 1995).

Clinical features

The bullae are tense, although rupture with the formation of erosions is common, and they often arise from an erythematous base. Both keratinized and non-keratinized skin may be involved (Fig. 5.29).

Histology

Histology shows subepidermal bullae, and direct IMF shows IgG at the basement membrane zone. The antigen is located in the basal epidermal cells. Indirect IMF shows a circulating IgG antibody.

EPIDERMOLYSIS BULLOSA ACQUISITA

Epidermolysis bullosa acquisita is a rare condition where clinical and histological findings, including those of IMF, are similar to those of BP. With salt-split skin preparations, however, the antibody binds to the floor of the blister, i.e. to dermal components. Park *et al.* (1997) reported an example in a six-year-old girl with genital involvement, and noted two similar previously reported examples.

CICATRICIAL PEMPHIGOID

In cicatricial pemphigoid (CP) the histological findings are identical to those of BP, as are those of direct and indirect IMF when they are positive; so the diagnosis is at present primarily a clinical one, although Setterfield *et al.* (1996a) have demonstrated that the DQB1* 0301 allele is found in a significant majority of patients with CP. However, evolution from BP to CP has been described (Banfield *et al.* 1997). The subjects are usually middle-aged but cases in children with genital involvement have been reported by Rosenbaum *et al.* (1984), who described a case in a boy and reviewed previous cases, and Marren *et al.* (1993). Cases that may have been drug induced have also been reported (van Joost *et al.* 1980, Shuttleworth *et al.* 1985).

Clinical features

The findings at the vulva range from a scarcely discernible obliteration of sulci to a gross distortion of the labia and introitus. Scarring is a prominent feature and the vagina is likely to be involved, as are also the eyes, mouth and larynx (Figs 5.30 & 5.31).

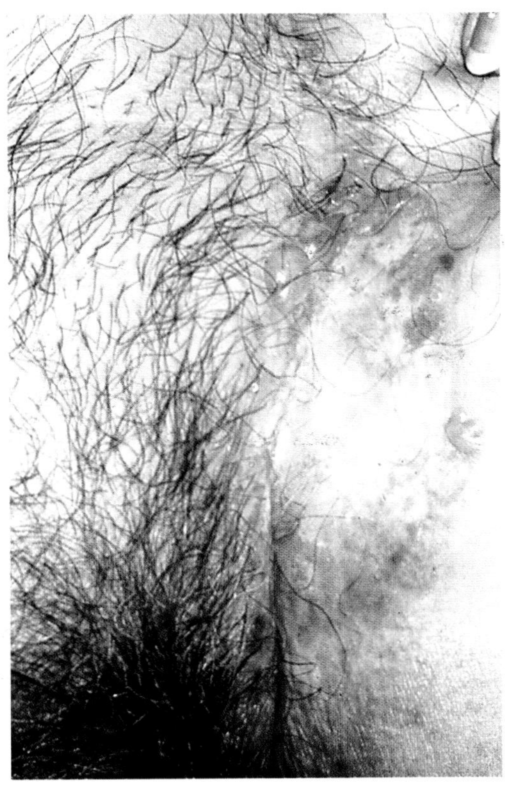

Fig. 5.30 Cicatricial pemphigoid: tense bullae with scarring in the genitocrural area.

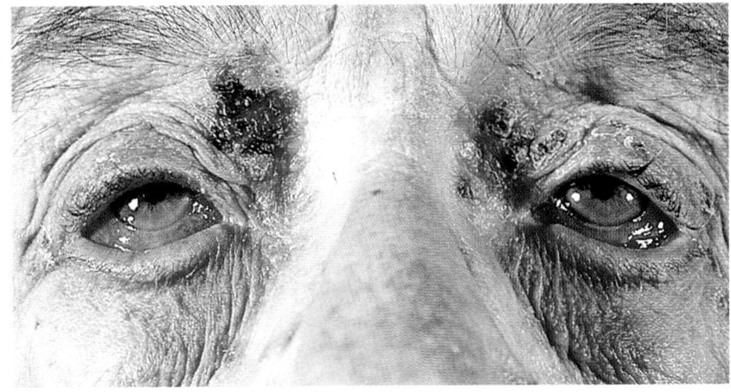

Fig. 5.31 Cicatricial pemphigoid: bullae on the face and obliteration of the conjunctival sulci.

LINEAR IgA DISEASE OF CHILDREN (CHRONIC BULLOUS DISEASE OF CHILDHOOD) AND OF ADULTS

Clinical features

These conditions present with tense bullae (Fig. 5.32). In children, where the vulval and perianal areas are sites of predilection, the blisters are often described as having a clustered appearance (Fig. 5.33). The condition sometimes, but not always, remits at puberty. At all ages scarring may ensue.

Histology

The histology is of a subepidermal bulla, and on IMF there is a linear band of IgA at the basement membrane zone. In children particularly, circulating IgA antibody may be found.

PEMPHIGUS VULGARIS

Pemphigus vulgaris is a rare disease of skin and mucosae often affecting the vulva. Ashkenazi Jewish subjects are par-

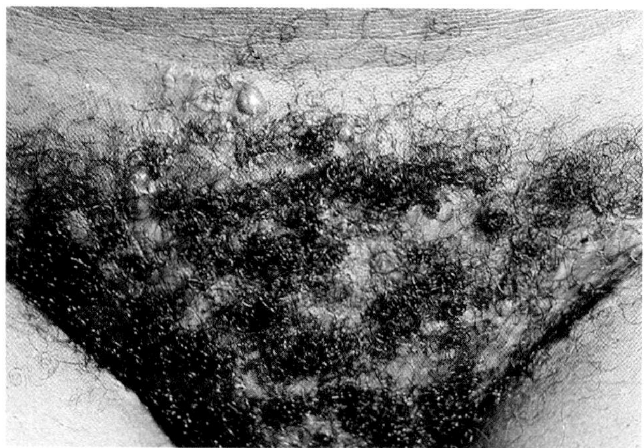

Fig. 5.32 Linear IgA disease in an adult: tense bullae of the pubic area.

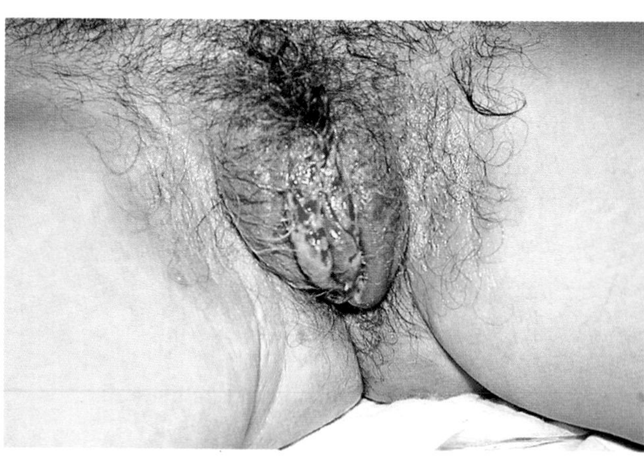

Fig. 5.34 Pemphigus vulgaris: confluent flaccid bullae of the vulva.

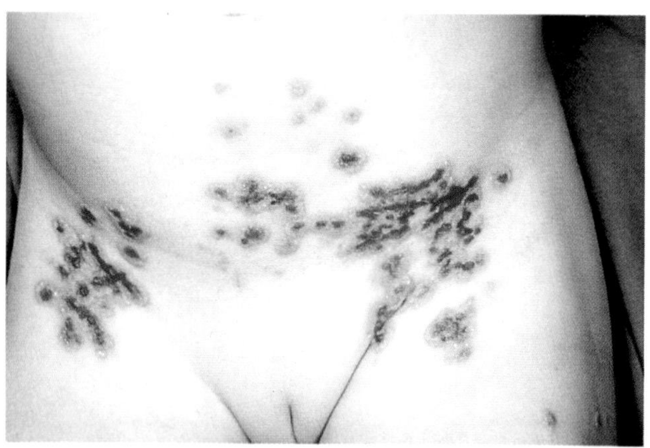

Fig. 5.33 Linear IgA disease in a child: clustered bullae of the lower abdomen and groins.

ticularly susceptible. In general, the condition begins in middle life. Although Sillevis Smitt (1985) in a review of 31 reports in the literature of pemphigus in children noted only one with specifically genital involvement, a boy, it has since been reported in male (Kanwar & Kaur 1991) and female (Marren *et al.* 1993) children in the genital area. Familial cases have also been described by Bhol *et al.* (1996). Lesions indistinguishable from pemphigus vulgaris are known to be precipitated by penicillamine (Troy *et al.* 1981) and an atypical form of the disease with vulval involvement was associated with angiofollicular lymph node hyperplasia (Castleman's syndrome) in a case reported by Coulson *et al.* (1986).

Clinical features

The bullae are painful, flaccid and easily eroded (Fig. 5.34). In pemphigus vegetans, a more benign and chronic variant,

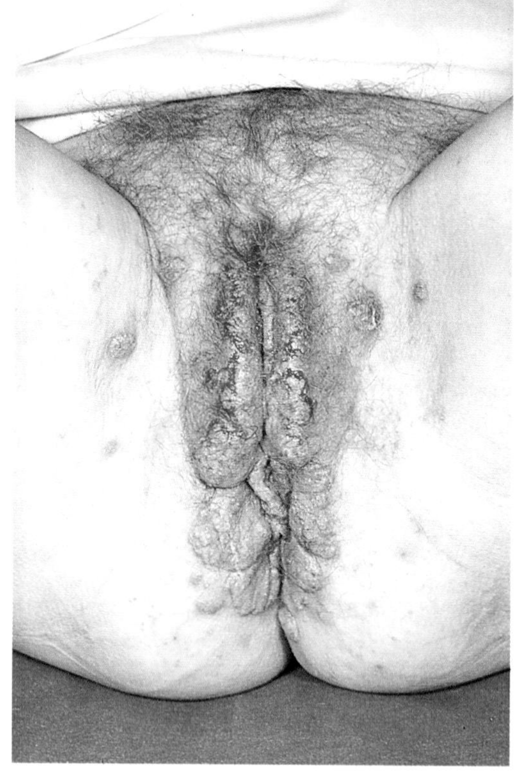

Fig. 5.35 Pemphigus vulgaris, vegetans type: confluent bullous masses.

heaped-up masses are a feature (Fig. 5.35). The vagina, and also the cervix (Mikhail *et al.* 1967, Friedman *et al.* 1971, Lonsdale & Gibbs 1998) may be affected.

Histology

Histology shows suprabasal acantholysis, and hence

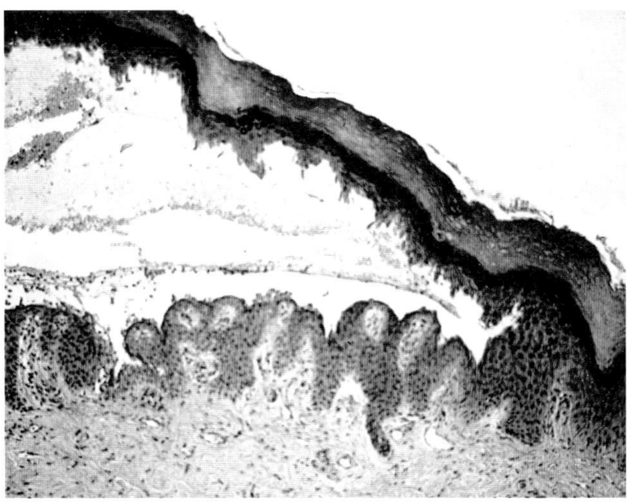

Fig. 5.36 Pemphigus vulgaris, intraepidermal bulla with acantholysis.

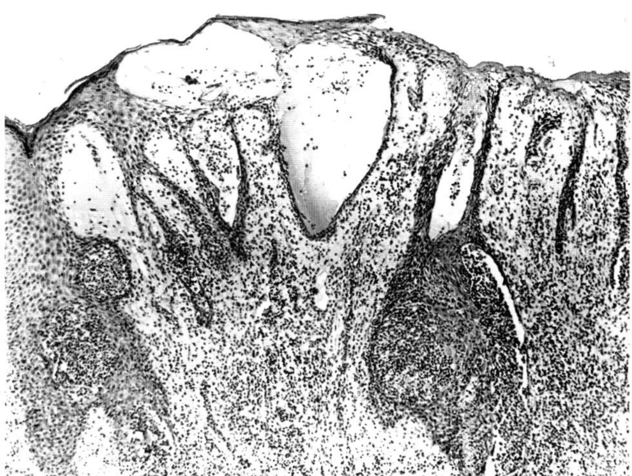

Fig. 5.37 Pemphigus vulgaris, vegetans type: intraepidermal bullae, acantholysis, acanthosis and an eosinophilic infiltrate.

intraepidermal bullae (Fig. 5.36). In pemphigus vegetans, downward proliferation of epithelial strands is associated with papillomatosis, acanthosis, hyperkeratosis and eosinophilic infiltration of the dermis (Fig. 5.37). Direct IMF shows deposition of the IgG antibody in the intercellular spaces and indirect IMF demonstrates circulating IgG antibodies

DIFFERENTIAL DIAGNOSIS OF THE IMMUNOBULLOUS DISORDERS

Apart from the exclusion of herpes simplex virus infections, where the lesions are usually acute, the main difficulty is in distinguishing these conditions from each other, and from lichen planus and lichen sclerosus. In children, sexual abuse must be borne in mind; conversely, whenever such abuse is suspected, confusion with these dermatological conditions should be considered. The distinction from lichen planus and lichen sclerosus may present difficulties since bullae are readily eroded and may therefore not be visible as such, and the histology may not always be diagnostic. The distinction can be particularly difficult with CP, where IMF findings tend to be negative. Repeat biopsies, IMF testing and careful observation over a period of time will often be required. The appearance of more easily recognized lesions at other sites can often give support to a provisional diagnosis.

MANAGEMENT OF IMMUNOBULLOUS DISORDERS

Detailed management is outside the scope of this account. It will often involve the care of patients with widespread disease and involve the use of potentially dangerous drugs, and it should always be under the supervision of a dermatologist, in cooperation as necesary with the gynaecologist and the ophthalmologist. The general principles of using bland emollients, soaks of potassium permanganate for open areas, appropriate agents for secondary infection and potent topical corticosteroids for eroded and blistered areas will apply. Whilst this may suffice for mild and localized manifestations, other patients will require systemic treatment. This is largely empirical and may include, singly or together, steroids, dapsone, sulphamethoxypyridazine, minocycline, nicotinamide, azathioprine and cyclosporin.

Inflammatory dermatoses

Intertrigo

Aetiology, clinical features and histology

This non-specific inflammation of the flexures, brought about by heat, sweating, obesity and friction, is common in the groins, genitocrural area and natal cleft. It is further encouraged by diabetes, incontinence and immobility. The ill-defined erythema is often malodorous and secondarily infected with mixed bacteria and *Candida*. In the case of *Candida*, small, outlying, scaly satellite lesions are often present and the main lesions tend to have a macerated sodden fringe. This infection is not necessarily associated with a *Candida* vulvovaginitis. The histology shows non-specific changes.

Differential diagnosis

Intertrigo must be distinguished from flexural psoriasis, where the border is sharper, from seborrhoeic dermatitis (in both of which there are often lesions elsewhere) and from erythrasma, which is brownish with well-defined edges and shows a coral-pink fluorescence under Wood's light.

Management

This depends on treating predisposing factors, the separation of folds by smooth, closely woven material such as cotton, and the use of mild topical corticosteroids combined with antibacterial or antifungal agents, for example miconazole/hydrocortisone.

Psoriasis

Aetiology and incidence

Although psoriasis is genetically determined, various trigger factors will provoke it in those with the diathesis, and friction or occlusion may initiate or perpetuate flexural lesions. Flexural psoriasis is less common than are lesions on extensor aspects, but nevertheless is not infrequently encountered.

Clinical features

The silvery scaling of psoriasis elsewhere is lost in these areas, but the bright erythema and sharp outline tend to remain (Fig. 5.38). A fissure in the natal cleft often bisects lesions there. The mons pubis is often involved and the appearance at that site is more scaly. Although psoriasis is not generally recognized to cause tissue loss, this does appear sometimes to happen (Fig. 5.39). Psoriasis, except in the rare pustular form and in that probably manifested in Reiter's disease, does not affect mucosal surfaces. However, some patients who have definite psoriasis elsewhere, and perhaps perianal lesions, complain of itching of the inner aspects of the vulva, with little to see; it is possible that this is caused by psoriasis.

Histology

There is parakeratosis, acanthosis with elongation of the rete ridges and a reduced or absent granular layer, often with collections of neutrophils in the epidermis; as well as papillary oedema and perivascular dermal inflammation (Fig. 5.40).

Differential diagnosis

The differential diagnosis includes intertrigo, seborrhoeic dermatitis and eczema, in all of which the margins are less well defined. The presence of more typical lesions elsewhere is often helpful.

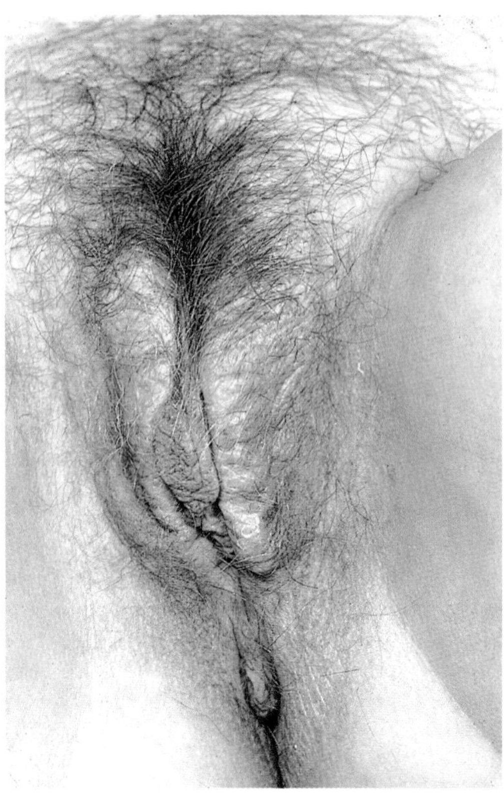

Fig. 5.38 Psoriasis: well-defined, bright erythema of the labia majora and perianal area.

Seborrhoeic dermatitis

Definition and clinical features

This common condition has eczematous and psoriasiform features and is probably caused by the yeast *Pityrosporum ovale*. As well as in the genitocrural area and natal cleft, lesions are likely to be found elsewhere, for instance on the scalp, behind the ears and on the face. They are orange-pink, slightly scaly, not well defined, and sometimes secondarily infected (Fig. 5.41).

Histology, differential diagonsis and management

The histology is non-specific or psoriasiform. The rash is often difficult or impossible to distinguish from psoriasis; lesions vary, resembling first one and then the other, and treatment and management are as for psoriasis.

Management of psoriasis and seborrhoeic dermatitis

Bland emollients, for example emulsifying ointment or aqueous cream, and a moderately potent topical corticosteroid are usually effective, but sometimes a very potent

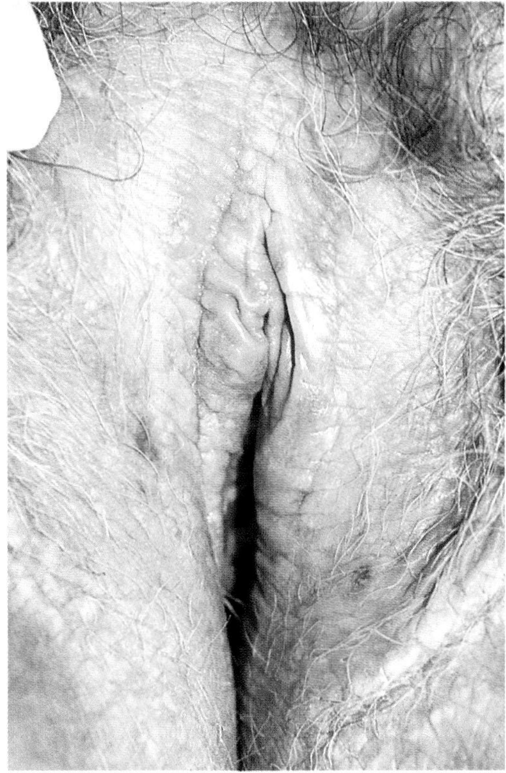

Fig. 5.39 Psoriasis: extensive and severe lesions, with some loss of architecture.

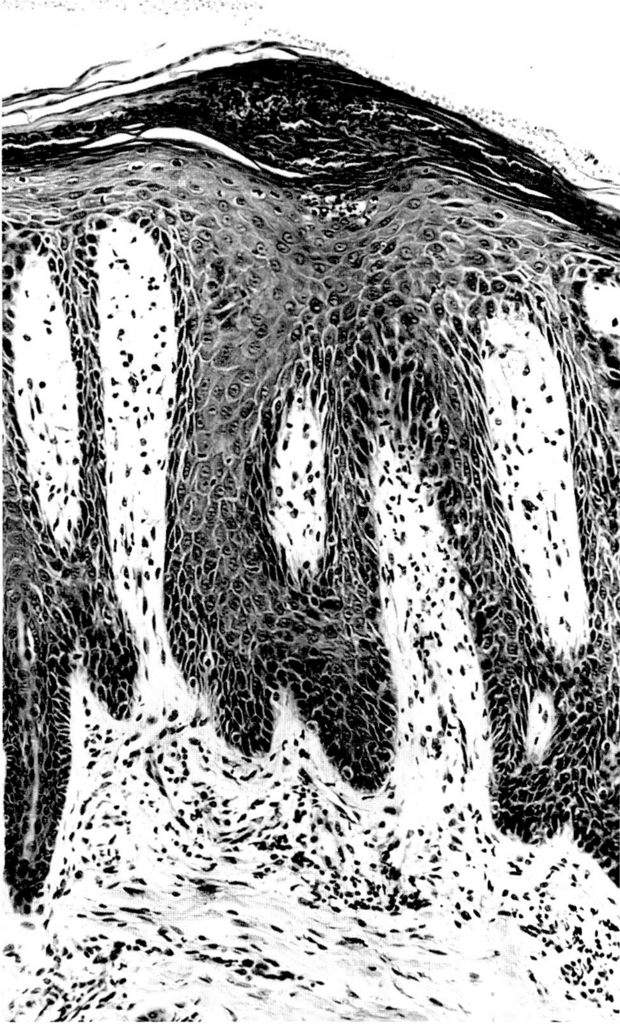

Fig. 5.40 Psoriasis: parakeratosis with small collection of neutrophils (Monro's abscess), elongation of rete ridges, oedema of papillae, dermal inflammatory infitrate.

type is required to begin with, particularly in so far as the lesions affect inner aspects of the vulva. Milder preparations, or instead the occasional use of the most potent, are options for maintenance. Tar, dithranol and calcipotriol, whilst good for psoriasis in other areas, are irritant in the genital area and should be avoided.

Reiter's disease

Definition and clinical features

The condition is defined as a non-suppurative polyarthritis of more than 1 month's duration following an enteric or more commonly a lower genital tract infection. Urethritis and/or cervicitis are common, as is conjunctivitis. Subjects with the HLA-B27 are particularly susceptible. Patients often have a psoriasiform rash on the feet and hands. Although this presents as a pattern which is clinically distinct from psoriasis, it may represent a form of it which has been precipitated by a chlamydial or other genital infection. In men, a circinate balanitis is common. The equivalent vulvitis is very rare but has been reported by Thambar *et al.* (1977), Daunt *et al.* (1982), Haake and Altmeyer (1988) and Edwards and Hansen (1992). The patient described by

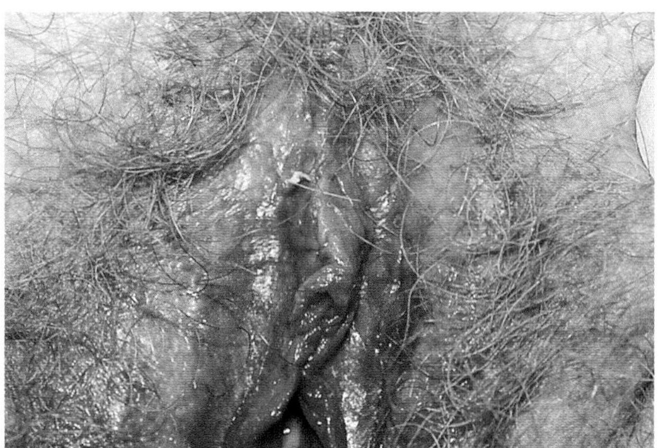

Fig. 5.41 Seborrhoeic dermatitis: diffuse, patchy erythema of the vulva.

Edwards and Hansen had striking lesions originally thought to be of mucocutaneous candidosis. In the genital area scaling and crusting involved the keratinized skin; she had a vaginal discharge and white papules on the cervix and, later, white papules that became eroded and affected the whole of the vulva including the mucosal aspects.

Histology

The histology is that of pustular psoriasis, with hyperkeratosis, parakeratosis, an absent granular layer and prominent polymorph microabscesses in the epidermis.

Differential diagnosis

The differential diagnosis is usually from candidosis, and from psoriasis with which it may constitute a spectrum. However, two rare conditions may sometimes have to be considered: IgA pemphigus and subcorneal pustulosis (see below).

Management

If a chlamydial infection is suspected as the initiating feature, the sexual partner should be screened and a course of a tetracycline given. Mild lesions can be controlled with topical corticosteroids; long-term treatment may, however, have to be complex, utilizing systemic agents such as methotrexate and retinoids as in severe psoriasis, and including measures for the joints. Supervision by a dermatologist and a rheumatologist will be indicated. Psoriasis and Reiter's disease are both significantly more severe and difficult to control in individuals who are HIV positive.

IgA pemphigus (intraepidermal IgA pustulosis)

Clinical and histological features

This condition is characterized (Wallach 1990) by widespread pustules and may affect the genital area. It appears to be essentially a neutrophilic disorder. Histologically there is acantholysis and an intraepidermal or subcorneal pustule, with intercellular IgA deposition on IMF. There may also be an IgA paraproteinaemia.

Subcorneal pustulosis (Sneddon–Wilkinson disease)

Clinical and histological features

This condition of unknown aetiology is characterized by waves of superficial pustules in a circinate pattern. It may affect the vulva. Its aetiology is unknown. Histologically the pustules are subcorneal and filled with neutrophils. IMF is negative.

Differential diagnosis

The clinical differential diagnosis of both these conditions includes pemphigus, pustular psoriasis and Reiter's disease. The histology, where the pustule of subcorneal pustulosis is more superficial and IgA pemphigus shows acantholysis, and the IMF findings, are helpful.

Management

Both respond well to dapsone.

Eczema

Definition

Eczema and dermatitis are synonymous terms, except when it so happens that the word 'dermatitis' has been incorporated in the name of some particular disease, for example acrodermatitis enteropathica, dermatitis herpetiformis. Eczema is characterized by epidermal spongiosis, with or without acanthosis, and a dermal perivascular lymphohistiocytic infiltrate. It appears in a wide variety of clinical patterns, at the genital area as elsewhere.

ATOPIC ECZEMA

Patients rarely complain of vulval involvement even when there is severe and widespread eczema elsewhere. However, in patients complaining of itching, with an atopic background and perhaps a few signs elsewhere, minimal erythema, which is often found between the labia, perianally and in the natal cleft is probably a manifestation of eczema; it responds to appropriate treatment.

IRRITANT AND ALLERGIC ECZEMATOUS REACTIONS

These can be difficult to distinguish, and indeed may coexist.

Irritant reactions

Irritant reactions are those where there is a direct effect on the tissues, without any allergic mechanism. Elsner *et al.* (1990) have noted the particular susceptibility of the vulval skin in this respect.

A wide variety of medicaments can be responsible, for example podophyllin or dequalinium; the latter has caused genital necrosis in both sexes (Tilsley & Wilkinson 1965).

Cosmetic preparations can be involved, for example deodorant sprays and tissues, which however are little used now, in the UK. Bubble baths are potentially irritant if the concentration is high. Rycroft and Penney (1983) incriminated bromination of swimming pools.

Allergic reactions (allergic contact dermatitis)

Here a true allergic response has arisen to a substance that is not an irritant. Figures for the incidence of contact dermatitis in the anogenital area are somewhat variable. Marren *et al.* (1992) found clinically relevant allergies in 39 out of 135 patients (35%) who had been referred for patch testing because response to treatment was slow or the diagnosis uncertain. The patients had a variety of underlying conditions, the largest groups being lichen sclerosus, eczema and those where the diagnosis was uncertain. The positive results were to substances found in scented products, medicaments and corticosteroids. Lewis *et al.* (1994b) reported results in 69 patients referred for testing, where 40 (58%) had positives considered relevant, i.e. medicaments, substances found in scented products, local anaesthetics and corticosteroids. Goldsmith *et al.* (1997), however, carried out a retrospective survey on 201 patients who had been referred for testing over a period of 14 years. Of these, 103 had involvement of the vulva, 42 of the perianal area, and 56 involvement of both sites. Those with vulval lesions alone had positive relevant findings in 19%, those with perianal disease alone in 33%, but those where both areas were involved 43%. The positives were to local anaesthetics, antibiotics, scents and the steroid marker tixolone pivalate. It seems therefore that patients with vulval lesions *per se* do not have frequent sensitivity reactions, but that these problems are commoner in those with perianal involvement or, particularly, with involvement of both areas. The explanation might be related to the greater extent of skin involvement, or could reflect differences in reactivity of the two sites.

Many individual cases have been reported. The preservative ethylene diamine is a potent sensitizer. Vaginal preparations and an intrauterine device have been held responsible (Robin 1978, Romaguera & Grimalt 1981, Corazza *et al.* 1992), as have perfumes and disinfectants in sanitary pads (Sterry and Schmoll 1985). Reactions to contraceptives are well recognized; in the report of Bircher *et al.* (1993) both partners were allergic to condoms. The antifungal agent nifuratel was responsible for another case of connubial contact dermatitis (di Prima *et al.* 1990). Lewis *et al.* (1994a) described a cello player with an unusual relevant allergy, to colophony, found in the resin used on the instrument. Seminal fluid may, rarely, produce a type IV reaction rather than the commoner immediate type I (Kint *et al.* 1994).

Clinical features

The end point of an irritant and of an allergic dermatitis is a diffusely oedematous erythema, often with flexural maceration secondarily infected with bacteria and *Candida*; in the latter case satellite scaly or eroded papules are a characteristic feature. Subsequent lichenification will render the area thick and pale.

Histology

There is spongiosis, sometimes acanthosis and parakeratosis, and some dermal inflammatory infiltrate.

Differential diagnosis

The differential diagnosis will include a *Candida* vulvovaginitis, where there is usually a vaginal discharge, and psoriasis or seborrhoeic dermatitis, where the distinction may be more difficult, much depending on the history, the presence of lesions elsewhere and the unfolding of events.

Management

In all cases of eczema, any known or suspected causative agent should be withdrawn. In the acute stage, bathing with potassium permanganate 1 in 10 000 is soothing. This can be carried out by sitting in a plastic bowl or small bath (the solution causes staining) or by the application of gauze or other soft material that has been soaked in the liquid. Bland emollients such as emulsifying ointment or aqueous cream are used for washing and as moisturizers. Topical corticosteroids, often requiring the addition of an antibacterial or antifungal agent (e.g. miconazole/hydrocortisone, or fusidic acid/betamethasone valerate, or a combination of clobetasol butyrate, oxytetracycline and nystatin, according to severity) are valuable. When the condition has settled, patch testing is indicated if an allergy is suspected.

Lichen simplex and lichenification

Definition

Lichen is a term used in describing many lesions that have an appearance of closely set papules as their main characteristic; hence lichen simplex and lichenification, lichen planus, lichen sclerosus. They have some resemblance to the mossy surface of lichen on a tree. However, the terms 'lichenoid' as in many drug rashes and 'lichenoides' as in an entity such as pityriasis lichenoides chronica stem from lichen planus only and imply resemblance to the distinctive features of lichen planus, rather than to those of lichen simplex and lichenification. In lichen planus and lichen sclerosus, genuine closely set papules are indeed to be found, but in lichen simplex and lichenification the appearance is a similitude only; the normal rhomboidal pattern of the skin, magnified as a result of uniform thickening, gives the impression of papulation. These terms, lichen simplex and lichenification, refer to a thickening of the skin, manifested histologically mainly as acanthosis and hyperkeratosis, which is the response to prolonged itching and subsequent rubbing. Some individuals are particularly likely to show this reaction. In lichen simplex, the change occurs on skin that was clinically normal, whereas in lichenification the change is superimposed on some underlying dermatosis, for example eczema or psoriasis.

It should be noted that there is a discrepancy here as regards the usage of dermatologists and that of pathologists. The latter do not recognize the term lichenification, employing only that of lichen simplex or lichen simplex chronicus to encompass all the aspects noted above; and this scheme may well be adopted by the International Society for the Study of Vulvovaginal Disease, i.e. the terms lichen simplex and lichenification will be used synonymously.

Clinical features

Underlying lesions are usually masked and the clinical picture is of thickened, slightly scaly, pale or earthy-coloured skin with accentuated markings and a diffuse outline. The tissues look soggy and tend to be fissured (Fig. 5.42).

Histology

The histology shows hyperkeratosis, parakeratosis, acanthosis, a prominent granular layer, lengthened rete ridges and a variable chronic inflammatory infiltrate (Fig. 5.43). There is lamellar thickening of the papillary dermis and sometimes perineural fibrosis. All the epidermal components are hyperplastic, and the labelling index is increased (Marks & Wells 1973a,b). There may be some evidence of an underlying dermatological condition.

The phenomenon called multinucleated atypia of the vulva by McLachlin *et al.* (1994), who reported 12 cases, has been ascribed by le Boit (1996) to a non-specific change found not uncommonly in lichenified skin, as noted by Tagami and Uehara (1981).

Differential diagnosis

The clinical diagnosis is usually straightforward, but it is important to ensure that an underlying skin condition is not missed.

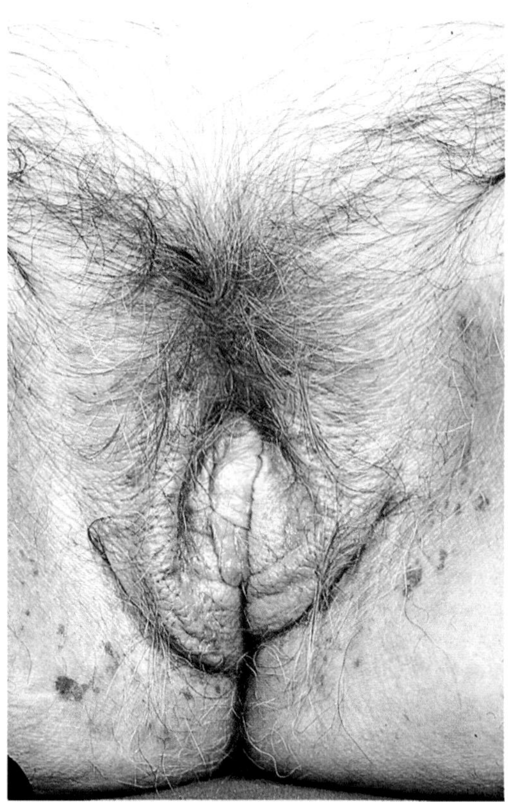

Fig. 5.42 Lichenified eczema: thick, pale, excoriated appearance.

Management

The treatment is essentially that of eczema, but the potent topical corticosteroids, e.g. betamethasone valerate 00.1% or even clobetasol propionate 0.05%, are often needed initially to break the cycle of itching and rubbing. A mildly anxiolytic antihistamine such as hydroxyzine at night is helpful.

Inflammatory conditions in infancy: napkin rashes

In infancy the napkin area is the site of a variety of eczematous rashes, classified (Atherton 1992) as primary irritant napkin dermatitis, seborrhoeic dermatitis (of which psoriasiform napkin rash is probably a variant) and intertrigo. Infantile gluteal granuloma is a rare condition. In addition, perianal dermatitis may affect the newborn.

PRIMARY IRRITANT NAPKIN DERMATITIS

Aetiology

Allergic contact dermatitis is very rare in infants, but this rash, related to irritants such as topical applications, urine and faeces, is common; it appears after the first few weeks of life. Conditions of warmth and occlusion favour it, as do

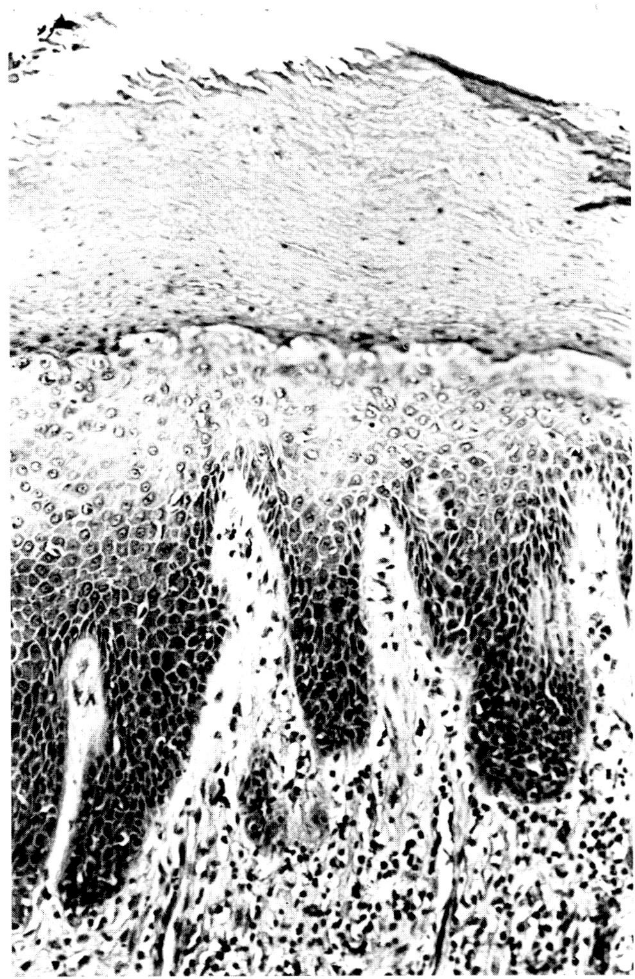

Fig. 5.43 Lichen simplex: hyperkeratosis, acanthosis, lengthened and broadened rete ridges, chronic inflammatory infiltrate.

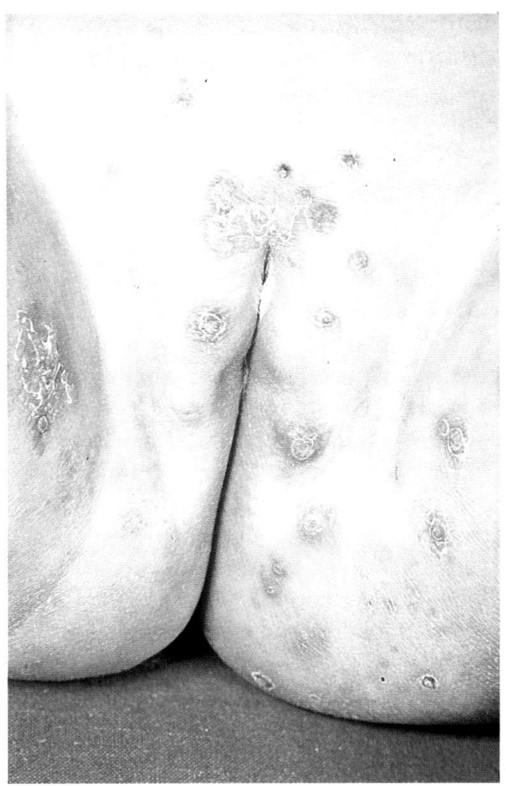

Fig. 5.44 Napkin rash: papules and small nodules.

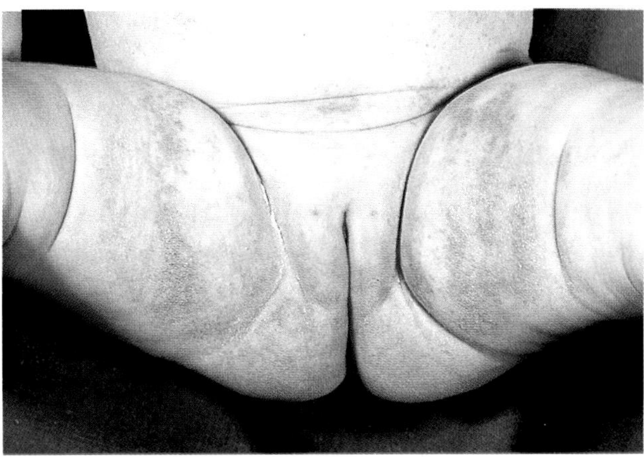

Fig. 5.45 Napkin rash: patchy erythema avoiding the flexures.

the inadequate sweating mechanisms in the very young, and it is commoner in bottle-fed compared with breast-fed babies. Ammonia from urine is not now thought to be causative, but urine of relatively high pH increases the activity of faecal proteases and this may be a relevant factor. Secondary infection is common, particularly with *Candida*, of which there may be intestinal carriage. It is seen with disposable as well as with washable napkins.

Clinical features

The confluent erythema is sometimes eroded and may become papular or even nodular (Fig. 5.44). It tends, except where *Candida* infection is predominant, to avoid the deep flexures of the area; sometimes it mainly affects its edges (Fig. 5.45).

PSORIASIFORM NAPKIN RASH

Aetiology and clinical features

This form has strikingly scaly and well-defined patchy lesions, and often similar lesions elsewhere (see Fig. 5.22). Most of these children probably do not have the psoriatic diathesis or, as noted by Skoven and Hjortshoj (1978), the

HLA pattern of the potential psoriatic patient; nevertheless, some do seem to be significantly liable to develop it later (Neville & Finn 1975).

SEBORRHOEIC DERMATITIS OF THE NAPKIN AREA

Clinical features

This is not related to adult seborrhoeic dermatitis. There is a fairly typical clinical picture of patchy, scaly erythema, often affecting also other areas, especially the scalp. Some of these children may be suffering from atopic dermatitis or may later develop this more troublesome form of eczema, which has a worse prognosis.

INTERTRIGO

Genital intertrigo may occur in plump babies, and will tend to become infected.

HISTOLOGY OF NAPKIN RASHES

The histology of all these rashes is rarely sought, but it is generally held that they have a similar mildly eczematous appearance; the psoriasiform variant may, however, show psoriasiform features.

DIFFERENTIAL DIAGNOSIS OF NAPKIN RASHES

Their differential diagnosis will include Langerhans cell histiocytosis and zinc deficiency; although in both of these there are likely to be typical lesions elsewhere, they may have to be borne in mind if response to treatment is unsatisfactory. Infections such as congenital syphilis, a primary *Candida* infection or herpes simplex are unlikely to present diagnostic difficulty.

MANAGEMENT OF NAPKIN RASHES

As regards management, probably the most important measure is to ensure frequent changes of the napkin, whatever its type. This should be followed by adequate cleansing, using water and a bland emulsifying preparation such as emulsifying ointment, and the application of a water-repellent ointment such as white soft paraffin. Proprietary oils for the daily bath are also useful. Topical corticosteroids are effective for the rash, and hydrocortisone is sufficiently strong; more potent preparations at this site can lead to significant absorption, atrophy and even wasting (Johns & Bower 1970). Hydrocortisone will often need to be combined with antibacterial or antifungal agents.

INFANTILE GLUTEAL GRANULOMA

Aetiology

Cases of this unusual condition, commoner in the male and arising on an irritant napkin rash (often as it is improving), were reported by Tappeiner and Pfleger (1971), Bonifazi *et al.* (1981), Uyeda *et al.* (1973) and Lovell and Atherton (1984). It appears to be an entity, and occlusion and fluorinated corticosteroids are thought to be involved. *Candida* is less likely to be culpable. Curiously, similar cases have been reported in incontinent elderly women, where corticosteroids were not a factor (Maekawa *et al.* 1978).

Clinical features

Oval, livid nodules with eroded surfaces affect the convexities of the whole napkin area. They regress after a few weeks, probably spontaneously, and may leave scars.

Histology

There is dermal oedema and a dense granulomatous plasma cell and lymphocytic infiltrate together with vascular dilatation, fibrinoid necrosis and haemosiderin deposits.

Management

The potency of topical corticosteroids, if relevant, should be reduced, and occlusion minimized.

PERIANAL DERMATITIS OF THE NEWBORN

This is a rather rare condition, and arises in the first week or so of life as an erythematous, often oedematous patch round the anus. It clears with simple measures in a few weeks and is thought to be an inflammatory response to faecal irritants. It may or may not be associated with a napkin rash.

Lichen sclerosus

Aspects of terminology

Some of the problems earlier surrounding the place of lichen sclerosus (LS) were noted briefly in the introduction to this chapter. It is appropriate here to discuss them in more detail because of their historical significance, because even today they may present difficulties in communication of practical importance, and because their study can yield much of value to our current views.

Historical. A welter of terms was applied from the end of the 19th century to describe those vulval lesions which were characterized by atrophy and shrinkage, which appeared to be associated with the development of carcinoma and which could not be clearly related to recognized skin conditions as seen elsewhere such as psoriasis or eczema. It is probable that they were all or almost all examples of LS, defined clinically by Hallopeau (1887, 1889) and histologically by Darier (1892); a few no doubt were lichen planus (LP).

The process begins with the descriptions of Weir (1875) of 'ichthyosis' of the tongue and vulva, of Schwimmer (1878) of 'leukoplakia' (a term used to imply potentially malignant change in white patches of mucosal or mucocutaneous tissues) and of Breisky (1885) of vulval 'kraurosis'. Shelley and Crissey (1953) supply a translation of this latter account:

> . . . the labia are apparently missing, in that they are plastered to the mucous surface of the labia majora, so that the edges alone remain indicated by narrow furrows. From the mons veneris to the urethral orifice the integument is drawn tight over the clitoris. . . . The general effect of this extensive shrivelling is a striking smallness and inflexibility of the vestibular portion of the vulva . . . which may indeed . . . offer abnormal resistance . . . in coitus . . . The skin . . . appears whitish and dry . . . while the adjacent skin parts involved are shiny and dry, pale reddish grey, covered also with faded whitish spots, and show ectatic vascular branching here and there.

Jayle (1906) considered that these changes could occur without leukoplakia. Although Perrin (1901) had pointed out the essential identity of kraurosis and 'leukoplasia vulvo-orale' (leukoplakia), Berkeley and Bonney (1909) and Bonney (1938) thought the lesions should be subdivided into 'kraurosis', which was characterized by an inflammatory and benign condition of the vestibule and introitus, and (entirely separate and distinct) 'leukoplakic vulvitis', which was characterized by white areas and had malignant potential.

The account by Berkeley and Bonney of leukoplakic vulvitis described vulval and perianal lesions and some on the thighs, appearing red, later white (hence the name), cracked, smooth and atrophic; histologically there was at first a thickened epidermis, with a dermal infiltrate, a subepidermal homogeneous zone and a loss of elastic tissue, culminating in a thin epidermis and dermal sclerosis with no inflammatory cells. The term 'leukoplakia' was used here to refer to changes in keratinized skin.

Kraurosis on the other hand they described as confined to the introitus, vestibule, urethral orifice and sometimes the clitoris. The tissue was red, shiny, later 'pale yellow and glistening'. There was vaginal stenosis, with disappearance of the labia minora and clitoris. Histologically there was striking atrophy, much inflammation and no subepidermal homogeneous zone.

The incidence of malignancy in kraurosis or leukoplakic vulvitis (in all, 19 cases in 10 years) was not stated but, in every case of carcinoma encountered by the authors (58 in 10 years), leukoplakic vulvitis was present. It was correlated with 'maximum hypertrophy of the interpapillar epithelial processes'.

As regards treatment of leukoplakic vulvitis, they found X-rays helpful (which may have been a factor in their incidence of malignancy). They advised excision if this failed—wide excision because of the risk of recurrence. In kraurosis they also advocated surgical removal of affected tissue. Darier (1928) retained the original definition of kraurosis, with its lack of thigh and perianal lesions. In the USA, Taussig (1929) also contributed to this debate; he described a leukoplakic vulvitis, which began as a hypertrophic condition but ended as an atrophic one, with an inflammatory infiltrate and a subepidermal 'collagenous' zone. He used the term kraurosis for the end stage of this leukoplakic vulvitis, whereas Berkeley and Bonney had totally separated the two.

The gynaecological and dermatological literature continued to develop along entirely separate paths. Ormsby and Mitchell (1922) clearly recognized vulval kraurosis as indistinguishable from LS in a patient with vulval and extragenital lesions; yet the connection was not realized by others for a considerable time.

Wallace and Whimster (1951), Wallace (1955) and Whimster (1959), in a series of accounts summarized by Wallace (1971), tried to overcome the confusion surrounding kraurosis, leukoplakic vulvitis and leukoplakia, and their relation to LS. They proposed that cases indisputably showing typical LS, clinically and histologically, should be noted as such, that the terms kraurosis and leukoplakic vulvitis should be dropped, and that where the appearance originally described by Breisky as kraurosis was seen without clear evidence of LS it should be termed 'primary atrophy'. Primary atrophy thus comprised cases with no extragenital LS, no perianal LS and no recognizable vulval LS papules. There was some potential for malignant change. Whereas Berkeley and Bonney had found no hyalinization histologically, but much inflammation, the picture of primary atrophy was described by Wallace and Whimster as an atrophic epidermis, reduced elastic tissue, hyalinized collagen and some inflammatory cells—changes that would all be compatible with LS. They wished to retain the term leukoplakia as a histological entity, characterized by marked dermal hyalinization, sometimes a dermal infiltrate, and a hyperkeratotic epidermis with lengthened, irregular and forked rete pegs with or without cellular atypia. It was distinguishable from lichenification by its lesser degree of acanthosis, spongiosis and parakeratosis, as well by the irregularity of the epidermal downgrowths and the marked hyalinization. They noted its presence adjacent to 20 squamous carcinomas, and regarded it as premalignant. In retrospect it seems as if they were describing something very similar to the 'maximum hypertrophy of the interpapillar epithelial processes' of Berkeley and Bonney. They differed from Taussig in viewing this change as a sequel rather than as a precursor of atrophy. Although usually to be found arising on LS or on primary atrophy, they believed that occasionally it developed on a vulva that was apparently otherwise normal or that showed just lichenification.

It was at this stage that Jeffcoate and Woodcock (1961) tried to simplify the situation; beginning with an analysis of all putative causes of vulval malignancy (and noting with perspicacity the possibility of a 'field change') they went on to consider leukoplakia and leukoplakic vulvitis. They commented that, ironically, the clinician expected the pathologist to give him or her the diagnosis of leukoplakia, while the pathologist felt it was a clinical diagnosis and would have no part in it. The authors analysed too the confusion noted above between the writings of Berkeley and Bonney and those of Taussig, and then turned to LS. Here they saw that between LS and (clinical) leukoplakia and kraurosis there was no essential difference. Their conclusion was that the same end point might come from different aetiological factors, and that 'the vulval and perianal regions are subject to chronic skin changes, the particular characteristics of which are probably conditioned by environment rather than causes' and '... irrespective of their appearances, all these intractable skin changes, for which a specific cause is not clear, are best given clinically an all-embracing and non-committal title such as "chronic epithelial dystrophy"'.

From this concept stemmed the 1976 ISSVD classification of non-malignant epithelial disorders as LS, hypertrophic and mixed dystrophy, which was noted in the introduction. Abolition of the terms lichen sclerosus et atrophicus, leukoplakia, neurodermatitis, leukokeratosis, Bowen's disease, erythroplasia of Queyrat, carcinoma simplex, leukoplakic vulvitis, hypoplastic vulvitis and kraurosis vulvae was recommended. The decision to refer to lichen sclerosus rather than to lichen sclerosus et atrophicus was not controversial. This was the case too as regards the other deletions, with the exception of Bowen's disease, which was to be retained only as Bowenoid papulosis, for a specific clinical picture; but Bowenoid vulval intraepithelial neoplasia (VIN) is a term still often used histologically, as is Bowen's disease for the clinical and histological picture in those vulval lesions which correspond exactly to lesions always known by this term in other parts of the body. In some respects this scheme, however, was the source of much misapprehension, which lasted at least until the classification of 1987 supplanted it and which to some extent persists. The view that skin changes at the vulva, representing so many different conditions, could only be categorized as 'dystrophy', something quite apart from skin disorders elsewhere, has done considerable harm. The current scheme of 1987 was noted in Table 5.1 and may soon itself become part of the historical background, being superseded by a simpler, more comprehensive listing such as is used in this chapter. The vulva will come to be recognized as it was rightly described by Weisfogel (1969): 'although the area involved is genital, the tissue concerned is skin'.

Correlation with the current position. However, it is worth trying to extract the essentials that remain helpful from these earlier accounts.

The kraurosis and leukoplakic vulvitis of Berkeley and Bonney appear to have been essentially unitary and quite compatible with the view that they were different patterns of LS. The same applies to Taussig's kraurosis and leukoplakic vulvitis, which he indeed regarded as stages in one disease process, although it would be generally considered now that the atrophic appearance is the precursor rather than the end result, embodying the primary nature of the condition.

Wallace and Whimster hoped by the term primary atrophy to avoid controversy when there was no incontrovertible evidence of LS. However, on the basis of their clinical and histological findings, the fact that many developed unequivocal LS (98 out of 120 of their cases were finally categorized as such) and the common clinical experience of how much the appearances can alter in patients with LS from one clinic visit to another, there seems little doubt that (with the proviso that perhaps some had lichen planus) all these patients could safely be said to have LS and the term primary atrophy dropped.

As regards the same authors' concept of leukoplakia, unfortunately the discrepancy between the implication in its name of a clinical picture and its definition as a histological entity has given rise to some confusion. Leukoplakia was one of the terms recommended for abolition in 1976, and there is no doubt that this was a wise decision; its continuing usage is to be deplored; it has overtones from the past which may incline a gynaecologist to an inappropriate vulvectomy.

Nevertheless, the histological appearance described by Wallace and Whimster as leukoplakia is recognized today as a manifestation of LS, i.e. LS with epithelial hyperplasia of a particular pattern. When it is accompanied by VIN 3, differentiated type, with atypia confined to the lower epidermis, it is probably the precursor of malignancy and not reversible; however, when it is found without atypia its malignant potential in LS is unknown. This aspect is discussed later, under the heading of LS and malignancy. There is therefore a thread running through these reports from the earliest times, which we can with profit catch hold of now and which may lead to fuller knowledge of LS.

Aetiology

Familial incidence is well recognized (Hunt 1954, Barket & Gross 1962, Hofs 1978, Friedrich & MacLaren 1984, Murphy *et al.* 1982); it may concern both sexes, for example father and daughter, and has been noted in identical (Meyrick Thomas & Kennedy 1986) and non-identical (Cox *et al.* 1986) twins. The link with autoimmune disease is also established (Goolamali *et al.* 1974, Harrington & Dunsmore 1981, Meyrick Thomas *et al.* 1988), although relatively weak; about 21% of patients have an autoimmune disease, 22% a family history and 44% one or more autoantibodies in significant concentration. Those with such a background do not differ significantly in clinical respects from those without (Meyrick Thomas *et al.* 1988). Until recently the HLA findings, which one would expect to be distinctive in some way, were inconclusive; they were summarized by Purcell *et al.* (1990). Marren *et al.* (1995), however, were able to study class II antigens (of which DR and DQ are known to be linked with other autoimmune conditions) and found a significant association of patients compared with controls as regards DQ7, and as regards DR7, DQ8 or DQ9, singly or together. There was also a suggestion that A2 might exert a protective role in that it tended to be absent in patients who had extensive extragenital lesions, and that linkage of DR4 with DQ8 was commoner in those without marked structural change of the anogenital area.

There is a great deal of somewhat fragmentary material pertaining to pathogenesis, reviewed in detail by Meffert *et al.* (1995), but most has lacked significant outcome. Lavery (1984), noting that some cases were associated with achlorhydria, speculated on interactions between urogastrone (epidermal growth factor) and somatostatin; Friedrich and Kalra (1984), believing that testosterone topically was effective, found lower levels of dihydrotestosterone in LS patients and suggested that the enzyme 5α-reductase might be involved. Various other abnormalities, unlikely to be of primary importance, include changes in synthesis and distribution of collagenase and elastin (Godeau *et al.* 1982, Barnes & Douglas 1985), and positive immunoreactivity for an intestinal polypeptide substance (Johansson & Nordlind 1986).

An infective agent has been sought. Cantwell (1984) described pleomorphic, variably acid-fast bacilli in LS and in the closely related morphoea. Others have suggested that the spirochaete *Borrelia burgdorferi* is concerned (Aberer & Stanek 1987, Ross *et al.* 1990, Schemmp *et al.* 1993), although findings have been conflicting (Abele & Anders 1990, Raguin *et al.* 1992). However, a recent study (Farrell *et al.* 1997) using vulval tissue has shown no spirochaetal forms, and coccoid bodies that were seen appeared to be mast cells rather than bacilli.

Studies of cell kinetics have accumulated more recently. Oikarinen *et al.* (1991) showed that active regeneration and synthesis of collagen, as well as concomitant loss of connective tissue, took place. S.M. Neill (personal communication, 1991) studied epidermal differentiation in LS; keratins 6 and 16, associated with increased cell turnover, were expressed suprabasally, and keratins 1 and 10, markers of cornifying epithelium, persisted in spite of the apparent atrophy of the epidermis. Soini *et al.* (1994) have shown, in a study of proliferating cell nuclear antigen, that vulval skin affected by LS has a wide range of proliferative capacity and that high levels are associated with overexpression of wild-type p53. Tan *et al.* (1994) also showed an altered p53 expression and epidermal cell proliferation in vulval LS, compared with normal vulval skin and with extragenital LS, and Newton *et al.* (1987), using flow cytometry, found both aneuploidy and a hyperproliferative pattern in some cases. Carli *et al.* (1991) found an increase of CD1a+ Langerhans cells at all stages of the disease, supporting the concept of an abnormality of the skin immunological system, and the study of Marren *et al.* (1997b), demonstrating a lack of correlation between duration of symptoms and histological appearances, suggests a continuing inflammatory process in which activated Langerhans cells may be involved.

Clinical features

LS is found at all ages and in all parts of the body, in both sexes. The female anogenital area is the most frequently affected site. Although there may be reporting discrepancies, it seems likely that it is more common in white racial groups than in others.

Lichen sclerosus in the male. Extragenital lesions are rare. In the genital area, the condition affects boys, where it is the commonest cause of acquired phimosis (Chalmers *et al.* 1984), and men, where it affects the prepuce and/or the glans and in advanced stages causes marked atrophy and sclerosis. At all ages in the male the natural history is uncertain. Ledwig and Weigand (1989) have suggested that early circumcision may protect, but this may be fallacious in the absence of knowledge as to why the circumcision was carried out. Many cases are dealt with by urologists, and most have been reported as balanitis xerotica obliterans. There appears to be a small risk of malignancy; the literature on this point is reviewed by Meffert *et al.* (1995).

Lichen sclerosus in women. About 11% of women with anogenital LS have extragenital lesions (Meyrick Thomas *et al.* 1996). The primary lesion is an ivory-white papule, flat, polygonal and often with a central plug or dell. The papules are scattered or confluent in plaques (Fig. 5.46).

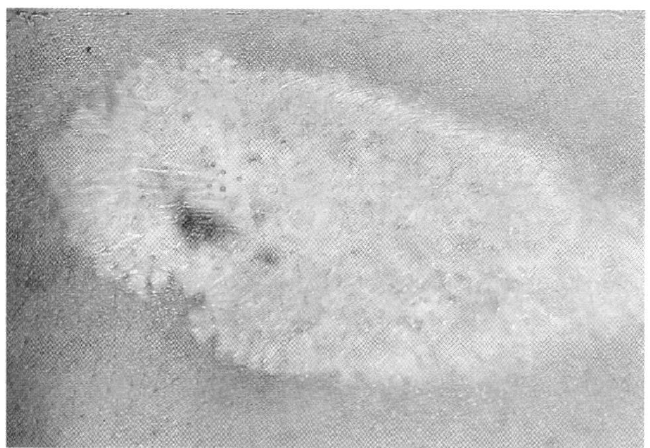

Fig. 5.46 Lichen sclerosus: large plaque on the back, showing confluent crinkly atrophy with some 'delling'.

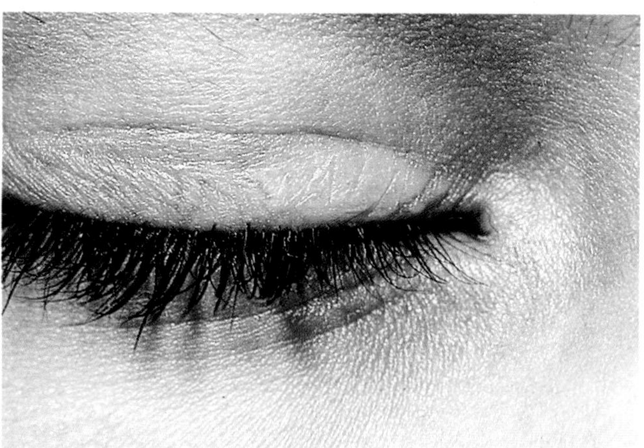

Fig. 5.47 Lichen sclerosus: smooth, white, crinkly plaque of the eyelid.

Bullae, purpura, marked atrophy and pallor are frequent features. The lesions occur anywhere, although scalp lesions are rare (Foulds 1980) and facial lesions unusual (Fig. 5.47). The Koebner phenomenon is often seen. Lesions occur at the site of straps or belts, in scars of various types including burn scars (Meffert & Grimwood 1994), and on skin previously treated with radiotherapy (Yates *et al.* 1985); in such patients with breast cancer the LS can be very firm in texture and may simulate malignant infiltration. Weigand (1993), prompted by finding histological features identical to those of LS in some large skin tags, has suggested that occlusion and pressure may be factors in the development of LS. Whimster (1973) noted that LS developed in a split skin graft transferred to the vulva from the thigh, whereas vulval LS skin reverted to normal when transferred to the thigh. LS may develop or recur not only in skin grafts (Foulds 1980, Ellis & Crow 1982) but in a myocutaneous graft (di Paola *et al.* 1982). It is well known clinically that it tends to recur at the edge of the resection after vulvectomy.

The frequency of oral lesions is uncertain. Miller (1957), in reporting a case with suggestive histology, reviewed previous reports; these numbered only six, and only one was supported by histology. The problem is twofold: histology is rarely carried out, or is indefinite (Brookes & Sarkany 1970), and in some of the cases coexisting Lichen planus or scleroderma may have accounted for the lesions (Dalziel *et al.* 1987, Marren *et al.* 1994). However, cases with convincing histology have been reported by Ravits and Welsh (1957), Kaminsky *et al.* (1974), Macleod and Soames (1991) and de Araújo *et al.* (1985); two personally encountered and histologically confirmed cases have been on the tongue.

Anogenital lesions in girls. Extragenital lesions are relatively infrequent. The vulval condition was originally regarded as rare, but this is no longer the case, perhaps because a changed cultural climate has led, at least in the UK, to more reporting. It may present at a very young age, for example at 1 year (Meyrick Thomas *et al.* 1988). The lesions are essentially the same as in adults, but more liable to be secondarily infected and even haemorrhagic, sometimes presenting with frank bleeding (Figs 5.48 & 5.49). Constipation may complicate perianal lesions, and its cause is often not recognized.

Anogenital lesions in adult women. The perineum, fourchette, labia minora and majora, and clitoris may all be affected. In some patients the architecture is preserved, the main signs being waxiness, pallor and ecchymosis (Fig. 5.50). In others there is gross obliteration of contours, with loss of the labia minora, burying of the clitoris and sclerosis of the introitus (Fig. 5.51). There is often a figure-of-eight-shaped perianal involvement, with extension into the natal cleft (Fig. 5.52). Fusion in the midline is seen in some patients, and may proceed inexorably to leave only a posteriorly situated pinhole opening (Fig. 5.53). However, the signs may be limited to tiny white patches, or to adhesion and pallor of the clitoral hood. Lesions of the genitocrural folds, thighs and buttocks are fairly common. It is generally accepted that vaginal lesions do not occur.

Histology

The epidermis may be thin and flat but is sometimes hyperkeratotic with some acanthosis and elongated rete pegs. The typical feature is hyalinization of the dermis, bordered inferiorly by an aggregation, usually band-like, of chronic inflammatory cells (Fig. 5.54). Extravasated red cells are commonly seen. IMF may show fibrin deposition at the epidermal junction (Bushkell *et al.* 1981, Dickie *et al.* 1982)

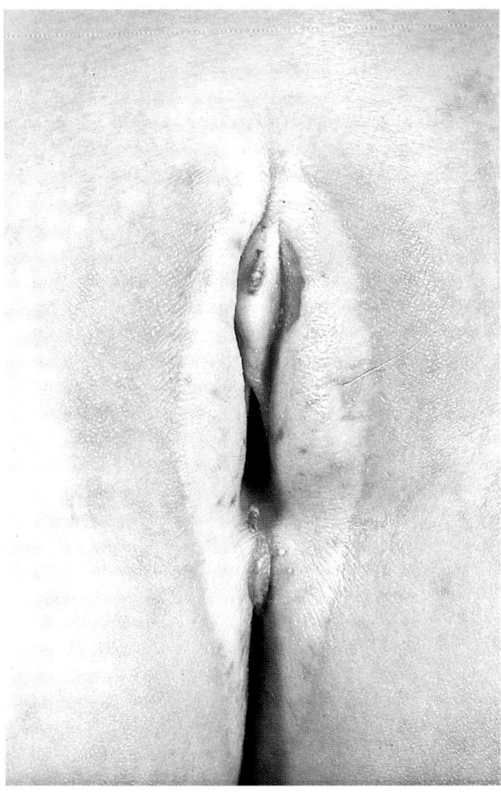

Fig. 5.48 Lichen sclerosus in a child: shiny, smooth pallor with some ecchymosis.

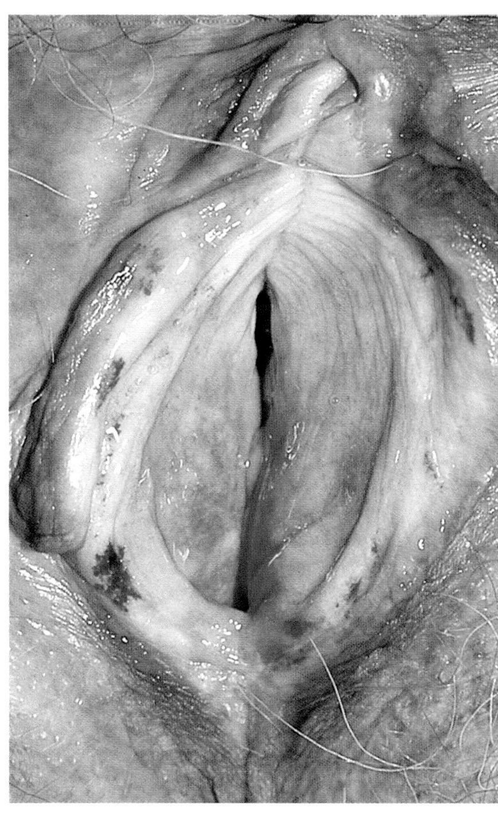

Fig. 5.50 Lichen sclerosus: pallor and ecchymosis at the vulva but no loss of substance.

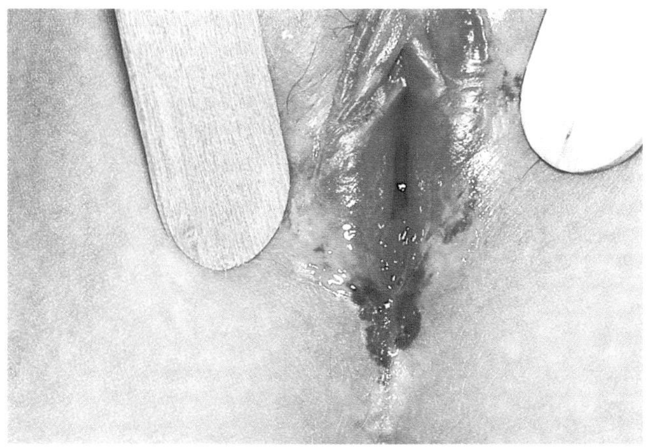

Fig. 5.49 Lichen sclerosus in a child: haemorrhagic appearance and loss of architecture.

but this is thought to be a non-specific phenomenon (Miller & Griffiths 1982). Marren *et al.* (1997a) have reported distortions of the basement membrane zone, which may be a cause or an effect of the disease. A searching study of the histology, with a system of grading, was carried out by Hewitt (1986).

Differential diagnosis

In children, sexual abuse may have to be considered, particularly when the lesions are haemorrhagic. Often LS is entirely responsible for the signs under discussion, but it must not be forgotten that LS and abuse can coexist. It has been speculated, but without general acceptance, that sexual abuse could precipitate LS as a Koebner phenomenon in a predisposed child (Warrington & de San Lazaro 1996). Scarring bullous disorders will also enter the differential diagnosis, but vitiligo is probably the commonest problem, since the textural changes expected in LS may be subtle.

In adults also, vitiligo sometimes presents a difficulty (Fig. 5.55); when signs of LS are minimal, they can easily be overlooked. Cicatricial pemphigoid is an important differential diagnosis; this will apply particularly to patients where fusion is extreme. Such cases (reported by, for example, Taylor 1941, Chuong & Hodgkinson 1984, Parkinson & Alderman 1984, Savona-Ventura 1985 and Kato *et al.* 1986) tend to be attributed to oestrogen deficiency, age or diabetes, but are likely all to be caused by cicatricial pemphigoid, LP or (most commonly) LS. IMF in cicatricial pemphigoid is often negative, and both IMF and

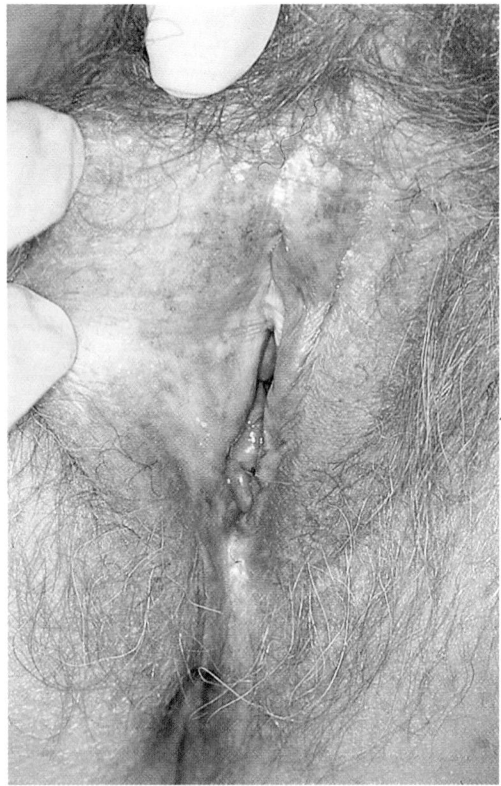

Fig. 5.51 Lichen sclerosus: pallor and atrophy, with loss of labia minora.

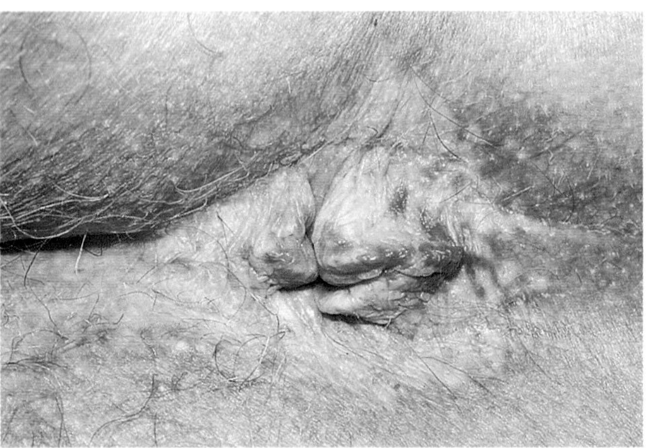

Fig. 5.52 Lichen sclerosus: typical perianal pallor and erosions.

histological examination may have to be repeated; vaginal, ocular or oral lesions are helpful if present and suggestive of that condition.

The main difficulty is usually to differentiate extragenital lesions of LS from morphoea, and genital ones from LP. The three conditions are indeed closely related; there is, for example, a close resemblance to each in the various stages of graft-versus-host disease. Connelly and Winkelmann (1985) reported cases where they were all combined.

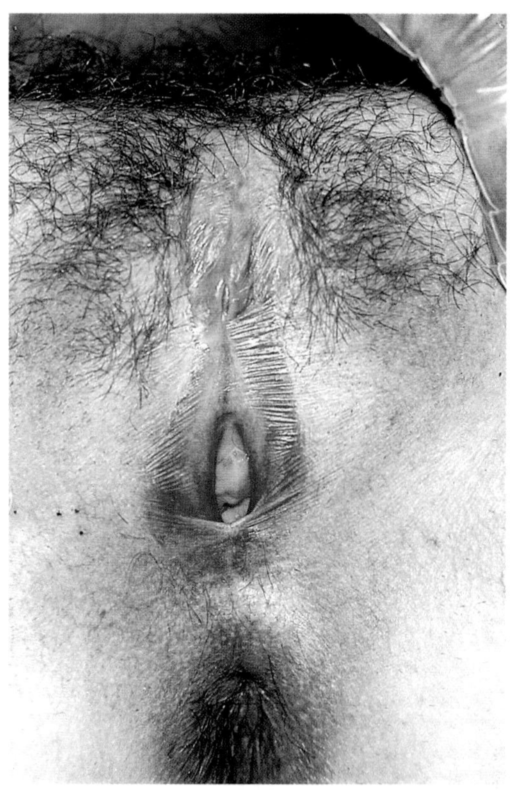

Fig. 5.53 Lichen sclerosus: loss of architecture and midline fusion.

Although purely genital lesions do not cause confusion with morphoea, elsewhere they may merge into one another. Morphoea tends to be firmer, with a violaceous halo, and resolves to leave brownish areas. Shono *et al.* (1991) showed some differences in the lectin staining patterns between the two, and Hacker (1994) found single-stranded DNA antibodies in many examples of morphoea but in none of (vulval) LS. Patterson and Ackerman (1984) concluded that the conditions were distinct, favouring as criteria for the diagnosis of LS a vacuolar change at the dermal–epidermal junction and a lichenoid lymphocytic infiltrate beneath the papillary dermis, whereas in (extragenital) morphoea the subcutis and reticular dermis show sclerosis and inflammatory infiltration. Nevertheless, it is difficult to accept them as entirely separate entities.

As regards LP, LS was indeed called, by Hallopeau, *lichen plan atrophique*, and by Darier *lichen plan scléreux*. The conditions have much in common, clinically and histologically. The vulval signs may be very similar if no typical papules of either, or the network associated with lichen planus, are to be seen. Oral lesions, even if typical of lichen planus, are not conclusive evidence of the similarity of vulval lesions. The vaginal involvement often found in

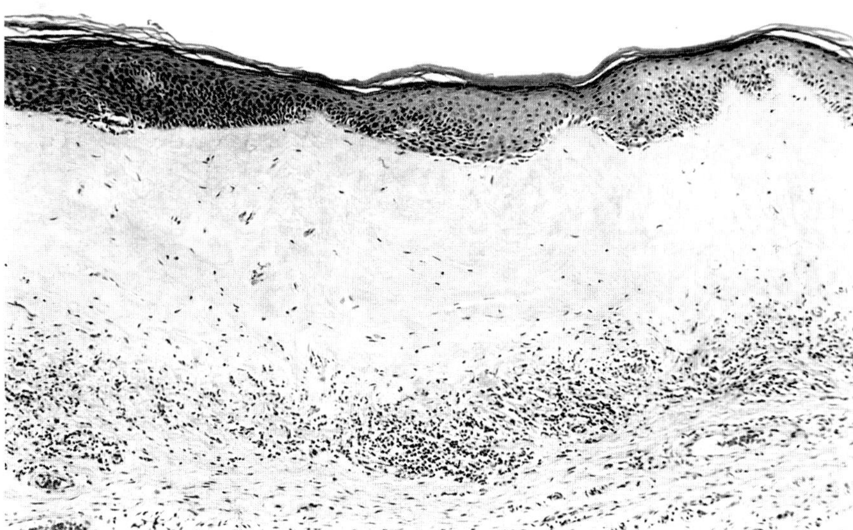

Fig. 5.54 Lichen sclerosus: thin epidermis, subepidermal hyalinization, band-like infiltrate in lower dermis.

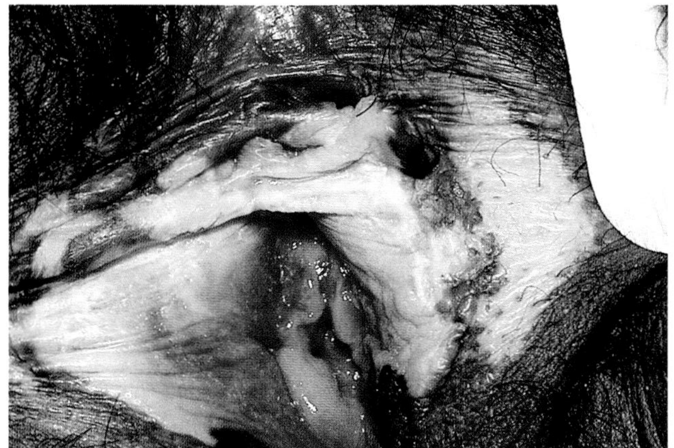

Fig. 5.55 Lichen sclerosus, here associated with vitiligo.

erosive LP is diagnostic, but the incidence of vaginal involvement in other forms is unknown since it is not commonly sought and, finally, LP may be underdiagnosed since those patients with vulval signs compatible with LS may not undergo vaginal examination. The histology can be difficult to interpret, with minimal hyalinization or interface dermatitis to differentiate the two; IMF is helpful if it shows the cytoid bodies associated with LP. Carli *et al.* (1997) have described higher expression of fibrogenic cytokines in LS as compared with LP, which may prove useful as a distinguishing feature. In some cases, however, differentiation may be wellnigh impossible, the clinical and histological features signs seeming to vary within the clinical course (Meyrick Thomas *et al.* 1996), and it may well be that the two conditions are part of a spectrum rather than two distinct entities.

Management and course

Children. Treatment in the past was as unsatisfactory in children as in adults and could even include vulvectomy. In conjunction with avoidance of irritants such as bubble baths, careful attention to hygiene and the use of bland emollients, topical corticosteroids are now the mainstay of therapy. Until the last few years, the mildest, i.e. hydrocortisone, was used and certainly this often relieves symptoms. In fact many children have few symptoms. It is now, however, generally accepted that treatment with the most potent corticosteroid, using basically the regimen in adults described below, is both wise and safe wise in that it arrests the process, and with it loss of tissue, and safe in that a tiny amount is required and can be stipulated by advising a longer period for the use of a given amount. Such treatment, employing a slightly less potent corticosteroid, has now been documented (Fischer & Rogers 1997). In many cases the appearance virtually returns to normal. This fact, incidentally, will render it even more difficult in the future to make a valid judgement of the natural history.

The course in children is towards improvement of signs and symptoms; however, previous suggestions that complete resolution occurs at puberty in most of them are not well founded. Very few clear completely, although it is admittedly difficult to distinguish between the inactive scarring remaining after destruction of tissue and continuing disease (Ridley 1993). In some the symptoms disappear, to recur later; in the series of Wallace (1971), of 32 patients presenting as young adults 19 had had symptoms as children, although in the larger series of Meyrick Thomas *et al.* (1996) only 11 had been similarly affected. Malignancy has been reported in adolescence in a few cases

(Wallace 1971, Cario *et al.* 1984, Pelisse 1987, Roman *et al.* 1991). In both the cases of Pelisse, the girls had previously undiagnosed, untreated LS. A malignant melanoma was reported in a girl of 14 with LS (Friedman *et al.* 1984). It has been noted that junctional and compound naevi may be mistaken for malignant melanoma when they are superimposed on LS in children and adolescents (Ackerman 1988).

Adults. Adult patients may present at any age, although most do so in the fifth and sixth decades. The condition is independent of whether or not the patient is taking hormone replacement therapy, and the patient may be assured that such therapy will have no effect on the disease process, for good or ill. An information sheet is useful for the patient's reference. As with all the epithelial disorders, bland emollients are advised. Aqueous cream is less greasy than the parent substance, emulsifying ointment, but contains preservatives that may make it less well tolerated. As definitive treatment, clobetasol propionate 0.05% ointment has now been used to good effect for several years, and its safety and efficacy have been recorded by Dalziel *et al.* (1991) and Dalziel & Wojnarowska (1993). Carli *et al.* (1992) demonstrated a response of the skin immune system in biopsies of patients so treated. It is important to use a quantitative regimen on a monitored basis. It appears that if not more than 30g is used in a period of 3 months there are no adverse local or systemic effects; most patients in fact use much less than this. Allergy or intolerance to the ointment (which is preferable to the cream as no preservatives are incorporated) may develop; if patch tests do not show true steroid allergy another very potent or potent steroid may be used. A steroid/antibacterial combination is useful for episodes of secondary infection.

It is known that there is no role for the use of oestrogen or testosterone creams in LS. Unfortunately, some gynaecologists continue to use them. Testosterone has been shown to be no better than petrolatum in treating LS (Sideri *et al.* 1994) and does not maintain the improvement brought about by clobetasol proprionate (Cattaneo *et al.* 1996). Since a retinoid has been shown to reduce connective tissue degeneration in LS (Niinimaki *et al.* 1989), these agents are worth considering in difficult cases. Although there are discrepancies between clinical and laboratory responses, etretinate (Niinimaki *et al.* 1989) and acitretin (Bousema *et al.* 1994) were beneficial when given orally. However, in view of the side effects of this drug it might be preferable to use it topically, as was done with good results in an open study by Virgili *et al.* (1995); the side effects did not induce patients to leave the trial. Laser treatment has recently been employed but does not seem likely to prove beneficial (Kartamaa & Reitamo 1997).

A few patients have no symptoms, the condition being found by chance. It would seem nevertheless wise to treat florid signs.

Many cases respond to treatment and have their signs as well as symptoms all but abolished, but in most some the signs remain, while symptoms are intermittent. Anxious patients may develop a superimposed dysaesthetic vulvodynia. Pregnancy and delivery are unlikely to be significantly affected by LS. Dyspareunia, however, is common, as is splitting at the introitus with intercourse. Attention to sexual technique and the liberal use of lubricants, with clobetasol propionate to heal the fissures if they have occurred, are usually effective; sometimes, however, minor surgery is required. Patients' concepts of sexual and obstetric disabilities were reviewed by Dalziel (1995).

Should symptoms recur or hyperkeratotic or eroded areas develop, the patient should be instructed to reattend at once if they do not respond promptly to a resumption of treatment, or to an increase in its frequency. It is difficult to advise on the optimal spacing of follow-up visits, since a carcinoma may appear with dramatic suddenness; moreover, there may be financial or geographical constraints as regards out-patient appointments. It is vital, however, that the patient should be aware of the possibility of malignancy, however small it may be.

In the absence of malignancy, the role of surgical procedures in LS is very limited but stenosis of the introitus and adhesions can be effectively treated (Chapter 11).

Vulvectomy was carried out prophylactically in the 1930s (Taussig 1929) and even in the 1970s it was being considered for those with persistent itching (Wallace 1971). Vulvectomy does not prevent carcinoma (three of the patients in one series who had undergone a vulvectomy for benign disease later developed a carcinoma (Meyrick Thomas *et al.* 1996)), symptoms are not always relieved and signs recur; the operation has significant morbidity and complications, both physical and psychosexual. Unfortunately, even in recent years, with good topical treatment available, such unnecessary surgery is still sometimes performed. In a recent series (Meyrick Thomas *et al.* 1996) 28 patients out of a total of 357 had undergone a vulvectomy for benign disease, 17 of them since 1960 and two as recently as the 1980s. To our knowledge, some women with LS are even now being subjected to this procedure.

LICHEN SCLEROSUS AND MALIGNANCY
(see also Chapter 10)

LS has been reported, presumably coincidentally, with malignant melanoma (Friedman, R.J. *et al.* 1984) and basal cell carcinoma (McAdams & Kistner 1958, Meyrick

Thomas *et al.* 1985). Several cases of verrucous carcinoma in LS have also been reported (Brisigotti *et al.* 1989).

As regards squamous cell carcinoma (SCC), that LS patients make up a significant proportion of affected women is not in doubt, but the likelihood of its development in any given patient is less clear. A few cases in girls have been reported, as noted above, but in the main it occurs in older age groups (Fig. 5.56).

In clinical reports, the incidence of SCC in LS is of the order of 4–6% (Wallace 1971, Meyrick Thomas *et al.* 1996). Radiotherapy may have been a relevant factor in some, since it was used extensively in the past for pruritus. These series, as others that have been reported, included patients who had presented with their carcinomas, not having been diagnosed as having LS previously.

When pathological specimens of SCC are examined, however, the incidence is much higher, figures varying from 4 to 25%, 53%, 61% and even 96% (McAdams & Kistner 1958, Zaino *et al.* 1982, Hewitt 1984, Punnonen *et al.* 1985, Leibowitch *et al.* 1990); the variation in figures reflects the thoroughness of examination of vulvectomy specimens and the criteria employed to diagnose LS; the confusion discussed earlier surrounding the question of terminology has been particularly frustrating in this field of study. Indeed, even in recent times, skin disease is not well assessed in SCC specimens (Zaki *et al.* 1997). Moreover, in recent years it has become gradually accepted that there are two aetiological patterns of incidence in vulval SCC. One applies to mainly younger women, and is often associated with the oncogenic types of human papillomavirus, and the other is relevant in older women, in whom many of the lesions are associated with LS (Crum 1992). In the latter group, reports have been to some extent conflicting (Leibowitch *et al.* 1990, Toki *et al.* 1991, Ansink *et al.* 1994, Haefner *et al.* 1995), but the human papillomavirus has not been considered relevant except in isolated cases (Ridley 1986). These differing patterns were not taken into account in earlier work. However, recent studies have tended to raise the possibility that ageing, mutations, the human papillomavirus and LS may all interact in the older group (Crum *et al.* 1997).

A related aspect is that of the histological precursor of malignancy. In the younger age group SCC appears to be a development of VIN 3 of undifferentiated type, often multifocal; in those of the older group without LS, it tends rather to arise from a solitary patch of VIN 3 of undifferentiated type on an otherwise normal vulva. However, in the case of the LS patient with an SCC, if VIN is found it is VIN 3 of differentiated type, and epithelial hyperplasia is usually a prominent feature (Leibowitch *et al.* 1990, Carli *et al.* 1995). The association of this type of VIN with SCC in LS was well described by Abell (1965). The epithelial hyperplasia may mask or replace histological evidence of LS in the vicinity of the tumour and so contribute towards a falsely low estimate of the incidence of LS in SCC. This epithelial hyperplasia is distinct from lichen simplex or lichenification and more akin to the 'leukoplakia' described by Wallace and Whimster (Fig. 5.57).

The clinical presentation is of an erythematous, ulcerated or hyperkeratotic plaque or nodule (Fig. 5.56). The carcinoma tends to arise on the clitoris or labia minora, sites of predilection for LS. It is striking how often a patient presents with an SCC on LS that has been undiagnosed, and usually untreated, and which may be entirely asymptomatic. Interest now centres on whether or not effective treatment of LS will prevent the development of SCC, and on this point there is as yet no firm evidence.

Added to this uncertainty must be the knowledge that an indeterminate number of women with LS never seek advice, or are never referred from primary care. Nevertheless, prospective surveys of women known to have LS would furnish valuable information, such as that of Carli *et al.* (1995), who made a longitudinal cohort study of 211 patients. The number of invasive SCCs significantly exceeded that in an age-matched group; the cumulative risk was 14.8% compared with 0.06% in the general population. If plans to form a national register (Tidy *et al.* 1996)

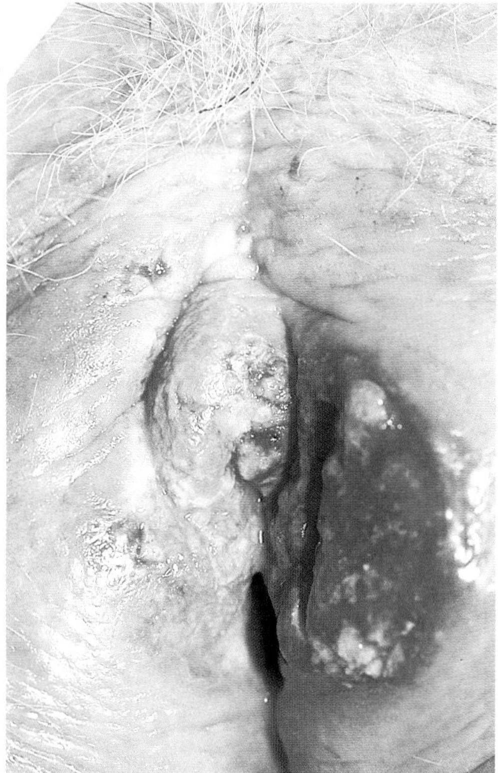

Fig. 5.56 Lichen sclerosus with a squamous cell carcinoma.

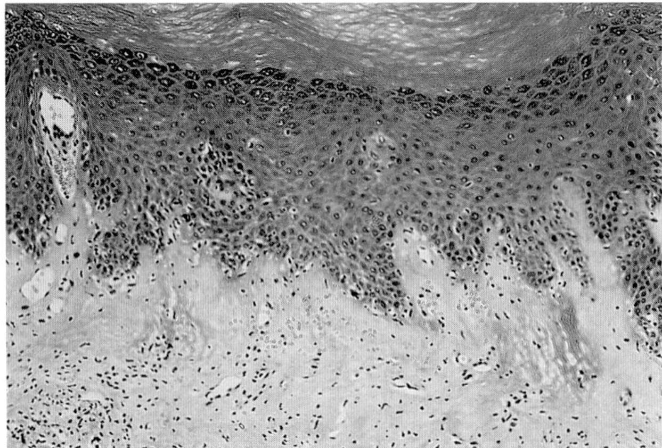

Fig. 5.57 Lichen sclerosus: hyperkeratosis, epithelial hyperplasia, pointed, forked rete ridges, subepidermal hyalinization.

come to fruition, a worthwhile prospective survey could be carried out in the UK. Meanwhile, it would seen reasonable to conclude that there is indeed an increased risk of malignancy and that therefore advice to the patients and their supervision should be very careful.

Lichen planus

Definition and aetiology

LP is a clinical entity characterized in its commonest manifestation by an eruption of shiny, flat, polygonal and violaceous papules, which, on keratinized skin, often show whitish striae (Wickham's striae), and by reticulate whitish lesions of the mucosae, commonly of the mouth. The histology is lichenoid, by which is understood a disturbance of the dermal–epidermal interface by a chronic inflammatory infiltrate (Black 1992). The pathogenesis is uncertain but probably of immunological origin, by which activated T cells are directed against basal keratinocytes. LP-like pictures can be produced by drugs and are seen in graft-versus-host reactions. Familial cases are well recognized, as is an association with autoimmune conditions. HLA findings are conflicting, but there may be an association with the HLA-DR1 (Powell *et al.* 1986, Valsecchi *et al.* 1988) and there may be some differences as regards HLA associations between clinical patterns of the disease (La Nasa *et al.* 1995, Setterfield *et al.* 1996b), immunogenetic studies suggesting that some at least constitute distinct entities.

Clinical features

In all cases it is important to make a full examination of the rest of the body surface, including the nails, scalp and mouth. Oesophageal lesions may occur, and should be looked for if there are suspicious symptoms. Conjunctival lesions have also been reported and, if sought, might be found more often. Anogenital lesions may, for convenience, be divided into a few groups according to their clinical presentation, although there is a considerable degree of overlap.

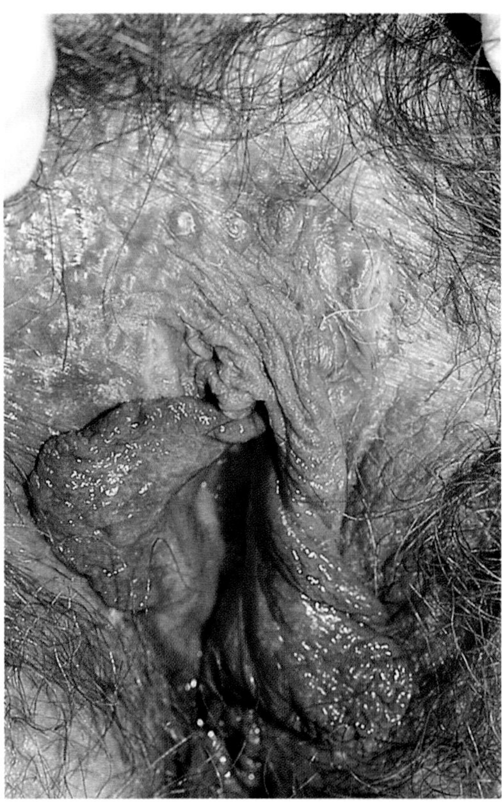

Fig. 5.58 Lichen planus: shiny polygonal papules on the anterior part of the vulva.

In the 'classical' form, typical papules will be found on the keratinized anogenital skin, with or without milky striae on the inner aspects of the vulva (Figs 5.58–5.60). As elsewhere, hyperpigmentation may following resolution, particularly in the dark-skinned subject (see Fig. 5.19). The lesions may not give rise to symptoms when they are, as is often the case, part of a generalized eruption, and vulval involvement is likely to be underdiagnosed since the area may not routinely be examined. Lewis *et al.* (1996) found vulval lesions in 19 of 37 women with LP, four of the 19 having had no symptoms. Vaginal lesions have not been systematically studied in these patients, but probably do not occur.

Hernando *et al.* (1992) have reported apparently the first case of the rare variant, lichen planus pemphigoides, at the vulva in a child aged 10, an unusual age since LP is rarely seen in childhood.

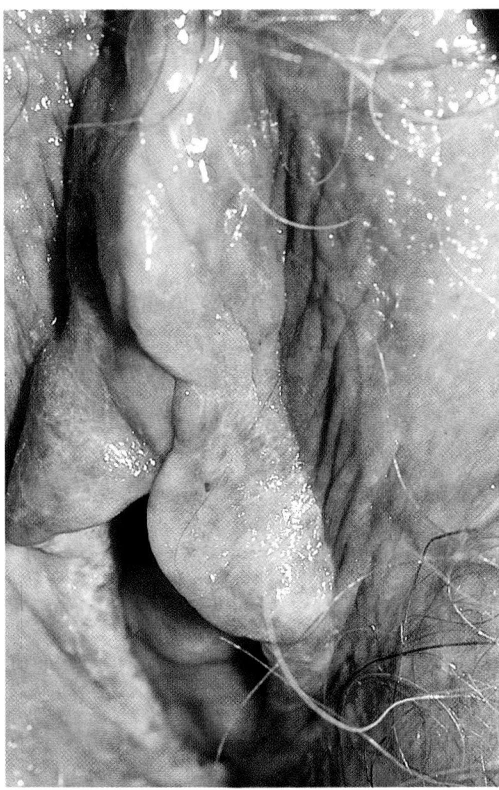

Fig. 5.59 Lichen planus: whitish network on the inner aspect of the right labium minus.

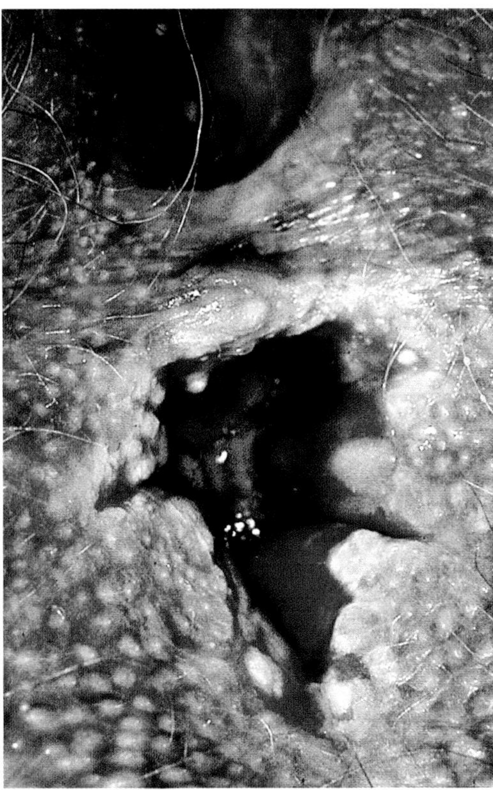

Fig. 5.60 Lichen planus: close-up view of the perianal area.

Hypertrophic lesions, where the surface is hyperkeratotic and roughened, are relatively rare and can be difficult to diagnose. They may become ulcerated, infected and painful, and may mimic malignancy (Fig. 5.61). They do not appear to be accompanied by vaginal lesions, although experience of this group is limited by its rarity. There is a tendency to affect the perineum and perianal area preferentially.

Mucocutaneous erosive lesions are perhaps the commonest form; and they affect the inner aspects of the vulva, and the vagina.

A distinctive pattern was categorized as the vulvovaginal–gingival form by Pelisse *et al.* (1982) and described in many subsequent accounts (Edwards & Friedrich 1988, Pelisse 1989, Edwards 1989, Bermejo *et al.* 1990, Ridley 1990, Eisen 1994). Some prefer the term plurimucosal LP (Bermejo *et al.* 1990). There may or may not be manifestations of LP on keratinized skin of the anogenital area or elsewhere. The lesions affecting the different mucosal sites need not necessarily appear contemporaneously. Recently (Setterfield *et al.* 1996b) it has been shown that this vulvovaginal–gingival syndrome is significantly associated with the HLA-DQB1* 0201 allele when the patients were compared with patients who had other clinical patterns of LP. A patient with striking familial involvement has been described (Walsh *et al.* 1995). It seems that patients with vulvovaginal–oral lesions represent a distinct genetic subset.

The gingivitis, which mainly affects the buccal surface, may be mild or marked, and is primarily erosive, although reticulate lesions may also be seen (Eisen 1994). Buccal lesions may also occur; the tongue is often affected, with whitish or bald patches along the sides (Figs 5.62 & 5.63).

The vulval lesions are chronic and painful and involve the inner aspects of the labia minora and the vestibule. They appear as frank erosions or as patches of glazed erythema on a vulva that is otherwise normal in appearance, or on one that shows marked atrophy, fusion and scarring of the clitoris and labia minora, the erythema being limited to the introitus. Striae are often visible at the margins of the lesions, and loss of architecture may be extreme (Fig. 5.64).

The vaginal lesions consist of friable telangiectasia and patchy erythema, sometimes with synechiae, and in severe cases there is stenosis of the vagina, which may be shortened to the extent that it barely admits the tip of a finger (Figs 5.18 & 5.65). Bleeding after intercourse, dyspareunia and variable degrees of discharge are common symtpoms. It is likely that they were the basis for earlier reports of 'desquamative vaginitis', for example those of Gray and Barnes (1965), Gardner (1969) and Lynch (1975).

A number of patients have involvement of the anal margin, and the cervix may also be involved (Gougerot & Burnier 1937, Eisen 1994, Pelisse 1996).

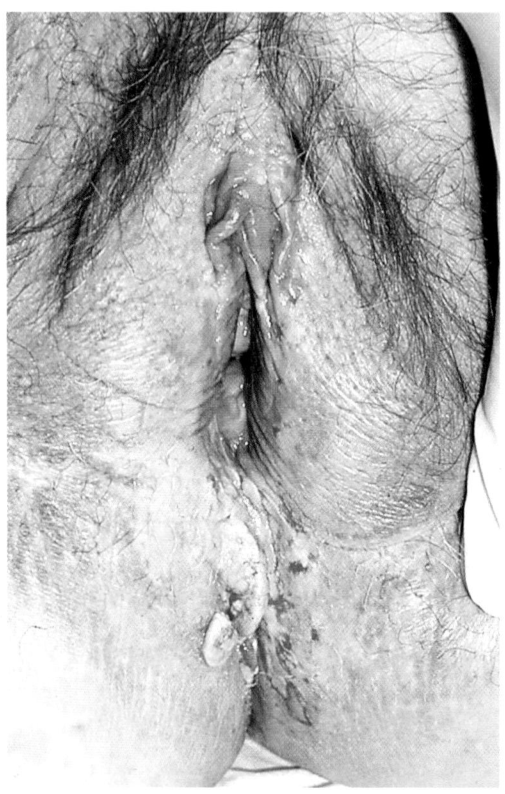

Fig. 5.61 Lichen planus: hypertrophic lesions of the perineum and perianal area.

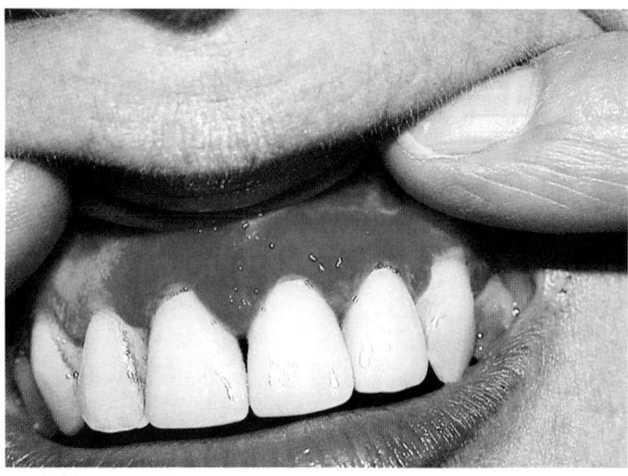

Fig. 5.62 Lichen planus: gingivitis in the vulvovaginal–gingival syndrome.

A patient reported with conjunctival lesions (Moyal-Barracco *et al.* 1993) had this syndrome, as did some but not apparently all of these reported with oesophageal LP (Sheehan-Dare *et al.* 1986, Dickens *et al.* 1990); that of Bousser *et al.* (1986), with probable oesophageal lesions, had 'kraurosis' bleeding on touch, but with no mention of the vagina.

With any form of LP the end result may be a striking atrophy and loss of architecture of the vulva, sometimes accompanied by erythema round the introitus. This picture is often virtually indistinguishable from LS clinically or histologically.

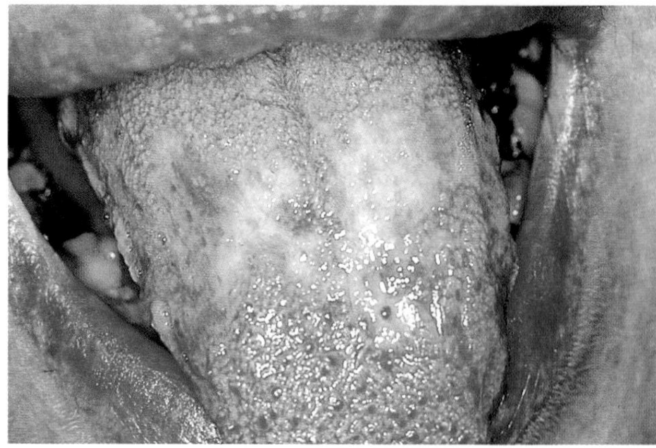

Fig. 5.63 Lichen planus: white plaques on the tongue.

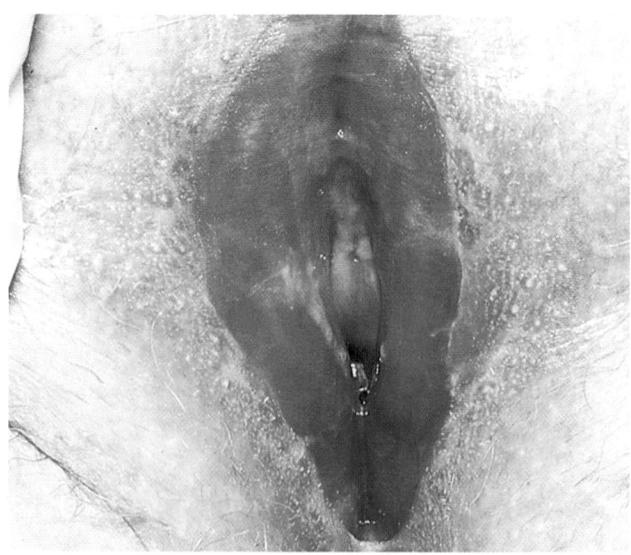

Fig. 5.64 Lichen planus: erosive lesions of the vulva, with a whitish network at the periphery and loss of architecture, in the vulvovaginal–gingival syndrome.

Histology

The histology of LP shows hyperkeratosis in areas of keratinized skin, acanthosis that is typically irregular with a saw-tooth appearance, an increased granular layer and basal cell liquefaction (Fig. 5.66). The hyperkeratosis and acanthosis are especially marked in the hypertrophic form. Sometimes there are apoptotic eosinophilic basal and prickle cells, the so-called colloid bodies. There is a band-like dermal infiltrate mainly composed of T cells and closely apposed to the dermis; in chronic hypertrophic lesions this feature is less evident. Immunofluorescence (Helander & Rogers 1994) reveals shaggy staining of the basement membrane zone for fibrinogen and IgM, cytoid bodies and sometimes granular IgG or IgA.

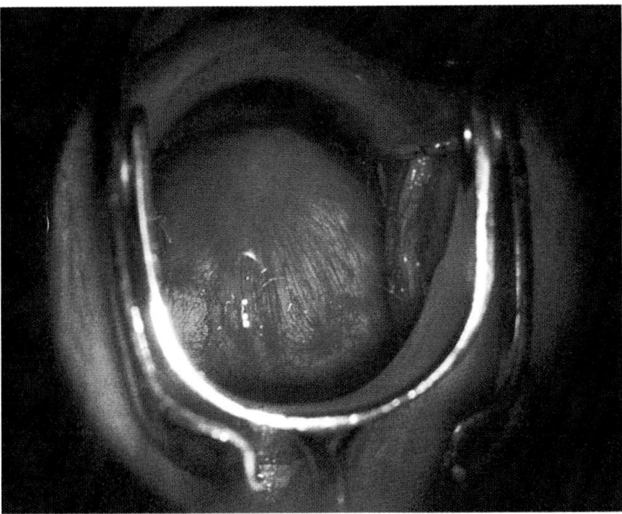

Fig. 5.65 Lichen planus: fiery and fragile appearance of the vaginal wall in the vulvovaginal–gingival syndrome.

Differential diagnosis

Apart from the hypertrophic variant, the differential diagnosis of LP at the vulva is mainly of the immunobullous diseases, especially those associated with scarring, and LS. If vaginal lesions are present, this excludes LS. Without vaginal lesions, the differentiation from LS can be difficult to make unless there is unequivocal histological evidence of subepidermal hyalinization to confirm LS, or interface changes and cytoid bodies to offer convincing evidence of LP. The presence of definite LP elsewhere by no means allows in itself a confident diagnosis of vulval LP, since overlap with LS is well recognized (Marren *et al.* 1994). IMF findings to support cicatricial pemphigoid are helpful, but often negative in that condition, the diagnosis of which is mainly clinical. A group of patients has been reported (Stewart *et al.* 1995) with the diagnosis of 'glazed erythema of the vulva'; it seems likely that in fact they could be considered as having LP. Lichenoid drug eruptions may occasionally have to be considered (van Voorst Vader *et al.* 1988), as may Zoon's vulvitis (see below).

Hypertrophic LP also presents diagnostic difficulty, particularly when overlaid by infection: with solitary or sparse lesions an SCC is often suspected; with more diffuse lesions a much lichenified LS or lichen simplex may be considered.

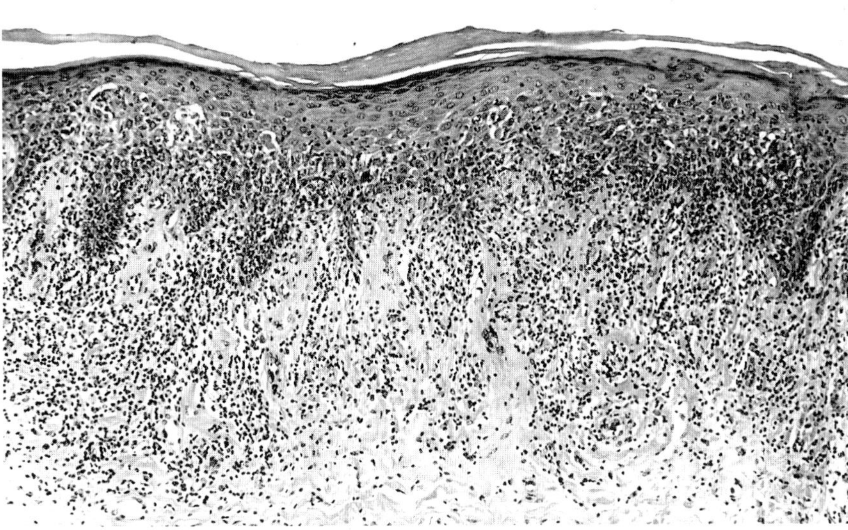

Fig. 5.66 Lichen planus: hyperkeratosis, prominent granular layer, irregular acanthosis, saw-tooth pattern of rete ridges, band-like infiltrate in apposition to the basal layer.

Management

The mainstays of topical therapy are, as well as bland emollients such as aqueous cream or emulsifying ointment, potent topical corticosteroids. The most potent is usually required, i.e. clobetasone propionate 0.05%, in a carefully monitored regimen (as described above). The preferred vehicle is the ointment. Intolerance is rare; allergy can occur and should be investigated by patch testing. Preparations in an adhesive base, as used in the mouth, are on the whole not tolerated well at the vulva. Where there is an element of secondary infection, combinations of a corticosteroid with an antibacterial or antifungal agent is helpful. In the vulvovaginal–gingival syndrome, topical cyclosporin and retinoic acid have been used but with little success, although Eisen (1994) found that both cyclosporin and retinoic acid were more helpful when combined with a corticosteroid than when used alone.

Delivery of corticosteroids to the vagina is not easy. A proprietary preparation containing hydrocortisone (Colifoam), introduced with an applicator, is useful. Prednisolone suppositories may be used in more severe cases. A regimen has been described by Walsh *et al.* (1995). This utilizes a prosthesis of silicone rubber, which occludes a steroid preparation. The latter is combined with a polycarbophil vehicle (Replens). In addition steroid iontophoresis is carried out at weekly intervals. Synechiae can be treated in a more conventional way by dilators in conjunction with corticosteroids, and this approach should always follow surgical attempts to remove adhesions or reduce stenosis; unfortunately many of these patients will present to gynaecologists who may be unaware of the true diagnosis and may carry out isolated surgical procedures, which will invariably lead to further sealing of the vagina. Regular sexual intercourse will help to preserve patency, but is often impracticable because of dyspareunia.

When LP does not respond to topical measures, oral steroids are used, for example prednisolone 40 mg/day, tapered off over a few weeks; courses can be repeated as necessary. In the vulvovaginal–gingival syndrome there is general agreement that azathioprine, dapsone, griseofulvin, chloroquine and minocycline, all tried empirically, are of little or no benefit; oral cyclosporin may be considered. Retinoids are of great value in hypertrophic cases. All these potentially dangerous therapies are best supervised by a dermatologist.

COURSE AND POTENTIAL FOR MALIGNANCY

Those lesions characterized by papules tend to clear completely. Where atrophy has developed, however, and in the mucocutaneous and hypertrophic forms, the course is chronic with perhaps some fluctuations but no remissions.

The potential for malignancy in oral LP, although sometimes disputed, is generally accepted, and in genital lesions there also appears to be an increased risk of malignancy, although its degree is uncertain. It appears that there have been no reported examples in the vulvovaginal–gingival syndrome, with the possible exception of that of Crotty *et al.* (1980), and those dermatologists with the widest current experience of such patients have yet to see a case. In other forms, however, a number have been reported (Jänner *et al.* 1967, Wallace 1971, Lewis & Harrington 1994, Dwyer *et al.* 1995, Zaki *et al.* 1997). The report of Zaki *et al.* (1997) dealt with the finding of three cases with LP in a retrospective survey of 61 women with vulval carcinoma; in none had the diagnosis of LP been made in life, and it is therefore likely that other cases associated with LP remain undiagnosed.

Zoon's vulvitis

Having earlier given the title plasma cell balanitis to erythematous lesions localized to the glans and prepuce, Zoon (1955) described a similar condition at the vulva, as did Garnier (1954, 1957). Further reports of examples in the male were given by Brodin (1980) and Stern and Rosen (1982), while Crosti and Riboldi (1975) and Mensing and Jänner (1981) described further cases in women. It appears that the condition is commoner in men, and of the 19 cases reported by Souteyrand *et al.* (1981) only one was a woman. These authors included, as examples of what they considered to be an entity, the cases reported by Jonquières and de Lutsky (1980) as lichenoid telangiectatic purpuric balanitis or vulvitis.

Clinical features

It is generally agreed that clinically the lesions in the male are striking, with glistening red areas, often speckled and haemorrhagic, affecting the glans and prepuce, while in the female they are similar but perhaps less well defined and are to be found in all areas of the vulva, although few have been reported on the clitoris (corresponding to the glans and prepuce). Symptoms are variable.

Histology

Souteyrand *et al.* (1981) described what they considered to be the essential histological features. The dermis was the site of a dense inflammatory cell infiltrate; plasma cells usually accounted for at least 50% of the cells, but were not thought to be a specific feature. The dermal vessels were dilated and dermal haemosiderin was prominent. There was epidermal thinning, absent horny and granular layers and lozenge-shaped keratinocytes with widened intercellular spaces. Further cases have been reported in women, for example by Davis *et al.* (1983) and Neri *et al.* (1995); these later reports have tended to stress the plasma cells and the haemosiderin rather than the epidermal changes, although the latter were noted by Kavanagh *et al.* (1993) and Scurry *et al.* (1993a). The report of Woodruff *et al.* (1989) mentions dermal–epidermal splitting and Russell bodies, not found by others.

Diagnosis

There remains some doubt as to whether or not Zoon's vulvitis is a definite entity, the diagnosis tending to be attached rather too easily to any purpuric lesion in which plasma cells and haemosiderin are histologically demonstrable, such as for example might be associated with LS or LP. Kossard and Shumack (1989) considered that there was an overlap with lichen aureus, and Scurry *et al.* (1993a) that in some cases the lesions may in fact be those of mucosal LP. It seems that a few cases may be distinctive, but that many if not most are more accurately categorized as other conditions. The term chronic vulval purpura was used by Kato *et al.* (1990) and may provide a more useful descriptive term.

Management

A trial of topical corticosteroids is worthwhile, and some patients appear to be improved by topical flamazine or clindamycin. Morioko *et al.* (1988) reported good results in an atypical case with intralesional interferon-α.

Plasma cell orificial mucositis (plasmocytosis circumorificialis)

Cases were reported under these titles by Schuermann (1960), White *et al.* (1986) and Aiba and Tagami (1989); lesions usually involved the lips but on occasion the vulva. There was a dense infiltrate of plasma cells but apparently no haemosiderin deposition. Although the authors grouped their cases with those reported as Zoon's balanitis or vulvitis, it seems possible, on clinical and histological grounds, that the condition is distinct.

Angiolymphoid hyperplasia with eosinophilia
(see also Chapter 8)

This angiomatous inflammatory condition, whose relationship to Kimura's disease is disputed (Kuo *et al.* 1988), presents as erythematous intradermal or subcutaneous nodules, and only very rarely affects the vulva or perianal area (Sanders *et al.* 1989, Aguilar *et al.* 1990, Scurry *et al.* 1995).

Management

Surgical removal may be effective (Sanders *et al.* 1989) and oral retinoids can also be helpful (Marcoux *et al.* 1991).

Lesions related to blood and lymphatic vessels

Varicose veins

Vulval varicosities, usually accompanied by varicosities in the leg veins, may be the consequence of chronic pelvic congestion, portal hypertension or obstructive pelvic lesions (Fig. 5.67). They are common in pregnancy when, in addition, increased pelvic blood flow is relevant, but when a hormonal factor may also be involved, since the veins often enlarge in the first trimester. After delivery, some lesions thrombose spontaneously. Where they do not do so, and where there are no varicosities of the leg, further investigation by venography and computed tomography scan is indicated.

Management

When the vulval varices are a problem, elevation of the foot of the bed during sleep and supporting garments are helpful. Active treatment includes ligation, sclerosing injections and the use of a pelvic support (Gallagher 1986, Ninia & Goldberg 1996, Fliegner 1997).

Oedema

Oedema, as presumably a passive transfer effect, has been reported in patients on abdominal dialysis, where the

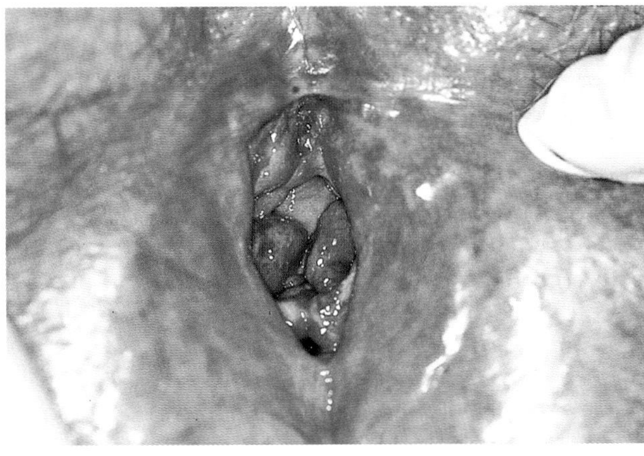

Fig. 5.67 Varicosities: engorged veins in the vestibular area, in a patient who also has lichen sclerosus.

channel can be a small hernia or a defect of the peritoneal fascia (Cooper *et al.* 1983, Kopecky *et al.* 1985).

In general, however, oedema results essentially from leakage through, or increased pressure in, the capillaries, and as such has multiple causes. The lax tissue of the vulva readily accumulates fluid, and oedema is a frequent accompaniment of *Candida* infections and of eczema.

Urticaria or angio-oedema, including hereditary angio-oedema, may affect the vulva. Dermographism has been suspected of being involved in vulval problems (Sherertz 1994, Lambiris & Greaves 1997) and pressure urticaria is also a possible cause.

Type I reactions to latex in condoms (Kint *et al.* 1994) and to surgical gloves are increasingly recognized, and are of great concern since potentially fatal reactions may occur if the patient is unaware of the problem and is examined by someone wearing latex-containing gloves. Diaz *et al.* (1996) described three cases where reactions occurred during delivery.

A further cause of this type of oedema is allergy to seminal plasma. This is undoubtedly an entity, but a rare one. Adequate investigation presents ethical and practical problems as regards controls. Fortunately, however, with many of those women who come suspecting that this is the problem a careful history will serve to rule it out; they are usually suffering from vestibulitis. Convincing cases have been reported by Chang (1976) noting familial incidence, Friedman, S.A. *et al.* (1984) and Freeman (1986). The mechanisms involved were reviewed fully by Jones (1991) and Kint *et al.* (1994), the latter authors reporting a case where type I allergy to seminal plasma was, unusually, possibly combined with a type IV reaction to it. The responsible agent is thought to be a glycoprotein. A recent case that was fully investigated was described by Poskitt *et al.* (1995). The patients are usually atopic. The reaction can start at the first intercourse, or begin later. There has been speculation that the occurrence at the first intercourse could be accounted for by intrauterine exposure to the relevant prostatic protein antigen from a male twin, the presence of whom may not always have been known; an alternative explanation is cross-sensitization. The signs may be local or may spread to other areas and even lead to anaphylaxis. Abstinence or the use of a condom is effective management; desensitization has variable results; intravaginal cromoglycate prior to intercourse may be helpful. The differential diagnosis includes reactions to drugs or even to dietary constituents that may be present in the fluid (Kint *et al.* 1994).

Vulval oedema has been reported in the ovarian hyperstimulation syndrome, a rare complication following ovulation in cases of infertility (Coccia *et al.* 1995, Luxman *et al.* 1996). The mechanism was thought to be fluid retention, decreased oncotic and increased hydrostatic pressure. Post-partum oedema has been reported following the use of a birthing chair (Davenport & Richardson 1986); fatal cases reported by Ewing *et al.* (1979) died of vascular collapse and may have had an infective origin. Trice *et al.* (1996) reviewed these and other cases and described pre-partum oedema in a woman with a twin pregnancy who was receiving tocolytic drugs to inhibit early labour. They postulated a combination of factors, involving glucocorticoids, terbutaline and magnesium sulphate, and noted that β-mimetic drugs such as terbutaline are recognized to cause pulmonary oedema and have been found in association with vulval oedema in one other reported case. Rainford (1970) noted gross vulval oedema in pre-eclamptic toxaemia.

OEDEMA RELATED TO LYMPHATIC PATHOLOGY

Lymphoedema may be primary, consequent upon congenital hypoplasia, or secondary.

Primary lymphoedema can sometimes be improved by surgery, and may be investigated by lymphangiography. Large amounts of fluid may be discharged locally. An immune deficit was associated, perhaps because of loss of lymphatic fluid into the gut, in the case of severe lymphoedema involving the genital area reported by Shelley and Wood (1981).

Secondary lymphoedema may follow chronic local disease such as hidradenitis suppurativa and Crohn's disease, chronic infections such as filariasis, obstruction by malignant deposits, surgery (especially if associated with lymphadenectomy) and radiotherapy given, for example, for carcinoma of the cervix or endometrium. The vulva becomes indurated and often verrucose; small lymphatic vesicles (lymphangiectases) may develop (Fig. 5.68).

Such vesicles, however, may also appear without overt clinical evidence of lymphoedema, as in the cases reported by Fisher and Orkin (1970) and Ambrojo *et al.* (1990), and indeed sometimes in the absence of any underlying cause (Cecchi *et al.* 1995). They may give rise to diagnostic difficulties, being mistaken for warts or other infections (Handfield-Jones *et al.* 1989, Harwood & Mortimer 1993).

The histology of lymphangiectases shows dilated lymphatic vessels lined by a single layer of endothelial cells, and can be difficult to distinguish from that of lymphangiomata circumscripta. It may be indeed that all lymphangiectases, whether arising spontaneously or induced by lymphatic blockage, should be regarded under the heading of lymphangioma circumscriptum (see also Chapter 9).

Management

Lymphangiectases respond to treatment with the carbon dioxide laser (Bailin *et al.* 1986, Landthaler *et al.* 1990).

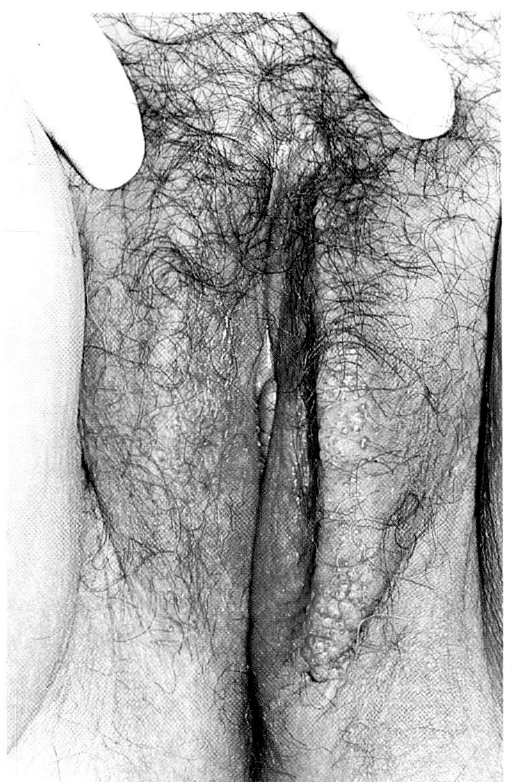

Fig. 5.68 Lymphangiectases: vesicular lesions along the edge of the labia majora.

The skills of a dedicated lymphoedema service nurse can be of great help. Massage, skin care and advice on support garments are important, particularly to the post-vulvectomy patient whose problems are unfamiliar and often acute, and some are benefited by referral to a patient support group.

In both types of lymphoedema, the affected tissue is subject to recurrent streptococcal infections, which in turn increase the obstruction and predispose to further attacks. The patient described by Buckley and Barnes (1995), who appeared to have the former type, developed extensive vesiculation following repeated attacks. The cellulitis is associ-ated with pain, fever and malaise. It is treated with phenoxymethyl penicillin plus flucloxacillin, or by co-amoxiclav, or by erythromycin if the subject is allergic to penicillin. Phenoxymethyl penicillin or erythromycin can also be given over long periods with benefit to prevent attacks.

In both types of lymphoedema, moreover, a lymphangiosarcoma or angiosarcoma may occasionally develop; a relevant example was reported by Huey *et al.* (1985). Selective localization of other malignancies to an area of lymphoedema, in their case a limb, was discussed by Tatnall and Mann (1985); an immune deficit may be responsible.

Vulval and vaginal lesions of traumatic and miscellaneous origin

Vaginal lesions are included here in so far as they touch upon vulval disease, but are not dealt with comprehensively; the reader is referred for fuller accounts of most aspects to Schmidt (1995).

Traumatic lesions (see also Chapter 7)

Artefactual, accidental, sexual, gynaecological, obstetric and surgical traumas lead to a variety of injuries. These may be life threatening, for example haematomas complicating delivery (Zahn *et al.* 1996). The patient of Rege and Shukla (1993) presented with a genital ulcer that proved to be connected by a sinus to a dislocated and osteomyelitic symphysis pubis. Injury may lead in due course to abscesses, keloids, cysts, neuromas and calculi (Onuigbo 1976, Aziz 1980, Junaid & Thomas 1981). In those of childbearing years there will sometimes be an increased risk of further problems in subsequent labours. Relatively easily managed examples of post-traumatic lesions are areas of endometriosis following surgery, or granulation tissue in episiotomy scars (Atia & Tidbury 1995). As regards severe injuries of any origin, Pokorny *et al.* (1992) have described in detail optimal procedures in examination and treatment.

Sexual abuse in children
(see also Chapters 4 and 7)

In considering the diagnosis of sexual abuse, invaluable sources of reference are the reviews of Bays and Chadwick (1993) and, particularly, the recent new edition of the *Report of the Working Party of the Royal College of Physicians* in London (Royal College of Physicians 1997). The latter provides full guidance on all aspects, including recommended terminology for physical findings, advice on examination techniques and notes on normal appearances. The most important evidence is considered to be a clear statement from the child. Physical signs alone are rarely sufficient for the diagnosis. Forensic evidence is helpful if it yields positive findings such as the presence of seminal fluid and/or of sexually transmitted disease, although as regards the latter even here caution must be exercised; genital warts, for example, are not incontrovertible evidence of abuse if found alone, since they are well recognized to occur in non-sexually abused children, and vertical transmission of *Chlamydia* and *Neisseria gonorrhoeae* is possible. While abuse does not necessarily result in abnormal physical signs, and while any such signs must be interpreted with care and in the light of other evidence, there are often signs and indeed injuries which if present must be noted in assessment. A scar or laceration of the hymen, or of the anal mucosa extending on to the perineal skin, is highly suggestive of abuse. A horizontal hymenal diameter of more than 1 cm is not diagnostic of abuse, nor is anal dilatation thought to be a reliable sign of anal abuse in the absence of other evidence. The utmost care in history taking and examination is essential, and the emergence of a small number of highly trained doctors in appropriately chosen centres is recommended.

Radiotherapy, laser treatment and cryotherapy can all damage the vaginal or vulva, with resulting scarring and inflammation. With radiotherapy there may be long-term sequelae of radiodermatitis, including malignancy and lymphatic obstruction.

Vulvovaginal adenosis

Adenosis in the upper vagina is well recognized as a result of *in utero* exposure to diethyl stilboestrol taken by the mother in pregnancy. It may also occur spontaneously, or after trauma, for example treatment with 5-fluorouracil (Goodman *et al.* 1991). It may be associated with the development of a clear-cell adenocarcinoma. Vulval and lower vaginal adenosis is rarer and appears usually to arise following trauma such as occurs in Stevens–Johnson syndrome (Marquette 1985, Wilson & Malinak 1988, Bonafe *et al.* 1990) and treatment with the laser (Sedlacek *et al.* 1990). Kranl *et al.* 1998 have described vaginal adenosis occurring spontaneously.

The pathogenesis is obscure, reflecting the uncertainties of the origin of the vagina in its different parts (Chapter 1). One explanation of the upper vaginal lesions is the unmasking of tissue of Mullerian (paramesonephric) origin. Vulval and lower vaginal lesions are even more difficult to explain; suggestions include the presence of mesodermal Mullerian tissue in the urogenital sinus area, and origin from Bartholin's glands. The adenosis is red and friable, and the main differential diagnosis is from endometriosis; the two can be distinguished histologically.

Vulvovaginitis in children

Vulvovaginitis in children can be caused by foreign bodies (Pokorny 1994) and this form can be particularly difficult to differentiate from child sexual abuse, since the history may be unreliable and the hymen disrupted, with recurrent bleeding, in both cases; this applies also when a foreign body has been spontaneously extruded, leaving hymenal changes and a granular reddening of the vaginal wall (which, if the diagnosis is firm, can be effectively treated with an oestrogen cream applied to the vulva for up to 2 weeks (Pokorny 1992)). The differential diagnosis includes also vulvovaginitis related to irritants and to infections, usually streptococcal (Chapter 4). When the child presents with intense vulval or perianal pruritus, threadworm (*Enterobius vermicularis*) infection is the most likely cause. Poor local hygiene, with resulting faecal contamination, is often a predisposing factor. Perianal streptococcal dermatitis has been described in children (Krol 1990) and occasionally in adults (Neri *et al.* 1996); the rash is pink, moist and tender but more superficial than in cellulitis. An underlying condition such as LS should be excluded. Resolution of vulvitis may be followed by the appearance of adhesions of the clitoral hood (Pokorny 1992). When the primary problem is a vaginitis, the child may present with few symptoms, the parents being concerned by discharge. A valuable sign indicating long-standing discharge is a pigmented and scaly rim on the inner dependent parts of the labia majora (Pokorny 1992). Investigation should include high vaginal swabs, which must be taken with due regard to the unoestrogenized mucosa and exclusion of foreign bodies, vaginal tumours and lower genital tract abnormalities; these measures will usually call for the help of an appropriately trained specialist.

Hormonal factors

Under the influence of maternal hormones, the vulva may appear swollen in the neonate, and there may be a vaginal discharge; the hymen may be thickened and pinkish white in colour up to the age of 4 years (Bays & Chadwick 1993). In children, labial adhesions are thought to be related at least in part to a hypo-oestrogenic state, in combination with mild inflammation (Fig. 5.69). They are fairly common in infancy, with a 1.4% incidence according to Christensen and Øster (1971). Leung *et al.* (1993) found them in 1.8% of children attending a paediatric clinic for various disorders, with a peak incidence of 3.3% at 13–23 months of age. Capraro and Greenberg (1972) found in 50 cases that the presentation was mainly before the age of 2 years and that all were pre-menarchal. None was seen before the age of 2 months; nevertheless, congenital abnormalities are an important differential diagnosis. In the case of adhesions, there is always a line of demarcation to be found between the clitoral hood and the labia minora (Pokorny 1992). Spontaneous resolution is common (Jenkinson & MacKinnon 1984) but treatment is advised if there are problems with micturition or with pooling of urine, or if fusion is almost complete, leaving only a pinhole aperture anteriorly. This may take the form of gentle separation by the mother, using a bland cream; improvement also follows the application of oestrogen cream, for up to a maximum of 2 weeks (Pokorny 1992). Surgical separation is not advised except in the older child if there is no eventual resolution (see Chapter 11).

Cyclical changes in the appearance of the hymen are also sometimes found in adult women.

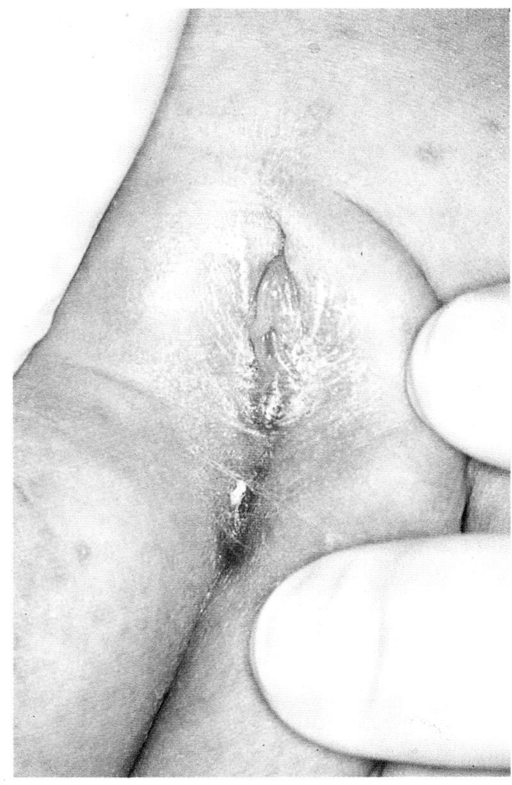

Fig. 5.69 Labial adhesions: midline fusion, leaving a small anteriorly placed opening.

Nutritional factors

Lack of riboflavine can produce an eczematous genital rash and was described in (male) prisoners of war (Whitfield 1947). Lack of zinc is relevant in acrodermatitis enteropathica. Haemorrhagic lesions of the mucosae, including the vulva and vagina, may be found in scurvy. Parks and Martin (1948) ascribed vulvitis to blood dyscrasia and anaemia, and Hunt (1954) commented on a vulvitis in iron deficiency. Gross (1941) used vitamin B and liver in 'kraurosis' and Jeffcoate (1949) hydrochloric acid and iron. It is difficult to assess the findings in these older reports in view of the very different states of nutrition encountered at that time. There is no evidence that vulvovaginitis in well-nourished subjects is related now to any such deficiency.

Drug-related factors

SYSTEMIC

Retinoids can cause vulvitis and vaginitis as part of their intensely drying effect on mucous membranes (Besa *et al.* 1986, Thomson 1986). Genital ulceration in patients taking foscarnet has been described in men, and now in an HIV-positive woman (Caumes *et al.* 1993); the ulcers healed when the drug was withdrawn, and did not recur when it was restarted and the area washed after micturition, as recommended by the manufacturer. It is likely that the effect is an irritant one, related to high levels in the urine. When an aperient containing anthraquinone was in use the urine, skin and vaginal secretions became brownish in colour (see above). A vaginitis possibly related to oral lithium was reported by Srebrnik *et al.* (1991). Cotrimoxazole in vaginal fluid has been reported as causing a fixed drug eruption on the penis (Gruber *et al.* 1997).

TOPICAL

Allergic contact dermatitis is discussed above. Oestrogen cream can be absorbed through the vagina (Rigg *et al.* 1978) while Donlan and Scutero (1975) attributed a rash accompanied by an eosinophilic pneumonia to a vaginal cream containing a sulphonamide, allantoin and aminacrine. Dextropropoxyphene suppositories have led to ulceration of the anus, rectum and vagina (Laplanche *et al.* 1984, Fenzy & Bogomoletz 1986). Eigler *et al.* (1986) reported four patients in whom anorectal ulceration seemed to be related to the abuse of ergotamine tartrate suppositories. Abortifacients can cause damage, and in one early report (Gellhorn 1901), where caustic suppositories were used to 'treat' fibroids, complete casts of the vagina were shed.

Immunological factors

Miller *et al.* (1994) reported cases of vulvovaginal erythema in women with graft-versus-host disease; they had symptoms and biopsies supported the diagnosis. The authors suspected that ovarian failure and medication were additional factors.

References

Abele, D.C. & Anders, K.H. (1990) The many faces and phases of borreliosis II. *Journal of the American Academy of Dermatology* **23**, 401–410.

Abell, M.R. (1965) Intraepithelial carcinoma of epidermis and squamous mucosa of vulva and perineum. *Surgical Clinics of North America* **46**, 1179–1198.

Aberer, E. & Stanek, G. (1987) Histological evidence for spirochetal origin of morphea and lichen sclerosus et atrophicans. *American Journal of Dermatopathology* **9**, 374–379.

Ackerman, A.B. (1972) Focal acantholytic dyskeratosis. *Archives of Dermatology* **106**, 65–67.

Ackerman, A.B. (1988) Melanocytic proliferation that simulates malignant melanoma histopathologically. In: *Pathology and Recognition and Malignant Melanoma* (eds M.C. Mihm, G.F. Murphy & N. Kaufman), pp. 166–167. Williams & Wilkins, Baltimore.

Ackroyd, J.F. (1985) Fixed drug eruptions. *British Medical Journal* **290**, 1533–1534.

Aguilar, A., Ambrojo, P., Requena, L., Olmos, L. & Sánchez Yus, E. (1990) Angiolymphoid hyperplasia with eosinophilia limited to the vulva. *Clinical and Experimental Dermatology* **15**, 65–67.

Aiba, S. & Tagami, H. (1989) Immunoglobulin-producing cells in plasma cell orificial mucositis. *Journal of Cutaneous Pathology* **16**, 207–210.

Alli, N., Karakayali, G., Kahraman, I. & Artüz, F. (1997) Local intralesional therapy with rh GM-CSF for a large genital ulcer in Behçet's disease. *British Journal of Dermatology* **136**, 639–640.

Altimari, A., Bhoopalam, N., O'Dorsio, T. *et al.* (1986) Use of a somatostatin analogue in the glucagonoma syndrome. *Surgery* **100**, 989–996.

Ambrojo, P., Cogolludo, E.F., Aguilar, A., Sánchez Yus, E. & Sánchez de Paz, F. (1990) Cutaneous lymphangiectases after therapy for carcinoma of the cervix—a case with unusual clinical and histological features. *Clinical and Experimental Dermatology* **15**, 57–59.

Ansink, A.C., Krul, M.R.L., de Weger, R.A. *et al.* (1994) Human papillomavirus, lichen sclerosus, and squamous cell carcinoma of the vulva: detection and diagnostic significance. *Gynecologic Oncology* **52**, 180–184.

Atherton, D.J. (1992) The neonate. In: *Textbook of Dermatology*, 5th edn (eds R.H. Champion, J.L. Burton & F.J.G. Ebling), pp. 381–443. Blackwell Scientific Publications, Oxford.

Atia, W.A. & Tidbury, P.J. (1995) Persistent episiotomy granulation polyps: a polysymptomatic clinical entity. *Acta Obstetrica Gynaecologica Scandinavica* **74**, 361–366.

Axiotis, C.A., Merino, M.J. & Duray, P.H. (1991) Langherhans cell histiocytosis of the female genital tract. *Cancer* **67**, 1650–1660.

Aziz, F.A. (1980) Gynecologic and obstetric complications of female circumcision. *International Journal of Gynaecology and Obstetrics* **17**, 560–563.

Bailin, P., Kantor, G.K. & Wheeland, R.G. (1986) Carbon dioxide laser vaporization of lymphangioma circumscriptum. *Journal of the American Academy and Dermatology* **14**, 257–262.

Ball, C.S., Wujanto, R., Haboubi, N.Y. & Schofield, P.F. (1988) Carcinoma in Crohn's disease: discussion paper. *Journal of the Royal Society of Medicine* **81**, 217–219.

Banerjee, A.K. (1992) Surgical treatment of hidradenitis suppurativa. *British Journal of Surgery* **79**, 863–866.

Banfield, C.C., Papadavid, E., Frith, P., Allen, J. & Wojnarowska, F.T. (1997) Bullous pemphigoid evolving into cicatricial pemphigoid? *Clinical and Experimental Dermatology* **22**, 30–33.

Barker, L.P. & Gross, P. (1962) Lichen sclerosus et atrophicus of the female genitalia. *Archives of Dermatology* **85**, 362–371.

Barnes, C.J. & Douglas, C.P. (1985) Preliminary findings on levels of collagenase and its tissue inhibitor in some vulval dystrophies. *Journal of Obstetrics and Gynaecology* **6**, 55–56.

Barnhill, R.L., Albert, L.S., Shama, S.K., Goldenhersh, M.A., Rhodes, A.R. & Sober, A.J. (1990) Genital lentiginosis: a clinical and histopathologic study. *Journal of the American Academy of Dermatology* **22**, 453–460.

Barrett, J.F.R., Murray, L.A. & Macdonald, H.N. (1989) Darier's disease localized to the vulva. Case report. *British Journal of Obstetrics and Gynaecology* **96**, 997–999.

Barth, J.H., Reshad, H., Darley, C.R. & Gibson, J.R. (1984) A cutaneous complication of Dorbanex therapy. *Clinical and Experimental Dermatology* **9**, 95–96.

Barth, J.H., Layton, A.M. & Cunliffe, W.J. (1996) Endocrine factors in pre- and post-menopausal women with hidradenitis suppurativa. *British Journal of Dermatology* **134**, 1057–1059.

Bays, J. & Chadwick, D. (1993) Medical diagnosis of the sexually abused child. *Child Abuse and Neglect* **17**, 91–110.

Berkeley, C. & Bonney, V. (1909) Leukoplakic vulvitis and its relation to kraurosis vulvae and to carcinoma vulvae. *Proceedings of the Royal Society of Medicine* **3**, 29–31.

Bermejo, A., Bermejo, M.D., Román, P., Botella, R. & Bagán, J.V. (1990) Lichen planus with simultaneous involvement of the oral cavity and genitalia. *Oral Surgery, Oral Medicine and Oral Pathology* **69**, 209–216.

Berth-Jones, J., Smith, S.G. & Graham-Brown, R.A.C. (1995) Benign familial chronic pemphigus (Hailey–Hailey disease) responds to cyclosporin. *Clinical and Experimental Dermatology* **20**, 70–72.

Besa, E.C., Hyzinski, M., Nowell, P. & Abrahm, J. (1986) Clinical trials and *in vitro* studies of 13-cis retinoic acid in the myelodysplastic syndrome. In: *Vitamins and Cancer. Human Cancer Prevention by Vitamins and Micronutrients* (eds F.L. Meyskens & K. Prasad), pp. 453–469. Human Press, Clifton, NJ.

Best, C.L., Walters, C. & Adelman, D.C. (1988) Fixed cutaneous eruptions to seminal-plasma challenge: a case report. *Fertility and Sterility* **50**, 532–534.

Betson, J.R., Chiffelle, T.L. & George, R.P. (1962) Pilonidal sinuses involving the clitoris. *American Journal of Obstetrics and Gynecology* **84**, 543–545.

Bhol, K., Yunis, J. & Ahmed, A.R. (1996) Pemphigus vulgaris in distant relatives of two families: association with major histocompatibility complex class II genes. *Clinical and Experimental Dermatology* **21**, 100–103.

Bircher, A.J., Hirsbrunner, P. & Langauer, S. (1993) Allergic contact dermatitis of the genitals from additives in condoms. *Contact Dermatitis* **28**, 125–126.

Blaauwgeers, J.L.G., Bleker, O.P., Veltkamp, S. & Weigel, H.M. (1993) Langerhans cell histiocytosis of the vulva. *European Journal of Obstetric, Gynaecological and Reproductive Biology* **48**, 145–148.

Black, M.M. (1992) Lichen planus and lichenoid disorders. In: *Textbook of Dermatology*, 5th edn (eds R.H. Champion, J.L. Burton & F.J.G. Ebling), pp. 1675–1679. Blackwell Scientific Publications, Oxford.

Bloch, K.J., Buchanan, W.W., Wohl, M.J. & Bunim, J.J. (1965) Sjögren's syndrome. *Medicine* **44**, 187–231.

Boer, J. & Weltevreden, E.F. (1996) Hidradenitis suppurativa or acne inversa. A clinicopathological study of early lesions. *British Journal of Dermatology* **135**, 721–725.

Bonafe, J.L., Thibaut, I. & Hoff, J. (1990) Introital adenosis associated with Stevens–Johnson syndrome. *Clinical and Experimental Dermatology* **15**, 356–357.

Bonifazi, E., Garofalo, L., Lospalluti M. *et al.* (1981) Granuloma gluteal infantum with atrophic scars. Clinical and histological observations in 11 cases. *Clinical and Experimental Dermatology* **6**, 23–29.

Bonney, V. (1938) Leukoplakic vulvitis and the conditions likely to be confused with it. *Proceedings of the Royal Society of Medicine* **31**, 1057–1060.

Bousema, M.T., Rompannen, U., Geiger, J-M. *et al.* (1994) Acitretin in the treatment of severe lichen sclerosus et atrophicus of the vulva: a double-blind placebo-controlled study. *Journal of the American Academy of Dermatology* **30**, 225–231.

Bousser, A.M., Nilias, G., Mosser, C. *et al.* (1986) Lichen plan et sténose oesophagienne. à propos d'un cas. *Annales de Dermatologie et de Vénéréologie* **113**, 938–939.

Boyce, D.C. & Valpey, J.M. (1971) Acute ulcerative vulvitis of obscure etiology. *Obstetrics and Gynecology* **38**, 440–443.

Brandrup, F., Petri, J. & Aegidius, J. (1990) Acantholytic lesions in the vagina. *British Journal of Dermatology* **123**, 691–692.

Breisky, D. (1885) Über Kraurosis Vulvae. *Zeitschrift für Heilkunde* **6**, 69–80.

Brisigotti, M., Moreno, A., Murcia, C., Matías-Giuiu, X. & Prat, J. (1989) Verrucous carcinoma of the vulva. A clinicopathologic and immunohistochemical study of 5 cases. *International Journal of Gynecological Pathology* **8**, 1–7.

Brodin, M.B. (1980) Balanitis circumscripta plasmacellularis. *Journal of the American Academy of Dermatology* **2**, 33–35.

Brookes, D. & Sarkany, I. (1970) Lichen sclerosus et atrophicus with mouth lesions. *British Journal of Dermatology* **83**, 422.

Brown, J. & Winkelmann, R.K. (1968) Acanthosis nigricans: a study of 90 cases. *Medicine* **47**, 33–51.

Brownstein, M.H., Mehregan, A.R., Bikowski, B., Lupulescu, A. & Patterson, J.C. (1979) The dermatopathology of Cowden's syndrome. *British Journal of Dermatology* **100**, 667–673.

Buchholz, F., Schubert, C. & Lehmann-Willenbrock, E. (1985) White sponge nevus of the vulva. *International Journal of Gynaecology and Obstetrics* **23**, 505–507.

Buckley, C.H. (1995) Interrelationships of non-gynaecological and gynaecological disease. In: *Haines and Taylor Obstetrical and Gynaecological Pathology*, 4th edn (eds H. Fox & M. Wells), pp. 1257–1278. Churchill Livingstone, Edinburgh.

Buckley, D.A. & Barnes, L. (1996) Vulvar lymphangiectasia due to recurrent cellulitis. *Clinical and Experimental Dermatology* **21**, 215–216.

Buckley, D.A. & Rogers, S. (1995) Cyclosporin-responsive hidradenitis suppurativa. *Journal of the Royal Society of Medicine* **88**, 289–290.

Buezo, G.F., Pěnas, P.F., Firaga, J., Alegre, A. & Aragües, M. (1996) Condyloma-like lesions as the presenting sign of multiple myeloma associated amyloidosis. *British Journal of Dermatology* **135**, 665–666.

Burgdorf, W. (1981) Cutaneous manifestations of Crohn's disease. *Journal of the American Academy of Dermatology* **5**, 689–695.

Burge, S.M., Frith, P.A., Juniper, R.P. & Wojnarowska, F.W. (1989) Mucosal involvement in systemic and chronic cutaneous lupus erythematosus. *British Journal of Dermatology* **121**, 727–741.

Burge, S.M. (1992) Hailey–Hailey disease: the clinical features, response to treatment and prognosis. *British Journal of Dermatology* **126**, 275–282.

Burge, S. (1994) Darier's disease—the clinical features and pathogenesis. *Clinical and Experimental Dermatology* **19**, 193–205.

Burge, S.M. & Wilkinson, J.D. (1992) Darier–White disease: a review of the clinical features in 163 patients. *Journal of the American Academy of Dermatology* **27**, 40–50.

Burke, D.A., Adams, R.M. & Arundell, F.D. (1969) Febrile ulceronecrotic Mucha–Habermann's disease. *Archives of Dermatology* **100**, 200–206.

Burnett, J.W., Goldner, R. & Calton, G.J. (1975) Cowden's disease: Report of 2 additional cases. *British Journal of Dermatology* **93**, 329–336.

Burrows, N.P. & Russell-Jones, R. (1992) Crohn's disease in association with hidradenitis suppurativa. *British Journal of Dermatology* **126**, 523–529.

Bushkell, L.L., Friedrich, E.G. & Jordon, R.E. (1981) An appraisal of routine immuno-fluorescence in vulvar disease. *Acta Dermato-venereologica (Stockholm)* **61**, 157–161.

Cantwell, A.R. (1984) Histologic observations of pleomorphic, variably acid-fast bacteria in scleroderma, morphoea, and lichen sclerosus et atrophicus. *International Journal of Dermatology* **23**, 45–52.

Capraro, V.J. & Greenberg, H. (1972) Adhesions of the labia minora: a study of 50 patients. *Obstetrics and Gynecology* **39**, 65–69.

Capriello, P., Barale, E., Cappelli, N., Lupo, S. & Teti, G. (1988) Sjögren's syndrome; clinical, cytological, histological and colposcopic aspects in women. *Clinical and Experimental Obstetrics and Gynaecology* **15**, 9–12.

Cario, G.M., House, M.J. & Paradinos, F.J. (1984) Squamous cell carcinoma of the vulva in association with mixed vulvar dystrophy in an 18 year old girl. *British Journal of Obstetrics and Gynaecology* **91**, 87–90.

Carli, P., Cattaneo, A., Pimpinelli, N. *et al.* (1991) Immunohistochemical evidence of skin immune system involvement in vulvar lichen sclerosus and atrophicus. *Dermatologica* **182**, 18–22.

Carli, P., Cattaneo, A. & Gianotti, B. (1992) Clobetasol propionate 0.05% cream in the treatment of vulvar lichen sclerosus: effect on the immunohistological profile. *British Journal of Dermatology* **127**, 542–543.

Carli, P., Cattaneo, A., de Magnis, A., Biggeri, A., Taddei, G. & Gianotti, B. (1995) Squamous cell carcinoma arising in lichen sclerosus: a longitudinal cohort study. *European Journal of Cancer Prevention* **4**, 491–495.

Carli, P., Moretti, S., Spallanzani, A., Berti, E. & Cattaneo, A. (1997) Fibrogenic cytokines in vulvar lichen sclerosus. An immunohistochemical study. *Journal of Reproductive Medicine* **42**, 161–165.

Cattaneo, A., Carli, P., de Marco, A. *et al.* (1996) Testosterone maintenance therapy. *Journal of Reproductive Medicine* **41**, 99–102.

Caughman, W., Stern, R. & Haines, H. (1983) Neutrophilic dermatoses of myeloproliferative disorders. *Journal of the American Academy of Dermatology* **9**, 751–758.

Caumes, E., Gatineau, M., Bricaire, F. *et al.* (1993) Foscarnet-induced vulvar erosion. *Journal of the American Academy of Dermatology* **28**, 799 (letter).

Cecchi, R., Bartoli, L., Brunetti, L., Pavesi, M. & Giomi, A. (1995) Lymphangioma circumscriptum of the vulva of late onset. *Acta Dermato-venereologica* **75**, 79–80.

Chalmers, R.J.G., Burton, P.A., Bennett, R.F., Goring, C.C. & Smith, J.B. (1984) Lichen sclerosus et atrophicus. A common and distinctive cause of phimosis in boys. *Archives of Dermatology* **120**, 1025–1027.

Chang, T.W. (1976) Familial allergic seminal vulvovaginitis. *American Journal of Obstetrics and Gynecology* **126**, 442–444.

Chen, K.T.K. & Hendricks, E.J. (1985) Malakoplakia of the female genital tract. *Obstetrics and Gynecology* **65**, 84S–87S.

Cho, H.K., Shin, K.S., Sohn, S.J., Choi, S.J. & Lee, Y.S. (1989) Behçet's disease with Sweet's syndrome-like presentation: a report of 6 cases. *Clinical and Experimental Dermatology* **14**, 20–24.

Chorzelski, T.P., Kudejko, J. & Jablonska, S. (1984) Is papular acantholytic dyskeratosis of the vulva a new entity? *American Journal of Dermatopathology* **6**, 557–560.

Christensen, E.H. & Øster, J. (1971) Adhesions of labia minora (synechia vulvae) in childhood. *Acta Paediatrica Scandinavica* **60**, 709–714.

Chuong, C.J. & Hodgkinson, C.P. (1984) Labial adhesions presenting as urinary incontinence in post-menopausal women. *Obstetrics and Gynecology* **64**, 81S–84S.

Coccia, M.E., Bracco, G.L., Cattaneo, A. & Scarselli, G. (1995) Massive vulvar edema in ovarian hyperstimulation syndrome. *Journal of Reproductive Medicine* **40**, 659–660.

Connelly, M.G. & Winkelmann, R.K. (1985) Coexistence of lichen sclerosus, morphea and lichen planus. Report of 4 cases and review of the literature. *Journal of the American Academy of Dermatology* **12**, 844–851.

Cooper, J.C., Nicholls, A.J., Simms, J.M. *et al.* (1983) Genital oedema in patients treated by continuous ambulatory peritoneal dialysis. *British Medical Journal* **286**, 1923–1924.

Cooper, P.H. (1989) Acantholytic dermatosis localized to the vulvocrural area. *Journal of Cutaneous Pathology* **16**, 81–84.

Corazza, M., Virgili, A. & Mantovani, L. (1992) Vulvar contact dermatitis from nifuratel. *Contact Dermatitis* **27**, 273–274.

Coulson, I.H., Cook, M.G., Bruton, J. & Penfold, C. (1986) Atypical pemphigus vulgaris associated with angiofollicular lymph node hyperplasia (Castleman's disease). *Clinical and Experimental Dermatology* **11**, 656–663.

Cox, N.H., Mitchell, J.N.S. & Morley, W.N. (1986) Lichen sclerosus et atrophicus in non-identical female twins. *British Journal of Dermatology* **115**, 743.

Creamer, J.D., Whittaker, S.J., Kerr-Muir, M. & Smith, N.P. (1996) Phenytoin-induced toxic epidermal necrolysis: a case report. *Clinical and Experimental Dermatology* **21**, 116–120.

Crosti, C. & Riboldi, A. (1975) Eritoplasia plasmacellular benigna vulvare. *Giornale Italiano di Dermatologia—Minerva Dermatologica* **110**, 386–389.

Crotty, C.P., Su, W.P.D. & Winkelmann, R.K. (1980) Ulcerative lichen planus. Follow up of surgical excision and grafting. *Archives of Dermatology* **116**, 1252–1256.

Crowe, F.W. (1964) Axillary freckling as a diagnostic aid in neurofibromatosis. *Annals of Internal Medicine* **61**, 1142–1143.

Crum, C.P. (1992) Carcinoma of the vulva: epidemiology and pathogenesis. *Obstetrics and Gynecology* **79**, 448–458.

Crum, C.P., McLachlin, C.M., Tate, J.E. & Mutter, G.L. (1997) Pathobiology of vulvar squamous neoplasia. *Current Opinion in Obstetrics and Gynecology* **9**, 63–69.

Dalziel, K.L. (1995) Effect of lichen sclerosus on sexual function and parturition. *Journal of Reproductive Medicine* **40**, 351–354.

Dalziel, K.L. & Wojnarowska, F. (1993) Long term control of vulvar lichen sclerosus after treatment with a very potent topical steroid (clobetasol propionate 0.05%) cream. *Journal of Reproductive Medicine* **38**, 25–27.

Dalziel, K., Reynolds, A.J. & Holt, P.J.A. (1987) Lichen sclerosus et atrophicus with ocular and maxillary complications. *British Journal of Dermatology* **116**, 735–737.

Dalziel, K.L., Millard, P. & Wojnarowska, F. (1991) The treatment of vulval lichen sclerosus with a very potent topical steroid (clobetasol propionate 0.05%) cream. *British Journal of Dermatology* **124**, 461–464.

Darier, J. (1892) Lichen plan scléreux. *Annales de Dermatologie et de Syphiligraphie* **3**, 833–837.

Darier, J.G. (1928) Kraurosis de la vulve. In: *Précis de Dermatologie*, 4th. edn, p. 465. Masson et cie, Paris.

Daunt, S.O'N., Kotowski, K.E., O'Reilly, A.P. & Richardson, A.T. (1982) Ulcerative vulvitis in Reiter's syndrome: a case report. *British Journal of Venereal Diseases* **58**, 405–407.

Davenport, D.M. & Richardson, D.A. (1986) Labial adhesions secondary to postpartum vulvar edema. Report of 2 cases. *Journal of Reproductive Medicine* **31**, 523–527.

Davidson, F., Guaanachelvank, K., Marsden, R.A. & Cooke, M. (1989) Deep and acute vulval ulceration. *British Journal of Obstetrics and Gynaecology* **96**, 1351–1354.

Davis, J., Shapiro, L. & Baral, J. (1983) Vulvitis circumscripta plasmacellularis. *Journal of the American Academy of Dermatology* **8**, 413–416.

de Araújo, V., Orsini, S.C., Marcucci, G. & de Araújo, N.S. (1985) Lichen sclerosus et atrophicus. *Oral Surgery Oral Medicine Oral Pathology* **60**, 655–657.

deCastro, P., Jorizzo, J.L., Rajaraman, S. *et al.* (1985) Localized vulvar pemphigoid in a child. *Pediatric Dermatology* **2**, 302–307.

Dégos, R. & Ebrard, G. (1958) Leukokératose papillomateuse bucco-génitale. *Bulletin de la Société Française de Dermatologie et Syphiligraphie* **65**, 242.

Delke, I., Veridiano, N.P., Tanger, M.L., Gomez, Z. & Diamond, I. (1981) Sweet syndrome with involvement of the female genital tract. *Obstetrics and Gynecology* **58**, 394–396.

de Oliveira Neto, M.P. (1972) Sarcoidose com lesoes da vulva. *Revista Brasileira de Medicina* **29**, 134–139.

Diaz, T., Martinez, Tx., Antépara, I. *et al.* (1996) Latex allergy as a risk during delivery. *British Journal of Obstetrics and Gynaecology* **103**, 173–175.

Dicken, C.H., Powell, S.T. & Spear, K.L. (1984) Evaluation of isotretinoin treatment of hidradenitis suppurativa. *Journal of the American Academy of Dermatology* **11**, 500–502.

Dickens, C.M., Heseltine, D., Walton, S. & Bennett, J.R. (1990) The oesophagus in lichen planus: an endoscopic study. *British Medical Journal* **300**, 84.

Dickie, R.J., Powell, S.T. & Spear, K.L. (1982) Direct evidence of localised immunological damage in vulvar lichen sclerosus et atrophicus. *Journal of Clinical Pathology* **35**, 1395–1397.

di Paola, G.R., Rueda-Leverone, N.G. & Becardi, M.G. (1982) Lichen sclerosus of the vulva recurrent after myocutaneous graft: a case report. *Journal of Reproductive Medicine* **27**, 666–668.

di Prima, T.M., de Pasquale, R. & Nigro, M.A. (1990) Connubial contact dermatitis from nifuratel. *Contact Dermatitis* **22**, 117–118.

Donlan, C.J. & Scutero, J.V. (1975) Transient eosinophilic pneumonia secondary to the use of a vaginal cream. *Chest* **67**, 232–233.

Duhra, P. & Paul, C.J. (1988) Metastatic Crohn's disease responding to metronidazole. *British Journal of Dermatology* **119**, 87–91.

Dupré, A. & Viraben, R. (1990) Laugier's disease. *Dermatologica* **181**, 183–186.

Dupree, E.L. & Lee, R.A. (1973) Histiocytosis X in the female genital tract. *Obstetrics and Gynecology* **42**, 201–204.

Duray, P.H., Merino, M.J. & Axiotis, C. (1983) Warty dyskeratoma of the vulva. *International Journal of Gynecological Pathology* **2**, 286–293.

Dwyer, C.M., Kerr, R.E.I. & Millan, D.W.M. (1995) Squamous

carcinoma following lichen planus of the vulva. *Clinical and Experimental Dermatology* 20, 171–172.

Edwards, L. (1989) Vulvar lichen planus. *Archives of Dermatology* 125, 1677–1680.

Edwards, L. & Friedrich, E.G. (1988) Desquamative gingivitis: lichen planus in disguise. *Obstetrics and Gynecology* 71, 832–836.

Edwards, L. & Hansen, R. (1992) Reiter's syndrome of the vulva. The psoriasis spectrum. *Archives of Dermatology* 128, 811–814.

Eigler, F.W., Schaarschmidt, K., Gross, E. & Richter, H.J. (1986) Anorectal ulcers as a complication of migraine therapy. *Journal of the Royal Society of Medicine* 79, 424–426.

Eisen, D. (1994) The vulvovaginal–gingival syndrome of lichen planus. *Archives of Dermatology* 130, 1379–1382.

Ellis, J.P. & Crow, K.D. (1982) A case of lichen sclerosus et atrophicus of the perineum with carcinomata of vulva and perianal area and recurrent lichen sclerosus in a full thickness skin graft. Case Presentation. *XVI Congressus Internationalis Dermatologiae* 212.

Elsner, P., Wilhelm, D. & Maibach, H.I. (1990) Multiple parameter assessment of vulvar irritant contact dermatitis. *Contact Dermatitis* 23, 20–26.

Estrada, R. & Kaufman, R. (1993) Benign vulvar melanosis. *Journal of Reproductive Medicine* 38, 5–8.

Ewing, T.L., Smale, L.E. & Elliott, F.A. (1979) Maternal deaths associated with postpartum vulvar edema. *American Journal of Obstetrics and Gynecology* 134, 173–179.

Farrell, A.M., Millard, P.R., Schomberg, K.H. & Wojnarowksa, F. (1997) An infective aetiology for lichen sclerosus: myth or reality? *British Journal of Dermatology* 137 (Suppl. 50), 25.

Fenzy, A. & Bogomoletz, W.V. (1986) Anorectal ulceration due to abuse of dextropropoxyphene and paracetamol suppositories. *Journal of the Royal Society of Medicine* 80, 62 (letter).

Finley, E.M. & Ratz., J.L. (1996) Treatment of hidradenitis suppurativa with carbon dioxide laser excision and secondary intention healing. *Journal of the American Academy of Dermatology* 34, 465–469.

Fischer, G. & Rogers, M. (1997) Treatment of childhood vulvar lichen sclerosus with a potent topical corticosteroid. *Pediatric Dermatology* 14, 235–238.

Fisher, I. & Orkin, M. (1970) Acquired lymphangioma. *Archives of Dermatology* 101, 230–234.

Fliegner, J.R.H. (1997) Vulval varicosities and labial reduction. *Australian and New Zealand Journal of Obstetrics and Gynaecology* 37, 129–130.

Forman, L. (1966) The skin and the colon. *Transactions of the St John's Hospital Dermatological Society* 52, 139–154.

Foulds, I.S. (1980) Lichen sclerosus et atrophicus of the scalp. *British Journal of Dermatology* 103, 197–200.

Freeman, S. (1986) Woman allergic to husband's sweat and semen. *Contact Dermatitis* 14, 110–112.

Friedman, D., Haim, S. & Paldi, E. (1971) Refractory involvement of cervix uteri in a case of pemphigus vulgaris. *American Journal of Obstetrics and Gynecology* 110, 1023–1024.

Friedman, R.J., Kopf, A.W.J. & Jones, W.B. (1984) Malignant melanoma in association with lichen sclerosus on the vulva of a 14 year old. *American Journal of Dermatopathology* 6 (Suppl. 1), 253–256.

Friedman, S.A., Bernstein, I.L., Enrione, M. & Marcus, Z.H. (1984) Successful long-term immunotherapy for human seminal plasma anaphylaxis. *Journal of the American Medical Association* 251, 2684–2687.

Friedrich, E.G. (1976) New nomenclature for vulvar disease. Report of the committee on terminology. *Obstetrics and Gynecology* 47, 122–124.

Friedrich, E.G. & Kalra, P.S. (1984) Serum levels of sex hormones in vulvar lichen sclerosus and the effect of topical testosterone. *New England Journal of Medicine* 310, 488–491.

Friedrich, E.G. & MacLaren, N.K. (1984) Genetic aspects of lichen sclerosus. *American Journal of Obstetrics and Gynecology* 150, 161–166.

Gallagher, P.G. (1986) Varicose veins of the vulva. *British Journal of Sexual Medicine* 13, 12–14.

Gardner, H.L. (1969) Desquamative vaginitis. A newly defined entity. *American Journal of Obstetrics and Gynecology* 102, 1102–1105.

Garnier, G. (1954) Vulvite érythémateuse circonscrite bénigne à type érythroplasique. *Bulletin de la Société Française de Dermatologie et de Syphilographie* 61, 102–103.

Garnier, G. (1957) Benign plasma cell erythroplasia. *British Journal of Dermatology* 69, 70–81.

Gellert, A., Green, E.S., Beck, E.R. & Ridley, C.M. (1983) Erythema nodosum progressing to pyoderma gangrenosum as a complication of Crohn's disease. *Postgraduate Medical Journal* 59, 791–793.

Gellhorn, G. (1901) A rare case of exfoliative vaginitis. *American Journal of Obstetrics and Gynecology* 44, 342.

Gerbig, A.W. & Hunziker, T. (1996) Idiopathic lenticular mucocutaneous pigmentation or Laugier–Hunziker syndrome with atypical features. *Archives of Dermatology* 32, 844–845.

Godeau, G., Frances, C., Hornebeck, W., Brechemier, D. & Robert, L. (1982) Isolation and partial characterization of an elastase-type protease in human vulva fibroblasts: its possible involvement in vulvar elastic tissue destruction of patients with lichen sclerosus et atrophicus. *Journal of Investigative Dermatology* 78, 270–275.

Goldsmith, P.C., Rycroft, R.J.G., White, I.R. *et al.* (1997) Contact sensitivity in women patients with anogenital dermatoses. *Contact Dermatitis* 36, 174–175.

Goltz, R.W. (1952) Systematized amyloidosis: a review of the skin and mucous membrane lesions and a report of 2 cases. *Medicine* 31, 381–409.

Goodman, A., Zukerberg, L.R., Nikrui, N. & Scully, R.E. (1991) Vaginal adenosis and clear cell carcinoma after 5-fluorouracil treatment for condyloma. *Cancer* 68, 1628–1632.

Goodman, R.M., Smith, E.W., Paton, D. *et al.* (1963) Pseudoxanthoma elasticum: a clinical and histological study. *Medicine* 42, 297–334.

Goolamali, S.K., Barbes, E.W., Irvine, W.J. & Shuster, S. (1974) Organ-specific antibodies in patients with lichen sclerosus. *British Medical Journal* iv, 78–79.

Gorodeski, I.G., Cordoba, M., Shapira, A. & Bahary, C.M. (1988) Primary localized cutaneous lichen amyloidosis of the vulva. *International Journal of Dermatology* 27, 259–260.

Gougerot, H. & Burnier, R. (1937) Lichen plan du col utérin, accompagnant un lichen plan jugal et un lichen plan stomacal. Lichen plan plurimuqueuse sans lichen cutané. *Bulletin de la Société Française de Dermatologie et Syphiligraphie* 44, 637–640.

Graham-Brown. R.A.C., Cochrane, G.W., Swinhoe, J.R., Sarkany, I. & Epsztejn, L.J. (1981) Vaginal stenosis due to bullous erythema multiforme (Stevens Johnson syndrome). *British Journal of Obstetrics and Gynaecology* **88**, 1156–1157.

Gray, L.A. & Barnes, M.L. (1965) Vaginitis in women, diagnosis and treatment. *American Journal of Obstetrics and Gynecology* **92**, 125–134.

Greaves, M.W. (1992) Pruritus. In: *Textbook of Dermatology*, 5th edn (eds R.H. Champion, J.L. Burton and F.J.G. Ebling), pp. 527–535. Blackwell Scientific Publications. Oxford.

Greene, S.L. & Muller, S.A. (1985) Netherton's syndrome. Report of a case and review of the literature. *Journal of the American Academy of Dermatology* **13**, 329–337.

Greenspan, A.H., Shupack, J.L., Foo, S.H. & Wise, A.C. (1985) Acanthosis nigricans like eruption hyperpigmentation secondary to triazinate therapy. *Archives of Dermatology* **121**, 232–235.

Greer, I.A. (1984) Orange periods. *British Medical Journal* **289**, 323.

Grimmer, H. (1968) Apokrine miliaria der Vulva (subcorneale Schweissdrüsen-retention). *Zeitschrift für Haut und Geslechts-Krankheit* **43**, 123–132.

Gross, P. (1941) Non-pellagrous eruptions due to deficiency of vitamin B complex. *Archives of Dermatology* **43**, 504–531.

Gruber, F., Stasić, A., Lenković, M. & Brajać, I. (1997) Postcoital fixed drug eruption in a man sensitive to trimethoprim–sulphamethoxazole. *Clinical and Experimental Dermatology* **22**, 144–145.

Guenther, L.C. & Shum, D. (1990) Localized childhood vulvar pemphigoid. *Journal of the American Academy of Dermatology* **22**, 762–764.

Haake, N. & Altmeyer, P. (1988) Vulvovaginitis circinata bei Morbus Reiter. *Hautarzt* **39**, 748–749.

Hackel, H., Hartmann, A.A. & Burg, G. (1991) Vulvitis granulomatosa and anoperineitis granulomatosa. *Dermatologica* **182**, 128–131.

Hacker, S.M. (1994) Absence of anti-single stranded DNA antibodies in vulvar lichen sclerosus and atrophicus. *Archives of Dermatology* **130**, 1454–1455.

Haefner, H.K., Tate, J.E., McLachlin, C.M. & Crum, C.P. (1995) Vulvar intraepithelial neoplasia: age, morphological phenotype, papillomavirus DNA, and coexisting invasive carcinoma. *Human Pathology* **26**, 147–154.

Hallopeau, H. (1887) Leçons cliniques sur les maladies cutanées et syphilitiques. *L'Union Médicale* **43**, 742–747.

Hallopeau, H. (1889) Lichen plan scléreux. *Annales de Dermatologie et de Syphiligraphie* (2nd series) **10**, 447–449.

Hamilton, P.A., Brown, P., Davies, J.D. & Salmon, P.R. (1977) Crohn's disease: an unusual cause of dyspareunia. *British Medical Journal* **ii**, 101.

Handfield-Jones, S.E., Prendiville, W.J. & Norman, S. (1989) Vulval lymphangiectasia. *Genitourinary Medicine* **65**, 335–337.

Harrington, C.I. & Dunsmore, I.R. (1981) An investigation into the incidence of autoimmune disorders in patients with lichen sclerosus et atrophicus. *British Journal of Dermatology* **104**, 563–566.

Harwood, C.A. & Mortimer, P.S. (1993) Acquired lymphangiomata mimicking genital warts. *British Journal of Dermatology* **129**, 334–336.

Hazelrigg, D.E. & Stoller, L.J. (1977) Isolated familial benign chronic pemphigus. *Archives of Dermatology* **113**, 1302.

Helander, S.D. & Rogers, R.S. (1994) The sensitivity and specificity of direct immunofluorescence testing in disorders of mucous membranes. *Journal of the American Academy of Dermatology* **30**, 65–75.

Hernando, L.B., Sebastian, F.V., Sanchez, J.H., Romero, P.O. & Diez, L.I. (1992) Lichen planus pemphigoides in a 10 year old girl. *Journal of the American Academy of Dermatology* **26**, 124–125.

Hewitt, J. (1984) Conditions étiologiques du carcinome invasif d'emblée de la vulve. Possibilité d'un traitement prophylactique? *Journal de Gynécologie, Obstétrique et Biologie de la Reproduction* **13**, 297–303.

Hewitt, J. (1986) Histologic criteria for lichen sclerosus of the vulva. *Journal of Reproductive Medicine* **31**, 781–787.

Highet, A.S., Warren, R.E., Staughton, R.C.D. & Roberts, S.O.B. (1980) *Streptococcus milleri* causing treatable infection in perineal hidradenitis suppurativa. *British Journal of Dermatology* **103**, 375–382.

Ho, K.K-L., Dervan, P., O'Loughlin, S. & Powell, F.C. (1993) Labial melanotic macule: a clinical, histopathologic, and ultrastructural study. *Journal of the American Academy of Dermatology* **28**, 33–39.

Hofs, von W. (1978) Familiärer Lichen sclerosus et atrophicans bei Vater, Mutter und 9 jahriger Tochter. *Dermatologische Monatsschrift* **164**, 633–639.

Hogan, D.J. & Light, M.J. (1988) Successful treatment of hidradenitis suppurativa with acitretin. *Journal of the American Journal of Dermatology* **19**, 355–356.

Huey, G.R., Stehman, F.B., Roth, L.M. & Ehrlich, C.E. (1985) Lymphangioma of the edematous thigh after radiation therapy for carcinoma of the vulva. *Gynecologic Oncology* **20**, 394–401.

Hughes, B.R., Holt, P.J.A. & Marks, R. (1987) Trimethoprim associated fixed drug eruption. *British Journal of Dermatology* **116**, 241–242.

Hunt, E. (1954) *Diseases Affecting the Vulva*, 4th edn, pp. 65–74. Henry Kimpton, London.

International Study Group for Behçet's disease (1990) *Lancet* **335**, 1078–1080.

Issa, P.Y., Salem, P.A., Brihi, E. *et al.* (1980) Eosinophilic granuloma with involvement of the female genitalia. *American Journal of Obstetrics and Gynecology* **137**, 608–612.

Jackson, R. (1984) Melanosis of the vulva. *Journal of Dermatologic Surgery and Oncology* **10**, 119–121.

James, W.D. & Lupton, G.P. (1988) Acquired dyskeratotic leukoplakia. *Archives of Dermatology* **124**, 117–120.

Jänner, M., Muissus, E. & Rohde, B. (1967) Lichen planus als fakultative Präkanzerose. *Dermatologische Wochenschrift* **153**, 513–518.

Jayle, F. (1906) Le kraurosis vulvae. *Revue de Gynécologie et de Chirurgie Abdominale* **10**, 633–668.

Jeffcoate, T.N.A. (1949) Pruritus vulvae. *British Medical Journal* **ii**, 1196–1200.

Jeffcoate, T.N.A. & Woodcock, A.S. (1961) Premalignant conditions of the vulva, with particular reference to chronic epithelial dystrophies. *British Medical Journal* **ii**, 127–134.

Jenkinson, S.D. & MacKinnon, A.E. (1984) Spontaneous separation of fused labia minora in prepubertal girls. *British Medical Journal* **289**, 160–161.

Johansson, O. & Nordlind, K. (1986) Immunoreactivity to material like vasoactive intestinal polypeptide in epidermal cells of lichen sclerosus et atrophicus. *American Journal of Dermatopathology* **8**, 105–108.

Johns, A.M. & Bower, B.D. (1970) Wasting of napkin area after repeated use of fluorinated steroid. *British Medical Journal* **i**, 347–348.

Jones, W.R. (1991) Allergy to coitus. *Australian and New Zealand Journal of Obstetrics and Gynaecology* **31**, 137–141.

Jonquières, E.D.L. & de Lutsky, F.K. (1980) Balanites et vulvites pseudo-érythroplasiques chroniques. Aspects histopathologiques. *Annales de Dermatologie et de Vénéréologie* **107**, 173–180.

Joosse, L.A., Koudstaal, J. & Oswald, F.H. (1964) Chromidrosis vulvae. *Tijdschrift voor Verloskunde und Gynecologie* **64**, 179–187.

Jordaan, H.F. (1989) Acute febrile neutrophilic dermatosis: histopathological study of 57 patients and review of the literature. *American Journal of Dermatopathology* **11**, 99–113.

Jorgenson, R.J. & Levin, L.S. (1981) White sponge nevus. *Archives of Dermatology* **117**, 73–76.

Joulia, P. & le Coulant, P. (1954) La maladie de Mucha, sa place actuelle dans la nosologie dermatologique. *Minerva Dermatologica* **29**, 172–178.

Junaid, T.A. & Thomas, S.M. (1981) Cysts of the vulva and vagina: a comparative study. *International Journal of Gynaecology and Obstetrics* **19**, 239–243.

Kaminsky *et al.* (1974) Cited by Macleod and Soames (1991).

Kanj, L.F., Rubeiz, N.G., Mrouett, A.M. & Kibbi, A.-G. (1992) Vulvar melanosis and lentiginosis: a case report. *Journal of the American Academy of Dermatology* **27**, 777–778.

Kanwar, A.J. & Kaur, S. (1991) Pemphigus in children. *International Journal of Dermatology* **30**, 343–346.

Kao, M.S., Paulson, J.D. & Askin, F.B. (1975) Crohn's disease of the vulva. *Obstetrics and Gynecology* **46**, 329–333.

Kartamaa, M. & Reitamo, S. (1997) Treatment of lichen sclerosus with carbon dioxide laser vaporization. *British Journal of Dermatology* **136**, 356–359.

Kasper, C.S. & McMurry, K. (1991) Necrolytic erythema without glucagonoma versus canine superfical necrolytic dermatitis: Is hepatic involvement a clue to pathogenesis? *Journal of the Academy of Dermatology* **25**, 534–541.

Kato, K., Kondo, A., Takita, T. & Mitsuya, H. (1986) Labial adhesions in a diabetic woman. *Urologica Internationalis* **41**, 455–456.

Kato, T., Kuramoto, Y., Tadaki, T., Hashimoto, K. & Tagami, H. (1990) Chronic vulvar porpura. *Dermatologica* **180**, 174–176.

Kavanagh, G.M., Burton, P.A. & Kennedy, C.T.C. (1993) Vulvitis chronica plasmacellularis (Zoon's vulvitis). *British Journal of Dermatology* **129**, 92–93.

Keefe, M., Wakeel, R.A. & Kerr, R.E.I. (1988) Sweet's syndrome, plantar pustulosis and vulval pustules. *Clinical and Experimental Dermatology* **13**, 344–346.

Kim, N.-I., Eom, J.-Y, Sim, W.-Y. & Haw, C.-R. (1992) Crohn's disease of the vulva. *Journal of the American Academy of Dermatology* **27**, 764–765.

Kingsland, C.R. & Alderman, B. (1991) Crohn's disease of the vulva. *Journal of the Royal Society of Medicine* **84**, 236–237.

Kint, B., Degreef, H. & Dooms-Goossens, A. (1994) Combined allergy to human seminal plasma and latex: case report and review of the literature. *Contact Dermatitis* **30**, 7–11.

Kissmeyer, A. & With, C. (1922) Clinical and histological studies on the pathological changes in the elastic tissue of the skin. *British Journal of Dermatology* **34**, 221–237.

Klostermann, G.F. (1972) Weibliche Gerschlechtsorgane. Vierter Teil: Vulva, Vagina, Urethra. In: *Handbuch der speziellen pathologischen Anatomie und Histologie* (ed. E. Vehling), p. 221. Springer-Verlag, Berlin.

Koo, S.-W., Suh, C.O. & Hann, S.K. (1996) Vitiligo following radiotherapy for carcinoma of the breast. *British Journal of Dermatology* **135**, 858–859.

Kopecky, R.T., Funk, M.M. & Kreitzer, P.R. (1985) Localized genital edema in patients undergoing continuous ambulatory peritoneal dialysis. *Journal of Urology* **134**, 880–884.

Kossard, S. & Shumack, S. (1989) Lichen aureus of the glans penis as an expression of Zoon's balanitis. *Journal of the American Journal of Dermatology* **21**, 804–806.

Kranl, C., Zelger, B., Kofler, H., Heim, K., Sepp, N. & Fritsch, P. (1998) Vulvar & vaginal adenosis. *British Journal of Dermatology* **139**, 128–131.

Krol, A.L. (1990) Perianal streptococcal dermatitis. *Pediatric Dermatology* **7**, 97–100.

Kübler, H.C., Kühn, W., Rummel, H.H., Kaufmann, I. & Kaufmann, M. (1987) Zur Karzinomentstehung (Vulvakarzinom) beim Netherton-Syndrom (Ichthyosis, Haaranomalien, atopische Diathese). *Geburtshilfe und Frauenheilkunde* **47**, 742–744.

Kuo, T.T., Shih, L.Y. & Chan, H.L. (1988) Kimura's disease: involvement of regional lymph nodes and distinction from angiolymphoid hyperplasia with eosinophilia. *American Journal of Surgical Pathology* **12**, 843–854.

Kuroda, K., Kojima, T., Fujita, M., Iseki, T. & Shinkai, H. (1995) Unusual cutaneous manifestations of the myelodysplastic syndrome. *British Journal of Dermatology* **133**, 483–486.

Lally, M.R., Orenstein, S.R. & Cohen, B.A. (1988) Crohn's disease of the vulva in an eight year old girl. *Pediatric Dermatology* **5**, 103–106.

Lambiris, A. & Greaves, M.W. (1997) Dyspareunia and vulvodynia: unrecognised manifestations of symptomatic dermographism. *Lancet* **349**, 28.

Lampert, A., Assier-Bonnet, H., Chevallier, B., Clerici, T. & Saiag, P. (1996) Lipschutz's genital ulceration: a manifestation of Epstein–Barr virus primary infection. *British Journal of Dermatology* **135**, 663–665.

La Nasa, G., Cattoni, F., Mulargia, M. *et al.* (1995) HLA antigen distribution in different clinical sub-groups demonstrates genetic heterogeneity in lichen planus. *British Journal of Dermatology* **132**, 897–900.

Lancet (editorial) (1990) Ligneous conjunctivitis. *Lancet* **335**, 84.

Landthaler, M., Hohenleutner, U. & Braun-Falco, O. (1990) Acquired lymphangioma of the vulva: palliative treatment by means of laser vaporization carbon dioxide. *Archives of Dermatology* **126**, 967–968.

Langenberg, A., Berger, T.G., Cardelli, M. *et al.* (1992) Genital benign chronic pemphigus (Hailey–Hailey disease) presenting as condylomas. *Journal of the American Academy of Dermatology* **26**, 952–955.

Laplanche, C., Grosshans, E. & Heid, G. (1984) Anorectal ulcerations after prolonged use of suppositories containing dextropopoxyphene. *Annales de Dermatologie et de Vénéréologie* **111**, 347–355.

Laugier, P., Hunziker, N. & Olmos, L. (1977) Pigmentation mélanique lenticulaire essentielle de la muqueuse jugale et des lèvres. *Annales de Dermatologie et de Vénéréologie* **104**, 181–184.

Lavery, H.A. (1984) Vulval dystrophies: new approaches. *Clinics in Obstetrics and Gynaecology* **11**, 155–169.

Lavery, H.A., Pinkerton, J.H.M., Roberts, S.D., Sloan, J. & Walsh, M. (1985) Dermatomyositis of the vulva—first reported case. *British Journal of Dermatology* **113**, 349–352.

Lebbe, C., Moulonguet-Michau, I., Perrin P. *et al.* (1992) Steroid-responsive pyoderma gangrenosum with vulvar and pulmonary involvement. *Journal of the American Academy of Dermatology* **27**, 623–625.

le Boit, P.E. (1996) Multinucleated atypia. *American Journal of Surgical Pathology* **20**, 507.

Ledwig, P.A. & Weigand, D.A. (1989) Late circumcision and lichen sclerosus et atrophicus of the penis. *Journal of the American Academy of Dermatology* **20**, 211–214.

Leibowitch, M., Neill, S., Pelisse, M. & Moyal-Barracco, M. (1990) The epithelial changes associated with squamous carcinoma of the vulva: a review of the clinical, histological and virological findings in 78 women. *British Journal of Obstetrics and Gynaecology* **97**, 1135–1139.

Leigh, I.M., Sanderson, K.V., Atherton, D.J. & Wells, R.S. (1979) Hypozincaemia in infancy. *British Journal of Dermatology* **101** (Suppl. 17), 73–75.

Leung, A.K.C., Robson, W.L.M. & Tay-Uyboco, J. (1993) The incidence of labial fusion in children. *Journal of Paediatrics and Child Health* **29**, 235–236.

Levine, V., Sanchez, M. & Nestor, M. (1992) Localized vulvar pemphigoid in a child misdiagnosed as sexual abuse. *Archives of Dermatology* **128**, 804–806.

Lewis, F.M. & Harrington, C.I. (1994) Squamous cell carcinoma arising in vulval lichen planus. *British Journal of Dermatology* **131**, 703–705.

Lewis, F.M., Gawkrodger, D.J. & Harrington, C.I. (1994a) Colophony: an unusual factor in pruritus vulvae. *Contact Dermatitis* **31**, 119.

Lewis, F.M., Harrington, C.I. & Gawkrodger, D.J. (1994b) Contact sensitivity in pruritus vulvae: a common and manageable problem. *Contact Dermatitis* **31**, 264–265.

Lewis, F.M., Shah, M. & Harrington, C.I. (1996) Vulval involvement in lichen planus: a study of 37 women. *British Journal of Dermatology* **135**, 89–91.

Lim, J. & Ng, S.K. (1992) Oral tetracycline rinse improves symptoms of white sponge nevus. *Journal of the American Academy of Dermatology* **26**, 1003–1005.

Lindskov R. (1984) Acute febrile neurophilic dermatosis with genital involvement. *Acta Dermato-venereologica (Stockholm)* **64**, 559–561.

Lipschutz, B. (1913) Über eine eigenartige Geschwürsform des Weiblichen Genitales (ulcus vulvae acutum). *Archiv für Dermatologie und Syphilis (Berlin)* **114**, 363–396.

Lonsdale, R.N. & Gibbs, S. (1998) Pemphigus vulgaris with involvement of the cervix. *British Journal of Dermatology* **138**, 363–365.

Lovell, C.R. & Atherton, D.J. (1984) Infantile gluteal granulomata: case report. *Clinical and Experimental Dermatology* **9**, 522–525.

Lurie, S., Manor, M. & Hagay, Z.J. (1998) The threat of type IV Ehlers–Danlos syndrome on maternal well-being during pregnancies: early delivery may make a difference. *Journal of Obstetrics and Gynaecology* **18**, 245–248.

Luxman, D., Cohen, J.R., Gordon, D., Wolman, I., Wolf, Y. & David, M.P. (1996) Unilateral vulvar edema associated with severe ovarian hyperstimulation syndrome. *Journal of Reproductive Medicine* **41**, 771–774.

Lyles, J.W., Knox, J.M. & Richardson, J.B. (1958) Atypical features in familial benign chronic pemphigus. *Archives of Dermatology* **78**, 446–453.

Lynch, P.J. (1975) Desquamative inflammatory vaginitis with oral lichen planus. *Proceedings of the Second International Congress, I.S.S.V.D.*, pp. 30–31.

McAdams, A.J. & Kistner, R.W. (1958) The relationship of chronic vulvar disease, leukoplakia and carcinoma *in situ* to carcinoma of the vulva. *Cancer* **11**, 740–757.

McCallum, D.I. & Gray, W.M. (1976) Metastatic Crohn's disease. *British Journal of Dermatology* **95**, 551–554.

McCallum, D.I. & Kinmont, P.D. (1968) Dermatological manifestations of Crohn's disease. *British Journal of Dermatology* **80**, 1–8.

McCalmont, C.S., Leshin, B., White, W.L., Greiss, F.C. & Jorizzo, J.L. (1991) Vulvar pyoderma gangrenosum. *International Journal of Gynecology and Obstetrics* **35**, 175–178.

McDonagh, A.J.G., Gawkrodger, D.J. & Walker, A.E. (1990) White sponge naevus successfully treated with topical tetracycline. *Clinical and Experimental Dermatology* **15**, 152–153.

Machnicki, S. (1953) Diphtheria of the vulva and of the vagina. *Zeitschrift für Haut und Geschlechtskrankenheiten* **86**, 368 (abstract from Polish).

McKenna, G., Edwards, S. & Cleland, H. (1994) Genital ulceration secondary to Epstein–Barr virus infection. *Genitourinary Medicine* **70**, 356–357.

McLachlin, C.M., Mutter, G.L. & Crum, C.P. (1994) Multinucleated atypia of the vulva. Report of a distinct entity not associated with human papillomavirus. *American Journal of Surgical Pathology* **18**, 1233–1239.

Macleod, R.I. & Soames, J.V. (1991) Lichen sclerosus of the oral mucosa. *British Journal of Oral and Maxillofacial Surgery* **29**, 64–65.

Maekawa, Y., Sakazaki, Y. & Hayashibara, T. (1978) Diaper area granuloma of the aged. *Archives of Dermatology* **114**, 382–383.

Marcoux, C., Bourland, A. & Decroix, J. (1991) Hyperplasie angio-lymphoïde avec éosinophilie (HALE). *Annales de Dermatologie et de Vénéréologie* **118**, 217–221.

Marks, R. & Wells, G.C. (1973a) Lichen simplex: morphodynamic correlates. *British Journal of Dermatology* **88**, 249–256.

Marks, R. & Wells, G.C. (1973b) A histochemical profile of lichen simplex. *British Journal of Dermatology* **88**, 557–562.

Marquette, E.P., Su, B. & Woodruff, R.D. (1985) Introital adenosis associated with Stevens–Johnson syndrome. *Obstetrics and Gynecology* **66**, 143–145.

Marren, P., Wojnarowska, F. & Powell, S. (1992) Allergic contact dermatitis and vulvar dermatoses. *British Journal of Dermatology* **126**, 52–56.

Marren, P., Wojnarowska, F., Venning, V., Wilson, C. & Nayar, M. (1993) Vulvar involvement in autoimmune bullous diseases. *Journal of Reproductive Medicine* **38**, 101–107.

Marren, P., Millard, P., Chia, Y. & Wojnarowska, F. (1994) Mucosal lichen sclerosus/lichen planus overlap syndromes. *British Journal of Dermatology* **131**, 118–123.

Marren, P., Yell, J., Charnock, F.M. *et al.* (1995) The association between lichen sclerosus and antigens of the HLA system. *British Journal of Dermatology* **132**, 197–203.

Marren, P., Dean, D., Charnock, M. & Wojnarowska, F. (1997a) The basement membrane zone in lichen sclerosus: an immunohistochemical study. *British Journal of Dermatology* **136**, 508–514.

Marren, P.M., Millard, P.R. & Wojnarowska, F. (1997b) Vulval lichen sclerosus: lack of correlation between duration of clinical symptoms and histological appearances. *Journal of the European Academy of Dermatology and Venereology* **8**, 212–216.

Martin, J. & Holdstock, G. (1997) Isolated vulval oedema as a feature of Crohn's disease. *Journal of Obstetrics and Gynaecology* **17**, 92–93.

Martini, P., Peonia, G., Benedetti, A. & Lorenzi, S. (1995) Darier–White syndrome and cyclosporin. *Dermatology* **190**, 174–175.

Masri-Fridling, G.D. & Turner, M.L.C. (1992) Necrolytic migratory erythema without glucagonoma. *Journal of the American Academy of Dermatology* **2**, 486.

Meffert, J.J. & Grimwood, R.E. (1994) Lichen sclerosus appearing in an old burn scar. *Journal of the American Academy of Dermatology* **31**, 671–673.

Meffert, J.J., Davis, B.M. & Grimwood, R.E. (1995) Lichen sclerosus. *Journal of the American Academy of Dermatology* **32**, 393–416.

Meneux, E., Paniel, B.J., Pouget, F. *et al.* (1997) Vulvovaginal sequelae in toxic epidermal necrolysis. *Journal of Reproductive Medicine* **42**, 153–156.

Mensing, H. & Jänner, M. (1981) Vulvitis plasmacellularis Zoon. *Zeitschrift für Hautkrankheiten* **56**, 728–732.

Mering, J.H. (1952) A surgical approach to intractable pruritus vulvae. *American Journal of Obstetrics and Gynecology* **64**, 619.

Meyrick Thomas, R.H. & Kennedy, C.T.C. (1986) The development of lichen sclerosus et atrophicus in monozygotic twin girls. *British Journal of Dermatology* **114**, 377–379.

Meyrick Thomas, R.H., McGibbon, D.H. & Munro, D.D. (1985) Basal cell carcinoma of the vulva in association with vulval lichen sclerosus et atrophicus. *Journal of the Royal Society of Medicine* **78** (Suppl. II), 16–18.

Meyrick Thomas, R.H., Ridley, C.M., McGibbon, D.H. & Black, M.M. (1988) Lichen sclerosus and autoimmunity—a study of 350 women. *British Journal of Dermatology* **118**, 41–46.

Meyrick Thomas, R.H., Ridley, C.M., McGibbon, D.H. & Black, M.M. (1996) Anogenital lichen sclerosus in women. *Journal of the Royal Society of Medicine*, **89**, 694–698.

Mikhail, G.R., Drukker, B.H. & Chow, C (1967) Pemphigus vulgaris involving the cervix uteri. *Archives of Dermatology* **95**, 496–498.

Mikhail, G.R., Fachnie, D'A.M., Drukker, B.H., Farah, R. & Allen, H.M. (1979) Generalised malignant acanthosis nigricans. *Archives of Dermatology* **115**, 201–202.

Miller, D.M., Lerner, K., Thompson, S.L. & Ehlen, T.G. (1994) Graft-versus-host disease of the female lower genital tract. *The Cervix and the Lower Genital Tract* **12**, 83–87.

Miller, R.A.M. & Griffiths, W.A.D. (1982) Experimentally induced complement and immunoglobulin deposition along the basement membrane zone (BMZ) and in dermal blood vessels. *British Journal of Dermatology* **106**, 275–279.

Miller, R.F. (1957) Lichen sclerosus with oral involvement. *Archives of Dermatology* **76**, 43–45.

Mizoguchi, M., Chikakane, K., Goh, K., Asahina, Y. & Masida, K. (1987) Acute febrile neutrophilic dermatosis (Sweet's syndrome) in Behçet's disease. *British Journal of Dermatology* **116**, 727–734.

Morgan, E.D., Laszlo, J.D.B. & Stumpf, P.G. (1988) Incomplete Behçet's syndrome in the differential diagnosis of genital ulceration and post-coital bleeding: a case report. *Journal of Reproductive Medicine* **33**, 844–846.

Morioko, S., Nakajima, S., Yaguchi, H. *et al.* (1988) Vulvitis circumscripta plasmacellularis treated successfully with interferon alpha. *Journal of the American Journal of Dermatology* **19**, 947–950.

Mortimer, P.S., Dawber, R.P.R., Gales, M.A. & Moore, R.A. (1986a) Mediation of hidradenitis suppurativa by androgens. *British Medical Journal* **292**, 245–248.

Mortimer, P.S., Dawber, R.P.R., Gales, M.A. & Moore, R.A. (1986b) A double-blind cross-over trial of cyproterone acetate in females with hidradenitis suppurativa. *British Journal of Dermatology* **115**, 263–268.

Moss, T.R. & Stevenson, C.J. (1981) Incidence of male genital vitiligo. Report of a screening programme. *British Journal of Venereal Diseases* **57**, 145–146.

Mountain, J.C. (1970) Cutaneous ulceration in Crohn's disease. *Gut* **11**, 18–26.

Moyal-Barracco, M., Lautier-Frau, M., Bechérel, P.A. *et al.* (1993) Lichen plan conjunctival: une observation. *Annales de Dermatologie et de Vénéréologie* **120**, 857–859.

Munro, C.S. (1992) The phenotypes of Darier's disease: penetrance and expression in adults and children. *British Journal of Dermatology* **127**, 126–130.

Muram, D. & Gold, S.S. (1993) Vulvar ulcerations in girls with myelocytic leukemia. *Southern Medical Journal* **86**, 293–294.

Murphy, F.R., Lipa, M. & Haberman, H.F. (1982) Familial vulvar dystrophy of lichen sclerosus type. *Archives of Dermatology* **118**, 329–331.

Nagano, T., Tani, M., Adachi, A. *et al.* (1994) Childhood bullous pemphigoid: immunohistochemical, immunoelectronmicroscopic and Western blot analysis. *Journal of the American Journal of Dermatology* **39**, 884–888.

Näher, H., Gissman, L., Freese, U.K., Petzoldt, D. & Helfrich, S. (1992) Subclinical Epstein–Barr virus infection of both the male and female genital tract—indication for sexual transmission. *Journal of Investigative Dermatology* **98**, 791–793.

Neill, S.M., Smith, N.P. & Eady, R.A.J. (1984) Ulcerative sarcoidosis: a rare manifestation of a common disease. *Clinical and Experimental Dermatology* **9**, 277–279.

Neri, I., Patrizi, A., Marzaduri, S., Marini, R. & Negosanti, M. (1995) Vulvitis plasmacellularis: two new cases. *Genitourinary Medicine* **71**, 311–313.

Neri, I., Bardazzi, F., Marzaduri, S. & Patrizi, A. (1996) Perianal streptococcal dermatitis in adults. *British Journal of Dermatology* **135**, 796–798.

Neville, E.A. & Finn, O.A. (1975) Psoriasiform napkin rash—a follow-up study. *British Journal of Dermatology* **92**, 279–285.

Newton, J.A., Camplejohn, R.S. & McGibbon, D.H. (1987) A flow cytometric study of the significance of DNA aneuploidy in cutaneous lesions. *British Journal of Dermatology* **117**, 169–174.

Nichols, G.E., Cooper, P.H., Underwood, P.B. & Greer, K.E. (1990) White sponge nevus. *Obstetrics and Gynecology* **76**, 545–548.

Niinimäki, A., Kallioinen, M & Oikarinen, A. (1989) Etretinate reduces connective tissue degeneration in lichen sclerosus et atrophicus. *Acta Dermato-venereologica (Stockholm)* **69**, 439–442.

Ninia, J.G. & Goldberg, T.L. (1996) Treatment of vulvar varicosities by injection compression and a pelvic support. *Obstetrics and Gynecology* **87**, 786–788.

Nisar, M., Gawkrodger, D. & Bax, D. (1995) Cyclosporin A in the treatment of rheumatoid associated pyoderma gangrenosum. *British Journal of Rheumatology* **34**, 182.

Norris, J.F.B. & Cunliffe, W.J. (1986) Failure of treatment of familial widespread hidradenitis suppurativa with isotretinoin. *Clinical and Experimental Dermatology* **11**, 579–583.

Northcutt, A.D. & Vanover, M.J. (1985) Nodular cutaneous amyloidois involving the vulva. *Archives of Dermatology* **121**, 518–521.

Oikarinen, A., Sandberg, M., Aurskainen T., Kinnnunen, T. & Kallioinen, M. (1991) Collagen biosynthesis in lichen sclerosus et atrophicus studied by biochemical *in situ* hybridization techniques. *Acta Dermato-venereologica Supplement (Stockholm)* **162**, 3–12.

O'Keefe, R., Dagg, J.H. & MacKie, R.M. (1987) The staphylococcal scalded skin syndrome in two elderly immunocompromised patients. *British Medical Journal* **295**, 179–180.

Onuigbo, W.I.B. (1976) Vulval epidermoid cysts in the Igbos of Nigeria. *Archives of Dermatology* **112**, 1405–1406.

Ormsby, O. & Mitchell, J.H. (1922) Lichen planus atrophicus et sclerosus and kraurosis vulvae. *Archives of Dermatology and Syphilology* **5**, 786.

Ostlere, L.S., Lanetry, J.A.A., Mortimer, P.S. & Staughton, R.C.D. (1991) Hidradenitis in Crohn's syndrome. *British Journal of Dermatology* **125**, 384–386.

Park, S.B., Cho, K.H., Youn, J.I. *et al.* (1997) Epidermolysis bullosa acquisita in childhood—a case mimicking chronic bullous disease of childhood. *Clinical and Experimental Dermatology* **22**, 220–222.

Parkinson, D.J. & Alderman, B. (1984) Vulval adhesions causing urinary incontinence. *Postgraduate Medical Journal* **60**, 634–635.

Parks, A.G., Morson, B.C. & Pegum, J.S. (1965) Crohn's disease with cutaneous involvement. *Proceedings of the Royal Society of Medicine* **58**, 241–242.

Parks, J. (1941) Diphtheritic vaginitis in the adult. *American Journal of Obstetrics and Gynecology* **41**, 714–715.

Parks, J. & Martin, S. (1948) Reactions of the vulva to systemic disease. *American Journal of Obstetrics and Gynecology* **55**, 117–130.

Patterson, J.A.K. & Ackerman, A.B. (1984) Lichen sclerosus et atrophicus is not related to morphea. A clinical and histological study of 24 patients in whom both conditions were reputed to be present simultaneously. *American Journal of Dermatopathology* **6**, 323–335.

Pelisse, M. (1987) Lichen sclerosus. *Annales de Dermatologie et de Vénéréologie* **114**, 411–419.

Pelisse, M. (1989) The vulvo-vaginal–gingival syndrome: a new form of erosive lichen planus. *International Journal of Dermatology* **28**, 381–384.

Pelisse, M. (1996) Erosive vulvar lichen planus and desquamative vaginitis. *Seminars in Dermatology* **15**, 47–50.

Pelisse, M., Leibowitch, M., Sedel, D. & Hewitt, J. (1982) Un nouveau syndrome vulvo-vagino-gingival. Lichen plan érosif plurimuqueux. *Annales de Dermatologie et de Vénéréologie* **110**, 797–798.

Perrin, L. (1901) Contribution à l'étude de la leucoplasie vulvo-anale, ses rapports avec le kraurosis vulvae, son traitement. *Annales de Dermatologie et de Syphiligraphie* **2**, 21–28.

Petersen, C.S., Brocks, K., Weisman, K., Kobayasi, T. & Thomsen, H.K. (1996) Pretibial epidermolysis bullosa with vulvar involvement. *Acta Dermato-venerologica (Stockholm)* **76**, 80–81.

Pokorny, S.F. (1992) Prepubertal vulvovaginopathies. *Obstetrics and Gynecology Clinics of North America* **19**, 39–58.

Pokorny, S.F. (1994) Longterm intravaginal presence of foreign bodies in children. A preliminary study. *Journal of Reproductive Medicine* **39**, 931–935.

Pokorny, S.F., Pokorny, W.J. & Kramer, W. (1992) Acute genital injury in the prepubertal girl. *American Journal of Obstetrics and Gynecology* **166**, 1461–1466.

Portnoy, J., Ahronheim, G.A., Ghibu, F., Clecner, B. & Joncas, J.H. (1984) Recovery of Epstein Barr virus from genital ulcers. *New England Journal of Medicine* **311**, 966–968.

Poskitt, B.L., Wojnarowska, F.T. & Shaw, S. (1995) Semen contact urticaria. *Journal of the Royal Society of Medicine* **88**, 108P–109P.

Powell, F.C., Rogers, R.S., Dickson, E.R. & Moore, S.B. (1986) An association between HLA DR1 and lichen planus. *British Journal of Dermatology* **114**, 473–478.

Powell, R.J. (1996) New roles for thalidomide. *British Medical Journal* **313**, 377.

Prezyna, A.P. & Kalyanaraman, B. (1977) Bowen's carcinoma in vulvo-vaginal Crohn's disease (regional enterocolitis): report of first case. *American Journal of Obstetrics and Gynecology* **128**, 914–915.

Punnonen, R., Soidinmäki, H., Kaupilla, O. & Pystynen, P. (1985) Relationship of vulvar lichen sclerosus et atrophicus to carcinoma. *Annales Chirurgiae et Gynecologiae* **74** (Suppl. 197), 23–26.

Purcell, K.G., Spencer, L.V., Simpson, P.M. *et al.* (1990) HLA antigens in lichen sclerosus et atrophicus. *Archives of Dermatology* **126**, 1043–1045.

Radman, H.M. & Bhagavan, B.S. (1972) Pilonidal disease of the female genitalia. *American Journal of Obstetrics and Gynecology* **114**, 271–272.

Raguin, G., Boisnic, S., Souteyrand, P. *et al.* (1992) No evidence for a spirochaetal origin of localized scleroderma. *British Journal of Dermatology* **127**, 218–220.

Rainford, D. (1970) Southey's tubes and vulval oedema. *British Medical Journal* **iv**, 538.

Ravits, H.G. & Welsh, A.L. (1957) Lichen sclerosus et atrophicus of the mouth. *Archives of Dermatology* **76**, 56–58.

Reed, O.M., Mellette, J.R. & Fitzpatrick, J.E. (1986) Cutaneous lentiginosis with atrial myxomas. *Journal of the American Academy of Dermatology* **15**, 398–402.

Rege, V.L. & Shukla, P. (1993) Osteomyelitis presenting as genital sore: a case report. *Genitourinary Medicine* **69**, 460–461.

Rendon, M.I., Cruz, P.D., Sontheimer R.D. & Bergstrasser, P.R. (1989) Acanthosis nigricans: a cutaneous marker of tissue resistance to insulin. *Journal of the American Academy of Dermatology* **21**, 461–469.

Reyman, L., Milano, A., Demopoulos, R., Mayron, J. & Schuster, S. (1986) Metastatic vulvar ulceration in Crohn's disease. *American Journal of Gastroenterology* **81**, 46–49.

Rhodes, A.R., Silverman, R.A., Harrist, T.J. & Perez-Atayde, A.R. (1986) Mucocutaneous lentigines cardiomuco-cutaneous myxomas and multiple blue nevi: the LAMB syndrome. *Journal of the American Academy of Dermatology* 10, 72–82.

Ricard-Rothiot, L., Ruiz-Hernandez, C.E. & Fernandez-Torres, E. (1979) Acquired vaginal atresia in Sjögren's syndrome. *Ginecologyica y Obstetricia de Mexico* 45, 217–222.

Ricci, J. (1945) *One Hundred Years of Gynaecology*. Blakiston, Philadelphia.

Ridley, C.M. (1982) Zinc deficiency developing in treatment for thalassaemia. *Journal of the Royal Society of Medicine* 75, 38–39.

Ridley, C.M. (1986) Genital warts with malignant transformation in association with lichen sclerosus in elderly women: a report of two cases. *Journal of Reproductive Medicine* 10, 984–985.

Ridley, C.M. (1990) Chronic erosive vulval disease. *Clinical and Experimental Dermatology* 15, 245–252.

Ridley, C.M. (1993) Genital lichen sclerosus (lichen sclerosus et atrophicus) in childhood and adolescence. *Journal of the Royal Society of Medicine* 86, 69–75.

Ridley, C.M. & Morgan, H. (1993) Ligneous conjunctivitis involving the Fallopian tube. *British Journal of Obstetrics and Gynaecology* 100, 791.

Ridley, C.M., Frankman, O., Jones, I.S.C. *et al.* (1989) New nomenclature for vulvar disease: report of the committee on terminology. *American Journal of Obstetrics and Gynecology* 160, 769.

Rigg, L.A., Hermann, H. & Yen, S.S.C. (1978) Absorption of estrogens from vaginal creams. *New England Journal of Medicine* 298, 195–197.

Robin, J (1978) Contact dermatitis to acetarsol. *Contact Dermatitis* 4, 309–310.

Rocamora, A., Santonja, C., Vives, R. & Varona, C (1986) Sebaceous gland hyperplasia of the vulva: a case report. *Obstetrics and Gynecology* 68, 63S–65S.

Romaguera, C. & Grimalt, F. (1981) Contact dermatitis from a copper containing IUD. *Contact Dermatitis* 7, 163–164.

Roman, L.D., Mitchell, M.D., Burke, T.W. & Silva, E.G. (1991) Unsuspected invasive squamous carcinoma of the vulva in young women. *Gynecologic Oncology* 41, 182–185.

Rosenbaum, M.M., Esterly, N.B., Greenwald, M.J. & Gerson, C.R. (1984) Cicatricial pemphigoid in a 6 year old child: report of a case and review of the literature. *Pediatric Dermatology* 2, 13–22.

Ross, S.A., Sánchez, J.L. & Taboas, J.G. (1990) Spirochaetal forms in the dermal lesions of morphea and lichen sclerosus and atrophicus. *American Journal of Dermatopathology* 12, 357–362.

Royal College of Physicians (1997) *Physical Signs of Sexual Abuse in Children. Report of the Working Party of the Royal College of Physicians*, 2nd edn. Royal College of Physicians, London.

Rubin, A., Buck, D. & MacDonald, M.R. (1989) Ligneous conjunctivitis involving the cervix. *British Journal of Obstetrics and Gynaecology* 96, 1228–1230.

Rudd, N.L., Nimrod, C., Holbrook, K.A. & Byers, P.H. (1983) Pregnancy complications in Type IV Ehlers–Danlos syndrome. *Lancet* i, 50–53.

Rycroft, R.J.G. & Penney, P.T. (1983) Dermatoses associated with brominated swimming pools. *British Medical Journal* 287, 462.

Saad, R.W., Domloge-Hultsch, N., Yancey, K.B., Benson, P.M. & James, W.D. (1992) Childhood localized vulvar pemphigoid is a true variant of bullous pemphigoid. *Archives of Dermatology* 128, 807–810.

Salem, O.S. & Steck, W.D. (1983) Cowden's disease (multiple hamartoma and neoplasia syndrome). A case report and review of the English literature. *Journal of the American Academy of Dermatology* 8, 686–696.

Salopek, T.G., Krol, A. & Jimbow, K. (1993) Case report of Darier's disease localized to the vulva in a 5 year old girl. *Pediatric Dermatology* 10, 146–148.

Samaratunga, H., Strutton, G., Wright, R.G. & Hill, B. (1991) Squamous cell carcinoma arising in a case of vulvitis granulomatosa or vulval variant of Melkersson–Rosenthal syndrome. *Gynecologic Oncology* 47, 263–269.

Sanders, C.J.G., Hulsmans, R.-F.H. & van Weersch-Rietjens, L.C.S.M. (1989) Angiolymphoid hyperplasia with eosinophilia. *British Journal of Dermatology* 121, 536–538.

Sarkany, I. (1959) Grenz ray treatment of familial benign chronic pemphigus. *British Journal of Dermatology* 71, 247–252.

Savona-Ventura, C. (1985) Labial adhesions in postmenopausal women with hip joint disease. *Australian and New Zealand Journal of Obstetrics and Gynaecology* 25, 303–304.

Schempp, C., Bocklage, H., Lange, R. *et al.* (1993) Further evidence for *Borrelia burgdorferi* infection in morphea and lichen sclerosus et atrophicus confirmed by DNA amplification. *Journal of Investigative Dermatology* 100, 717–720.

Schmidt, W.A. (1995) Pathology of the vagina. In: *Haines and Taylor Obstetrical and Gynaecological Pathology*, Vol. 1, 4th edn (eds H. Fox & M. Wells), pp. 135–223. Churchill Livingstone, Edinburgh.

Schuermann, H. (1960) Plasmocytosis circumorificialis. *Deutsche Zahnärztliche Zeitschrift* 15, 601–610.

Schwimmer, E. (1878) Die idiopathischen Schleimhaut der Mundhöle; Leukoplakia buccalis. *Vierteljahresschrift für Dermatologie und Syphilis* 5, 53–114.

Scully, C. (1992) The oral cavity. In: *Textbook of Dermatology*, 5th edn (eds R.H. Champion, J.L. Burton & F.J.G. Ebling), pp. 2689–2760. Blackwell Scientific Publications, Oxford.

Scully, R.E. (1989) Case records of the Massachussetts General Hospital (case 26-1989). *New England Journal of Medicine* 320, 1741–1747.

Scurry, J., Dennerstein, G., Brenan, J. *et al.* (1993a) Vulvitis circumscripta plasmacellularis. A clinicopathological entity? *Journal of Reproductive Medicine* 38, 14–18.

Scurry, J., Planner, R., Fortune, D.W., Lee, C.S. & Rode, J. (1993b) Ligneous (pseudomembranous) inflammation of the female genital tract. A report of two cases. *Journal of Reproductive Medicine* 38, 407–412.

Scurry, J., Dennerstein, G. & Brennan, J. (1995) Angiolymphoid hyperplasia of the vulva. *Australian and New Zealand Journal of Obstetrics and Gynaecology* 35, 347–348.

Sedlacek, T.V., Riva, J.M., Magen, A.B., Mangan, C. & Cunnane, M.F. (1990) Vaginal and vulvar adenosis. An unsuspected side effect of carbon dioxide laser vaporization. *Journal of Reproductive Medicine* 35, 995–1001.

Sehgal, V.H. & Gangwan, O.P. (1986) Genital fixed drug eruptions. *Genitourinary Medicine* 62, 56–58.

Setterfield, J., Bhogal, B., Shirlaw, P. *et al.* (1996a) A comprehensive study of the clinical immunopathological and immunogenetic findings in cicatricial pemphigoid. *British Journal of Dermatology* 135 (Suppl. 47), 13.

Setterfield, J., Neill, S., Ridley, M. *et al.* (1996b) The vulvo-vaginal syndrome is associated with the HLA DQB1*0201 allele. *British Journal of Dermatology* 135, Suppl. 47, 43.

Shackleford, G.D., Bauer, E.A., Graviss, E.R. & McAlister, W.H.

(1982) Upper airway and external genital involvement in epidermolysis bullosa dystrophica. *Radiology* **143**, 429–432.

Sheehan-Dare, R.A., Cotterill, J.A. & Simmons, A.V. (1986) Oesophageal lichen planus. *British Journal of Dermatology* **115**, 729–730.

Shelley, W.B. & Crissey, J.T. (1953) *Classics in Clinical Dermatology*, pp. 194–195. Thomas, Springfield, IL.

Shelley, W.B. & Wood, M.G. (1981) Transformation of the common wart into squamous cell carcinoma in a patient with primary lymphoedema. *Cancer* **48**, 820–824.

Sherertz, E.F. (1994) Clinical pearl: symptomatic dermatographism as a cause of genital pruritus. *Journal of the American Academy of Dermatology* **31**, 1040–1041.

Shono, S., Imura, M., Ota, M. *et al.* (1991) Lichen sclerosus et atrophicus, morphea, and coexistence of both diseases. Histological studies using lectins. *Archives of Dermatology* **127**, 1352–1356.

Shum, D.T. & Guenther, L. (1990) Metastatic Crohn's disease. *Archives of Dermatology* **126**, 645–648.

Shuttleworth, D., Graham-Brown, G.A.C., Hutchinson, P.E. & Joliffe, D.S. (1985) Cicatricial pemphigoid in D-penicillamine treated patients with arthritis—a report of three cases. *Clinical and Experimental Dermatology* **10**, 392–397.

Sideri, M., Origoni, M., Spinaci, L. & Ferrari, A. (1994) Topical testosterone in the treatment of vulvar lichen sclerosus. *International Journal of Gynecology and Obstetrics* **46**, 53–56.

Sillevis Smitt, J.H. (1985) Pemphigus vulgaris in childhood; clinical features, treatment and prognosis. *Pediatric Dermatology* **2**, 185–190.

Sinha, M.R. (1982) Fixed genital drug eruption due to dapsone. A case report. *Leprosy in India* **54**, 152–154.

Sison-Torre, E.Q. & Ackerman, A.B. (1985) Melanosis of the vagina. *American Journal of Dermatopathology* **7**, 51–60.

Skoven, I.G. & Hjortshoj, A. (1978) HLA antigens and psoriasiform napkin dermatitis. *Dermatologica* **157**, 225–228.

Soini, Y., Paako, P., Vahakangas, K., Vuopala, S. & Lehto, V.-P. (1994) Expression of p53 and proliferating cell nuclear antigen in lichen sclerosus et atrophicus with different histological features. *International Journal of Gynecological Pathology* **13**, 199–204.

Sorrow, J.M. & Hitch, J.M. (1963) Dyskeratosis congenita. *Archives of Dermatology* **88**, 340–347.

Souteyrand, P., Wong, E. & MacDonald, D.M. (1981) Zoon's balanitis (balanitis circumscripta plasmacellularis). *British Journal of Dermatology* **105**, 195–199.

Sparks, M.K., Kuhlman, D.S., Prieto, A. & Callen, J.P. (1985) Hypercalcemia in association with cutaneous squamous cell carcinoma; occurrence as a late complication of hidradenitis suppurativa. *Archives of Dermatology* **121**, 243–246.

Srebrnik, A., Bar-Nathan, G.A., Ilie, B., Peyser, R. & Brenner, S. (1991) Vaginal ulceration due to lithium carbonate therapy. *Cutis* **48**, 65–66.

Starink, T.M. & Hausman, R. (1984) The cutaneous pathology of facial lesions in Cowden's disease. *Journal of Cutaneous Pathology* **11**, 331–337.

Steinkampf, M.P., Reilly, S.D. & Ackerman, A.B. (1987) Vaginal agglutination and hematometra associated with epidermolysis bullosa. *Obstetrica and Gynecology* **69**, 519–521.

Stern, J.K. & Rosen, T. (1982) Balanitis plasmacellularis circumscripts (Zoon's balanitis plasmacellularis). *Cutis* **25**, 57–60.

Sterry, W. & Schmoll, M. (1985) Contact urticaria and dermatitis from self-adhesive pads. *Contact Dermatitis* **13**, 284–285.

Stewart, E.J.C., Wojnarowska, F. & Marren, P. (1995) Glazed erythema of the vulva. *British Journal of Dermatology* **133** (Suppl. 45), 31.

Stewart, W.D. & Light, M.J. (1984) Successful treatment of hidradenitis suppurativa with etretinate. *Dermatologica* **169**, 258.

Sutton, R.L. (1935) *Diseases of the Skin*, Vol. 2, 9th edn, p. 1386. Mosby, St Louis.

Sweet, R.D. (1979) Acute febrile neutrophilic dermatosis. *British Journal of Dermatology* **100**, 93–99.

Szymanski, F.J. & Caro, M.R. (1955) Pseudoxanthoma elasticum. Review of its relationship to internal disease and report of an unusual case. *Archives of Dermatology* **71**, 184–189.

Tagami, H. & Uehara, M. (1981) Multinucleated epidermal giant cells in inflammatory skin diseases. *Archives of Dermatology* **117**, 23–25.

Tan, S.-H., Derrick, E., McKee, P.H. *et al.* (1994) Altered p53 expression and epidermal cell proliferation is seen in vulval lichen sclerosus. *Journal of Cutaneous Pathology* **21**, 316–323.

Tappeiner, J. & Pfleger, L. (1971) Granuloma gluteale infantum. *Hautarzt* **22**, 383–388.

Tatnall, F.M. & Mann, B.S. (1985) Non-Hodgkin's lymphoma of the skin associated with chronic limb oedema. *British Journal of Dermatology* **113**, 751–756.

Tatnall, F.M., Barnes, H.M. & Sarkany, I. (1985) Sarcoidosis of the vulva. *Clinical and Experimental Dermatology* **10**, 384–385.

Taussig, F.J. (1929) Leukoplakic vulvitis and cancer of the vulva (etiology, histopathology, treatment, five-year results). *American Journal of Obstetrics and Gynecology* **18**, 472–503.

Taylor, S.C., Baker, E. & Grossman, M.E. (1991) Nodular vulvar amyloid as a presentation of systemic amyloidosis. *Journal of the American Academy of Dermatology* **24**, 139.

Taylor, W.N. (1941) Vulvar fusion: two cases with urological aspects. *Journal of Urology* **45**, 710–714.

Thambar, I.V., Dunlop, R., Thin, R.N. & Huskisson, E.C. (1977) Circinate vulvitis in Reiter's syndrome. *British Journal of Venereal Diseases* **53**, 260–262.

Thiers, H., Moulin, G., Rochet, Y. & Lieux, J. (1968) Maladie de Haïley–Hailey à localisation vulvaire prédominante. Étude génétique et ultrastructurale. *Bulletin de la Société Française de Dermatologie et de Syphiligraphie* **75**, 352–355.

Thomson, J. (1986) Etretinate and vulvitis. *Retinoids Today and Tomorrow* **5**, 49.

Tidman, M.J. & Eady, R.A.J. (1990) Diagnosis and diagnostic techniques. In: *Management of Blistering Disease* (eds F. Wojnarowska & R.A. Briggaman), pp. 163–172. Chapman and Hall, London.

Tidy, J.A., Soutter, W.P., Luesley, D.M. *et al.* (1996) Management of lichen sclerosus and intraepithelial neoplasia of the vulva in the United Kingdom. *Journal of the Royal Society of Medicine* **89**, 699–701.

Tilsley, D.A. & Wilkinson, D.S. (1965) Necrosis and dequalinium. II. Vulval and extra-genital ulceration. *Transactions of the St John's Hospital Dermatological Society* **51**, 49–54.

Toki, T., Kurman, R.J., Park, J.S. *et al.* (1991) Probable non-HPV etiology of squamous cell carcinoma of the vulva in older women: a clinicopathologic study using *in situ* hybridization and polymerase chain reaction. *International Journal of Gynecological Pathology* **10**, 107–125.

Trice, L., Bennert, H. & Stubblefield, P.G. (1996) Massive vulvar edema complicating tocolysis in a patient with twins. *Journal of Reproductive Medicine* **41**, 121–124.

Tromovitch, T.A., Jacobs, P.H. & Kem, S. (1964), Acanthosis nigricans-like lesions from nicotinic acid. *Archives of Dermatology* **89**, 222–223.

Troy, J.L., Sivers, D.N., Grossman, M.E. & Jaffe, I.A. (1981) Penicillamine-related pemphigus: is it really pemphigus? *Journal of the American Academy of Dermatology* **4**, 545–547.

Uyeda, K., Nakayasu, K., Takaishi, Y. & Sotomatsu, S. (1973) Kaposi sarcoma-like granuloma on diaper dermatitis. *Archives of Dermatology* **107**, 605–607.

Václavínková, V. & Neumann, E. (1982) Vaginal involvement in familial benign chronic pemphigus (morbus Hailey–Hailey). *Acta Dermato-venereologica (Stockholm)* **62**, 80–81.

Vakilzadeh, F. & Kolde, G. (1985) Relapsing linear acantholytic dermatosis. *British Journal of Dermatology* **112**, 349–355.

Valsecchi, R., Bontempelli, M., Rossi, A. *et al.* (1988) HLA-DR and DQ antigens in lichen planus. *Acta Dermato-venereologica (Stockholm)* **68**, 77–80.

van Furth, M., van't Wout, J.W., Wertheimer, P.A. & Zwartendijk, J. (1992) Ciprofloxin for treatment of malakoplakia. *Lancet* **339**, 148–149.

van Joost, T., Faber, W.R. & Manuel, H.R. (1980) Drug induced anogenital cicatricial pemphigoid. *British Journal of Dermatology* **102**, 715–718.

van Joost, Th., Vuzevski, V.D., Tank, B. & Menke, H.E. (1991) Benign persistent papular acantholytic and dyskeratotic eruption: a case report and review of the literature. *British Journal of Dermatology* **124**, 92–95.

van Voorst Vader, P.C., Kardaun, S.H., Tupker, R.A. *et al.* (1988) Orogenital lichenoid (drug) reaction. *British Journal of Dermatology* **118**, 836–838.

Verbov, J.L. (1973) The skin in patients with Crohn's disease and ulcerative colitis, *Transactions of the St John's Hospital Dermatological Society* **59**, 30–36.

Verburg, D.J., Burd, L.I., Hoxtell, E.O. & Merrill, L.K. (1974) Acrodermatitis enteropathica in pregnancy. *Obstetrics and Gynecology* **44**, 233–237.

Viljoen, D.L., Beatty, S. & Beighton, P. (1987) The obstetric and gynaecological implications of pseudoxanthoma elasticum. *British Journal of Obstetrics and Gynaecology* **94**, 884–888.

Virgili, A., Corazzo, M., Bianchi, A., Mollica, G. & Califano, A. (1995) Open study of topical 0.025% tretinoin in the treatment of vulvar lichen sclerosus. *Journal of Reproductive Medicine* **40**, 614–618.

Wagenberg, H.R. & Downham, T.F. (1981) Chronic edema of the vulva: a condition similar to cheilitis granulomatosa. *Cutis* **27**, 526–527.

Wakelin, S.H., Allen, J. & Wojnarowska, F. (1995) Childhood bullous pemphigoid. Report of a case with dermal fluorescence on salt split skin. *British Journal of Dermatology* **133**, 615–618.

Wallace, H.J. (1955) Vulval atrophy and leukoplakia. In: *Modern Trends in Obstetrics and Gynaecology* (ed. R.K. Bowes), pp. 386–394. Butterworth, London.

Wallace, H.J. (1971) Lichen sclerosus et atrophicus. *Transactions of the St John's Dermatological Society* **57**, 9–30.

Wallace, H.J. & Whimster, I.W. (1951) Vulval atrophy and leukoplakia. *British Journal of Dermatology* **63**, 241–257.

Wallach, D. (1990) Editorial: intra-epidermal immunoglobulin A pustulosis. *Dermatologica* **181**, 261–263.

Walsh, D.S., Dunn, C.L., Kinzelman, J., Sau, P. & James, W.D. (1995) A vaginal prosthetic device as an aid in treating ulcerative lichen planus of the mucous membrane. *Archives of Dermatology* **131**, 265–267.

Ward, G.D. & Sutherst, J.R. (1975) Pruritus vulvae: treatment by multiple intradermal alcohol injections. *British Journal of Dermatology* **93**, 201–204.

Warrington, S.A. & de San Lazaro, C. (1996) Lichen sclerosus et atrophicus and sexual abuse. *Archives of Diseases of Childhood* **75**, 512–516.

Wechsler, B. & Piette, J.C. (1992) Behçet's disease. *British Medical Journal* **304**, 1199–1200.

Weigand, D.A. (1993) Microscopic features of lichen sclerosus et atrophicus in achrocordons: A clue to the cause of lichen sclerosus et atrophicus? *Journal of the American Academy of Dermatology* **28**, 751–754.

Weir, R.F. (1875) Cited by Ricci, J. (1945).

Weisfogel, E. (1969) Aims of joint gynecologic, dermatologic and pathologic vulvar clinics. *New York State Journal of Medicine* **69**, 1184–1186.

Werlin, S.L., Esterly, N.B. & Oechler, H. (1992) Crohn's disease presenting as unilateral labial hypertrophy. *Journal of the American Academy of Dermatology* **27**, 893–895.

Wermers, R.A., Fatourechi, V., Wynne, A.G., Kvols, L.K. & Lloyd, R.V. (1996) The glucagonoma syndrome. Clinical and pathologic features in 21 patients. *Medicine (Baltimore)* **75**, 53–63.

Westermark, P. & Henriksson, T. (1979) Granulomatous inflammation of the vulva and penis. *Dermatologica* **158**, 269–274.

Whimster, I.W. (1959) The nature of leukoplakia. *Nederlandsch Tidjdschrift voor Geneeskunde* **103**, 2469–2473.

Whimster, I.W. (1973) The natural history of endogenous skin malignancy as a basis for experimental research. *Transactions of the St John's Hospital Dermatological Society* **59**, 195–224.

White, J.D., Olsen, K.D. & Banks, P.M. (1986) Plasma cell orificial mucositis. *Archives of Dermatology* **122**, 1321–1324.

Whitfield, R.G.S. (1947) Anomalous manifestations of malnutrition in Japanese prison camps. *British Medical Journal* **ii**, 164–168.

Whitlock, F.A. (1976) Psychophysiological aspects of skin disease. In: *Major Problems in Dermatology 8*, pp. 110–117. Saunders, London.

Wilson, E.E.B. & Malinak, L.R. (1988) Vulvovaginal sequelae of Stevens–Johnson syndrome and their management. *Obstetrics and Gynecology* **71**, 478–480.

Woodruff, J.D., Sussman, J. & Shakfeh, S. (1989) Vulvitis circumscripta plasmacellularis. A report of 4 cases. *Journal of Reproductive Medicine* **34**, 369–372.

Work, B.A. (1980) Pyoderma gangrenosum of the perineum. *Obstetrics and Gynecology* **62**, 126–128.

Yates, V.M., King, C.M. & Dave, V.K. (1985) Lichen sclerosus et atrophicus following radiation therapy. *Archives of Dermatology* **121**, 1044–1047.

Yu, C.C.-W. & Cook, M.G. (1990) Hidradenitis suppurativa: a disease of follicular epithelium, rather than apocrine glands. *British Journal of Dermatology* **122**, 763–769.

Zahn, C.M., Hawkins, G.D.V. & Yeomans, E.R. (1996) Vulvovaginal hematomas complicating delivery. Rationale for drainage of the hematoma cavity. *Journal of Reproductive Medicine* **41**, 569–574.

Zaino, R.J., Husseinzadeh, N., Nahhas, W. & Mortel, R. (1982) Epithelial alterations in proximity to invasive squamous carcinoma of the vulva. *International Journal of Gynecological Pathology* **1**, 173–184.

Zaki, I., Dalziel, K.L., Solomonsz, F.A. & Stevens, A. (1997) The under-reporting of skin disease in association with squamous cell carcinoma of the vulva. *Clinical and Experimental Dermatology* **21**, 334–337.

Zoon, J.J. (1955) Balanitis und Vulvitis plasmacellularis. *Dermatologica* **111**, 157.

Chapter 6: Vulvodynia

S.M. Neill & C.M. Ridley

Historical aspects

For about the last 20 years, chronic vulval pain, soreness or burning (as opposed to itching) has become a frequently encountered complaint and one which, when there is no obvious cause, is often baffling and frustrating to the various doctors to whom the patient may present as well as to the patient herself. A brief account of how views of the subject have developed and are continuing to evolve, and then of how our current experience relates to past reports, will set the stage for its more detailed consideration.

In 1982 the International Society for the Study of Vulvovaginal Disease (ISSVD) set up a committee to study the problem (McKay *et al.* 1984). The term used for the complaint of chronic pain, soreness or burning, when there was no obvious cause for the symptoms, had been at the preliminary stage 'the burning vulva syndrome'. In the report it was proposed to continue this designation, but to use the term 'vulvodynia' to cover all examples of such chronic symptomatology, i.e. including those cases where it could be clearly attributed to some straightforward cause such as an inflammatory dermatosis. In due course, however, 'the burning vulva syndrome' was discarded, as being unappealing, with 'vulvodynia' remaining as the overall term. In practice, however, 'vulvodynia' tends to be used to refer to the group without an obvious cause; it should always be made clear in which sense it is being employed.

Between that time and the early 1990s, emphasis on the human papillomavirus in the genital area, chiefly in terms of its suspected oncogenicity, was marked; the finding of vestibular papillomatosis, further discussed below, was held to account for symptoms and attributed to the virus. Neither of these views is now accepted, and the condition is now recognized to be a variant of normal. A second report (McKay *et al.* 1991) noted this point, and listed what was then felt to represent some valid clinical groupings. The most clearly recognized was vestibulitis, as defined by the criteria of Friedrich (1987), i.e. severe pain on vestibular touch or attempted vaginal entry, tenderness to pressure localized within the vestibule, and physical findings confined to erythema of varying degrees. Essential vulvodynia, later termed dysaesthetic vulvodynia, was the term used for patients without abnormal physical signs but who complained of constant localized burning pain; these patients tended to be postmenopausal and were helped by small doses of tricyclic antidepressants. Cyclic vulvitis or vulvovaginitis was used for those patients where symptoms were intermittent and often accompanied by erythema of the labia and sensations of swelling. It was again emphasized that these categories were not applicable to cases where the symptoms were adequately accounted for by an inflammatory condition such as an infection or dermatosis.

During the ensuing years, vestibulitis and dysaesthetic vulvodynia emerged as being of the greatest significance, and it has been realized that, while generally distinct, they yet have much in common.

When, in the 1970s, attention began to be paid to patients with such symptoms, they were reported under such titles as 'psychosomatic vulvovaginitis' (Dodson & Friedrich 1978); but Weisfogel (1976) was astute in her plea for serious thought on the problem rather than its relegation to the category, as she put it, of a myth, like the unicorn. In retrospect, it is ironical that on the same occasion Pelisse and Hewitt (1976) were presenting cases they termed 'erythematous vulvitis en plaques', later to be recognized as part of the symptom complex now known as vestibulitis.

There are indeed accounts in much earlier texts which suggest that, again as regards vestibulitis, the problem was being seen at that time. Thus, Skene (1888) writes of 'hyperaesthesia' of the vulva:

> Pruritus is absent, and on examination of the parts affected no redness or other external manifestation of the disease is visible. When, however, the examining finger comes in contact with the hyperaesthetic part, the patient complains of pain, which is sometimes so great as to cause her to cry out. Indeed, the sensitiveness is occasionally so exaggerated as to keep

> the patient from consulting her physician until it becomes absolutely unbearable. Sexual intercourse is equally painful, and becomes in aggravated cases impossible. This affection must not be confounded with vaginismus, or with other conditions of increased sensitiveness of the vulva due to inflammatory conditions.

Thomas and Mundé (1891) also used the term 'hyperaesthesia', writing:

> The disease . . . constitutes, on account of its excessive obstinacy, and the great influence which it obtains over the mind of the patient, a malady of a great deal of importance. It consists in an excessive sensibility of the nerves supplying the mucous membrane of some portion of the vulva; sometimes the area of tenderness is confined to the vestibule, at other times to one labium minus, at others to the meatus urinarius; and again a number of these parts may be affected. . . . So commonly is it met with at least that it becomes a matter of surprise that it has not been more generally and fully described. . . . No inflammatory action affects the tender surface, no pruritus attends the condition, and physical examination reveals nothing except occasional spots of erythematous redness scattered here and there. . . . The slightest friction excites intolerable pain and nervousness; even a cold and unexpected current of air produces discomfort; and any degree of pressure is absolutely intolerable. For this reason sexual intercourse becomes a source of great discomfort, even when the ostium vaginae is large and free from disease. . . . it will be observed that her mind is disproportionately disturbed and depressed by this. In some cases it seems to absorb all the thoughts and to produce a state bordering upon monomania.

Kelly (1928) clearly distinguishes the condition from vaginismus, noting 'Exquisitely sensitive deep-red spots in the mucosa of the hymeneal ring are a fruitful source of dyspareunia—tender enough at times to make a vaginal examination impossible.'

Skene and Thomas and Mundé noted the inefficacy of surgical and caustic destructive measures, the latter saying 'My observation of the results of caustics and the knife is not such as to inspire me with confidence in them', and both favouring, although not it seems with great conviction, general measures such as tonics and change of air. Kelly suggested excision of the tender spots, as he did also of caruncles, but admitted '. . . the hope is greater when the cause lies more obviously in the caruncles'.

These accounts could be those of the patients with vestibulitis seen today. It is curious that the complaint was not noted thereafter in the literature until the 1970s. Were women during the intervening period really free of the problem, or were they less articulate, or were the doctors not sufficiently attentive? Another strange feature is that Mundé, enlarging and revising in 1891, for its sixth edition, the work of Thomas quoted above, adds a footnote to the section on 'hyperaesthesia': 'I have never seen an instance of this disease, but Dr Thomas assures me of its undoubted occurrence in his practice. Hence I reproduce this section unchanged.'

Current situation

An ever-increasing number of patients with chronic vulval pain is being seen by gynaecologists, urologists, genitourinary physicians, dermatologists and psychiatrists. Many of these specialists do not have either a particular interest in vulval problems or an expert knowledge of pain problems. Consequently these patients are not accurately diagnosed even after many of them have been subjected to extensive and invasive investigations. The final outcome is unsatisfactory for both the patient and the doctor. There have been major advances in our understanding of pain over the last 10 years with the recognition of chronic pain syndromes.

Complex regional pain syndromes

Definition

Chronic pain is defined as pain lasting more than 3 months. There are now a number of musculoskeletal conditions whose aetiopathology is not understood that have been defined as chronic pain syndromes. These pain syndromes have been further subdivided into two categories causing either diffuse pain, for example fibromyalgia, or regional pain, for example low back pain and repetitive strain injury. Vestibulitis and dysaesthetic vulvodynia are currently regarded as further examples of complex regional pain syndromes.

The physiology of acute and persistent pain

Pain has been defined (International Association for the Study of Pain 1986) as 'an unpleasant sensory and emotional experience associated with actual or potential tissue damage, or described in terms of such damage'. Pain has an important role in protecting tissues while they are being repaired after damage. The persistence of pain after such damage despite adequate repair leads to significant physical and mental morbidity.

The skin possesses pain receptors, nociceptors, that respond to mechanical, thermal or chemical stimulation. A painful signal is carried to the spinal cord via the dorsal root either by fast, myelinated Aδ fibres transmitting localized, short-lived, sharp pain or by slow, unmyelinated C fibres, which are responsible for the transmission of diffuse, dull, aching pain. The Aδ fibres carry signals predominantly from mechanical nociceptors, while the C fibres are sensitive to mechanical, thermal and chemical nociceptors.

The cell bodies of the peripheral sensory neurones lie in the dorsal root ganglia and these connect with internuncial neurones in the substantia gelatinosa of the same level. The fibres of the internuncial neurones then cross over the spinal cord to the opposite side and travel up the spinal cord in the lateral spinothalamic columns to the posteroventral nucleus of the thalamus. Signals from the thalamus are then sent to the post-central gyrus of the parietal lobe where the quality and site of the pain are recognized. Further connections to the frontal, hypothalamic and limbic systems result in a complex mixture of perception, arousal, interpretation, emotion and memory. Transmission is mediated by a large number of neuropeptides not all of which have been identified. Those transmitters that are known to be involved currently include β-endorphin, enkephalin, substance P, calcitonin gene-related peptide, histamine, vasoactive intestinal peptide, somastatin, serotonin and other catecholamines.

The gate theory of pain proposed by Melzack and Wall (1965) explains the processing of pain in the dorsal horn. There are neural mechanisms that control the transmission of pain signals within the dorsal horn by acting like a gate either facilitating or inhibiting the pain impulses that are coming in from the periphery. There is also a descending pathway of neurones to the dorsal horn cells from the brain that can also dampen down incoming pain impulses, providing one type of analgesia by 'closing' the gate.

Sensations of fine touch and proprioception are carried via Aβ fibres in the afferent nerve, and these fibres synapse with short neurones in the substantia gelatinosa that are inhibitory and can block the transmission of impulses carried by both the Aδ and C fibres, thereby 'closing' the gate. This is the principle behind the use of transcutaneous electric nerve stimulation (TENS). The nervous system is 'plastic' in that it can modulate type and quantity of neurotransmitters released, receptor sensitivity can alter and new synapses be developed.

Peripheral and central neurones can become sensitized, leading to an amplification of the signal; this phenomenon is known as 'wind-up'. The affected area may become hyperaesthetic, i.e. hypersensitive to touch, and hyperalgesic, i.e. hypersensitive to painful stimuli. There are two types of mechanical hyperalgesia: stroking hyperalgesia (dynamic hyperalgesia or allodynia) and punctate hyperalgesia. The sympathetic nervous system may also be involved.

Persistent pain falls into three groups.

1 Nociceptive. This pain is a result of excessive and continuous stimulation of pain receptors due to diseased tissue. The nervous system is intact.
2 Neuropathic. Here the pain is a result of damage to the nervous system, for example peripheral nerve injury, postherpetic neuralgia.
3 Psychogenic. No organic basis can be found.

Pain is exceedingly difficult to treat effectively once it has persisted for a year or more (Melzack 1982) and it may become permanent once established.

Vulval dermatoses

Any dermatosis that results in fissuring or erosions of the vulval epithelium will understandably result in pain, which will resolve once the damage is repaired with the appropriate treatment (Fig. 6.1). Inflammation without erosions or breaks in the vestibular epithelium may also result in pain. In some instances residual pain may be experienced even after the inflammation has settled and the epithelium has returned to normal. The conditions frequently associated with fissuring and erosion are infected eczema or psoriasis, herpes simplex, erosive lichen sclerosus or lichen planus and any of the blistering disorders. These diseases are all fully discussed in Chapters 4 and 5.

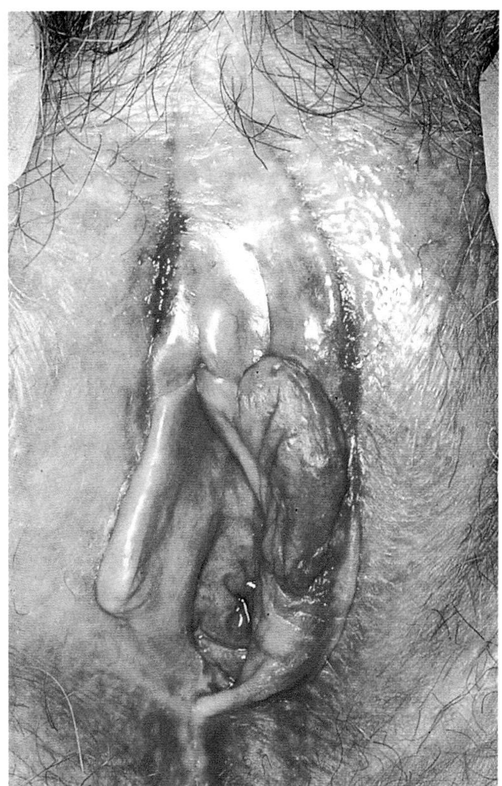

Fig. 6.1 Lichen sclerosus with fissuring.

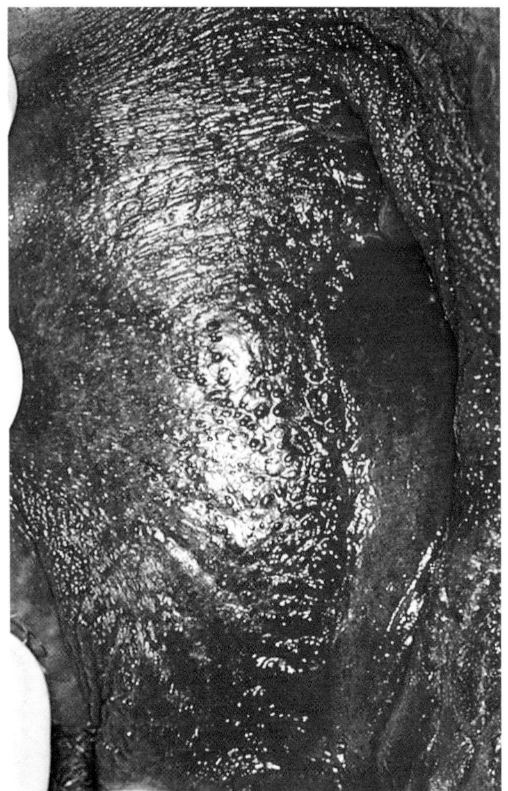

Fig. 6.2 Hart's line demarcating the junction of the skin of the labia minora and the mucosa of the vestibule.

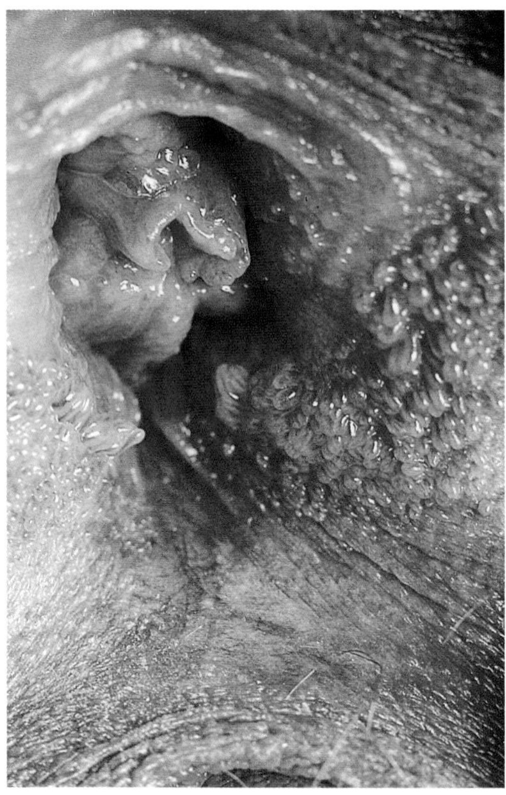

Fig. 6.3 Confluent sheets of tiny filamentous projections of the vestibular epithelium.

Vestibular papillomatosis

Vestibular papillomatosis is not a cause of vulval pain and it is now recognized as a variant of normal. It was described by Friedrich in 1987 and is an asymptomatic and insignificant entity. It has been included in this chapter on pain as historically it was originally believed to be one of the subsets of vulvodynia (McKay 1989).

Vestibular papillomatosis is the term used to describe the not infrequent finding of a myriad of tiny filamentous projections of the epithelium lining the vestibule and the inner parts of the labia minora. The vestibule is a mucosa and it is covered with non-cornifying, stratified epithelium and its boundaries extend from the hymenal ring to the inner, inferior aspects of the labia minora. In some patients there may be a distinct line, Hart's line, demarcating the junction of the cornified stratified squamous epithelium of the labium minus and the vestibular mucosa (Fig. 6.2). There have been many other terms used for this papillomatous appearance including papillomatosis labialis, hirsuties papillaris vulvae, hirsutoid papillomas of the vulva, pseudocondylomas, vulvar squamous papillomatosis (Growdon *et al.* 1985) (Fig. 6.3).

It has been proposed that human papillomavirus infection is an aetiological factor in the development of these papillae (Growdon *et al.* 1985, di Paola & Rueda 1986, Wang *et al.* 1991). However, there is now good evidence that the condition is unrelated to human papillomavirus (Bergeron *et al.* 1990, Moyal-Barracco *et al.* 1990). It is believed that vestibular papillomatosis is the female equivalent of the tiny symmetrical projections found around the coronal sulcus known as penile pearly papules or hirsutoid papules of the penis (Altmeyer *et al.* 1982).

Clinically they can be distinguished from viral warts as they are symmetrically distributed in an orderly fashion with each papilla arising from a solitary base and of the same colour as the rest of the vestibular epithelium. The histological features include papillomatosis, acanthosis and occasionally parakeratosis (Fig. 6.4). The application of 5% acetic acid does not produce acetowhitening confined to the lesions.

There has been a tendency over the last 20 years to attribute many vulval conditions to infection with the human papillomavirus, the diagnosis often being made on the finding of koilocytes in the histological specimens. The significance of koilocytes in the vulval epithelium is clearly uncertain in the light of a recent study that has shown that changes resembling koilocytic atypia can be found in

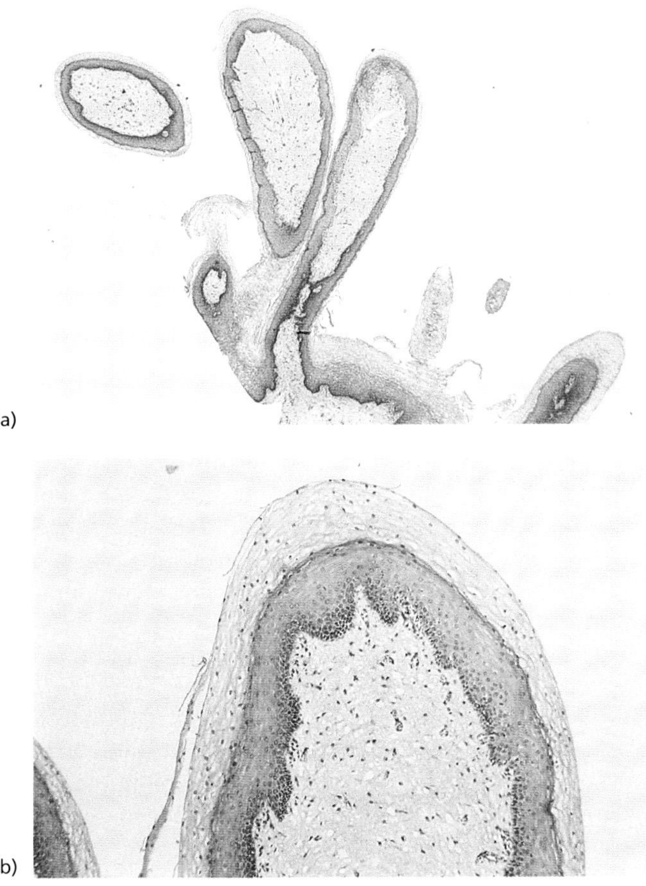
(a)

(b)

Fig. 6.4 (a) Histology of vestibular papillomatosis. Low-power magnification showing the papillary projections of the epithelium. (b) Higher-power magnification showing normal epithelium with a central core of connective tissue.

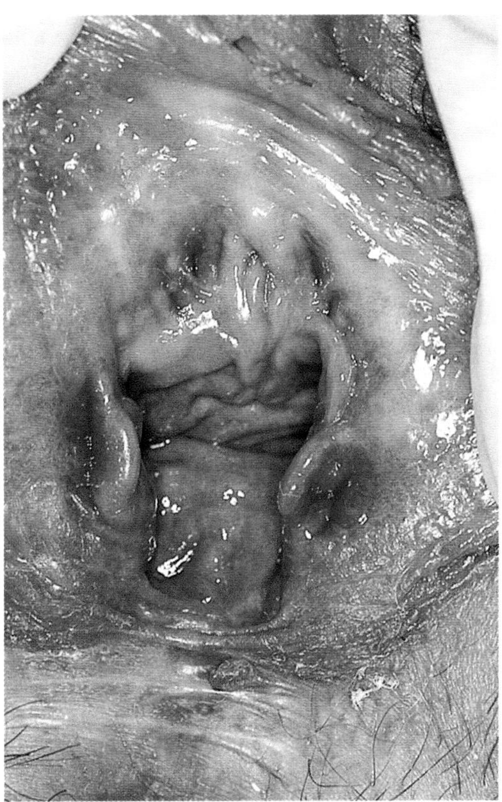

Fig. 6.5 Vestibule showing the openings of the Bartholin's gland ducts posteriorly and the ductal orifices of the minor vestibular glands around the urethra.

inflamed vulval epithelium in the absence of papillomavirus infection (Dennerstein *et al.* 1994).

There is also a problem of overdiagnosis of koilocytosis as the heavily glycogenated cells of the vestibular epithelium become clear in the processing of the specimens and these clear cells may be mistaken for koilocytes.

Vestibulitis

Vestibulitis is defined as a constellation of symptoms and signs, which includes entry dyspareunia, vestibular erythema and vestibular tenderness. It is not a diagnosis *per se* but a clinical syndrome of this triad of symptoms and signs (Friedrich 1987). The term vestibulitis is not used in those cases where there is an inflammatory condition present that accounts for these symptoms and signs, for example lichen planus affecting the vestibule or Sjögren's syndrome (Bloch *et al.* 1965, Capriello *et al.* 1988). The term vestibulitis is reserved for those cases where there is not an active dermatosis or disorder that would explain the findings. In this 'idiopathic' vulval vestibulitis the erythema and maximal tenderness are usually located at 5 and 7 o'clock in the posterior part of the vestibule close to the hymenal ring. These areas are where the major vestibular glands, Bartholin's glands, open on to the surface. The openings of the minor vestibular glands if present may appear as tiny pits and are found most frequently in the posterolateral aspects of the vestibule (Fig. 6.5). The number of minor vestibular glands present is very variable ranging from one to 100 with an average of two to 10 (Robboy *et al.* 1978). It has been suggested that the secretions from these glands are important in coital lubrication. However, it is now believed that the minor vestibular glands are not implicated in the aetiology of vulval vestibulitis. The histological changes found include a non-specific mixed inflammatory cell infiltrate without eosinophils, metaplasia of the vestibular glands forming clefts, and no evidence, despite special stains, to demonstrate bacterial or fungal organisms (Pyka *et al.* 1988). Despite the name, vestibulitis, and the finding of inflammatory cells it is not essentially an inflammatory condition. A non-specific inflammatory infiltrate has been demonstrated in healthy vestibular tissue (Friedman *et al.* 1993, Nylander Lundqvist *et al.* 1997).

In the majority of patients with this syndrome the posterior part of the vulva is affected and these patients should only complain of the discomfort with intercourse or the insertion of tampons. In a small proportion of patients the anterior vestibule is also tender, particularly over the openings of the paraurethral glands. These patients will complain of the additional symptoms of dysuria and strangury and a few are diagnosed as having interstitial cystitis. The association of vestibulitis and interstitial cystitis has raised the question as to whether the two conditions could be a disorder of the epithelium derived from the urogenital sinus (McCormack 1990, Fitzpatrick *et al.* 1993). Once the pain becomes continuous and occurs independent of touch the problem is more appropriately categorized as dysaesthetic vulvodynia.

Vestibulitis notably occurs in young white or Asian women and rarely if ever in African or Caribbean woman and is unrelated to socioeconomic factors. The incidence of vestibulis in an American private gynaecological practice was 15% but it was also noted in this study that 20% of asymptomatic women had some point tenderness to vestibular touch (Goetsch 1991).

There is usually a history of a precipitating event such as a severe episode of thrush or a reaction to an antifungal cream. The patients complain of discomfort after using many of the topical medications prescribed for their vulval problem and admit to a history of skin sensitivity at extragenital sites, particularly the face and hands, to highly perfumed soaps and cosmetics. The patients will often complain of being unable to tolerate the metal in costume jewellery. However, patch testing does not always reveal a relevant positive reaction, which would suggest that the problem may be a low-grade irritant reaction and not an allergic contact problem (Marinoff & Turner 1986). There are rare reports of allergic type I contact sensitivity to seminal fluid, which might mimic the symptoms of vestibulitis (Halpern *et al.* 1967). However, most of these reactions to seminal fluid are urticarial (Poskitt *et al.* 1995) with the characteristic symptoms of localized itching, swelling and erythema with associated bronchospasm and angio-oedema. In some instances there may be anaphylaxis. The history is very important in these cases as usually there is no problem if a condom is used. There are also reports of reactions to the drugs that the male partner is taking, which are secreted in the seminal fluid (Schimkat *et al.* 1993). Contact allergy has also been described to the latex in condoms (Turjanmaa & Reunala 1989) (see also Chapter 5).

The human papillomavirus (di Paola & Rueda 1986, Turner & Marinoff 1988, Umpierre *et al.* 1991) and *Candida* have been suggested as causative agents, as they are frequently associated in the history of the onset of the problem. However, the appropriate treatment for these conditions does not result in the eradication of the symptoms. Furthermore, several sound studies have failed to demonstrate evidence of any of the known human papillomavirus types (Wilkinson *et al.* 1993, Bergeron *et al.* 1994, Prayson *et al.* 1995). Genitourinary screening for other sexually transmitted diseases is invariably negative. Many of the patients are very health-conscious non-smokers who often verge on hypochondriasis as they consult frequently for other problems, the commonest of which include low back pain, migraine, irritable bowel syndrome and lassitude (Lynch 1986). There is initially a strong denial that there could be any underlying stressful problems in their lives either precipitating or exacerbating their vestibulitis. There are claims that their relationship with their partner is good and the partners are described as supportive and understanding with the additional comment that this state of affairs may not last indefinitely. In one study, vulvodynia patients were found to be more anxious and somatizing than women attending a vulval clinic for other vulval pathology (Stewart *et al.* 1994).

Vulval vestibulitis remains a syndrome of unexplained aetiology but in the light of what is currently known it is best categorized as a chronic pain syndrome (Bergeron *et al.* 1997). It may occur as a result of peripheral or central sensitization of nociceptors following some painful initiating event, which then leaves the patient with a frictional allodynia.

The anxiety engendered by these symptoms combined with the inevitable strain and stress of the inability to function sexually tends to intensify and reinforce the abnormal sensation of burning.

Management

Spontaneous resolution may occur but is unusual, although one report has cited a remission rate as high as 50% (Peckham *et al.* 1986).

There is no one effective treatment and often the consultation alone may prove to be therapeutic in those with minor symptoms. A careful consultation with an interested physician who clearly recognizes the problem will reassure the anxious patient that she has not been imagining her symptoms and that her condition has at long last been given a name.

Further medical measures include the use of a soap substitute and the topical local anaesthetic, 5% lignocaine ointment. Lignocaine is to be preferred to other local anaesthetics because of the low risk of sensitization. Topical steroids are unhelpful unless there is an associated skin condition such as eczema or psoriasis. If topical agents have not helped then a trial of a tricyclic antidepressant may be tried. The most frequently used is amitriptyline. This is used predominantly for its central effect on pain and not as an antidepressant, although many of these patients are secondarily depressed. The starting dose is low, at 10 mg each night, and each week the dose is increased by 10 mg each night until pain relief is experienced. The final dose required is usually 75–150 mg/day. Once the effective dose is reached the patient remains on the medication for at least 2 months and then the dose is gradually tapered down. The reason for the small doses initially is that many of these patients are very sensitive to the side effects, which may well be a reflection of their heightened awareness state. Oral steroids have no effect and have no role to play in the treatment of this condition. Calcium citrate tablets and a low oxalate diet proved effective for one woman with vestibulitis (Solomons *et al.* 1991). Recently however, Baggish *et al.* 1997 failed to show any significant relationship.

Intralesional interferon-α and -β have been reported as effective treatment for vestibulitis (Kent & Wisniewski 1990, Marinoff & Turner 1992, Bornstein *et al.* 1993). However, the rationale for this treatment is now uncertain in the light of recent evidence that infection with human papillomavirus is unlikely to be implicated in the aetiology of this syndrome. Furthermore, controlled trials need to be conducted before interferon can be recommended. A small proportion of women have pelvic floor muscle hypertonia, which results in vaginismus, and successful biofeedback techniques studying pelvic floor muscle function have resulted in improvement in women who have evidence of such muscle dysfunction (Glazer *et al.* 1995).

Surgical treatment is reportedly successful in the management of some patients with vulval vestibulitis, although there is no good clinical explanation or rationale why this should be a therapeutic option. In the past, surgical management has included excision of the posterior vestibule with advancement of the vaginal mucosa (Woodruff *et al.* 1981), perineoplasty (Friedrich 1983, 1987) and vestibuloplasty, which entails incising the distal perimeter of the vestibule, undermining the vestibule and then securing it back into position without any tissue advancement or excision.

Perineoplasty has proved to be the more effective of the two procedures (Bornstein *et al.* 1995). These authors emphasize that surgical success depends on the selection of those patients who fulfil the strict criteria laid down for the definition of vestibulitis. More recently a simple skinning dissection of the affected tissue in those patients who lose their tenderness to touch after the application of topical lignocaine has been described (Goetsch 1996). This procedure is not mutilating and can be performed under local anaesthetic with a successful outcome that is equal to that reported from the more extensive surgical procedures. However, it should be stressed that any surgical management should be reserved solely for those desperate patients who have failed to improve with all other treatments (Weijmar Schultz *et al.* 1996). It is also particularly important that these patients have a psychological assessment prior to surgery to ascertain their suitability for such a procedure (Schover *et al.* 1992). One long-term follow-up study showed that over half the women who had undergone a perineoplasty were still symptomatic and had been psychologically traumatized by their experience (de Jong *et al.* 1995). These authors felt that surgery was not the answer. Indeed, in the current state of our knowledge that vestibulitis is a chronic pain syndrome, surgery would seem to be an inappropriate option.

Carbon dioxide laser has been reported to be successful in the management of anterior vestibulitis but follow-up was only for 1 year (Friedrich 1983).

The majority of patients who are affected with vestibulitis are probably no more or less abnormal psychologically than any other comparable group but they do have significantly higher anxiety and somatization scores (van Lankveld *et al.* 1996). However, the stress, anxiety or depression associated with vestibulitis can lead to an exacerbation of any underlying psychological or personality disorder but it also has to be acknowledged that stress and depression arising in the patient's life from other causes may exacerbate and exaggerate pain. It is therefore important to address these problems in case stress is contributing to the perpetuation of their symptoms, as these patients may be offered referral for appropriate professional help if necessary. Behavioural therapy has proved beneficial in one group of patients (Weijmar Schultz *et al.* 1996). However, psychiatric intervention with psychologically normal patients is ineffective and not indicated. Although vestibulitis leads to difficulties with sexual intercourse because of complaints of poor lubrication and dyspareunia, there is no good evidence to date to support that there is marital dissatisfaction in either the patients themselves or their partners (van Lankveld *et al.* 1996). The prevalence of sexual abuse in patients with vestibulitis is similar to or lower than that of the normal population (Edwards *et al.* 1997, Friedrich 1987, Schover *et al.* 1992).

Dysaesthetic vulvodynia

Dysaesthetic vulvodynia may be defined as diffuse vulval pain that occurs with or without provocation and is usually constant and unremitting. The pain is described as being dull and burning with episodes of paroxysmal lancinating pain that radiates up into the pelvis or rectal area. The patients with dysaesthetic vulvodynia are usually elderly or postmenopausal and are not often still sexually active. However, those patients who are still sexually active deny any dyspareunia. There is often a complaint that even the lightest touch from underwear will initiate sharp, shooting pains, i.e. allodynia. The pain is usually confined to the vulval area but there may be some urethral or rectal discomfort. On examination the vulval skin and architecture are normal and there are no associated neurological abnormalities.

In a study of 17 patients with chronic perineal pain 13 were found to have sacral meningeal cysts using magnetic resonance imaging (MRI). Ten of these patients went on to surgical treatment of the cysts with resolution of the pain in nine patients (van der Kleft & van Vyve 1991). However, a further study of a group of patients with dysaesthetic vulvodynia showed no evidence of sacral cysts on MRI examination of the lumbosacral spine (Lewis & Harrington 1997).

Patients with dysaesthetic vulvodynia in addition to being older than the group with vulval vestibulitis seldom give a history of an initiating event. However, the symptoms of dysaesthetic vulvodynia may occur as a sequel to inflammatory conditions involving the vestibular epithelium. Despite the resolution of the inflammation patients will still complain of discomfort and tenderness, which will not respond to their usual anti-inflammatory treatment. Dysaesthetic vulvodynia may also develop as a complication in patients with vestibulitis so that they experieince pain independent of introital touch. These patients have an overlap problem with a mixture of symptoms and signs due to both vestibulitis and dysaesthetic vulvodynia.

Many of the patients that develop idiopathic dysaesthetic vulvodynia have a history of other chronic pain problems, most commonly glossodynia, temporomandibular joint dysfunction, facial or dental neuralgia and chronic low back pain. Depression is frequently associated with dysaesthetic vulvodynia but it is difficult to discern whether this is a primary event or a consequence of the chronic pain. It is well recognized that chronic pain is a disabling condition both physically and psychologically, leading to depression, which to some extent is dictated by the patient's lifestyle and pre-morbid personality.

It is uncertain whether women with dysaesthetic vulvodynia have a higher psychiatric morbidity than women with other vulval pathology. One study showed that although there was a higher overall psychiatric prevalence rate in women attending a vulval clinic, comparable to that seen in other out-patient clinics, there was not a higher prevalence rate in the vulvodynia group (Jadresic *et al.* 1993). This study did not specify whether the patients had dysaesthetic vulvodynia or vestibulitis. However, the mean age of the patients was 52.5 years, which is the age most likely to be associated with dysaesthetic vulvodynia. Another study did show that women with dysaesthetic vulvodynia had significant psychological distress (Stewart *et al.* 1994).

Many of these patients will stop their usual social activities and become housebound. Their disorder becomes so debilitating that there may be a risk of suicide.

Management

The management is essentially that used in the treatment of chronic pain syndromes in other medical specialities. Opioids are usually ineffective in the treatment of dysaesthesia. Patients who develop dysaesthesia following an inflammatory dermatosis such as lichen planus often improve dramatically with the simple measure of using topical 5% lignocaine as and when required.

The majority of patients with dysaesthetic vulvodynia will need to have treatment directed at the down-regulation of either the peripheral or central neuronal wind-up. Medications that block the reuptake of biogenic amines are effective in a significant number of patients. The tricyclic antidepressant amitriptyline is one of the most widely used medications for chronic pain syndromes, exerting an analgesic effect that is believed to be unrelated to its antidepressant action (Davar & Maaciewicz 1989). It has been shown that amitriptyline produces significant pain relief compared with placebo in patients who develop central pain syndrome following a stroke (Leijon & Boivie 1989). Tricyclic antidepressants are used in other chronic pain syndromes, for example fibromyalgia, atypical facial pain and temperomandibular joint dysfunction, and is of proven benefit in post-herpetic neuralgia (Volmink *et al.* 1996). The exact mechanism of action is unknown. The starting dose is usually 10 mg each night and the dose is increased weekly by an extra 10 mg per night until there is a response. The dose required may be anywhere between 30 mg and 100 mg a day. The patient should be warned that she will experience a dry mouth and drowsiness. If amitriptyline is too sedating, desipramine or nortryptiline can be used instead. The serotonin reuptake blockers alone do not seem to be as effective, although some patients have reported an improvement and they may be tried in those patients that cannot tolerate the side effects of the tricyclics. Carbamazepine and other anticonvulsants have been shown to have a beneficial effect on neuropathic pain syndromes, although their mechanism of action is not clear. These anticonvulsants are used widely for the treatment of trigeminal neuralgia, and the starting dose is 100 mg/day of carbamazepine, which may be gradually increased to 600 mg/day. Close monitoring of the full blood count and liver function tests is required. The other modalities of treatment, including regional nerve blocks, acupuncture, TENS and topical capsaicin, which acts by depleting the C fibres of substance P, have all been tried with inconsistent results. There is still very little published on the treatment of dysaesthetic vulvodynia. A solitary report of the successful treatment of dysaesthetic vulvodynia using a flashlamp-excited dye laser has been published (Reid *et al.* 1995), but further trials need to be done to establish whether this treatment is truly beneficial, as previous experience has shown that dysaesthetic vulvodynia may unfortunately develop as a postoperative complication of carbon dioxide laser treatment for other conditions.

Unfortunately a number of patients, particularly those with a long history of well-established pain, remain resistant to all modalities of treatment, and a strategy has to be devised to help them adjust and cope with their chronic pain. Pain clinics in the UK are well established and have management programmes for patients with back pain and pelvic pain syndromes but few as yet have experience with patients with vulvodynia. However, a pain clinic is important for patients with vulvodynia as the anaesthetists who run these clinics are experienced in the use of the medications that are used for other chronic pain syndrome and combinations of various drugs may achieve a positive result. The psychologists who are involved in the pain management programmes of these clinics may be able to offer help to these patients by using cognitive and behavioural techniques, which educate and distract the patient from her pain and help her to achieve the optimal adjustment to coping and living with a chronic pain syndrome.

References

Altmeyer, P., Chilf, G.N. & Holtzman, H. (1982) Hirsuties papillaris vulvae (Pseudokondylome der vulva). *Hautarzt* **33**, 281–283.

Baggish, M.S., Sze, E.H.M. & Johnson, R. (1997) Urinary oxalate excretion and its role in vulvar pain. *American Journal of Obstetrics and Gynecology* **177**, 507–511.

Bergeron, C., Ferenczy, A., Richart, R.M. & Guralnick, M. (1990) Micropapillomatosis labialis appears unrelated to human papillomavirus. *Obstetrics and Gynecology* **76**, 281–286.

Bergeron, C., Moyal-Barracco, M., Pelisse, M. & Lewin, P. (1994) Vulvar vestibulitis. Lack of evidence for a human papillomavirus etiology. *Journal of Reproductive Medicine* **39**, 936–938.

Bergeron, S., Binik, Y.M., Khalifé, S. & Pagidas, K. (1997) Vulvar vestibulitis syndrome: A critical review. *The Clinical Journal of Pain* **13**, 27–42.

Bloch, K.J., Buchanan, W.W., Wohl, M.J. & Bunim, J.J. (1965) Sjogren's syndrome. *Medicine* **44**, 187–231.

Bornstein, J., Pascal, B. & Abramovici, H. (1993) Intramuscular B interferon treatment for severe vulvar vestibulitis. *Journal of Reproductive Medicine* **38**, 117–120.

Bornstein, J., Zarfati, D., Goldik, Z. & Abramovici, H. (1995) Perineoplasty compared with vestibuloplasty for severe vulvar vestibulitis. *British Journal of Obstetrics and Gynaecology* **102**, 652–655.

Capriello, P., Barale, E., Cappelli, N., Lupo S. & Teti, G. (1988) Sjögrens syndrome: clinical, cytological, histological and colposcopic aspects in women. *Clinical and Experimental Obstetrics and Gynecology* **15**, 9–12.

Davar, G. & Maaciewicz, R.J. (1989) Deafferentation pain syndromes. *Neurological Clinics* **7**, 289–304.

de Jong, J.M.J., van Lunsen, R.H.W., Robertson, E.A., Stam, L.N.E. & Lammes, F.B. (1995) Focal vulvitis: a psychosexual problem for which surgery is not the answer. *Journal of Psychosomatic Obstetrics and Gynecology* **16**, 85–91.

Dennerstein, G.J., Scurry, J.P., Garland, S.M. *et al.* (1994) Human papilloma virus vulvitis: a new disease or an unfortunate mistake? *British Journal of Obstetrics and Gynaecology* **101**, 992–998.

di Paola, G.R. & Rueda, N.G. (1986) Deceptive vulvar papillomavirus infection: a possible explanation for certain cases of vulvodynia. *Journal of Reproductive Medicine* **31**, 966–970.

Dodson, M.G. & Friedrich, E.G. (1978) Psychosomatic vulvovaginitis. *Obstetrics and Gynecology* **51**, (Suppl) 23s–25s.

Edwards, L., Mason, M., Phillips, M., Norton, J. & Boyle, M. (1997) Childhood sexual and physical abuse. Incidence in patients with vulvodynia. *Journal of Reproductive Medicine* **42**, 135–139.

Fitzpatrick, C.C., DeLancey, J.O.L., Elkins, T.E. & McGuire, E.J. (1993) Vulvar vestibulitis and interstitial cystitis: a disorder of urogenital sinus derived epithelium? *Obstetrics and Gynecology* **81**, 860–861.

Friedman, M., Siegler, E. & Kerne, H. (1993) Clinical and histopathological changes of the vulvar vestibulum in healthy subjects and in patients with vulvar vestibulitis. In: *Abstracts of the XII International Congress of the International Society for the Study of Vulvovaginal Disease*, p. 21.

Friedrich, E.G. (1983) The vulvar vestibule. *Journal of Reproductive Medicine* **28**, 773–777.

Friedrich, E.G. (1987) Vulvar vestibulitis syndrome. *Journal of Reproductive Medicine* **32**, 110–114.

Glazer, H.I., Rodke, G., Swencionis, C., Hertz, R. & Young, A.W. (1995) Treatment of the vulvar vestibulitis syndrome with electromyographic biofeedback of pelvic floor musculature. *Journal of Reproductive Medicine* **40**, 283–290.

Goetsch, M.F. (1991) Vulvar vestibulitis: prevalence and historic features in a general gynecologic practice population. *American Journal of Obstetrics and Gynecology* **164**, 1609–1616.

Goetsch, M.F. (1996) Simplified surgical revision of the vulvar vestibule for vulvar vestibulitis. *American Journal of Obstetrics and Gynecology* **174**, 1701–1707.

Growdon, W.A., Fu, Y.S., Lebhertz, T.B. *et al.* (1985) Pruritic vulvar squamous papillomatosis: evidence for human papilloma virus etiology. *Obstetrics and Gynecology* **66**, 564–568.

Halpern, B.N., Ky, T. & Robert, B. (1967) Clinical and immunological study of an exceptional case of reagenic type sensitisation to human seminal fluid. *Immunology* **12**, 2457–2458.

International Association for the Study of Pain; Subcommittee on Taxonomy (1986) Classification of chronic pain: descriptions of chronic pain syndromes and definitions of pain terms. *Pain* **3** (Suppl.), S1–S226.

Jadresic, D., Barton, S., Neill, S., Staughton, R. & Marwood, R. (1993) Psychiatric morbidity in women attending a clinic for vulval problems: is there a higher rate in vulvodynia? *International Journal of STD and AIDS* **4**, 237–239.

Kelly, H.A. (1928) Dyspareunia. In: *Gynecology*, p. 23. Appleton, New York.

Kent, H.L. & Wisniewski, P.M. (1990) Interferon for vulvar vestibulitis. *Journal of Reproductive Medicine* **12**, 1138–1140.

Leijon, G. & Boivie, J. (1989) Central post stroke pain—a controlled trial of amitriptyline and carbamazepine. *Pain* **36**, 27–36.

Lewis, F.M. & Harrington, C.I. (1997) Use of magnetic resonance imaging in vulvodynia. *Journal of Reproductive Medicine* **42**, 169.

Lynch, P. (1986) Vulvodynia: a syndrome of unexplained vulvar pain, psychologic disability and sexual dysfunction. *Journal of Reproductive Medicine* **31**, 773–780.

McCormack, W.M. (1990) Two urogenital sinus syndromes. *Journal of Reproductive Medicine* **35**, 873–876.

McKay (1984) Burning vulva syndrome. Report of the ISSVD task force. *Journal of Reproductive Medicine* **29**, 457.

McKay, M. (1989) Vulvodynia. A multifactorial clinical problem. *Archives of Dermatology* **125**, 256–262.

McKay, M., Frankman, O., Horowitz, B.J. *et al.* (1991) Vulvar vestibulitis and vulvar papillomatosis. Report of the ISSVD Committee on vulvodynia. *Journal of Reproductive Medicine* **36**, 413–415.

Marinoff, S.C. & Turner, M.L.C. (1986) Hypersensitivity to vaginal candidiasis or treatment vehicles in the pathogenesis of minor vestibular gland syndrome. *Journal of Reproductive Medicine* **31**, 796–799.

Marinoff, S.C. & Turner, M.L.C. (1992) Vulvar vestibulitis syndrome. *Dermatologic Clinics* **10**, 435–444.

Melzack R. (1982) *The Challenge of Pain*. Basic Books, New York.

Melzack, R. & Wall, P.D. (1965) Pain mechanisms; A new theory. *Science* **150**, 971–979.

Moyal-Barracco, M., Leibowitch, M. & Orth, G. (1990) Vestibular papillae of the vulva. Lack of evidence for human papillomavirus etiology. *Archives of Dermatology* **126**, 1594–1598.

Nylander Lundqvist, E., Hofer, P.-A., Olofsson, J.I. & Sjoberg, I. (1997) Is vulvar vestibulitis an inflammatory condition? A comparison of histological findings in affected and healthy women. *Acta Dermato-venereologica (Stockholm)* **77**, 319–322.

Peckham, B.M., Maki, D.G., Patterson, J.J. & Hafez, G.-R. (1986) Focal vulvitis: a characteristic syndrome and cause of dyspareunia. *American Journal of Obstetrics and Gynecology* **154**, 855–864.

Pelisse, M. & Hewitt, J. (1976) Erythematous vulvitis 'en plaques'. *Proceedings of the 3rd International Congress of the International Society For the Study of Vulvar disease* pp. 34–37.

Poskitt, B.L., Wojnarowska, F.T. & Shaw, S. (1995) Semen contact urticaria. *Journal of the Royal Society of Medicine* **88**, 108–109.

Prayson, R.A., Stoler, M.H. & Hart, W.R. (1995) Vulvar vestibulitis. A histopathologic study of 36 cases including human papillomavirus *in situ* hybridization analysis. *American Journal of Surgical Pathology* **19**, 157–160.

Pyka, R.E., Wilkinson, E.J., Friedrich, E.G. & Croker, B.P. (1988) The histopathology of vulvar vestibulitis syndrome. *International Journal of Gynecological Pathology* **7**, 249–257.

Reid, R., Omoto, K.H., Precop, S.L. *et al.* (1995) Flashlamp-excited dye laser therapy of idiopathic vulvodynia is safe and efficacious. *American Journal of Obstetrics and Gynecology* **172**, 1684–1701.

Robboy, S.J., Ross, J.S., Prat, J., Keh, P.C. & Welch, W.R. (1978) Urogenital sinus origin of mucinous and ciliated cysts of the vulva. *Obstetrics and Gynecology* **51**, 347–351.

Schimkat, H.G., Meynadier, J.M. & Meynadier, J. (1993) Contact urticaria. In: *Vulvovaginitis* (eds P. Elsner & J. Martius), pp. 83–110. Marcel Dekker, New York.

Schover, L.R., Youngs, D.D. & Cannata, R. (1992) Psychosexual aspects of the evaluation and management of vulvar vestibulitis. *American Journal of Obstetrics and Gynecology* **167**, 630–636.

Skene, A.J.C. (1888) Diseases of the external organs of generation. In: *Treatise on Diseases of Women*. Appleton, New York, pp. 76–98. (1890, H.K. Lewis, London.)

Solomons, C., Melmed, M.H. & Heitler, S.M. (1991) Calcium citrate for vulval vestibulitis. A case report. *Journal of Reproductive Medicine* **36**, 879–882.

Stewart, D.E., Reicher, A.E., Gerulath, A.H. & Boydell, K.M. (1994) Vulvodynia and psychological distress. *Obstretrics and Gynecology* **84**, 587–590.

Thomas, T.G. & Mundé, P.F. (1891) *A Practical Treatise on the Diseases of Women*, p. 143. Lea Brothers, Philadelphia.

Turjanmaa, K. & Reunala, T. (1989) Condoms as a source of latex allergen and cause of contact urticaria. *Contact Dermatitis* **20**, 360–364.

Turner, M.L.C. & Marinoff, S.C. (1988) Association of human papillomavirus and vulvodynia and the vulvar vestibulitis syndrome. *Journal of Reproductive Medicine* **33**, 533–537.

Umpierre, S.A., Kaufman, R.H., Adam, E., Wood, K.V. & Adler-Storth, Z.K. (1991) Human papillomavirus DNA in tissue biopsy specimens of vulvar vestibulitis patients treated with interferon. *Obstetrics and Gynecology* **78**, 693–695.

van der Kleft, E. & van Vyve, M. (1991) Chronic perineal pain related to sacral meningeal cysts. *Neurosurgery* **29**, 223–226.

van Lankveld, J.J.D.M., Weijenborg, P.T.M. & Ter Kuile, M.M. (1996) Psychologic profiles of and sexual function in women with vulvar vestibulitis and their partners. *Obstetrics and Gynecology* **88**, 65–70.

Volmink, J., Lancaster, T., Gray, S., Silagy, C. (1996) Treatments of postherpetic neuralgia. A systemic review of randomised controlled trials. *Family Practice* **13**, 84–91.

Wang, A.C., Hsu, J.J., Hsueh, S., Sun, C.F. & Tsao, K.C. (1991) Evidence of human papillomavirus deoxyribonucleic acid in vulvar squamous papillomatosis. *International Journal of Gynecological Pathology* **10**, 44–50.

Weijmar Schultz, W.C.M., Gianotten, W.L., van der Meijden, W.I. *et al.* (1996) Behavioural approach with or without surgical intervention to the vulvar vestibulitis syndrome: a prospective randomized and non-randomized study. *Journal of Psychosomatic Obstetrics and Gynecology* **17**, 143–148.

Weisfogel, E. (1976) Battle with a unicorn: The burning vulva. *Proceeding of the 3rd International Congress of the International Society for the Study of Vulvar Disease* pp. 38–40.

Wilkinson, E.J., Guerrero, E., Daniel, R. *et al.* (1993) Vulvar vestibulitis is rarely associated with human papillomavirus infection types 6, 11, 16, or 18. *International Journal of Gynecological Pathology* **28**, 134–141.

Woodruff, J.D., Geandry, R. & Poliakoff, S. (1981) Treatment of dyspareunia and vaginal outlet distortions by perineoplasty. *Obstetrics and Gynecology* **57**, 750–754.

Chapter 7: Psychiatric disorders and the vulva

J.J. Bradley

General aspects

The genitalia and secondary sexual characteristics loom large in the body image of both sexes and it is hardly surprising that the vulva, representing an area of the body that is a source of pleasure, guilt, pride, embarrassment and procreation, should be a focus for anxieties, preoccupations, delusions and even hallucinations.

It follows that the physical examination of such a psychologically sensitive area should be conducted with gentleness, tact and perceptive awareness in a relaxed but thorough manner. The physical examination, and even physical contact by attempts to shake hands, of Asian, especially Muslim, women by a male doctor may cause embarrassment, offence or a total refusal to cooperate. If a woman doctor is not available, the examination must be carried out with a chaperon. Women frequently complain of feeling embarrassed, humiliated or demeaned by a genital examination, but the presence of a chaperon, explanation and reassurance will minimize distress and may be positively therapeutic.

In spite of a climate of sexual liberation and what amounts to an information explosion on sexual matters in the popular press and women's magazines, a surprisingly large number of women are ignorant of their genital anatomy and may be helped by explanation and diagrams. Instruction in formal self-examination may also be useful (Lawhead & Majmudar 1990).

Efforts have been made by anonymous questionnaire surveys to assess how widespread sexual contact is within the confines of an apparently professional doctor/patient relationship. Indecent assaults ranging from embracing, kissing, fondling of breasts or genitalia to rape are alleged to occur in consulting rooms and also in patients' homes. A comprehensive Dutch survey of 595 gynaecologists and 380 ENT surgeons gave a response rate of 74%. In both groups, perhaps surprisingly, 4% admitted sexual contact with their patients at some time (Wilbers *et al.* 1992). Indecent assault and rape are of course criminal offences and could lead to custodial sentences in addition to erasure from the Medical Register. However, many of the allegations are not pursued by complainants. Certainly a proportion will be realized on reflection to be misinterpretations of legitimate examinations. In others there will be a lack of corroborative evidence and in a great many a reluctance of the victim to risk giving evidence in court, which might increase her distress.

Significance of symptoms

Any vulval symptom, pain, irritation or observable lesion is likely to give rise to anxiety, the degree of which will be dependent on the disability it causes, the patient's personality, the context in which it occurs and the reactions of the sexual partner. Relatively minor disorders may become a focus for displaced anxiety and guilt, particularly that relating to sexuality and sexual relationships. When taking a history it is important to allow a woman sufficient time and sympathetic interest to talk about personal problems, which will give the doctor an opportunity for further exploration of her lifestyle and relationships, which might have a bearing on the presenting symptom. It is debatable whether any vulval symptoms (apart from some cases of pain and hallucinatory experiences) are purely psychogenic, although they may be perpetuated by psychological mechanisms (Whitlock 1976). On the other hand, the stress of adverse life events such as bereavement and divorce may induce white-cell dysfunction, allowing the patient to be more prone to fungal or viral infection. It is well recognized that dermatoses may be precipitated by stress, and existing disease exacerbated. Bartrop *et al.* (1977) reported depression of the mitotic response of lymphocytes in 29 subjects whose spouses had died 6 weeks earlier, and similar results have been reported by other workers (Kronfol *et al.* 1983, Schliefer *et al.* 1983). A review of emotion and immunity (*Lancet* 1985) concluded that the relationship between them may prove to be another strong argument for a return to 'whole person medicine', but the matter is not simple; Hall (1985) points out that there has been no evidence of any significant increase in illness that could be attributed to defects in immunity in air crews who survived the stresses of the Second World War. The field of psychosomatic interrelationships has been fraught with difficulties, not least because of problems with communication between clinicians, psychologist and immunologists (*Lancet* 1987).

A new concept, psychoneuroimmunology, now links the immune system with the nervous system and the endocrine system. It regards them as making up an integrated system of defence within which neural, endocrine and behavioural factors all modulate immune reactions. Ader *et al.* (1995) reviewed the evidence that cytokines and neurotransmitters, which are expressed and perceived by both the nervous and the immune system, engage in two-way transmissions, and that hormones, endorphins and psychological stress can affect the production of B cells and natural killer cells. There are indeed therefore good grounds for believing that emotional factors can influence the onset and outcome of infections, neoplastic and autoimmune disease.

Almost any genital symptom may be interpreted by a patient as being due to sexually transmitted disease and a high proportion of patients will be self-referred to genitourinary medicine (GUM) clinics. Some will indeed be suffering from such a disease and all (except perhaps some habitual attenders) will need an opportunity to express their feelings and be given appropriate reassurance and treatment, or referral to a gynaecologist, dermatologist or psychiatrist. Although it has been estimated that 30% of patients attending GUM clinics probably have an underlying psychiatric disorder, based on the General Health Questionnaire (GHQ) (Pedder & Goldberg 1970), compared with 12% of the general population (Goldberg *et al.* 1976), the patient's presenting symptoms may, of course, be due to organic disease, the psychiatric disorder being incidental. The psychiatric morbidity uncovered by the GHQ is generally mild to moderate anxiety or depression, which would usually not warrant referral to a psychiatrist. Frost (1985) has shown that only 0.4% of new attenders in a GUM clinic are thought to have overt psychiatric illness, based on referral rates to psychiatrists. Fitzpatrick *et al.* (1986) in a study of 381 patients attending a GUM clinic have found that, while 43% had GHQ scores indicating that there were psychiatric factors, only 4% of the total number appeared to have abnormal or inappropriate levels of distress in relation to their presenting complaint.

The majority of emotional and psychiatric problems relating to the vulva are likely to be of relatively minor severity in psychiatric terms. Nevertheless, sensitive psychological management, which will include explanation, reassurance and above all time to listen to the patient, may ease or cut short unnecessary suffering. Misinterpretations of physical symptoms or signs by a patient may lead her to believe, for example, that a benign vulval wart is malignant, but she may be reluctant to express her anxiety. Anticipation of her fears and encouragement to express them followed by firm reassurance should provide relief, whereas failure to do so may result in prolonged distress and rumination. Patients with serious vulval disease, such as carcinoma, have also been shown to benefit from pre- and postoperative counselling (Andersen & Hacker 1983, Crowther *et al.* 1994).

Hypochondriasis

A woman with a fear or conviction of disease that is unresponsive to a simple psychotherapeutic approach, and that dominates her life and leads her from doctor to doctor, may justifiably be regarded as suffering from hypochondriasis (Barksy & Klerman 1983). This may be a symptom of an obsessional neurosis in which the patient may be able to accept reassurance for a short period, but then rapidly returns to her ruminations of serious disease and rejects any psychological interpretation of the symptom. There may be a degree of associated clinical depression, which will respond to treatment with antidepressant drugs. Hypochondriasis may also be the presenting feature of severe depression, schizophrenia and monosymptomatic hypochondriasis, all of which may be grouped together as 'psychotic' disorders.

Psychotic disorders

The term 'psychosis' is applied to those illnesses in which patients suffer from delusions, hallucinations or other disorders of the thought processes or mood that cause them to be out of touch with reality. The more florid forms of schizophrenia, mania or endogenous depression will be readily recognizable as frank mental illness and, although some patients may complain of vulval symptoms, they will be incidental to the overall picture. Categorization as 'psychotic' is purely descriptive and does not have specific aetiological significance, apart from the organic psychoses caused by disease of the nervous system, metabolic disorders and drug intoxication or withdrawal. However, the so-called 'functional psychoses' (such as schizophrenia or endogenous depression) are syndromes which, once initiated, render the patient inaccessible to logical argument as regards certain ideas or symptoms, although insight may be retained in other respects. In practical terms, the patient is likely to be deeply distressed and bewildered by her symptoms, and may become suicidal or, more rarely, a danger to others.

A proportion of patients suffering from psychoses will present with vulval symptoms to general practitioners, physicians in GUM, gynaecologists or dermatologists, without appearing to be obviously mentally ill. Superficially the presenting complaint may seem to be a straightforward one such as discomfort, irritation, anxiety about anatomical structure, fear of venereal disease, unpleasant discharges or odours. The doctor may be initially alerted to the possibility of psychosis by the unusual quality of the complaint. There may be a discrepancy between its apparent trivial nature and the emotional response (or vice versa) or a bizarre way of describing pain or sensations. After thorough physical examination the patient will be unable to accept assurances that no abnormality has been found. The more the woman is allowed to talk about her complaints, the more the diagnosis will become clear. It is important to encourage the patient to say what she believes to be the cause of her symptoms and to express her ideas about its outcome and what she feels can be done to help her.

It is essential to recognize the presence of major psychiatric illness, without necessarily being able to make a precise psychiatric diagnosis, so that referral for appropriate psychiatric treatment can be made. There is understandable reluctance on the part of some physicians (Cotterill 1983) to alarm a patient who believes she has a physical disorder by referring her to a psychiatrist and thus risking the patient's refusing all medical care. Some doctors may feel confident in undertaking psychiatric management themselves; but where this is not the case it is usually possible to persuade the patient to accept a psychiatric consultation and at the same time to offer a further appointment with the referring doctor.

Schizophrenia

Symptoms relating to the vulva are not common, although about one-fifth of schizophrenic patients do suffer from hypochondriacal delusions (Lucas *et al.* 1962). The complaint is usually bizarre. The patient may feel that the appearance of her vulva has changed in a strange way, even to the extent that she fears she may be changing sex. Further questioning may reveal that she believes that it is due to some outside influence. Some schizophrenic patients experience tactile hallucinations in the genital area, or orgasmic sensations. Elaborate delusional explanations of these feelings may be elicited, such as the patient believing that she is being raped in her sleep. A hypochondriacal preoccupation, short of frank delusions, may be a prodromal symptom of late-onset schizophrenia (Kenyon 1976).

Endogenous depression

Endogenous depression is characterized by the well-recognized syndrome of gloom, early morning waking, weight loss, morning exacerbation of symptoms, loss of libido and self reproach. Ideas of hopelessness and suicide may occur from adolescence to old age. A preoccupation with bodily health and functions is a frequent concomitant to the extent that it may be the major symptom, and any mood changes noted may appear to be the effect rather than the cause of it.

The vulva may be the sole focus of symptoms, from a vague feeling of itch to clearly defined localized persistent pain (Bradley 1963). However, it is well recognized that chronic pain can lead to a secondary depression and this may make it difficult to decide whether the patient's depression is a primary or secondary event. In Chapter 6 the subject of pain is discussed further. The patient may often have fears of unspecified malignant or venereal disease, remaining unreassured by examination and negative investigations, or a conviction that an unpleasant odour that must be obvious to others emanates from the vulva. There may be soreness because of excessive use of deodorants and disinfectants. Following encouragement to speculate about the cause of her distress she may admit to feelings of guilt about masturbation or sexual indiscretions. Delusional ideas that the vulva has 'dried up' and that the vagina or urethra have been closed or obliterated may be encountered, and efforts to demonstrate that this is not so will be met with disbelief.

Given adequate time, the patient will give a clear indication of the emotional component of her symptoms. Fixed ideas of punishment, shame and the hopelessness of her case will emerge and the examining doctor should not avoid enquiring into whether she has considered suicide. Depressed patients are often relieved to be told that their illness is well recognized and that it can be treated. Depressive illnesses may be self limiting, but the judicious use of antidepressant drugs and, in special circumstances, electroconvulsive therapy, will shorten the period of suffering and may even prevent suicide.

Monosymptomatic hypochondriacal psychosis

Hypochondriacal ideas of delusional intensity, unresponsive to repeated reassurance by a series of doctors often unknown to each other, may occur without signs of schizophrenia or depression. The symptoms may be centred solely on the vulva and are generally vague ones such as discomfort, feeling 'not quite right' or dysmorphophobia. Dysmorphophobia is a disorder of perception of the body image in which the patient believes that the anatomical appearance is ugly or in some way abnormal. These patients generally have a pre-existing obsessional or paranoid personality disorder and the irrational belief may persist for many years despite investigations, reassurance and even appropriate psychiatric treatment.

Dysmorphophobia does not normally progress to a full psychosis, but a significant number of patients ultimately commit suicide (Bebbington 1976, McKenna 1984).

Delusional parasitosis is an allied condition, which is well recognized by dermatologists, although it is relatively rare and an individual dermatologist may see only three to four cases in a professional lifetime (Lyell 1983). The syndrome occurs most commonly in middle-aged women who believe that they are infested with parasites, usually involving the whole body but sometimes only the genitalia. The delusion will dominate the woman's life and often that of her family. The secondary effects of repeated washing and use of strong antiseptics may be seen on examination. Psychiatric referral may be strongly resisted. Neuroleptic drugs that are effective in the treatment of hypochondriacal psychosis and schizophrenia may result in a dramatic remission within a few weeks (Monro 1980). The patient rarely develops full insight into the delusional nature of the symptoms, but is no longer preoccupied by them. Unfortunately, to avoid relapse long-term treatment is usually necessary.

Epilepsy

Reports of vulval sensations or orgasm as part of an epileptic aura, or equivalent, are uncommon, although isolated cases are to be found (Scott 1978). A distinction must be made between an aura with a sexual component, which may have temporal lobe origin, and ictal genital sensory phenomena, which may have parietal lobe origin (Spencer *et al.* 1983).

Mutilation (see also Chapter 11)

Mutilation is an emotive term. Necessary surgery for malignant disease and episiotomy, for example, may be perceived by the patient, if not by the surgeon, as mutilation.

Mutilation may be accidental, or occur as a result of sexual violence and this elicits the appropriate concern and action. Sexual reassignment surgery is condemned by those who see it as tampering with nature, but it is sought eagerly by those who feel it will offer them greater fulfilment.

Ritual and cultural mutilation

Cultural pressures force millions of children and young women to submit to traditional rituals such as infibulation, which may be life threatening or disabling. Those involved usually accept these practices as an inevitable part of their lives, even though those outside these cultures regard them with horror.

Mutilation for cultural, religious or aesthetic reasons is now unusual in Western society, although the fashion trend for adornment with metal rings has spread from the ears to other parts of the body, including the vulva (Healey 1978). However, in the 19th century resection of the pudendal nerve and removal of the clitoris were sometimes carried out. Clitoridectomy was practised by Baker-Brown. He believed that masturbation led to a variety of organic neurological problems and that clitoridectomy could be curative (Black 1997).

There are reports of African tribes who measure female sexuality in terms of clitoral length and labial hypertrophy and whose girls are deliberately manipulated to stimulate enlargement of the clitoris and labia minora (Gelfand 1973).

The practice of what has been loosely termed 'female circumcision' has been carried on for many generations in more than 20 countries in Africa, from Nigeria in the West to Somalia and the Sudan in the East. It is also practised in Oman, South Yemen and the United Arab Emirates and among the Muslim population of Indonesia and Malaysia (Black & Debelle 1995). It has been estimated that as many as 127 million women are involved (Macready 1996). Christian missionaries have strongly deplored the practice over the last 100 years, but it is only in the last two decades that concern has been expressed by the international community and by outspoken women in those countries affected, who see these mutilations as a way of maintaining female subjugation. There is a widespread belief that female circumcision is a requirement of the Islamic faith, although this has been repudiated by Muslim theologians; it is apparently viewed as an 'embellishment' rather than an ordinance like male circumcision (Shandall 1967). It is not practised in a number of Muslim countries, including Saudi Arabia. The custom is perpetuated by other religious groups, including Catholics, Protestants, Copts and Animists, and seems to be related more to cultural tradition than to religion. The Prohibition of Female Circumcision Act (1985) banned the procedure in the UK but it continues in immigrant communities, being carried out illegally in the UK or achieved by sending the child temporarily back to the country of origin. The procedure was officially banned in the USA in 1997 (Macready 1996) and efforts are being made to curb it in France (Gallard 1995) and Egypt (Wiens 1996).

Three types of operation are carried out.

1 Circumcision, which involves the removal of the prepuce of the clitoris (Sunna circumcision).

2 Excision—clitoridectomy and excision of the labia minora.

3 Infibulation, which involves clitoridectomy, excision of the labia minora and the anterior two-thirds or the whole of the medial part of the labia majora. The vaginal introitus is obliterated by sutures, apart from a very small opening for menstrual blood and urine. After this operation the girl's legs are bound together for up to 40 days to allow for formation of scar tissue.

The type of operation and ritual surrounding it varies according to the country and culture. The operation is usually performed by older women, in some places with elaborate ceremony and in others without. No form of anaesthetic is used except when the operation is performed in hospital. The age at which it occurs varies from a few days old to late adolescence, or just before marriage.

The ritual is usually carried out in unhygienic surroundings and it is not surprising that there is a significant mortality from haemorrhage and infection, although accurate statistics are not available. Damage is often sustained to the urethra, bladder and vagina as the girl struggles to free herself. Haematocolpos and urinary problems occur as a result of obliteration of the vaginal introitus, and keloidal scars and calculi (Onuigbo 1976, Aziz 1980, Junaid & Thomas 1981) have also been reported. Sexual enjoyment is lost except in the most minor operations. In infibulated women, intercourse is impossible until the husband opens the vagina, often with a knife. The resulting tissue fibrosis leads to obstructed labour or makes vaginal delivery difficult with consequent tearing of the perineum and its associated structures. The social pressures are so great that despite the obvious psychological trauma of the operation and its sequelae, a girl and her parents will conform because of the danger of rejection, ridicule or unmarriageability (McLean 1980).

It is difficult to account for the continuation of this custom which to Western eyes appears to be wholly repugnant. The reasons advanced include initiation into adulthood, preservation of virginity, hygiene and aesthetic aspects. By its apologists it is seen as a way of maintaining tribal cohesion, and by its critics as a means by which men subjugate women, perpetuated out of spite by women who have undergone mutilation themselves. Anthropologists have suggested that female circumcision may be partly the result of male ambivalence towards female sexuality, and partly a reaction of women to male circumcision (Bettelheim 1954). In some cultures it is believed that the masculine element of a woman is her clitoris and that a man's femininity is represented by his foreskin; so in order to avoid sexual ambiguity both structures must be removed.

Self mutilation

Patients with learning difficulties and those with psychoses may injure the vulva with their fingernails or with various foreign bodies, as part of a masturbatory act or as a response to delusions or hallucinations. The mental disorder in such cases is usually obvious. Injuries are sometimes caused by clumsy efforts to procure abortion. It will be the apparently 'normal' young woman who presents with atypical excoriation, ulcers or even haematuria who will be a diagnostic problem when investigations all prove negative. Reports of self mutilation of the female genitalia are uncommon in the literature, and relatively common among males, although self mutilation, in general, is much commoner in women than in men (French & Nelson 1972).

Such a patient will often give a vague account of how and when the lesion began and, although consulting a doctor about it, she may seem inappropriately composed and phlegmatic. In fact, the lesion will have been caused by the patient herself using her nails, a needle or a cigarette, although this may be very hard to demonstrate. Straightforward conscious malingering is relatively unusual, although in a young woman held on remand in prison it may be used as a means of obtaining sympathy or hospital admission. The majority of patients who produce artefacts fall into a category that is neither truly malingering, nor truly unconscious behaviour. Lyell (1979) sums it up neatly: 'it is done consciously perhaps, but with a consciousness that is made to act in that way by forces that are outside the patient's control'.

When suspicion has been aroused, a closer look at the patient's personality and current life situation is indicated. Such women are emotionally immature and not necessarily young. There may be a history of early emotional deprivation, due to parental loss or discord, or an overdependence on parents. The patient may admit to sexual frigidity and yet present in a flirtatious way, or like a coy child. She may give a history of past sexual abuse. She may express disappointment with a sexual partner and an inability to form stable relationships. A history of overdoses, cut wrists or drug abuse may be obtained and she may have been in trouble with the law. 'Blackouts', amnesias or illnesses suggestive of hysterical conversion may be elicited during the course of taking her history.

A proportion of patients who produce self-inflicted lesions may appear to be superficially stable—a student nurse devoted to her profession, a devout religious postulant or a middle-aged spinster caring for a cantankerous elderly mother—but under the apparent stability is a bewildered child reacting to some intolerable situation by a need to be 'ill'. Gentle enquiry into current tensions, frustrations or disappointments may be very revealing. Confrontation with the suspicion that she is causing the lesion herself will not succeed, and the temptation to view the encounter in an adversarial way, by trying to 'catch the patient out', should be resisted. Judging the point at which to refer the patient to a psychiatrist can be difficult. If a good rapport has been established it may be possible, without accusing her of self mutiliation, to suggest that the lesion may be the effect of emotional problems and subsequently to share her care with a social worker. It is important that the two therapists should maintain good communication with each other, as there may well be a tendency for the patient to play one off against the other.

Sexual violence

Rape

The Sexual Offences Act 1956 and Sexual Offences (Amendment) Act 1976 define rape as 'unlawful sexual intercourse with a woman without her consent and at that time the man knows that she does not consent to intercourse, or is reckless as to whether or not she consents to it'. It is further defined as sexual intercourse by fraud or threats, or carried out when a woman is asleep, unconscious or mentally handicapped, or so young (under 16) as to be unable to understand the nature of the act. No age group from childhood to extreme old age is exempt. In practice, at least in the UK, probably most cases of rape go unreported by the victim because of fear of further distress caused by questioning, court appearances and reactions of relatives.

Injuries to the vulva may include bruising, fingernail scratches on the labia, dilatation of the introitus and sometimes rupture of the fourchette and perineum in young girls. Genital examination must be conducted with particular care because of the medicolegal implications (Knight 1976).

Trauma to the genitalia and other parts of the body, sexually transmitted disease and pregnancy will be anticipated complications, but the psychological trauma engendered by the experience of rape will, for most women, be the most serious effect, and one which can affect their lives for many years. At the time of the attack a woman may be literally paralysed by terror, fearing for her life. Others may resist violently, and perhaps suffer more physical injury thereby. The state of shock following the event may be shown by an immediate emotional response with a need to talk about it, while others will feel emotionally numb and be unable to communicate their distress. Surprisingly, some women carry on a normal life without telling anyone of their terrifying experience, but most will suffer nightmares, depression, feelings of unjustified guilt and shame, humiliation and anger. Reactions of relatives and friends, police and courts, and sometimes even doctors, may reinforce such feelings. The experience may lead to a temporary or long-lasting revulsion towards intercourse or any form of physical intimacy.

Many large towns and cities in the UK now have rape crisis centres with a 24-hour emergency service. They offer invaluable advice to both women and the doctors treating them at the time of the crisis, and also provide continuing psychological support (London Rape Crisis Centre 1984).

There is a widespread belief that false allegations of rape are common. However, there is little evidence to support this view, although rarely an allegation may be based on a sincerely held but mistaken belief on the part of the victim. In such cases the alleger has interpreted or experienced a sexual experience as coercive rather than consensual. Such women may have been survivors of childhood sexual and physical abuse who find it difficult in adulthood to protect themselves from further abuse or exploitation (Adshead 1996).

Post-traumatic stress disorder

All women who have experienced rape will be deeply distressed and the majority will suffer from some psychological symptoms for 3–6 months after the traumatic event. About 30% will suffer from a longer-lasting response characterized by 'flashback' episodes when the trauma is re-experienced, dreams of the event, intrusive distressing recollections, distress at reminders of the event and avoidance of such stimuli, and a generally increased arousal. They may also suffer from depression of mood, a feeling of emotional numbness and a sense of a foreshortened future. The onset of symptoms may be delayed for several months after the initial traumatic event. A combination of skilled psychological counselling and possibly antidepressant drugs will be the treatment of choice (Duddle 1991).

Sexual abuse in children (see also Chapters 4 and 5)

Epidemiological studies have yielded prevalence estimates of child sexual abuse between 6 and 62% for females (Finkelhor 1994), which highlights the difficulty in obtaining reliable statistics; the population sampled and the definitions used will lead to variations. Nevertheless, it is generally recognized that sexual abuse of children is underreported.

The Royal College of Physicians set up a working party on physical signs of abuse in 1988 in response to the enquiry into child abuse in Cleveland in 1987, and a new edition of their first report has now been published (Royal College of Physicians 1997). This gives invaluable guidelines on how the physical examination should be conducted when sexual abuse is alleged or suspected. A substantial proportion of sexually abused children will have no abnormal physical signs, but absence of signs does not imply absence of abuse. Anal signs may be prominent (Hobbs & Wynne 1986) with or without vulval signs. The question of abuse will arise when anogenital warts and mollusca are found, although in many cases there is probably no sexual connotation (see also Chapters 4 and 5). Moreover, sexual factors may be wrongly invoked when some naturally occurring vulval condition is not recognized or misinterpreted, for example lichen sclerosus et atrophicus (Handfield-Jones *et al.* 1987) or Crohn's disease (Hey *et al.* 1986).

It is recommended that physical examination should be

performed by a doctor, usually a paediatrician trained in forensic techniques. Alleged or proven sexual abuse will have far-reaching psychological, social and legal implications and it follows that history taking from the child, parent or carer will need to be done with great sensitivity, as will the physical examination.

Despite the popular anxiety that a child might be sexually molested by a stranger, abuse takes place more commonly in the home. Fathers, stepfathers, uncles and trusted family friends are commonly the culprits and abuse may be a regular occurrence for a child over a number of years from early childhood to adolescence. Threats, bribery and reassurance that it is 'normal' or 'educational' for a little girl to have sexual contact with an adult may be made and she may be persuaded to keep it as a 'secret' either from fear of some reprisal, withdrawal of love, or guilt. The traumatic impact of sexual abuse may result in behavioural problems at home or at school, depression, suicidal attempts or delinquency. If a child eventually tells someone, perhaps a teacher, what is going on, she may have the added burden of feeling responsible for putting her abuser in prison.

There is a positive correlation between reported sexual abuse and personality and mental health problems in adult life. However, it has been noted that childhood sexual abuse is more frequent in women coming from disrupted homes as well as in those who have been exposed to physical abuse or inadequate parenting. There is an overlap between the possible effects of sexual abuse and the effects of the background of disadvantage and doubts have been raised as to how often in practice sexual abuse operates as an independent causal element (Mullen *et al.* 1993).

Accidental injury: haematomas

While similar lesions may follow rape, coital injury, non-accidental injury in children and indeed any form of trauma, many such cases are the result of falls on to sharp objects, damage from inrush of water in water skiing, and similar episodes (see Chapters 11 and 12).

Surgical procedures

Sexual reassignment

Female to male transsexualism is rare. It has been estimated that of about 10 000 transsexuals in the USA 4000 are female to male. About 400 female to male reassignment operations were performed in 1980 in the USA (Lothstein 1982). Hoenig and Kenna (1974) estimated from a survey in the Manchester region that the incidence of transsexualism in England and Wales is one in 34 000 for males and one in 108 000 for females, suggesting that there are 181 female to male transsexuals in this population.

Inevitably such cases attract publicity out of proportion to the incidence of the condition, and complex social, psychological, ethical and legal issues are involved. It is controversial whether surgical attempts at constructing something approaching male genitalia are in the patient's interest, although, in spite of the dearth of adequate follow-up studies, it might be justified in a small number of cases.

The typical patient has a conviction from childhood that she is psychologically a male trapped in a female body. She will be erotically attracted to women and will have the ambition to be a faithful husband. Masturbation is rarely practised because of a feeling of revulsion towards her genitalia, which are a constant reminder of femininity. Many such patients will live as men without resorting to surgery. Some will feel more relaxed by regular use of androgens, which will suppress menses, cause deepening of the voice and growth of facial hair. Marked enlargement of the clitoris occurs and its erotic sensitivity increases. It is generally recommended that no surgical intervention is made until the subject has undergone regular psychotherapy and lived as a male for 2 years. Some patients will be content with mastectomy, hysterectomy and oophorectomy; others will wish to proceed, in spite of the hazards of multiple operations, to the construction of an artificial phallus from skin grafts with a urinary tube. The clitoris is retained to allow orgasm (Money & Ambinder 1978). Davies (1985) has described these procedures.

Kuiper and Cohen-Kettenis (1988) evaluated the therapeutic effect of sex reassignment surgery on 36 female to male and 105 male to female transsexuals. Only 50% of the female to male patients were traced. Most had not received a phalloplasty, but felt generally happier and better adjusted in their new role. The authors point out that in addition to surgery they need frequent psychosocial aid and support during and after the process of reassignment.

Cosmetic procedures

Reduction of the labia minora is sometimes requested, as is enhancement of the fat pads of the labia majora.

Episiotomy

Between 1965 and 1973 the incidence of the use of episiotomy was found to have doubled from 24.4 to 46.7% in a study of obstetric practice in residents of Wales (Chalmers *et al.* 1976), and episiotomy was performed in 62.5% of vaginal deliveries in the USA in 1979 (National Center for Health Statistics 1981). Thakar and Banta (1983) summarized both the benefits and risks of episiotomy in a comprehensive review of the literature. Despite undeniable benefit in ease of delivery in a proportion of cases, the risk of infection, blood loss, poor anatomical results, post-partum pain and dyspareunia may well outweigh the benefits, and the authors concluded that arguments for the widespread use of episiotomy do not withstand scientific scrutiny. An Australian Study (East & Webster 1995) found a decline in episiotomy rate from 65% in 1986 to 36% in 1992. The Argentine Episiotomy Trial Collaborative Group carried out a randomised controlled trial of selective vs routine episiotomy between 1990 and 1992 involving 2,606 women. The group concluded that routine episiotomy should be abandoned and that rates above 30% cannot be justified (Argentine Episiotomy Trial Collaborative Group 1993).

Uncomplicated pregnancy entails many psychological adjustments to change of body image and episiotomy is seen as a further (and in many cases unnecessary) insult, which leaves a women feeling scarred both physically and psychologically. However small the actual cut may be, delays in suturing can interfere with the mother's first interaction with her baby, and pain and discomfort in the puerperium may disturb the establishment of breast feeding. Dyspareunia shortly after delivery may cause a woman to lose confidence in her ability to have satisfying intercourse, which may persist long after any physical cause can be found for discomfort, which may in turn lead to marital disharmony and depression (Kitzinger 1981). However, antenatal and post-partum counselling about episiotomy may facilitate psychological adjustment (Reading *et al.* 1983).

Vulvectomy

There have been few studies of the psychosocial and sexual adjustment of patients who have undergone this severely disfiguring surgery. Di Saia *et al.* (1979) reported on 18 patients treated with wide local excision rather than radical vulvectomy and found that all the patients maintained sexual responsiveness. A more detailed study has been made by Andersen and Hacker (1983) of 15 patients, aged between 50 and 70 years, who had undergone either total or partial vulvectomy. Psychological testing showed scores of depression comparable with other patients who had any form of cancer. Physical disabilities caused by leg oedema and urinary problems curtailed some social activities and there was a reduction of sexual activity and arousal. Numbness of the perineum and a loss of, or failure to maintain, orgasm, whether or not the clitoris has been excised, contributed to this, and led in some cases to marital distress, disruption of body image and sexual anxiety.

A study by Moth *et al.* (1983) of 14 women (aged between 32 and 60 years) who had undergone vulvectomy, and of nine of their sexual partners, revealed that although all the patients had satisfactory sexual relationships before the operations about two-thirds reported dyspareunia and almost all some form of sexual dysfunction after the operation. The women disliked the appearance of the operation area and half of the men felt differently towards their partners' bodies. The women experienced reduced libido, depression and loss of self confidence. The authors underlined the need for pre- and postoperative counselling for the patient and her partner to prepare them for the sexual problems likely to be encountered.

These points have been further stressed in a report by the same authors (Andreasson *et al.* 1986) on a larger group; 25 women and 15 partners have now been studied following vulvectomy. More than half the women had both sexual dysfunction and psychological problems, while almost half the men had psychological problems. Corney *et al.* (1993) reviewed, amongst others who had gynaecological surgery for cancer, 28 patients who had undergone a vulvectomy. Psychosexual dysfunction was found to be related to both physical and psychological causes, and to be most marked in the younger and single women. The authors advocated prospective surveys, and noted the need for more imparting of information preoperatively. A further general account of this problem was given by Crowther *et al.* (1994). The assumption that patients in the older age group will not wish to remain sexually active has been shown to be untrue, and it is noteworthy that many patients in these studies attempted to maintain a sexual life despite physical loss and emotional disruption. The current trend towards individualization of treatment for vulval carcinoma will reduce the incidence of such extensive mutilating surgery.

Sexual dysfunction

The commonest form of sexual dysfunction leading to a woman seeking help is lack or loss of sexual feeling. It may be an expression of problems in a relationship, a symptom of depressive or debilitating physical illness, or related to a dermatological condition (Dalziel 1995). Sexual arousal disorders, orgasmic dysfunction, sexual aversion, vaginismus and dyspareunia may also be presenting symptoms, all of which will require full psychological and physical assessment. For those cases where a major psychiatric or organic illness has been excluded, various psychotherapeutic techniques may be applied ranging from individual counselling, joint counselling with a sexual partner or group therapy. Treatments may be carried out by organizations such as Relate, by psychologists, psychiatrists and by specially trained nurses or social workers. The sexual problems of victims of sexual abuse in childhood often require a treatment programme based on cognitive behavioural principles together with general counselling focusing on interpersonal relationships over a prolonged period (Hawton 1995).

References

Ader, R., Cohen, D. & Felten, D. (1995) Psychoneuroimmunology: interaction between the nervous system and the immune system. *Lancet* **345**, 99–103.

Adshead, G. (1996) Psychological trauma and its influence on genuine and false complaints of sexual assault. *Medical Science and the Law* **36**, 95–99.

Andersen, B.L. & Hacker, N.F. (1983) Psychosexual adjustment after vulval surgery. *Obstetrics and Gynaecology* **62**, 457–462.

Andreasson, B., Moth, I., Jensen, S.B. & Bock, J.E. (1986) Sexual function partners. *Acta Obstetrica et Gynaecologica Scandinavica* **65**, 7–10.

Argentine Episiotomy Trial Collaborative Group (1993) Routine vs selective episiotomy: a randomised controlled trial. *Lancet* **342**: 1517–1518.

Aziz, F.A. (1980) Gynaecologic and obstetric complications of female circumcision. *International Journal of Gynaecology and Obstetrics* **17**, 560–563.

Barsky, A.J. & Klerman, G.L. (1983) Overview: hypochondriasis, bodily complaints and somatic styles. *American Journal of Psychiatry* **140**, 273.

Bartrop, R.W., Lazarus, L., Luckhurst, E., Kilah, L.G. & Penny, R. (1977) Depressed lymphocyte function after bereavement. *Lancet* i, 835–836.

Bebbington, P.E. (1976) Monosymptomatic hypochondriasis, abnormal illness behaviour and suicide. *British Journal of Psychiatry* **128**, 475–478.

Bettelheim, B. (1954) *Meaning of Initiation Symbolic Wounds: Puberty Rites and the Envious Male*, pp. 104–127. Free Press, Glencoe, IL.

Black, J. (1997) Female genital mutilation: a contemporary issue, and a Victorian obsession. *Journal of the Royal Society of Medicine* **90**, 402–405.

Black, J.A. & Debelle, G.D. (1995) Female genital mutilation in Britain. *British Medical Journal* **310**, 1590–1592.

Bradley, J.J. (1963) Severe localised pain associated with the depressive syndrome. *British Journal of Psychiatry* **109**, 741–745.

Chalmers, I. Zlosnik, J.E., Johns, K.A. *et al.* (1976) Obstetric practice and outcome of pregnancy in Cardiff residents. *British Medical Journal* **1**, 735.

Corney, R.H., Crowther, M.E., Everett, H., Howells, A. & Shepherd, J.H. (1993) Psychosexual dysfunction in women with gynaecological cancer following radical surgery. *British Journal of Obstetrics and Gynaecology* **100**, 73–78.

Cotterill, J.A. (1983) Psychiatry and skin diseases. In: *Recent Advances in Dermatology*, Vol. 6 (eds A.J. Rook & H.I. Maibach). Churchill Livingstone, Edinburgh.

Crowther, M.E., Corney, R.H. & Shepherd, H.H. (1994) Psychosexual implications of gynaecological cancer. *British Medical Journal* **310**, 1592–1593.

Davies, D.M. (1985) Plastic and reconstructive surgery: cosmetic surgery 11. *British Medical Journal* **290**, 1499–1501.

Dalziel, K.L. (1995) Effect of lichen sclerosus on sexual function and parturition. *Journal of Reproductive Medicine* **40**, 351–354.

Di Saia, P.J., Cressman, W.T. & Rich, W.M. (1979) An alternative approach to early cancer of the vulva. *American Journal of Obstetrics and Gynaecology* **133**, 825.

Duddle, M. (1991) Emotional sequelae of sexual assault. *Journal of the Royal Society of Medicine* **84**, 26–28.

East C., Webster J. (1995) Episiotomy at the Royal Women's Hospital, Brisbane: A comparison of practices in 1986 and 1992. *Midwifery* **11(4)**: 195–200.

Finkelhor, D. (1994) The international epidemiology of child sexual abuse. *Child Abuse and Neglect* **18**, 409–417.

Fitzpatrick, R., Frost, D. & Ikkos, C. (1986) Survey of psychological disturbance in patients attending a sexually transmitted diseases clinic. *Genitourinary Medicine* **62**, 111–115.

French, A.P. & Nelson, H.L. (1972) Genital self-mutilation in women. *Archives of General Psychiatry* **27**, 618–621.

Frost, D.P. (1985) Recognition of hypochondriasis in a clinic for sexually transmitted disease. *Genitourinary Medicine* **61**, 133–137.

Gallard, C. (1995) Female genital mutilation in France. *British Medical Journal* **310**, 1592–1593.

Gelfand, M. (1973) Gross enlargement of the labia minora in an African female. *Central African Journal of Medicine* **19**, 101.

Goldberg, D.P., Kay, C. & Thompson, L. (1976) Psychiatric morbodity in general practice and in the community. *Psychological Medicine* **656**, 5–9.

Graham, H. (1950) *Eternal Eve*. Heinemann, London.

Hall, J.G. (1985) Emotion and immunity (correspondence). *Lancet* **ii**, 326–327.

Handfield-Jones, S.E., Hinde, F.J.R. & Kennedy, C.T.C. (1987) Lichen sclerosus et atrophicus in children misdiagnosed as sexual abuse. *British Medical Journal* **294**, 1404–1405.

Hawton, K. (1995) Treatment of sexual dysfunction by sex therapy and other approaches. *British Journal of Psychiatry* **167**, 307–314.

Healey, T. (1978) Those little perforations. *World Medicine* **14**, 99–102.

Hey, F., Bucham, P.C., Littlewood, J.M. & Hall, R.I. (1986) Differential diagnosis in child sexual abuse. *Lancet* i, 792–796.

Hobbs, C.J. & Wynne, J.M. (1986) Buggery in childhood—common syndrome of child abuse. *Lancet* ii, 792–796.

Hoenig, J. & Kenna, J.C. (1974) The prevalence of transsexualism in England and Wales. *British Journal of Psychiatry* **124**, 181–190.

Junaid, T.A. & Thomas, S.M. (1981) Cysts of the vulva and vagina: a comparative study. *International Journal of Gynaecology and Obstetrics* **19**, 239–243.

Kenyon, F.E. (1976) Hypochondriacal states. *British Journal of Psychiatry* **129**, 1–14.

Kitzinger, S. (ed.) (1981) Emotional aspects of episiotomy and postnatal sexual adjustment. In: *Episiotomy, Physical and Emotional Aspects*, pp. 45–53. National Childbirth Trust, London.

Knight, B. (1976) *Sexual Offences in Legal Aspects of Medical Practice*, pp. 160–168. Churchill Livingstone, London.

Kronfol, Z., Silca, J., Greden, J. *et al.* (1983) Impaired lymphocyte function in depressive illness. *Life Science* **33**, 241–247.

Kuiper, B. & Cohen-Kettenis, P. (1988) Sex reassignment surgery: a study of 141 Dutch transsexuals. *Activities of Sexual Behaviour* **17**, 439–457.

Lancet (editorial) (1985) Emotion and immunity. *Lancet* **ii**, 133–134.

Lancet (editorial) (1987) Depression, stress and immunity. *Lancet* i, 1467–1468.

Lawhead, R.A. & Majmudar, B. (1990) Early diagnosis of vulvar neoplasia as a result of vulvar self-examination. *Journal of Reproductive Medicine* **35**, 1134–1137.

London Rape Crisis Centre (1984) *Sexual Violence*. Women's Press Handbook Series, London.

Lothstein, L.M. (1982) Sex reassignment surgery: historical, bioethical and theoretical issues. *American Journal of Science* **139**, 417–426.

Lucas, C.J., Sainsbury, P. & Collins, J.C. (1962) A social and clinical study of delusions in schizophrenia. *Journal of Science* **108**, 747–758.

Lyell, A. (1979) Cutaneous artefactual disease. A review amplified by personal experience. *Journal of the American Academy of Dermatology* **1**, 391–407.

Lyell, A. (1983) The Michelson Lecture: Delusions of parasitosis. *British Journal of Dermatology* **108**, 485–499.

McKenna, P.J. (1984) Disorders with overvalued ideas. *British Journal of Psychiatry* **145**, 579–585.

McLean, S. (1980) *Female Circumcision, Excision and Infibulation: The Facts and Proposals for Change*. Minority Rights Group Report, No. 47. London.

Macready, N. (1996) Female genital mutilation outlawed in United States. *British Medical Journal* **313**, 1103.

Money, J. & Ambinder, R. (1978) Two year, real life diagnostic test rehabilitation versus cure. In: *Controversy in Psychiatry* (eds J.P. Brady & H.K.H. Brodie), pp. 833–845. Saunders, Philadelphia.

Monro, A. (1980) Monosymptomatic hypochondriacal psychosis. *British Journal of Hospital Medicine* **24**, 34–38.

Moth, I., Andreasson, B., Jensen, S.B. & Bock, J.E. (1983) Sexual dysfunction and somato-psychic reactions after vulvectomy: a preliminary report. *Danish Medical Bulletin* **30**, 27–30.

Mullen, P., Martin, J., Anderson, J., Romans, S. & Herbison, G. (1993) Childhood sexual abuse and mental health in adult life. *British Journal of Psychiatry* **163**, 721–732.

National Center for Health Statistics (1981) *Data from the Hospital Discharge Survey* (furnished by Eileen McCarthy). Hyattsville, ML.

Onuigbo, W.I.B. (1976) Vulval epidermoid cysts in the Igbos of Nigeria. *Archives of Dermatology* **112**, 1405–1406.

Pedder, J.R. & Goldberg, D.P. (1970) A survey by questionnaire of psychiatric disturbance in patients attending a venereal disease clinic. *British Journal of Venereal Diseases* **46**, 58–61.

Reading, A.E., Sledmere, C.M., Cox, D.N. & Campbell, S. (1983) How women view post-episiotomy pain. *British Medical Journal* **284**, 243–246.

Royal College of Physicians (1997) *Physical Signs of Sexual Abuse in Children. Report of the Royal College of Physicians*, 2nd edn. Royal College of Physicians, London.

Schliefer, S.J., Keller, S.E., Camerino, M., Thornton, J.C. & Stein, M. (1983) Suppression of lymphocyte stimulation following bereavement. *Journal of the American Medical Association* **250**, 374–377.

Scott, D. (1978) Psychiatric aspects of sexual medicine. In: *Epilepsy 1978: Perspectives on Epilepsy*, pp. 89–97. Compiled by the British Epilepsy Association, Woking.

Shandall, A.A. (1967) Circumcision and infibulation of females. A general consideration of the problem and a clinical study of the complications of Sudanese women. *Sudan Medical Journal* **5**, 178–212.

Spencer, S.S., Spencer, D.D., Williamson, P.D. & Mattson, R.H. (1983) Sexual automatisms in complex partial seizures. *Neurology* **33**, 527–533.

Thakar, S.B. & Banta, H.D. (1983) Benefits and risks of episiotomy: an interpretative review of the English language literature 1860–1980. *Obstetrical and Gynaecological Survey* **38**, 322–338.

Whitlock, F.A. (1976) Psychophysiological aspects of skin diseases. *Major Problems in Dermatology*, Vol. 8. WB Saunders, London, pp. 110–127.

Wiens, J. (1996) Female circumcision is curbed in Egypt. *British Medical Journal* **313**, 249.

Wilbers, D., Vennstra, G., Van de Wiel, H. & Schultz, W. (1992) Sexual contact in the doctor patient relationship in the Netherlands. *British Medical Journal* **304**, 1531–1534.

Chapter 8: Cysts and non-neoplastic swellings of the vulva

H. Fox & C.H. Buckley

Cysts

Cysts of the vulval region may arise in developmental remnants, can form following blockage of gland ducts or may be the result of epithelial inclusions; they may also develop in endometriotic foci.

Bartholin's gland duct cysts

These cysts develop as a consequence of obstruction to the main duct of Bartholin's gland, which results in the retention of secretions. Most occur between the ages of 20 and 50 years (Azzaz 1978) and the duct obstruction is usually due to previous infection. The cysts are found in the posterior part of the labium majora and may measure anything from 1 to 10 cm in diameter. They contain clear watery or mucoid fluid and are lined by transitional epithelium (Fig. 8.1), which frequently undergoes partial or complete squamous metaplasia. Compressed mucus-secreting glandular acini may be found in the cyst wall. These cysts are prone to repeated infection and this may result in a Bartholin's gland abscess. It has to be borne in mind that a carcinoma of Bartholin's gland duct may, because of ductal obstruction, first present as a Bartholin's cyst or abscess; excision of the entire cystic gland is therefore to be recommended, particularly in the older patient.

Epidermoid cysts

Epidermoid cysts of the vulva may develop from epithelial implants following surgical trauma, from epidermal inclusions occurring at fusion sites during embryogenesis or from obstructed sebaceous gland ducts that have undergone squamous metaplasia. They may be single (Fig. 8.2) or multiple and occur most commonly in the labia majora, where they are usually tethered to the overlying skin. They are lined by squamous epithelium and contain yellowish or greyish-white, flaky or greasy, laminated keratinous debris (Fig. 8.3). Partial rupture with leakage of cyst contents may elicit a foreign-body inflammatory response in the surrounding stroma, and this may eventually lead to local scarring of the skin.

Cysts of sebaceous glands

These cysts result from blockage of one or more of the numerous sebaceous glands of the labia majora and minora. They are commonly confused with epidermoid cysts because of the similarity of their clinical appearance and distribution but differ in being often surmounted by a punctum through which the cyst contents may leak, this leading to crusting. The cysts are lined by squamous epithelium showing sebaceous differentiation and contain greasy yellow material. It is not unusual for these cysts to become infected.

Mucinous cysts

Mucinous cysts of the vulva are not uncommon and whilst occurring mainly in adults are occasionally seen in adolescent girls (Friedrich & Wilkinson 1973). They are usually found in the vestibule where they develop secondary to obstruction of the duct of one of the many minor vestibular mucus-secreting glands; the cysts are therefore of urogenital sinus origin and not, as was once thought, of Mullerian origin (Robboy *et al.* 1978, Oi & Munn 1982). The cysts are lined by a mucinous epithelium similar to that seen in the endocervix (Fig. 8.4); this may show patchy squamous metaplasia.

Mesonephric (Gartner's duct) cysts

Cysts developing from remnants of the mesonephric duct arise in the lateral part of the vulva (Fig. 8.5). They are thin walled, contain clear, colourless fluid and are lined by cuboidal or low columnar epithelial cells; smooth muscle can be identified within their walls (Fig. 8.6).

Cysts of mammary-like glands

Van der Putte and van Gorp (1995) have described a vulval

cyst that originated in the collecting duct of a mammary-like gland (see below). The cyst lining was characterized by a basal layer of myoepithelial cells and a luminal layer of cuboidal to columnar cells with discrete cytoplasmic 'snouts'.

Cysts of the canal of Nuck

These arise from peritoneal extensions carried down into the labium majus by the round ligament as it passes from the abdominal cavity through the inguinal canal. The cysts

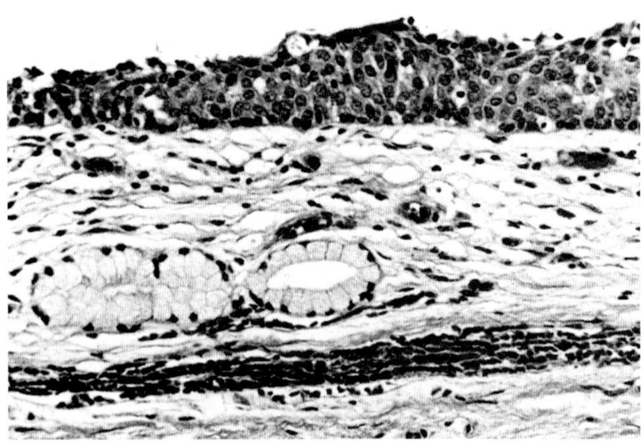

Fig. 8.1 A cyst of Bartholin's gland duct. The cyst is lined (above) by transitional epithelium, and mucus-secreting glandular acini are present in the wall.

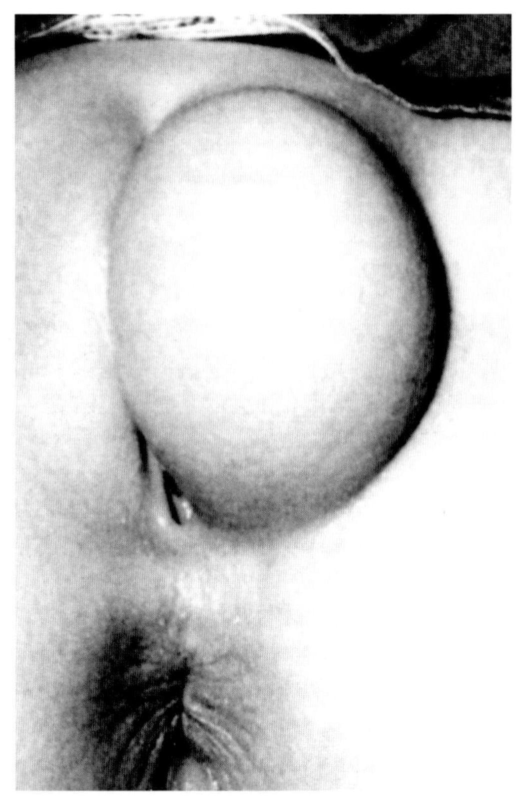

Fig. 8.2 An epidermoid cyst of the vulva.

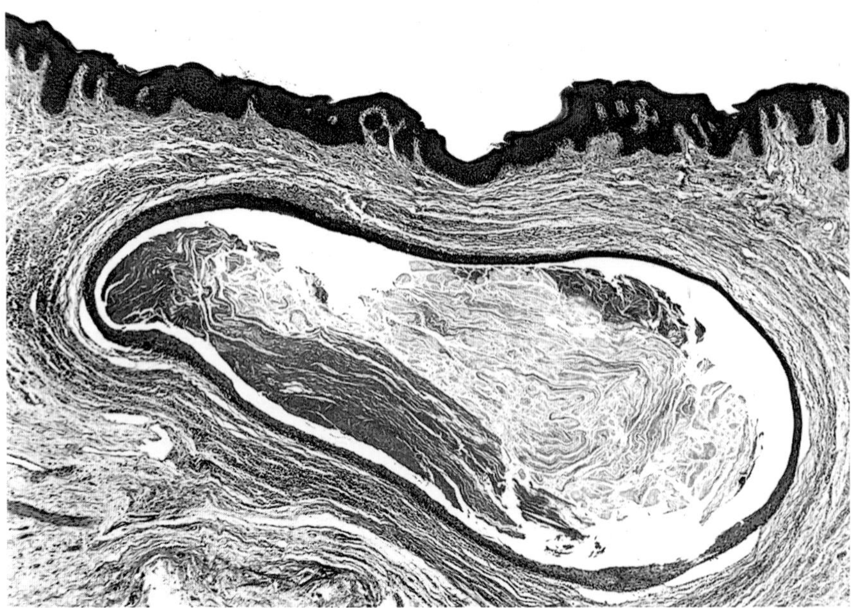

Fig. 8.3 Histological appearances of an epidermoid cyst of the vulva. The cyst is lined by squamous epithelium and contains keratinous material.

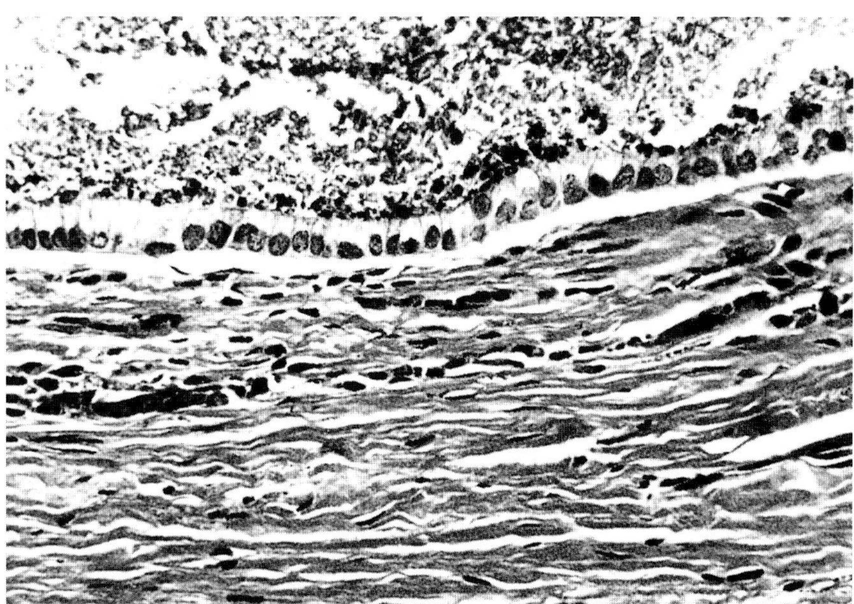

Fig. 8.4 A mucinous cyst of the vulva. The cyst is lined by columnar mucus-secreting cells and the cyst cavity contains inspissated mucinous material.

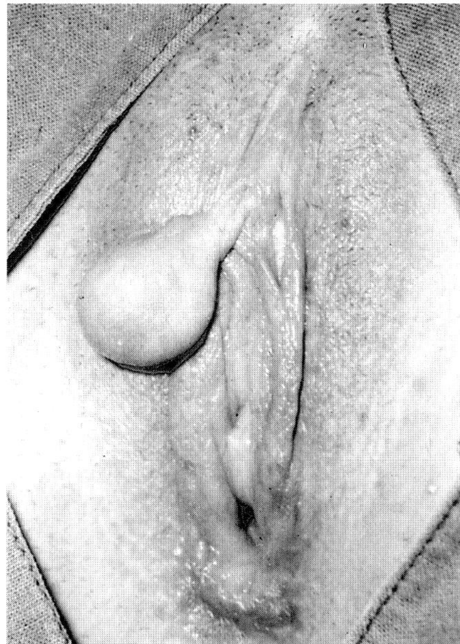

Fig. 8.5 A mesonephric (Gartner's) duct cyst.

occur in the upper part of the labia majora and are lined by a single layer of flattened mesothelium.

Steatocystoma

This lesion occasionally presents as a solitary cyst in the vulval region (Brownstein 1982). The cyst wall is intricately folded and the lining consists of squamous epithelium, which presents an apocrine appearance (Fig. 8.7). The cyst differs from a simple epidermal cyst by the presence of sebaceous glands in the cyst wall.

Non-neoplastic swellings

Included under this heading are a number of conditions linked only by the fact that they can present as a vulval mass, nodule or ulcer that can, clinically, be mistaken for a neoplasm.

Ectopic breast tissue

It has traditionally been thought that mammary tissue can occur in the vulva as a result of incomplete atresia of the mammary ridges (Levin & Diener 1968, Garcia *et al.* 1978, Reeves & Kaufman 1980, Gugliotta *et al.* 1983). This view has, however, recently been challenged by van der Putte (1991, 1993, 1994), who maintains that there is no embryological evidence to support the concept of mammary ridges in humans and that the structures generally regarded as ectopic, or accessory, breast tissue in the vulva are, in reality, mammary-like anogenital glands (Fig. 8.8). The evidence marshalled by van der Putte is impressive and, whilst there is no doubt that true ectopic mammary glands, complete with nipples, can very occasionally occur in the vulval region (Green 1936), it does appear that most cases of 'ectopic breast tissue' in the vulva are indeed mammary-like anogenital glands, which contain oestrogen and progesterone receptors and can show lactatory activity.

These glands may become clinically overt in young non-pregnant women who complain of cyclical swelling in the

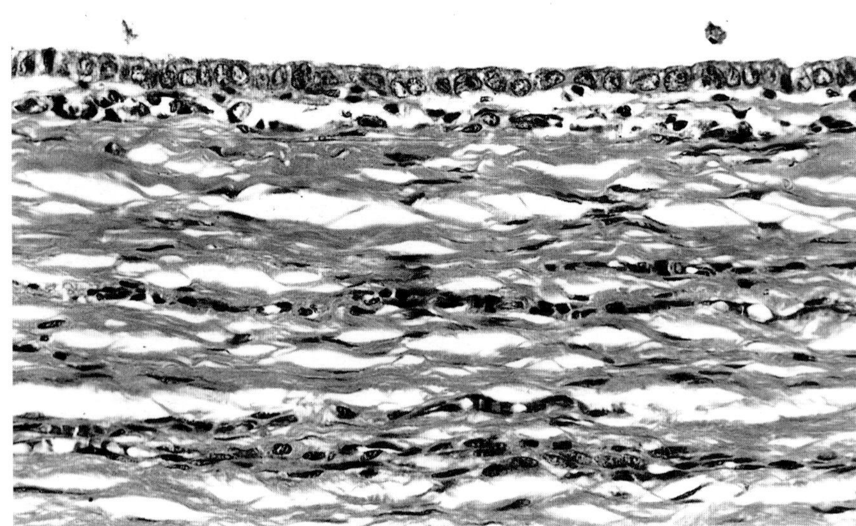

Fig. 8.6 A mesonephric (Gartner's) duct cyst. The cyst is lined (above) by tall cuboidal epithelial cells, and smooth muscle is present in the cyst wall.

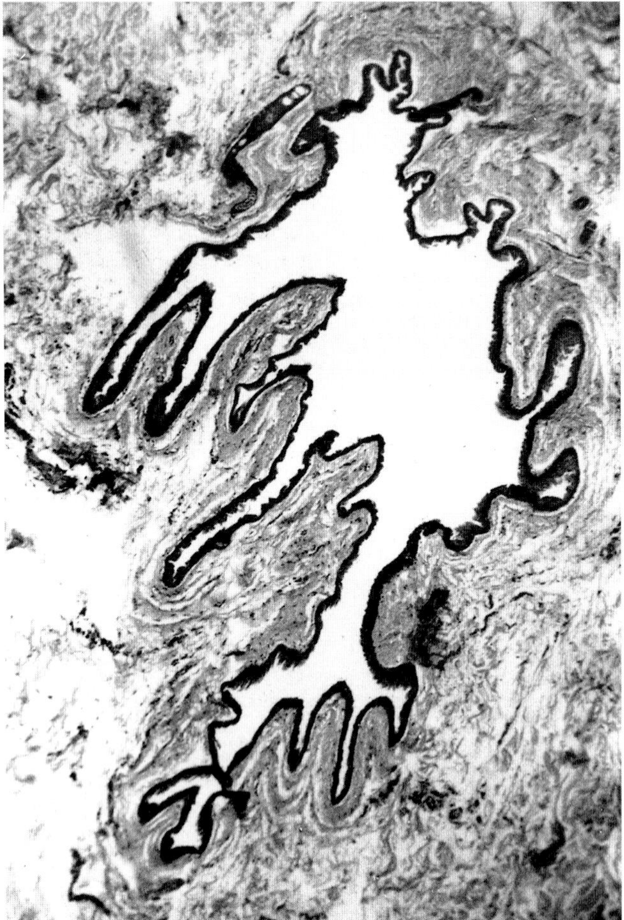

Fig. 8.7 Steatocystoma: the intricately folded cyst wall is composed of squamous epithelium showing apocrine differentiation.

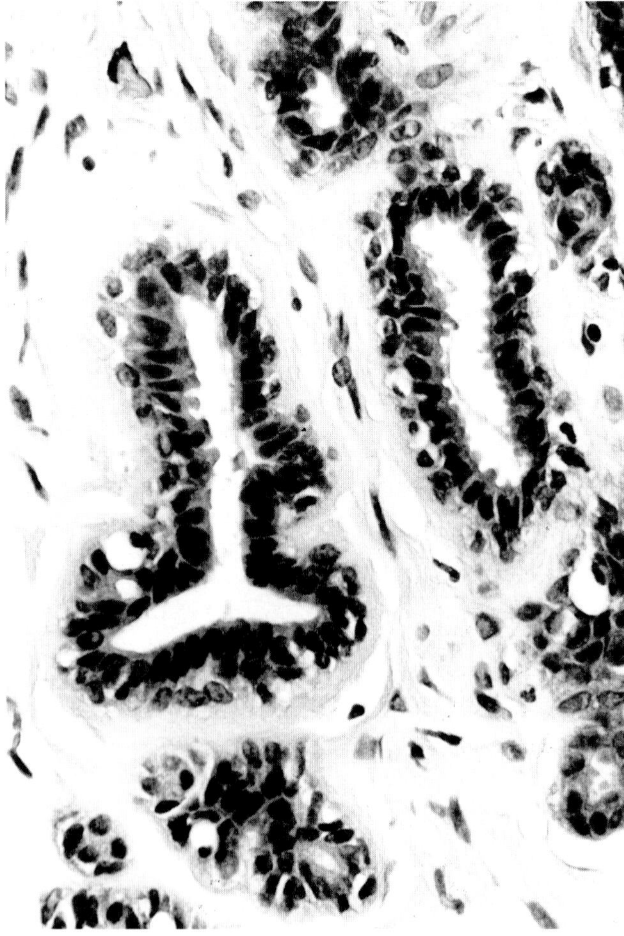

Fig. 8.8 Mammary-like anogenital glands in the vulva.

vulval region during the luteal phase of the menstrual cycle. Such cases are, however, exceptional and most patients present with a vulval swelling during the later months of pregnancy, this usually occurring, curiously, not in their first pregnancy but in subsequent gestations. The swelling is nearly always in the labia majora and is bilateral in about half the cases. Histologically the appearances are virtually identical to those of normal lactatory breast tissue.

Ectopic salivary tissue

An example of salivary gland tissue presenting as a vulval mass has been described (Marwah & Berman 1980). The salivary tissue was regarded as being ectopic in nature but, as it was associated with respiratory-type epithelium and cartilage, the true nature of this lesion is uncertain.

Endometriosis

Endometriosis of the vulva is uncommon. It can occur in an episiotomy scar (Brougher 1947, Catherwood & Cohen 1951), can complicate uterine curettage (Dutta 1987) and may follow implantation of menstrual fragments into a vulval surgical wound (Duson & Zelenik 1954); when occurring on the labia it has been postulated that endometrial fragments have migrated along the canal of Nuck (Janovski & Douglas 1972).

The lesion may be blue/purple and cystic, form a deep-seated, ill-defined, firm or fluctuant mass or appear as a painful nodule, which sometimes enlarges during menstruation. The histological appearances are characteristic of endometriosis.

Langerhans cell histiocytosis (see also Chapter 5)

Langerhans cell histiocytosis can involve the vulva either as a localized lesion or as one component of a multisystem disease (Curtis & Cawley 1947, McKay *et al.* 1953, Kierland *et al.* 1957, Borglin *et al.* 1966, Milodovnik *et al.* 1979, Issa *et al.* 1980, Lechner *et al.* 1983, Rose *et al.* 1984, Thomas *et al.* 1986, Schwartz & Zich 1989, McLelland & Chu 1990, Otis *et al.* 1990, Quiel *et al.* 1990, Axiotis *et al.* 1991, Saurel *et al.* 1992, Blaauwgeers *et al.* 1993, Voelklein *et al.* 1993, Savell *et al.* 1995). The patients are commonly in their third decade, although one patient with vulval Langerhans histiocytosis was 76 years old, and the vulval lesion may present as an area of local induration, as a nodule or as an ulcer (Fig. 8.9). Histologically there is characteristically a mixed cellular infiltrate of the dermis which extends into the epidermis; histiocytic cells predominate within this infiltrate but there are also a variable number of eosinophils, a few polymorphonuclear leucocytes and occasional lymphocytes and plasma cells. The histiocytes may be multinucleated or contain lobulated nuclei. Ultrastructural examination reveals the typical Birbeck's granules and the histiocytes stain positively for S100, Leu 6 and Leu M3.

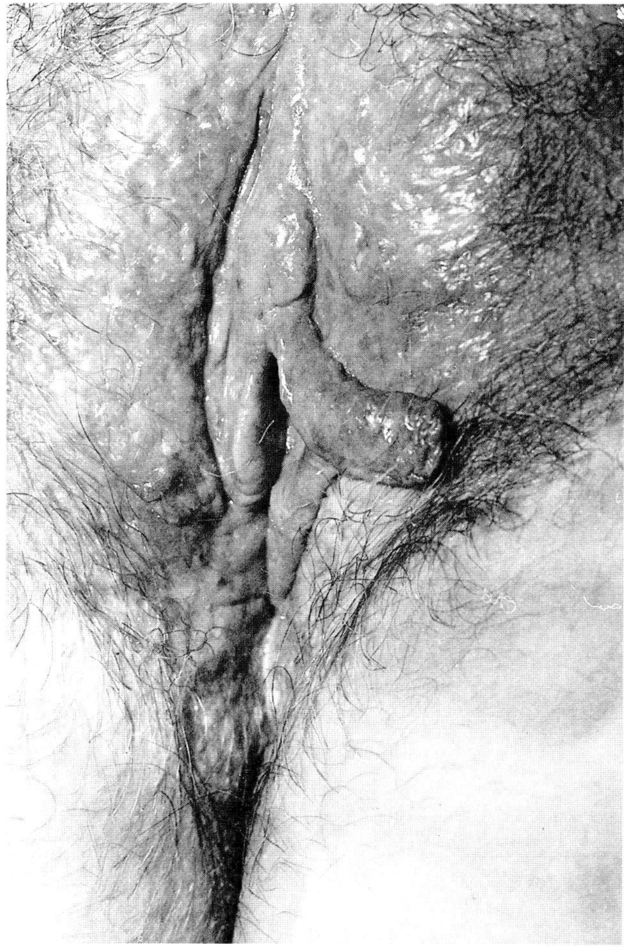

Fig. 8.9 Langerhans cell histiocytosis: diffuse nodulation, some superficial ulceration.

Nodular amyloidosis (see also Chapter 5)

The nodular cutaneous form of amyloidosis can involve the skin of the vulva where it may appear as an ulcerated nodule, which closely mimics the appearances of a squamous cell carcinoma (Northcutt & Vanover 1985, Gorodeski *et al.* 1988). Very occasionally vulval nodular amyloidosis has been the presenting feature of a systemic amyloidosis (Taylor *et al.* 1991).

Calcinosis

Calcinosis of the vulva is extremely rare (Jamaleddine *et al.* 1988, Balfour & Vincenti 1991, Fukaya & Veda 1991). Its pathogenesis is uncertain, although its development may possibly be linked to trauma. The condition presents as painless nodules, which appear on histological examination as homogeneous basophilic masses in the papillary dermis; they are usually surrounded by a lymphohistiocytic infiltrate, a few foreign-body-type giant cells and some haemosiderin. Von Kossa staining is positive.

Nodular fasciitis

Only 10 cases of nodular fasciitis of the vulva have been fully documented (Roberts & Daly 1981, Gaffney *et al.* 1982, LiVolsi & Brooks 1987, O'Connell *et al.* 1997), whilst one case has been briefly alluded to in a review of this lesion (Allen 1972).

The patients with vulval nodular fasciitis have ranged in age from 7 to 51 years, have presented with a short history of a vulval mass and have had mobile subcutaneous nodules, which measured 1.5–3.5 cm in diameter. The lesions had the typical histological features of this condition, namely plump fibroblasts arranged in bundles and fascicles set in a myxoid stroma with a mild or moderate lymphocytic infiltrate, intercellular clefts, numerous small blood vessels and a generous sprinkling of mitotic figures; multinucleated osteoclast-like cells may be present. Wide local excision was curative in all cases but there was a local recurrence in one patient in whom excision had been incomplete.

Postoperative spindle-cell nodule

These, as their name implies, develop within weeks or months of an operative procedure on the vulva and present as a rapidly growing mass (Proppe *et al.* 1984, Manson *et al.* 1995). Histologically they resemble a fibrosarcoma with sheets of spindle-shaped cells growing in a fascicular pattern and containing many mitotic figures. Despite their alarming appearances these nodules are a form of reactive response to tissue injury and will eventually resolve.

Rheumatoid nodule

Rheumatoid nodules occur in 20–30% of patients with rheumatoid arthritis and are usually located in the subcutaneous tissues over extensor surfaces. Histologically, they consist of a central area of necrosis surrounded by macrophages and fibrous tissue containing chronic inflammatory cells. A single example has been described of an ulcerating rheumatoid nodule in the vulva (Appleton & Ismail 1996): this occurred in a 76-year-old woman with rheumatoid arthritis and the appearances of the ulcerated mass, which was associated with inguinal lymphadenopathy, led to a clinical diagnosis of invasive carcinoma.

Desmoid tumor

Desmoid tumours are a form of local fibromatosis and, although histologically bland, can attain a large size, infiltrate neighbouring tissues and recur. They are formed of elongated, slender, spindle-shaped cells, which are separated from each other by abundant collagen. Only one desmoid tumour of the vulva has been recorded (Kfuri *et al.* 1981), this forming an indurated mass, 7 cm in diameter, in the labium majus of a 19-year-old woman. The patient was treated successfully by wide local excision.

Verruciform xanthoma

This non-neoplastic lesion can mimic a carcinoma, presenting as a cauliflower-like, verrucous or papillomatous nodule. It is characterized histologically by acanthosis and an accumulation of foamy xanthomatous cells within the papillary dermis between the acanthotic rete ridges. Santa Cruz and Martin (1979) described two examples of verruciform xanthoma of the vulva, one presenting as multiple warty lesions and the other as a single sessile mass.

Angiolymphoid hyperplasia with eosinophilia (see also Chapter 5)

This angiomatous inflammatory condition appears as intradermal or subcutaneous nodules; only very rarely is the vulva involved (Sanders *et al.* 1989, Aguilar *et al.* 1990, Scurry *et al.* 1995). Histologically, there is a dermal proliferation of thick- and thin-walled blood vessels with plump endothelial cells, which may focally obliterate the lumen; there is a stromal inflammatory infiltrate of eosinophils and lymphocytes.

The relationship between focal lesions of this type and eosinophilic lymphofolliculosis of the skin (Kimura's disease) is still a matter of dispute (Kuo *et al.* 1988).

Malacoplakia (see also Chapter 5)

This condition is thought to be the result of an inadequate, or atypical, inflammatory reponse to *Escherichia coli* and although involvement of the female genital tract by malacoplakia is well documented (Chen & Hendricks 1985) vulval lesions are extremely rare (Arul & Emmerson 1977, Bessim *et al.* 1991). Malacoplakia at this site may present as a nodule or as an ulcer. Two patients with malacoplakia of Bartholin's gland have also been recorded (Paquin *et al.* 1986) with, in both instances, the disease presenting as a cyst that contained a purulent exudate.

Histologically (Fig. 8.10), the lesion is formed predominantly by histiocytes, which contain variable numbers of cytoplasmic periodic acid–Schiff stain (PAS)-positive granules; there is usually an admixture of lymphocytes and plasma cells. The diagnosis is dependent upon the finding of Michaelis–Gutmann bodies, which may be intra- or extracellular and stain positively for iron and calcium.

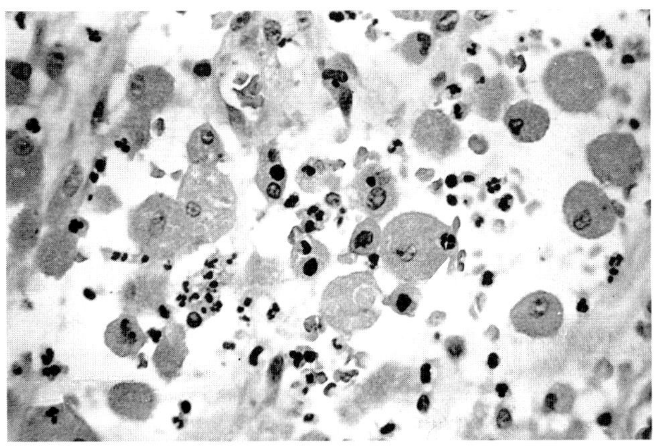

Fig. 8.10 Malacoplakia of the vulva: numerous large histiocytes are seen, some containing dense calcified Michaelis–Gutmann bodies.

Urethral caruncle

A urethral caruncle occurs in postmenopausal women as a red, fleshy, sessile or polypoid excrescence at the urethral meatus: it may measure from a few millimetres to a few centimetres in diameter. A caruncle is often asymptomatic but may cause dysuria or bleeding if ulcerated.

A urethral caruncle is simply a chronically inflamed everted portion of urethral mucosa and histologically (Fig. 8.11) there is highly vascular connective tissue heavily infiltrated by lymphocytes and plasma cells. Enmeshed in this inflamed stroma are varying quantities of glandular structures or solid islands of urethral epithelium, which is frequently ulcerated to display underlying granulation tisue.

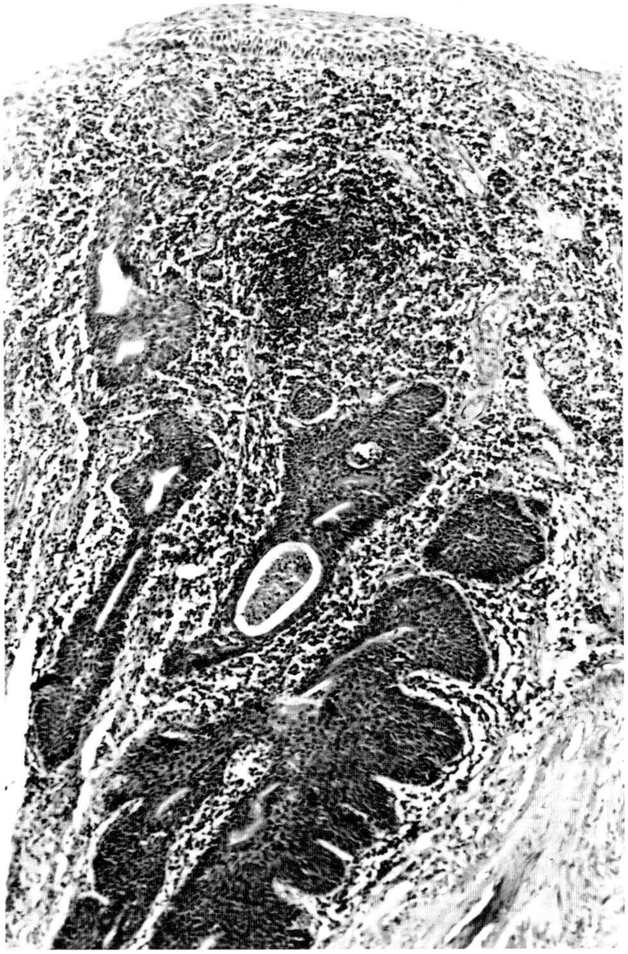

Fig. 8.11 A urethral caruncle. There is a marked inflammatory cell infiltrate, and separated islands and clefts of transitional epithelium are present.

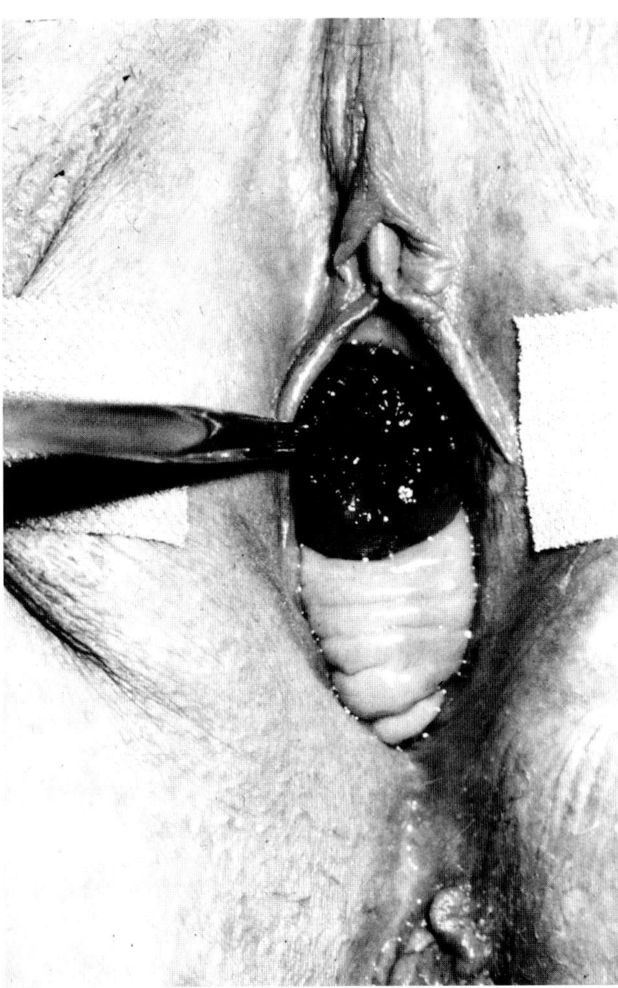

Fig. 8.12 Prolapsed urethral mucosa.

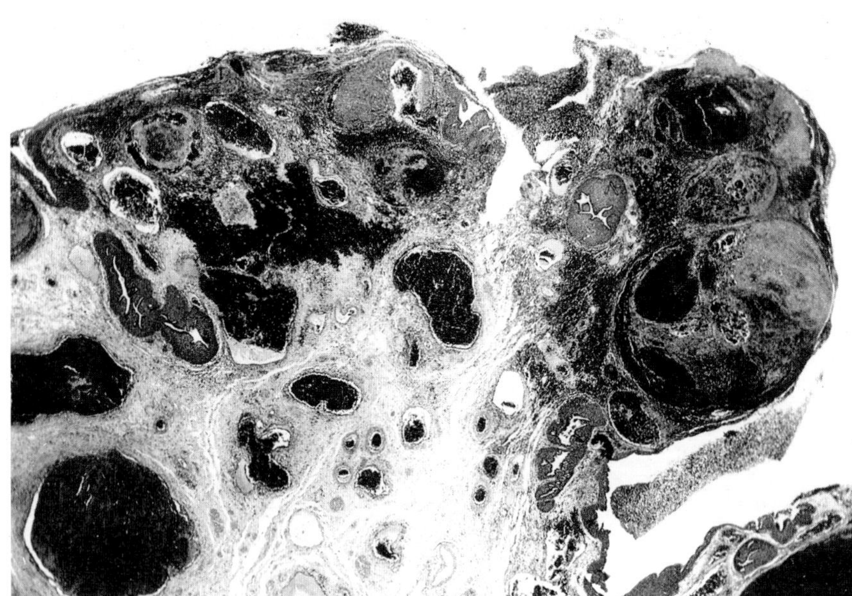

Fig. 8.13 Prolapsed urethral mucosa. The stroma contains markedly dilated vessels, some of which are thrombosed.

Urethral prolapse

Prolapse of the urethra may occur at any age and can be mistaken for a neoplasm (Fig. 8.12). Histologically, oedematous connective tissue is covered by urethral mucosa, which may be focally ulcerated. The underlying stroma shows marked vascular distension and engorgement, often with thrombosis (Fig. 8.13). The epithelial inclusions typically seen in a urethral caruncle are not present.

References

Aguilar, A., Ambrojo, P., Requena, L. *et al.* (1990) Angiolymphoid hyperplasia with eosinophilia limited to the vulva. *Clinical and Experimental Dermatology* **15**, 65–67.

Allen, P.W. (1972) Nodular fasciitis. *Pathology* **4**, 9–26.

Appleton, M.A. & Ismail, S.M. (1996) Ulcerating rheumatoid nodule of the vulva. *Journal of Clinical Pathology* **49**, 85–87.

Arul, K.J. & Emmerson, R.W. (1977) Malacoplakia of the skin. *Clinical and Experimental Dermatology* **2**, 131–135.

Axiotis, C.A., Merino, M.J. & Duray, P.H. (1991) Langerhans cell histiocytosis of the female genital tract. *Cancer* **67**, 1650–1660.

Azzaz, B.B. (1978) Bartholin's cyst and abscess: a review of treatment of 53 cases. *British Journal of Clinical Practice* **32**, 101–105.

Balfour, P.J.T. & Vincenti, A.C. (1991) Idiopathic vulvar calcinosis. *Histopathology* **18**, 183–184.

Bessim, S., Heller, D.S., Dottino, P., Deligdisch, L. & Gordon, R.E. (1991) Malakoplakia of the female genital tract causing urethral and ureteral obstruction: a case report. *Journal of Reproductive Medicine* **36**, 691–694.

Blaauwgeers, J.L., Bleker, O.P., Veltkamp, S. & Weigel, H.M. (1993) Langerhans cell histiocytosis of the vulva. *European Journal of Gynaecology Obstetrics and Reproductive Biology* **48**, 145–148.

Borglin, N.E., Sodestrom, J. & Wehlin, L. (1966) Eosinophilic granuloma histiocytosis X) of the vulva. *Journal of Obstetrics and Gynaecology of the British Commonwealth* **73**, 478–486.

Brougher, J.C. (1947) Endometrial cyst in an episiotomy scar. *American Journal of Obstetrics and Gynecology* **54**, 127–128.

Brownstein, M.H. (1982) Steatocystoma simplex. *Archives of Dermatology* **118**, 409–411.

Catherwood, A.E. & Cohen, E.S. (1951) Endometriosis with decidual reaction in episiotomy scar. *American Journal of Obstetrics and Gynecology* **62**, 1364–1366.

Chen, K.T.K. & Hendricks, E.J. (1985) Malakoplakia of the female genital tract. *Obstetrics and Gynecology* **65**, 84s–87s.

Curtis, A.C. & Cawley, E.P. (1947) Eosinophilic granuloma of bone with cutaneous manifestation. *Archives of Dermatology* **55**, 815–818.

Duson, C.K. & Zelenik, J.S. (1954) Vulvar endometriosis apparently produced by menstrual blood. *Obstetrics and Gynecology* **3**, 76–79.

Dutta, P. (1987) Vulval endometriosis. *Journal of the Indian Medical Association* **85**, 237–238.

Friedrich, E.G. & Wilkinson, E.J. (1973) Mucous cysts of the vulvar vestibule. *Obstetrics and Gynecology* **42**, 407–414.

Fukaya, Y. & Veda, H. (1991) A case of idiopathic vulvar calcinosis: the first in Japan. *Journal of Dermatology* **18**, 680–683.

Gaffney, E.F., Majmudar, B. & Bryan, J.A. (1982) Nodular (pseudosarcomatous) fasciitis of the vulva. *International Journal of Gynecological Pathology* **1**, 307–312.

Garcia, J.J., Verkauf, B.S., Hochberg, C.K. & Ingram, J.M. (1978) Aberrant breast tissue of the vulva: a case report and review of the literature. *Obstetrics and Gynecology* **52**, 225–228.

Gorodeski, I.G., Cordoba, M., Shapira, A. & Bahary, C.M. (1988) Primary localized cutaneous lichen amyloidosus of the vulva. *International Journal of Dermatology* **27**, 259–260.

Green, H.J. (1936) Adenocarcinoma of supernumary breasts of the labia majora in a case of epidermoid carcinoma of the vulva. *American Journal of Obstetrics and Gynecology* **31**, 660–663.

Gugliotta, P., Fibbi, M., Fessia, L., Canevini, P. & Bussolati, C. (1983) Lactating supernumary mammary gland tissue in the vulva. *Applied Pathology* **1**, 61–65.

Issa, P.Y., Saleem, P.A., Brihi, E. *et al.* (1980) Eosinophilic granuloma with involvement of the female genitalia. *American Journal of Obstetrics and Gynecology* **137**, 608–612.

Jamaleddine, F.N., Salman, S.M., Sabaklo, Z., Kibbi, A.G. & Zaynoun, S. (1988) Idiopathic vulvar calcinosis: the counterpart of idiopathic scrotal calcinosis. *Cutis* **41**, 273–275.

Janovski, N.A. & Douglas, C.P. (1972) *Diseases of the Vulva*. Harper & Row, Hagerstown, MD.

Kfuri, A., Rosenhein, N., Durfman, H. & Goldstein, P. (1981) Desmoid tumor of the vulva. *Journal of Reproductive Medicine* **26**, 272–273.

Kierland, R.B., Epstein, J.G. & Weber, W.E. (1957) Eosinophilic granuloma of skin and mucous membrane. *Archives of Dermatology* **75**, 45–54.

Kuo, T.T., Shih, L.Y. & Chan, H.L. (1988) Kimura's disease: involvement of regional lymph nodes and distinction from angiolymphoid hyperplasia with eosinophilia. *American Journal of Surgical Pathology* **12**, 843–854.

Lechner, W., Ortner, A., Thoni, A. *et al.* (1983) Histiocytosis X in gynecology. *Gynecologic Oncology* **15**, 253–260.

Levin, N. & Diener, R.L. (1968) Bilateral ectopic breast of the vulva. *Obstetrics and Gynecology* **32**, 274–276.

LiVolsi, V.A. & Brooks, J.J. (1987) Nodular fasciitis of the vulva: a report of two cases. *Obstetrics and Gynecology* **69**, 513–516.

McKay, D.G., Street, R.B., Benirschke, K. & Duncan, C.J. (1953) Eosinophilic granuloma of the vulva. *Surgery Gynecology and Obstetrics* **96**, 437–447.

McLelland, J. & Chu, A.C. (1990) Multisystem Langerhans cell histiocytosis in adults. *Clinical and Experimental Dermatology* **15**, 79–82.

Manson, C.M., Hirsch, P.J. & Coyne, J.D. (1995) Post-operative spindle cell nodule of the vulva. *Histopathology* **26**, 571–574.

Marwah, S. & Berman, M.L. (1980) Ectopic salivary gland in the vulva (choristoma): report of a case and review of the literature. *Obstetrics and Gynecology* **56**, 389–391.

Milodovnik, M., Adatto, R., Adoni, A. *et al.* (1979) Vulval eosinophilic granuloma. *Acta Obstetricia et Gynecologica Scandinavica* **58**, 565–567.

Northcutt, A.D. & Vanover, M.J. (1985) Nodular cutaneous amyloidosis involving the vulva: case report and literature review. *Archives of Dermatology* **121**, 518–521.

O'Connell, J.X., Young, R.H., Nielsen, G.P. *et al.* (1997) Nodular fasciitis of the vulva: a study of six cases and literature review. *International Journal of Gynecological Pathology* **16**, 117–123.

Oi, R.H. & Munn, R. (1982) Mucous cysts of the vulvar vestibule. *Human Pathology* **13**, 584–586.

Otis, C.N., Fischer, R.A., Johnson, N., Kelleher, J.F. & Powell, J.L. (1990) Histiocytosis X of the vulva: a case report and review of the literature. *Obstetrics and Gynecology* **75**, 555–558.

Paquin, M.L., Davis, J.R. & Weiner, S. (1986) Malakoplakia of Bartholin's gland. *Archives of Pathology and Laboratory Medicine* **110**, 757–758.

Proppe, K.H., Scully, R.E. & Rosai, J. (1984) Postoperative spindle cell nodules of the genitourinary tract resembling sarcomas: a report of eight cases. *American Journal of Surgical Pathology* **8**, 101–108.

Quiel, V., Sieg, U. & Ehrhardt, G. (1990) Genitale Manifestation einer Histiozytose X. *Zentralblatt für Gynäkologie* **112**, 1189–1191.

Reeves, K.O. & Kaufman, R.H. (1980) Vulvar ectopic breast tissue mimicking periclitoral abscess. *American Journal of Obstetrics and Gynecology* **137**, 509–511.

Robboy, S.J., Ross, J.S., Part, J., Keh, P.C. & Welch, W.R. (1978) Urogenital sinus origin of mucinous and ciliated cysts of the vulva. *Obstetrics and Gynecology* **51**, 347–351.

Roberts, W. & Daly, J.W. (1981) Pseudosarcomatous fasciitis of the vulva. *Gynecologic Oncology* **11**, 383–386.

Rose, P.G., Johnston, G.C. & O'Toole, R.V. (1984) Cutaneous histiocytosis X of the vulva. *Obstetrics and Gynecology* **64**, 587–590.

Sanders, C.J.G., Hursman, R.-F.H.J. & van Weersch-Rietjens, L.C.S.M. (1989) Angiolymphoid hyperplasia with eosinophilia. *British Journal of Dermatology* **121**, 536–538.

Santa Cruz, D.J. & Martin, S.A. (1979) Verruciform xanthoma of the vulva. *American Journal of Clinical Pathology* **71**, 224–228.

Saurel, J., Savin de Larclause, A.M., Mercier, M. *et al.* (1992) Histiocytose à cellules de Langerhans de la vulve: revue générale à propos d'une observation. *Journal de Gynécologie Obstétrique et Biologie de la Reproduction (Paris)* **21**, 897–901.

Savell, V., Hanna, R., Benda, J.A. & Argenyi, Z.B. (1995) Histiocytosis X of the vulva with a confusing clinical and pathologic presentation: a case report. *Journal of Reproductive Medicine* **40**, 323–326.

Schwartz, A. & Zich, P. (1989) Eosinophilic histiocytic granuloma of the vulva and cervix. *Sbornik Lekarsky (Praha)* **91**, 1–4.

Scurry, J., Dennerstein, G. & Brenan, J. (1995) Angiolymphoid hyperplasia with eosinophilia of the vulva. *Australian and New Zealand Journal of Obstetrics and Gynaecology* **35**, 347–348.

Taylor, S.C., Baker, E. & Grossman, M.E. (1991) Nodular vulvar amyloid as a presentation of systemic amyloidosis. *Journal of the American Academy of Dermatology* **24**, 139.

Thomas, R., Barnhill, D., Bibro, M. *et al.* (1986) Histiocytosis X in gynecology: a case presentation and review of the literature. *Obstetrics and Gynecology* **67**, 46s–49s.

van der Putte, S.C.J. (1991) Anogenital 'sweat' glands: histology and pathology of a gland that may mimic mammary glands. *American Journal of Dermatopathology* **13**, 557–565.

van der Putte, S.C.J. (1993) Ultrastructure of the human anogenital 'sweat' gland. *Anatomical Record* **235**, 583–590.

van der Putte, S.C.J. (1994) Mammary-like glands of the vulva and their disorders. *International Journal of Gynecological Pathology* **13**, 150–160.

van der Putte, S.C.J. & van Group, L.H.M. (1995) Cysts of mammarylike glands in the vulva. *International Journal of Gynecological Pathology* **14**, 184–188.

Voelklein, K., Horny, H.P., Marzusch, K. & Dietl, J. (1993) Histiozytosis X (Langerhanszell-Granulomatose) der Vulva. *Geburtshilfe und Frauenheilkunde* **53**, 198–200.

Chapter 9: Non-epithelial tumours of the vulva

H. Fox & C.H. Buckley

Mesenchymal neoplasms

All mesenchymal neoplasms of the vulva are either rare or extremely uncommon. Virtually all, whether benign or malignant, present as enlarging, but otherwise asymptomatic, vulval masses, which usually defy specific clinical diagnosis. Indeed, the clinical appearance of these tumours can be very misleading, for benign neoplasms, which are often pedunculated because of the effects of gravity, may become ulcerated and secondarily infected, a not unexpected outcome in view of the effects of local moisture and warmth together with friction from tight underclothing. A benign tumour with an ulcerated surface and secondary infection producing reactive enlargement of regional lymph nodes can clearly impart a false impression of malignancy.

Accurate identification of many malignant mesenchymal neoplasms on purely histological grounds can be very difficult or even impossible, but until recently the only other aid available to the histopathologist was electron microscopy, which is of only limited value in many of these neoplasms. The introduction of immunocytochemistry allowed, however, for much greater diagnostic accuracy to be attained in many sarcomas, whilst molecular genetic and cytogenetic studies have shown that many sarcomatous entities are characterized by specific translocations.

Tumours of smooth muscle

LEIOMYOMA

Vulval leiomyomas are relatively uncommon, and fewer than 100 examples have been documented (Lovelady *et al.* 1941, Palermino 1964, Riedel 1964, Tavassoli & Norris 1979, Smit *et al.* 1984, Yokoyama *et al.* 1987, Newman & Fletcher 1991, Neri *et al.* 1993, Nielsen *et al.* 1996a), although the majority of such neoplasms now pass unrecorded. There is no known association with uterine leiomyomas and it is far from clear whether these tumours originate from the smooth muscle of the vulval erectile tissue, from the muscular elements of the round ligament or from the myoepithelial cells of Bartholin's gland; most arise, however, in the labia majora and leiomyomas limited to the clitoris (Stenchever *et al.* 1973) or Bartholin's gland (Tavassoli & Norris 1979, Katenkamp & Stiller 1980) are distinctly rare.

Vulval leiomyomas occur during the reproductive years and have a tendency to enlarge during pregnancy; their size may also increase in women receiving hormonal treatment and these features, together with their content of progesterone and oestrogen receptors, suggest that they are, to some extent at least, hormone dependent (Siegle & Cartmell 1995). Leiomyomas usually present as well-circumscribed, painless, non-tender nodules or swellings in the labia: they are formed of firm, white, whorled tissue.

Histologically, leiomyomas of the vulva are generally similar to their more commonly occurring counterparts in the uterine body. They have, by definition, well-circumscribed, non-infiltrating margins, show little or no pleomorphism or atypia, and contain fewer than two mitotic figures per 10 high-power fields (Tavassoli & Norris 1979). Cellular (Kaufman & Gardner 1965), epithelioid (Tavassoli & Norris 1979, Aneiros *et al.* 1982, Newman & Fletcher 1991), symplastic and neurolemmoma-like variants can all occur at the vulva. The histological criteria, discussed below, for recognizing those vulval smooth-muscle neoplasms that are likely to behave as low-grade leiomyosarcomas are far from absolute and hence all require wide local excision.

LEIOMYOSARCOMA

Malignant smooth-muscle neoplasms of the vulva take two forms. One is that of a clearly sarcomatous tumour with considerable pleomorphism and mitotic activity whilst the other closely resembles a leiomyoma but nevertheless behaves in a malignant fashion. The clearly malignant neoplasms may or may not be easily recognizable as being of smooth-muscle origin and in doubtful cases a positive staining reaction for smooth-muscle actin and/or desmin is of considerable diagnostic value.

Easily recognizable leiomyosarcomas of the vulva, showing unmistakable histological evidence of malignancy, are rare (DiSaia *et al.* 1971, Pandhi *et al.* 1975, Davos & Abell 1976, Verhaegh *et al.* 1977, Audet-Lapointe *et al.* 1980, Smit *et al.* 1984, Guidozzi *et al.* 1987, Lenaz *et al.* 1987, Krag-Moller *et al.* 1990, Kuller *et al.* 1990, Patel *et al.* 1993, Nirenberg *et al.* 1995). These tumours have occurred in women aged from 35 to 84 years, although the mean age at initial presentation was just over 50 years. Patients with a neoplasm of this type usually have a history of less than 12 months of an enlarging vulval mass and most leiomyosarcomas arise in the labia. In most reported cases initial treatment was by local excision and the true diagnosis was only recognized on histological examination; nearly all patients treated solely by local excision alone suffer tumour recurrence. Other patients have been treated by radical surgery, often supplemented by radiotherapy or chemotherapy, and about 50% of such patients have died, the length of survival ranging from 6 months to 16 years and death being usually due to pulmonary, hepatic or skeletal metastases.

All the tumours discussed so far were overtly malignant and can be regarded as leiomyosarcomas of high-grade malignancy. Tavassoli and Norris (1979) looked at the question of malignancy in vulval smooth-muscle neoplasms from a quite different viewpoint. They studied 32 vulval neoplasms, which were quite clearly of smooth-muscle nature, and attempted to define criteria for the recognition of those neoplasms which, whilst not having any obvious potential for metastasis, would tend nevertheless to behave as low-grade leiomyosarcomas and recur locally after initial resection. They concluded that those neoplasms measuring more than 5 cm in diameter, having infiltrating margins and containing more than five mitotic figures per 10 high-power fields are very likely to recur and that tumours showing all these three features should be regarded, and treated, as leiomyosarcomas, irrespective of the degree, if any, of cellular atypia. They considered that neoplasms showing any two of these features should be regarded as low-grade leiomyosarcomas.

Nielsen *et al.* (1996a) generally agreed with these criteria but added a fourth, namely moderate to severe cytological atypia. They considered that if only one of these criteria was present the neoplasm should be regarded as a leiomyoma whilst if two were noted the tumour should be classed as an atypical leiomyoma. They considered that both leiomyomas and atypical leiomyomas should be excised conservatively whilst neoplasms classed by their criteria as leiomyosarcomas should be excised with wide negative margins. Smooth-muscle tumours of the vulva can, however, recur in the absence of all the morphological features suggestive of aggressive behaviour and all leiomyomatous neoplasms should therefore be treated by relatively wide local excision rather than by enucleation.

A few myxoid leiomyosarcomas of the vulva have been recorded (Salm & Evans 1985), although this is not a particular site of predilection for such neoplasms.

Tumours of striated muscle

RHABDOMYOMA

Vulvovaginal rhabdomyomas are well recognized, although there is some dispute as to whether these are a form of fetal rhabdomyoma or represent a specific and discrete entity of genital rhabdomyoma. Most occur in the vagina and only two have arisen at the vulva (Di Sant Agnese & Knowles 1980); one was an incidentally discovered nodule in a 24-year-old woman and the other presented as a nodule of 3 years' duration in an episiotomy scar. These benign neoplasms, if indeed they are neoplasms rather than hamartomas or examples of reactive hyperplasia, are formed of relatively mature elongated spindle-shaped or strap-like rhabdomyoblasts with distinct cross-striations; these cells are separated from each other by varying amounts of myxoid stroma and collagen and stain positively for both desmin and myoglobin.

RHABDOMYOSARCOMA

Three forms of rhabdomyosarcoma are recognized: embryonic, alveolar and pleomorphic, the first two occurring principally in children and young adults and the last mainly in adults. Desmin and muscle actin expression serve as markers for rhabdomyosarcomas whilst immunocytochemical demonstration of the *MyoD1* gene product is highly specific for striated muscle differentiation (Wesche *et al.* 1995).

Embryonal rhabdomyosarcomas tend to form oedematous polypoidal masses and usually have a myxoid stroma in which pleomorphic spindle-shaped or rounded cells are characteristically widely scattered. Two such neoplasms of the vulva in young children have been reported (James *et al.* 1969, Talerman 1973), although the diagnosis in both cases was not proved and was largely a matter of presumption.

DiSaia *et al.* (1971) reported three rhabdomyosarcomas of the vulva in adults but no histological details of these neoplasms were given and the criteria for their recognition as rhabdomyosarcomas were not detailed. Curtin *et al.* (1995) also reported two vulval rhabdomyosarcomas without giving any histological details; both patients died.

Alveolar rhabdomyosarcomas are formed principally of rounded cells that are separated into nodules by fibrous septa; central necrosis within these lobules imparts an alveolar pattern to the tumour. Five cases of alveolar rhabdomyosarcoma of the vulva have been reported (Copeland

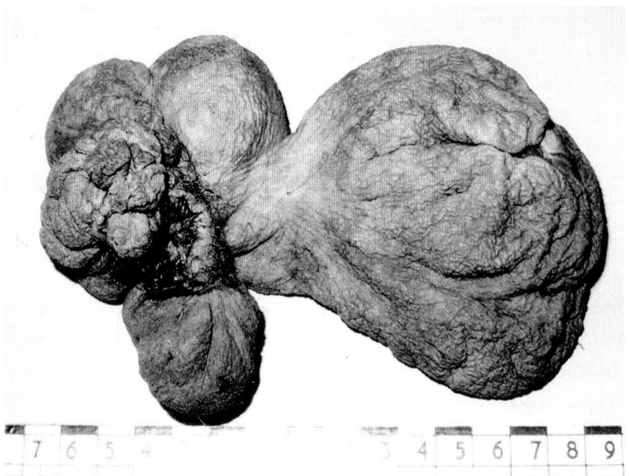

Fig. 9.1 An extirpated fibroma of the vulva.

et al. 1985, Imachi *et al.* 1991, Bond *et al.* 1994), one being confined to the clitoris. All occurred in patients aged between 4 and 17 years and three proved rapidly fatal; two patients survived after surgery, radiotherapy and chemotherapy.

Tumours of fibrous tissue

FIBROMA

Vulval fibromas, probably better considered as dermatofibromas, are similar to those elsewhere in the body and, whilst presenting as vulval masses (Fig. 9.1), probably arise from deeper connective tissue structures, particularly those surrounding the introitus and perineal body. They usually occur on the labia majora, are often pedunculated or pendulous, may be superficially ulcerated and can attain a very large size.

FIBROSARCOMA

The diagnosis of a fibrosarcoma is essentially one of exclusion, and stains for S-100, epithelial membrane antigen, cytokeratins and desmin should be negative. Only a few vulval fibrosarcomas have been described (Keller 1951, Woodruff & Brack 1958, DiSaia *et al.* 1971, Davos & Abell 1976, Hall & Amin 1981, Nirenberg *et al.* 1995) and it is far from certain that all these would currently be acceptable as true fibrosarcomas. These tumours have occurred in women aged between 30 and 67 years with a mean age of 44 years; most were in the labia majora, although one was confined to the clitoris and two involved the entire vulval area. Most of the tumours were between 6 and 8 cm in diameter but one was a huge mass measuring 25 cm in diameter. The histological features of vulval fibrosarcomas do not differ from those encountered elsewhere in the body: the tumours are formed of spindle cells with poorly delineated cytoplasm and elongated tapering nuclei, which are characteristically arranged in a 'herring bone' fascicular fashion. Fifty per cent of the reported patients with vulval fibrosarcoma died from their disease, all in less than 2 years from initial presentation and death being usually due to a combination of local recurrence and pulmonary metastases. Only one of the women who died had been treated by radical surgery whilst all those who survived, being alive and well at periods ranging from 4 to 9 years, had been treated by radical vulvectomy together with either pelvic lymphadenectomy or bilateral inguinal node dissection.

Tumours of fibrohistiocytic origin

The concept of fibrohistiocytic tumours has recently undergone considerable criticism and it is widely conceded that none of the neoplasms in this category shows true histiocytic differentiation, the term 'fibrohistiocytic' being a misnomer and bringing together a group of heterogeneous lesions, many of which are probably unrelated (Fletcher 1995). Nevertheless 'fibrohistiocytic' neoplasms will probably continue to be described as such until their true nature is determined.

DERMATOFIBROSARCOMA PROTUBERANS

Although doubt exists as to the histogenesis and nature of this dermal tumour it is probably best considered as a 'fibrohistiocytic' or fibroblastic neoplasm of low-grade malignancy (Brooks 1994). Only a few cases have been recorded at the vulva (Davos & Abell 1976, Soltan 1981, Agress *et al.* 1983, Bock *et al.* 1985, Barnhill *et al.* 1988, Leake *et al.* 1991, Panidis *et al.* 1993, Nirenberg *et al.* 1995, Karlen *et al.* 1996). These tumours have occurred in both pre- and postmenopausal women and have usually presented as slow-growing, painless, non-tender, mobile lumps, most commonly in the labia majora, which measure anything up to 8 cm in diameter; the overlying skin may be ulcerated. Histologically (Fig. 9.2), the tumour is infiltrative and formed of plump fibroblastic cells arranged in a distinctly storiform pattern; there is little pleomorphism and mitotic figures are sparse. All patients with vulval dermatofibrosarcoma protuberans have been treated initially by wide local excision, but recurrence occurred, often after a prolonged time interval, in nearly 50% of cases, this sometimes necessitated more radical surgery. There has been no reported instance of metastasis or tumour-related death, although a focal area of fibrosarcoma was noted in one neoplasm (Leake *et al.* 1991).

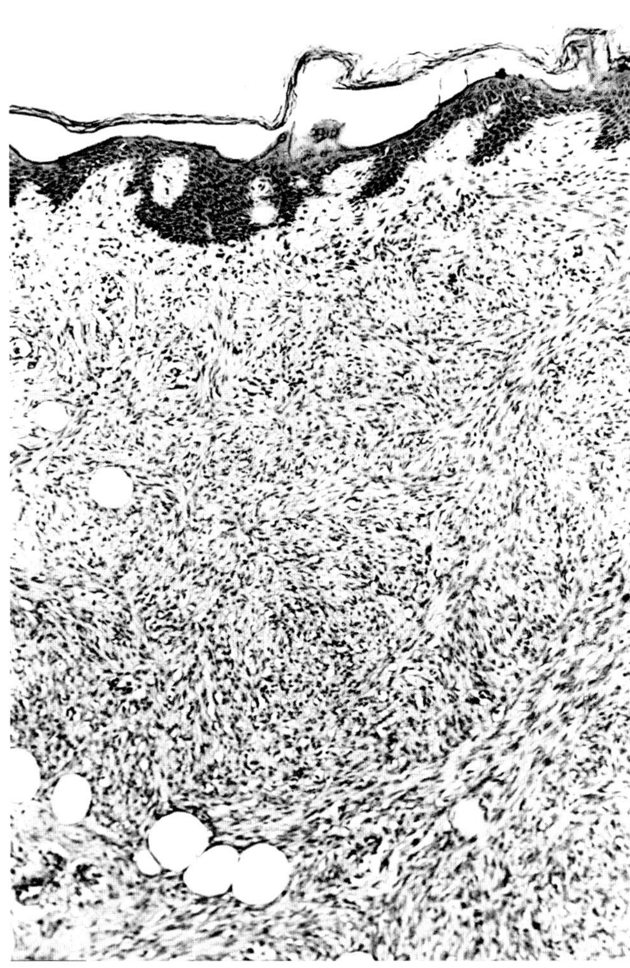

Fig. 9.2 A dermatofibrosarcoma of the vulva. There is a well-marked storiform pattern and the tumour is infiltrating fat.

MALIGNANT FIBROUS HISTIOCYTOMA

Some consider that malignant fibrous histiocytoma is a 'wastepaper basket' diagnosis, neoplasms classed as such being, in reality, either pleomorphic variants of liposarcoma, leiomyosarcoma or rhabdomyosarcoma, or, in some cases, pleomorphic spindle-celled carcinomas or melanomas (Fletcher 1995). Others, whilst maintaining that malignant fibrous histiocytoma is a distinct entity, albeit of unknown origin, consider the tumour to be greatly overdiagnosed (Brooks 1994). There is currently no specific immunocytochemical marker for these neoplasms.

Very few examples of a malignant fibrous histiocytoma of the vulva have been recorded, six as such (Davos & Abell 1976, Taylor *et al.* 1985, Santala *et al.* 1987, Elchalal *et al.* 1991, Nirenberg *et al.* 1995) and one as a 'malignant fibroxanthoma' (Hensley & Friedrich 1973). These neoplasms arose in women aged between 39 and 79 years who presented with a history, varying in length from 2 to 12 months, of an enlarging vulval mass, which, in two cases, was painful. One tumour involved the vulva and vagina and one the labium minus but the remainder were confined to the labia majora and ranged from 2.5 to 6 cm in diameter: two were ulcerated.

Histologically, these tumours are formed of plump spindle cells arranged in short fascicles in a storiform fashion around slit-like vascular spaces. These are admixed with 'histiocytic' cells and with larger, pleomorphic fibroblastic cells arranged in a haphazard fashion. Xanthomatous cells and multinucleated giant cells are often present and mitotic figures are a conspicuous feature.

Patients with a vulval malignant fibrous histiocytoma have been variously treated by local excision, hemivulvectomy, radical vulvectomy, and combined chemotherapy and radiotherapy, but only two patients suffered tumour recurrence and death, this despite initial treatment with radical vulvectomy and pelvic and groin node dissection, supplemented in one case by chemotherapy and radiotherapy.

Tumours of fat

LIPOMA

Benign lipomatous neoplasms of the vulva are relatively common and present either as soft, rounded, lobulated masses (Fig. 9.3) or as soft, pedunculated tumours (Lovelady *et al.* 1941, Kaufman & Gardner 1965). They can, on occasion, be extremely large and attain a diameter of nearly 20 cm. Most vulval lipomas develop from the fatty tissue of the labia majora but examples have been noted of clitoral localization (Haddad & Jones 1960); they can occur at any age and one has been described in a neonate (Fukaminzu *et al.* 1982). Histologically these neoplasms are formed of mature fat cells, which are often admixed with strands of fibrous tissue.

LIPOSARCOMA

Reports of vulval liposarcoma are extremely rare, with only three reasonably persuasive and fully described accounts of such a neoplasm. One liposarcoma developed in the labium majus of a 29-year-old woman (Taussig 1937); despite hemivulvectomy with inguinal and femoral node dissection the patient died 5 months later with pulmonary and skeletal metastases. Brooks and LiVolsi (1987) described a large myxoid liposarcoma in a 15-year-old girl that involved the vulva and perineum; following local excision the tumour recurred 20 months later, the patient dying from local disease 31 months after initial presentation. The patient reported by Genton and Maroni (1987) was a 60-year-old woman who presented with a slow-growing, sharply circumscribed lump in the labium majus; the tumour appeared encapsulated macroscopically and histologically was a well-differentiated liposarcoma. The patient was alive and well 10 months later.

Recently, Nucci and Fletcher (1997) briefly reported a series of six cases of vulval liposarcomas. The age range of their patients was 28–69 years and the neoplasms, which ranged in size from 0.8 to 8 cm in diameter, presented as slowly enlarging vulval masses, which had been present for between 2 and 5 years. Four of the six tumours had the typical histological appearances of a well-differentiated liposarcoma, being distinguished from a lipoma only by some variation in adipocyte cell size, a degree of adipocyte nuclear atypia and the presence of occasional lipoblasts. Two of the neoplasms showed an unusual appearance with an admixture of bland spindle-shaped cells, atypical adipocytes and numerous bivacuolated lipoblasts. All the patients were treated only by wide local excision and follow-up data were available for four cases; three patients were alive and well without recurrence at periods up to 18 months, whilst one woman, whose tumour was incompletely excised, suffered recurrence over a 10-year period but was alive and well 31 months after re-excision.

Tumours of vascular tissue

HAEMANGIOMA

Haemangiomas of the vulva occur primarily in infancy and childhood, this possibly indicating their hamartomatous, rather than neoplastic, nature. The lesions may be of capillary or cavernous type.

Clinically significant haemangiomas of the vulva are uncommon (Lovelady *et al.* 1941, Gerbie *et al.* 1955, Darnalt-Restrepo 1957, Giannone & Avezzi 1959, Gulienetti 1959, Mobius & Krause 1974); such cases are usually reported because the haemangioma is large and unsightly and there can be little doubt that most vulval haemangiomas either pass unrecorded or are insufficiently large for the parents of the child to seek medical aid. Those which have been described have usually been of the cavernous type and have involved the labia, usually unilaterally but sometimes bilaterally.

Some cavernous haemangiomas (Fig. 9.4) have been localized to the clitoris (Lovelady *et al.* 1941, Haddad & Jones 1960, Kaufmann-Friedman 1978); such lesions produce marked clitoromegaly and may lead to the patient being investigated for an intersex state or for congenital adrenal hyperplasia.

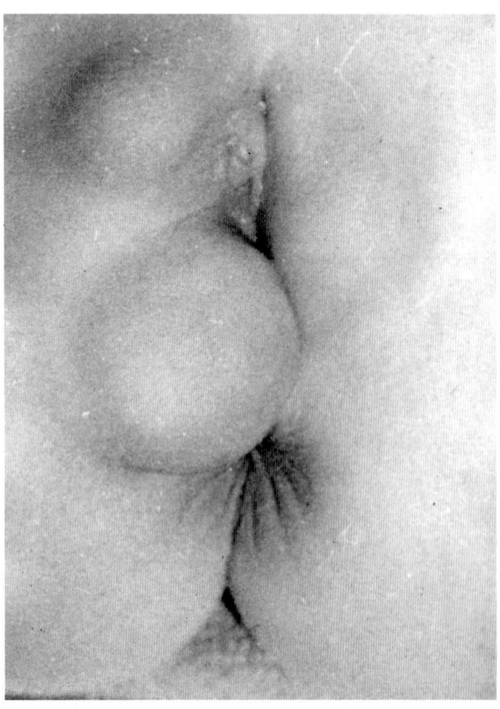

Fig. 9.3 A lipoma of the vulva.

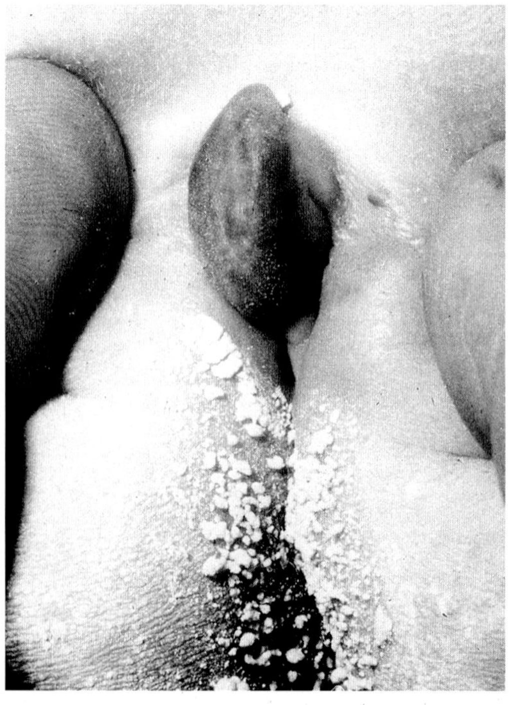

Fig. 9.4 A haemangioma of the clitoris in a neonate.

ANGIOKERATOMA

An angiokeratoma is often thought of as a variant of a haemangioma but its true nature is debatable; it is certainly not clearly neoplastic.

Vulval angiokeratomas are more common than their rather sparse coverage in the literature would suggest (Imperial & Helwig 1967, Blair 1970, Verbov & Manglabruks 1978, Uhlin 1980, Novick 1985, Dotters *et al.* 1986, Clark & Wheelock 1988, Cohen *et al.* 1989); the vulva is by no means the only area in which these lesions occur but it is certainly a site of predilection. Angiokeratomas develop principally in women aged between 20 and 40 years and the vast majority arise in the labia majora, although localization to the clitoris has been described (Yamazaki *et al.* 1992). They may be single but are, in 50% of cases, multiple; as many as 24 separate angiokeratomas having been noted in the vulva of one woman (Uhlin 1980). The lesions (Fig. 9.5) usually measure between 2 and 10 mm in diameter and may assume a papular, globular or warty appearance. In the early stages of their development angiokeratomas are commonly cherry red in colour but as they age their tint darkens to brown or black.

Histologically (Fig. 9.6), greatly dilated capillary vessels, often converted into a solitary, sinusoidal vascular channel, are present in the papillary dermis: the overlying epidermis shows a variable degree of hyperkeratosis and acanthosis with elongated rete ridges growing down to surround, almost embrace, the dilated vascular channels in the dermis.

Angiokeratomas are often asymptomatic but may cause pruritus, and bleeding from the lesion is not uncommon: the bleeding is usually of a relatively trivial degree but can occasionally be quite severe. The presence of a black, warty, bleeding lesion can arouse suspicions of a malignant melanoma, which are, however, rapidly dispelled by histological examination of the locally resected lesion, a procedure that is curative.

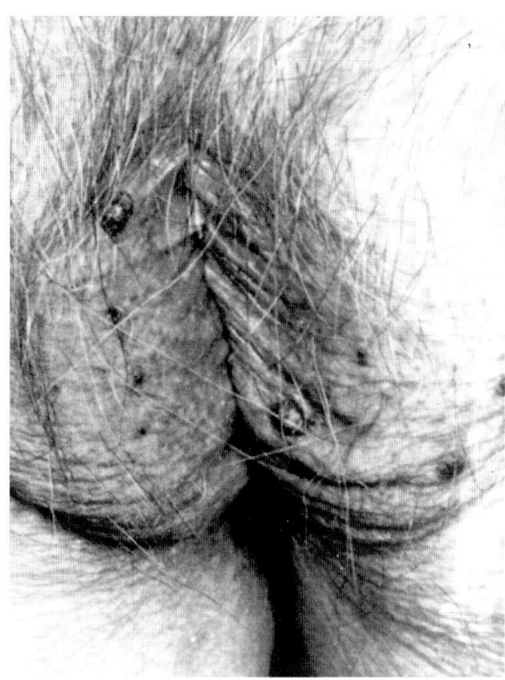

Fig. 9.5 Angiokeratomas of the vulva.

GLOMUS TUMOUR

This benign neoplasm, derived from modified smooth-muscle cells in the walls of arteriovenous anastomoses involved in temperature regulation, presents as a small blue-red, tender nodule and histologically consists of clusters of capillary-type vessels surrounded by cuffs of glomus cells. Vulval glomus tumours are very rare. Kohorn *et al.* (1986) reported a histologically confirmed lesion on the left labium minus causing severe introital dyspareunia and long-standing vulval pain in a woman aged 45 years and Katz *et al.* (1986) reported a similar lesion at the same site in a woman aged 29 years. Local excision is curative.

HAEMANGIOPERICYTOMA

The existence of these neoplasms as a true entity has been questioned (Fletcher 1994) but a few vulval neoplasms that appear to have fulfilled the usual diagnostic morphological criteria of a haemangiopericytoma have been reported (de Sousa & Lash 1959, Davos & Abell 1976, Reymond *et al.* 1972, Ambrosini *et al.* 1980, Guercio *et al.* 1982, Zakut

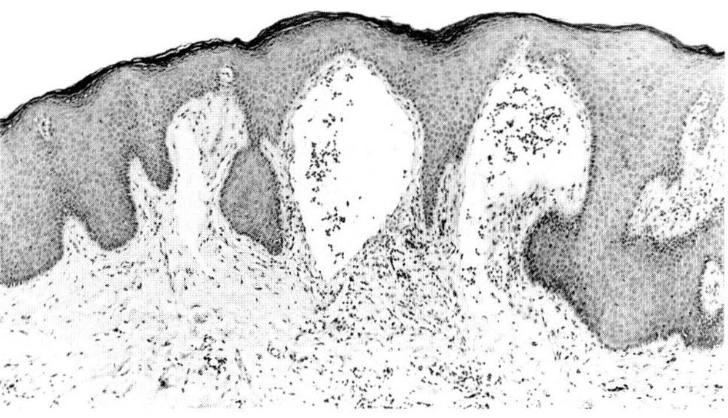

Fig. 9.6 An angiokeratoma of the vulva. Sinusoidally dilated vascular channels are present in the papillary dermis; they are embraced by elongated rete ridges.

et al. 1985). The ages of the patients ranged from 15 to 60 years, although the majority was aged under 25 years. All patients complained of an enlarging vulval mass, sometimes painful, usually present for less than 6 months. The tumour was in the labium majus in all cases except one in which there was a predominantly clitoral localization. Histologically, vulval haemangiopericytomas have the same appearance as those seen more commonly elsewhere in the body with multiple vascular channels set amidst tightly packed cells arranged in trabeculae, clumps and sheets; sometimes the tumour cells are disposed concentrically around the vessels in an 'onion skin' pattern. The vessels range from those of capillary calibre to wide sinusoids and form a ramifying network; very typically the dividing sinusoidal vessels have a 'stag horn' appearance.

Most of the patients with this tumour have remained alive and well after local excision, but one patient, aged 15, died after 5 months with widespread metastases that did not respond to radiotherapy or chemotherapy. A further patient suffered a skeletal metastasis 14 years after treatment by radical vulvectomy. In neither of these cases was there any overt histological evidence of malignancy.

ANGIOMYOFIBROBLASTOMA

These recently described neoplasms have a marked predilection for the vulval soft tissues (Fletcher *et al.* 1992, Katenkamp *et al.* 1993, Hisaoka *et al.* 1995, Toti *et al.* 1995, Nielsen *et al.* 1996b). The patients' ages ranged from 25 to 54 years and they presented with an otherwise asymptomatic vulval mass, nearly always in the labium majus, which had been present for periods ranging from 10 weeks to 8 years. The tumours are well circumscribed, range from 0.5 to 12 cm in diameter and have a partially myxoid appearance on section. Histologically, they are characterized by alternating hypercellular and hypocellular oedematous zones in which abundant blood vessels, predominantly of capillary type, are irregularly distributed. Spindled, plump spindled and oval stromal cells are aggregated around the blood vessels, sometimes forming solid compact foci, or are loosely dispersed in the hypocellular areas: binucleate or multinucleate cells may be present. There is an admixture of collagen, either as thin wavy strands or as thick bundles. The stromal cells stain positively for vimentin and desmin but are negative for cytokeratins, actins and S-100.

These tumours are fully benign and are cured by local excision. They can, however, be very easily confused with an aggressive angiomyxoma: points of distinction from an aggressive angiomyxoma include the circumscribed borders, greater cellularity, absence of vessels with thick or hyalinized walls, presence of plump stromal cells and the lack of extravasation of erythrocytes: it had previously been thought that positive staining of the stromal cells for desmin was also a distinguishing feature but it is now recognized that this is not the case (Granter *et al.* 1997).

AGGRESSIVE ANGIOMYXOMA

These tumours occur in the vulva, perineum and pelvis, most commonly in young patients in their third or fourth decade (Steeper & Rosai 1983, Begin *et al.* 1985, Hilgers *et al.* 1986, Mandai *et al.* 1990, Elchalal *et al.* 1992, Habeck 1992, Simo *et al.* 1992, Cheah *et al.* 1993, Skalova *et al.* 1993, Fetsch *et al.* 1996, Granter *et al.* 1997). The vulval lesion presents as an enlarging painless mass and the history is usually only of a few months. The neoplasms are nearly always more than 5 cm in diameter, commonly larger than 10 cm and can attain a diameter of 60 cm; they often extend into the pelvis, ischiorectal fossa and retroperitoneum. They are smooth, lobulated and, despite their infiltrative nature, may appear deceptively encapsulated; their cut surface has a myxoid appearance. The histological appearance is bland with many blood vessels set in a loose myxoid stroma, which also contains a small population of stellate or thin spindled cells with delicate cytoplasmic processes. The vessels vary in size but commonly some are relatively large and have thick muscular or hyalinized walls, whilst others may have an angiomatoid appearance; extravasation of erythrocytes into the stroma is a frequent finding. There is a variable amount of stromal collagen. Mitotic figures are usually absent. The stromal cells stain positively for vimentin, desmin, smooth-muscle actin and, generally, for oestrogen and progesterone receptors.

The appearances of an aggressive angiomyxoma differ significantly from those of an angiomyofibroblastoma but Granter *et al.* (1997) have described a few aggressive angiomyxomas that showed a transition, in some areas, to a pattern more characteristic of an angiomyofibroblastoma.

Because aggressive angiomyxomas infiltrate in such an insidious fashion, complete surgical removal is difficult and recurrences, often repetitive, occur in 70% of cases, usually within 2 years, although some are delayed for longer periods. Metastasis does not occur.

The presence in many of these neoplasms of hormone receptors, and the description of one case in which growth occurred during pregnancy, suggests a possible hormone dependency for at least some aggressive angiomyxomas (Htwe *et al.* 1995).

KAPOSI'S SARCOMA

The true nature and origin of this tumour is still open to debate, as, although often considered as a vascular neoplasm, it is more probably a multifocal viral-induced reactive vascular process. Vulval Kaposi's sarcoma appears to have the same gross and histological features as does the lesion elsewhere in the body, although there have been only two reported instances of this tumour involving the vulva. One (Hall *et al.* 1979) arose in a 69-year-old woman who had a large, raised, scaling lesion involving the entire right labium majus; satellite nodules were present in the skin of the groin, buttocks and thigh. The patient responded well to chemotherapy but died of renal disease 1 month later: no residual tumour was found at autopsy. LiVolsi & Brooks (1987) refer briefly to a multifocal Kaposi's sarcoma of the vulva and perineum in an elderly woman; following radiotherapy she was alive 15 years later.

EPITHELIOID HAEMANGIOENDOTHELIOMA

This is a vascular tumour of intermediate malignancy, which is characterized by cords and nests of large polygonal cells with abundant eosinophilic cytoplasm, some of the cells showing intracytoplasmic vacuolation. Immunohistochemically most neoplasms of this type express endothelial markers and many are also positive for cytokeratins; they react negatively for epithelial membrane antigen. Strayer *et al.* (1992) described a neoplasm of this type which presented as a small clitoral nodule, which had been present for a year. After radical vulvectomy and inguinal node dissection the patient was alive and well 27 months later.

ANGIOSARCOMA

Reports of vulvar angiosarcomas have been sparse and rather unsatisfactory. Davos & Abell (1976) described one case in an 83-year-old woman; the tumour was treated by local excision and no follow-up information was provided. Bo *et al.* (1976) also reported a vulval angiosarcoma, although this diagnosis was not convincingly supported by the illustrations of the histology. The only fully described and acceptable case was reported by Nirenberg *et al.* (1995): the tumour arose in an 87-year-old woman, formed an ulcerated, poorly circumscribed, bluish mass measuring 8 cm in diameter, and histologically was composed of irregular vascular channels lined by plump to cuboidal endothelial cells that focally formed solid nests. Stains for Factor VIII were negative but a positive staining reaction for UEAI was obtained. This neoplasm was treated by wide excision and radiotherapy but metastasized to bone and led to death within 2 years.

Tumours of lymphatic origin

LYMPHANGIOMAS (see also Chapter 5)

Two types of lymphangioma can occur in the vulva. The more common is the lesion known as lymphangioma simplex or lymphangioma circumscriptum, in which localized groups of small, thin-walled vesicles are present (Abu-Hamad *et al.* 1989, Johnson *et al.* 1991, Sood *et al.* 1991, Murugan *et al.* 1992, Akimoto *et al.* 1993, Harwood & Mortimer 1993); microscopically these consist of irregular dilated lymphatic channels, which may communicate with deeper lymphatic cisterns. These lesions typically develop after surgery or radiotherapy for cervical carcinoma but may arise spontaneously in the absence of predisposing factors. Some assume a warty appearance because of reactive acanthosis of the overlying epithelium. Lymphangioma circumscriptum is treated by laser therapy or local excision.

Much less common are cavernous lymphangiomas, which present as soft, compressible masses, usually in the labia minora but sometimes involving the entire vulva, and can attain a considerable bulk (Lovelady *et al.* 1941, Kaufman & Gardner 1965, Brown & Stenchever 1989, Bartels *et al.* 1995). Lymphangiomas of this type usually occur in childhood, and local excision is curative, but complete removal is not always easy to achieve and recurrence may occur. Treatment with carbon dioxide laser may well be a better therapeutic approach (Bartels *et al.* 1995).

Tumours of neural origin

SCHWANNOMA

Schwannomas are benign tumours that arise from peripheral nerve sheaths. A few Schwannomas of the vulva have been reported, most arising in the labia (Bryan 1955, Bianco & Samuel 1958, Dini 1959, Yamashita *et al.* 1996), but one being localized to the clitoris (Migliorini & Amato 1978). Schwannomas of the vulva show the admixture of Antoni A and B areas characteristic of these neoplasms in other sites, although one has been described which consisted almost entirely of Antoni A areas (Lawrence & Shingleton 1978); this particular neoplasm was classed, almost certainly incorrectly, as a 'malignant Schwannoma', largely because of its high content of mitotic figures, a finding that is not indicative of malignancy in an otherwise typical Schwannoma.

One example has been described of a vulval plexiform Schwannoma, a neoplasm resembling a plexiform neurofibroma (Woodruff *et al.* 1983); this tumour presented as a large mass in the labium majus of a 26-year-old woman and recurrences appeared at 18 months and 22 months after local excision, with the patient, however, being alive and well 42 months after initial diagnosis.

MALIGNANT SCHWANNOMA

These are extremely rare vulval tumours and only two reasonably convincing examples have been recorded (Davos & Abell 1976, Terada *et al.* 1988), both of which appeared to have arisen in a pre-existent solitary neurofibroma. One of the two patients died despite radical excision, whilst the other was alive and well 2 years after a hemivulvectomy.

BENIGN GRANULAR CELL TUMOUR

This neoplasm is currently thought to be derived from Schwann cells and occurs with modest frequency at the vulva (Birch & Sondag 1961, Radman & Bhagavan 1969, Coates & Hales 1973, Dgani *et al.* 1978, Chambers 1979, King *et al.* 1979, Lieb *et al.* 1979, Zenetta *et al.* 1981, Morris 1982, Lesoin *et al.* 1983, Void & Jerve 1984, Altaras *et al.* 1985, Raju & Naraynsingh 1987, Majmudar *et al.* 1990, Wolber *et al.* 1991, Guenther & Shum 1993, Horowitz *et al.* 1995). In most instances the vulval lesion has been an isolated occurrence but occasionally it has formed one component of a syndrome in which multiple granular cell tumours arise, either sequentially or synchronously, in various parts of the body (Powell 1946, Gifford & Birch 1973, Majmudar *et al.* 1990). The vulval neoplasms can occur at any age and usually arise in the labia (Fig. 9.7), although some have been confined to the clitoris (Doyle & Hutchinson 1968, Degefu *et al.* 1984, Wolber *et al.* 1991).

The tumour, which develops in the dermis or immediately subcutaneous tissue, presents as a slow-growing, painless, non-tender lump or nodule; the history usually extends over months or years and the tumour rarely exceeds 4 cm in diameter. The lump is commonly mobile but some tumours situated in the upper dermis show skin tethering. The elevated, overlying skin may be depigmented and occasionaly ulcerated. The tumour is poorly circumscribed and yellowish or yellow-grey on section.

Histologically (Fig. 9.8), the neoplasm is formed of rounded or polygonal cells with indistinct margins, central vesicular nuclei and abundant, coarsely granular cytoplasm. There is little pleomorphism and mitotic figures are either absent or extremely sparse. The tumour cells are usually arranged in ribbons or clumps, which are separated from each other. Sometimes a desmoplastic reaction can largely engulf the tumour cells, which then appear as scattered nests set in a dense fibrous stroma. In the case of those granular cell tumours set in the dermis, the overlying squamous epithelium often shows a pronounced pseudoepitheliomatous hyperplasia (Fig. 9.9), which is not infrequently misdiagnosed as a squamous cell carcinoma. The neoplastic cells stain positively, but weakly, with periodic acid–Schiff stain (PAS) both before and after diastase, and stain strongly for S-100, neurone-specific enolase and NK1-C3.

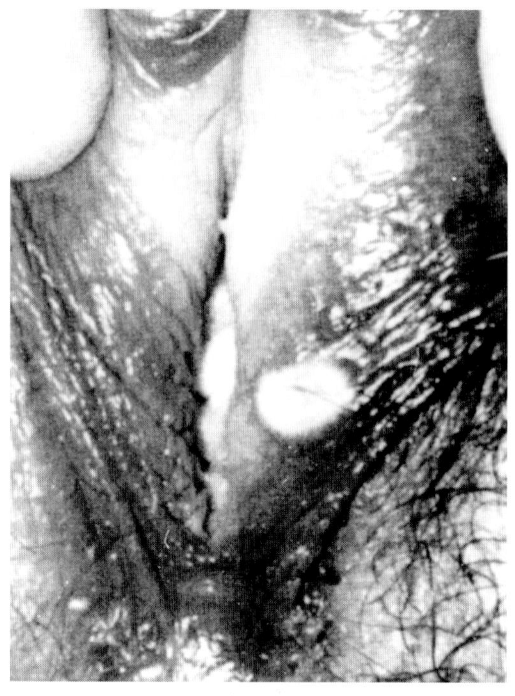

Fig. 9.7 A granular cell tumour of the vulva. This had a yellowish appearance.

The overwhelming majority (98%) of granular cell tumours are benign (the rare exceptions are discussed below) and the patient is cured by local excision, which has to be quite wide because of the common occurrence of groups of tumour cells beyond the apparent macroscopic limits of growth.

MALIGNANT GRANULAR CELL TUMOUR

Only two malignant granular cell tumours of the vulva have been reported. Magori and Szegvari (1973) described a 49-year-old woman who had a histologically benign granular cell tumour removed from her vulva; she subsequently suffered local recurrence and inguinal node metastasis but was well and tumour-free following further surgery. Robertson *et al.* (1981) reported a 33-year-old woman who developed right inguinal node metastases 5 years after removal of a histologically benign granular cell tumour; following block dissection of the right groin the patient was tumour-free 6 months later.

PARAGANGLIOMA

Only one paraganglioma of the vulva has been reported (Colgan *et al.* 1991): this presented as a painful, small

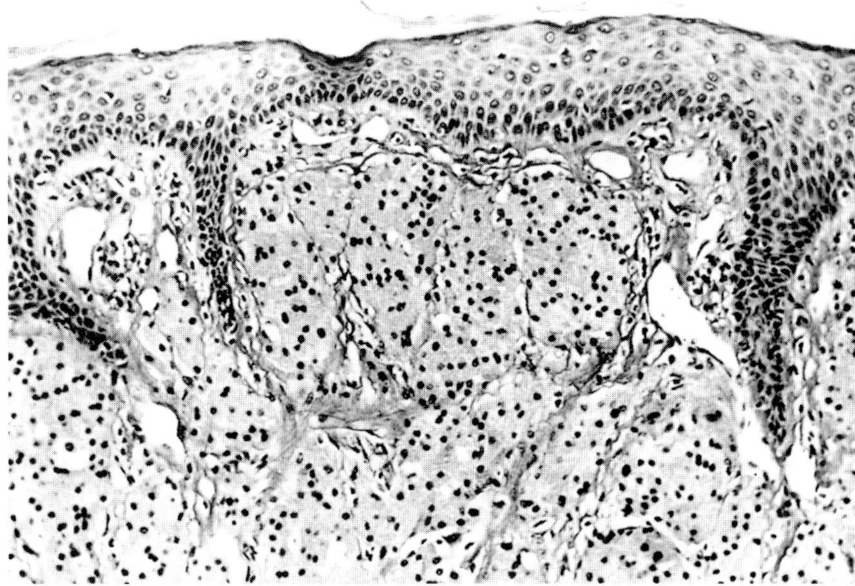

Fig. 9.8 Granular cell tumour of the vulva with granular cells in the dermis.

subepithelial nodule in the labium minus in a 58-year-old woman, was cured by local excision and was thought to arise from a peripheral component of the parasympathetic nervous system.

NEUROFIBROMA

A modest number of vulval neurofibromas have been described; a few of these were solitary lesions in women with no other features of von Recklinghausen's disease (Venter *et al.* 1981) but most have occurred in patients with clear-cut evidence of generalized neurofibromatosis. Vulval neurofibromas have also been described as one component of a localized neurofibromatosis of the female genitourinary tract (Gersell & Fulling 1989). Figure 9.10 shows a similar personal case, with lesions confined to the vulva and vagina. In both cases, the appearance was initially mistaken for warts.

In some instances the tumours have been confined to the labia (Miller 1979, Friedrich & Wilkinson 1985, Gomez-Bravo-Topete *et al.* 1993), but in others the clitoris has been the site of a plexiform neurofibroma, the resulting clitoromegaly in some instances being an isolated phenomenon but in others being associated with labial tumours (Petsche & Radinger 1954, Haddad & Jones 1960, Hoffmann 1962, Kenny *et al.* 1966, Labardini *et al.* 1968, Messina & Strauss 1976, Greer & Pederson 1981, Schepel & Tolhurst 1981, Milia *et al.* 1982, Craven & Bresnahan 1983, Ravikumar & Lakshmanan 1983). Not surprisingly, patients, usually children, with clitoral enlargement due to a plexiform neurofibroma tend to be initially diagnosed as cases of intersex, this being particularly the case if accompanying labial tumours are incorrectly taken to be testes. It is highly probable, however, that such cases tend to be selectively reported and thus place undue emphasis on clitoral neurofibromas.

A solitary neurofibroma of the vulva is adequately treated by local excision but in many cases of neurofibromatosis the large number of lesions limits surgical treatment to those which are large or painful; unfortunately, the poorly delineated nature of these neoplasms means that surgical removal is often incomplete and that recurrences are common.

EWING'S SARCOMA

Extraosseous Ewing's sarcoma is now considered to be a primitive neuroectodermal tumour. Nirenberg *et al.* (1995) described a neoplasm that they considered to be a Ewing's sarcoma of the vulva. This presented as a rapidly growing 12-cm mass in the labium majus of a 20-year-old girl. The histological pattern of sheets of small round cells with uniform nuclei, little cytoplasm and numerous mitoses was consistent with a diagnosis of Ewing's sarcoma, but positive staining for the MIC-2 gene product could not be demonstrated, this deficiency casting some doubt on the diagnosis. This neoplasm was treated by radical surgery, chemotherapy and radiotherapy but the patient died with lung metastases within 10 months.

Mesenchymal tumours of uncertain origin

EPITHELIOID SARCOMA

This is a neoplasm of unknown histogenesis, although it has been suggested, not too convincingly, that it is of synovial origin. Tumours classed as epithelioid sarcomas have only

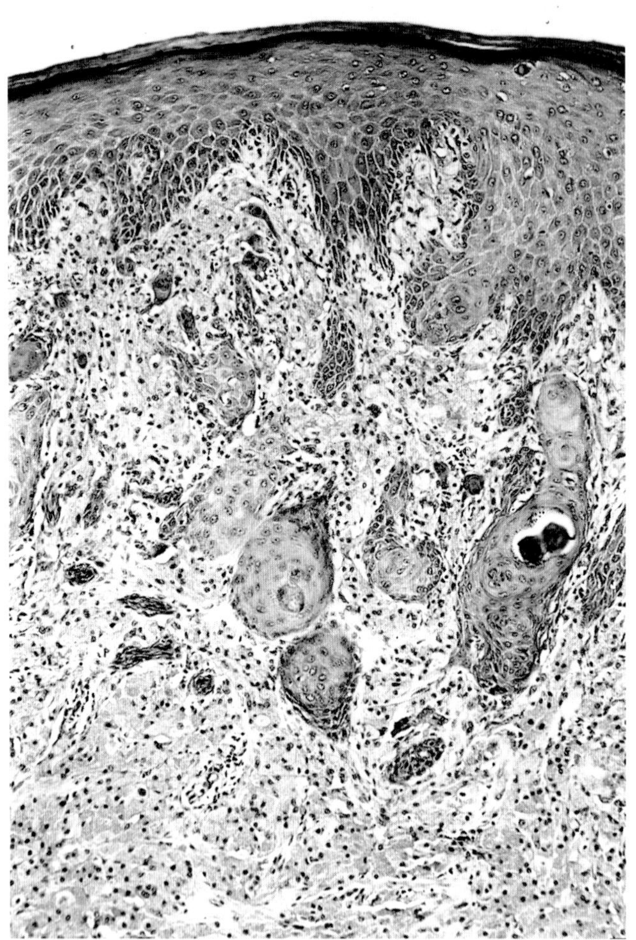

Fig. 9.9 Pseudocarcinomatous hyperplasia associated with a granular cell tumour of the vulva.

rarely been reported as occurring in the vulva (Piver *et al.* 1972, Gallup *et al.* 1976, Hall *et al.* 1980, Ulbright *et al.* 1983, Tan *et al.* 1989). It has been suggested that most of these, possibly all, were in fact malignant rhabdoid tumours (Perrone *et al.* 1989), this suggestion being based upon the overlap of histological features between these two neoplasms and the unusually aggressive nature of vulval epithelioid sarcomas; in fact two out of six patients with vulval epithelioid sarcomas have survived, a survival rate comparable to, and indeed better than, that noted by Wevers *et al.* (1989) in a large series of epithelioid sarcomas in more conventional sites.

The vulval lesions tend to occur in relatively young women as a slowly enlarging, painless, nodular mass, most commonly in the labium majus; the length of the history varies from 2 to 24 months. Histologically, the vulval neoplasms have the same appearance as those occurring elsewhere, with their deceptive resemblance to a carcinoma or a granuloma. The tumour cells are grouped into nodules that commonly show central necrosis; the cells are polygonal or fusiform with abundant strongly eosinophilic cytoplasm. Spindle-shaped cells are often also present and tend to aggregate at the periphery of the nodules. The tumours show consistent positivity for cytokeratins, vimentin and epithelial membrane antigen. Two of six patients have survived and, curiously, both these were treated only by local excision.

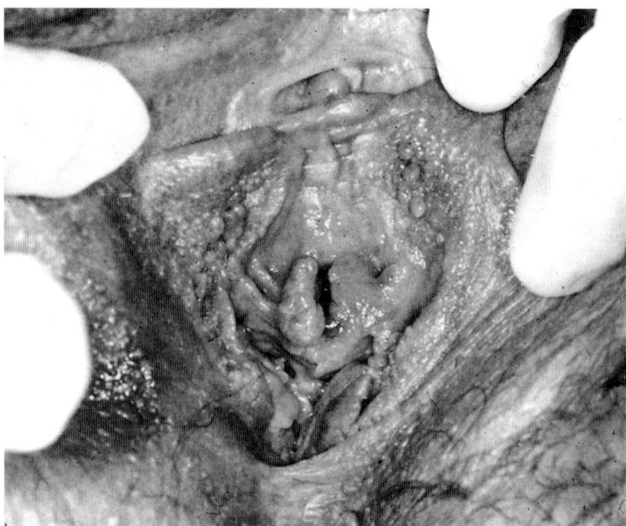

Fig. 9.10 Neurofibromatosis localized to the vulva and vagina: papilliferous lesions.

ALVEOLAR SOFT-PART SARCOMA

The histogenesis of this neoplasm is obscure, although there has been support for the belief that it arises from specific nerve endings or chemoreceptors; an alternative view, based on immunocytochemistry and expression of *MyoD*, is that it is of striated muscle origin. It has a characteristic organoid, pseudoalveolar arrangement of large, rounded or polygonal cells with central nuclei, distinct limiting membranes and abundant granular eosinophilic cytoplasm; it contains PAS-positive, diastase-resistant granules and crystalline rods. Alveolar soft-part sarcoma occurs with extreme rarity at the vulva, only two cases having been recorded (Kondratiev & Kurillov 1971, Shen *et al.* 1982); one patient was apparently cured by radical vulvectomy and the other suffered recurrence after local excision.

MALIGNANT RHABDOID TUMOUR

Malignant rhabdoid tumours occur most commonly as renal neoplasms during childhood but have been described in extrarenal sites in adults. Very few malignant rhabdoid tumours of the vulva have been reported (Perrone *et al.* 1989, Matias *et al.* 1990, Lupi *et al.* 1996), these having the same histological appearances as do extrarenal rhabdoid tumours elsewhere and pursuing a similarly aggressive course. As already noted, distinction between these tumours, with their content of epithelioid and spindle cells, from an epithelioid sarcoma may be difficult and even impossible.

Non-mesenchymal, non-epithelial neoplasms

Germ-cell neoplasms

YOLK SAC TUMOURS

Yolk sac tumours of the vulva are rare, only six cases having been fully documented (Ungerleider *et al.* 1978, Castaldo *et al.* 1980, Krishnamurphy & Sampat 1981, Dudley *et al.* 1983, Penkar *et al.* 1992, Craighead & du Toit 1993). It is assumed, but certainly not proven, that these neoplasms arise from germ cells which, during embryogenesis, have gone astray during their migration from the yolk sac to the developing gonad.

Yolk sac tumours of the vulva have had exactly the same appearance as their more commonly occurring ovarian counterparts and have arisen in infants, children and young adults. The patients present with a short history, usually of only a few months, of a painless, enlarging vulval mass, usually in the labium majus but in one case confined to the clitoris. A majority of the reported patients with a vulval yolk sac tumour have died, but these were treated before the advent of effective chemotherapy for this neoplasm and more recently reported patients have had a much more optimistic prognosis.

Lymphoma and leukaemia

The vulva can be the site of an apparently primary extranodal lymphoma. Most of the reported cases have been non-Hodgkin's lymphomas (Taussig 1937, Ramioul 1952, Buckingham & McClure 1955, Iliya *et al.* 1968, Wishart 1973, Verhaegh *et al.* 1977, Bagella *et al.* 1990, Chalubinski *et al.* 1992, Marcos *et al.* 1992, Nam *et al.* 1992, Klein *et al.* 1993, Bai & Sun 1995) but there have also been occasional examples of Hodgkin's disease (Hahn 1958) and of post-transplantation T-cell lymphoma (Kaplan *et al.* 1993). There has been one case of an immunoblastic lymphoma of the vulva arising in an HIV-positive woman (Kaplan *et al.* 1996).

Presentation of a disseminated lymphoma as a vulval lesion is very rare (Schiller & Madge 1970, Egwuatu *et al.* 1980); presentation of a myeloid leukaemia with vulval ulceration of uncertain nature (Muram & Gold 1993) or as a granulocytic sarcoma of the vulva has also been recorded (Joswig & Joswig-Priewe 1974, Gardaise *et al.* 1974, Laricchia *et al.* 1977).

References

Abu-Hamad, A., Provencher, D., Ganjei, P. & Penalver, M. (1989) Lymphangioma circumscripta of the vulva: case report and review of the literature. *Obstetrics and Gynecology* 73, 496–499.

Agress, R., Figge, D.C., Tamimi, H. & Greer, B. (1983) Dermatofibrosarcoma protuberans of the vulva. *Gynecologic Oncology* 16, 288–291.

Akimoto, K., Nogita, T. & Kawashima, M. (1993) A case of acquired lymphangioma of the vulva. *Journal of Dermatology* 20, 449–451.

Altaras, M., Jaffe, R., Bernheim, J. & Ben Aderet, M. (1985) Granular cell myoblastoma of the vulva. *Gynecologic Oncology* 22, 352–355.

Ambrosini, A., Becagli, L. & de Bastiani, B.M. (1980) Hemangiopericytoma of the vulva: a study of two cases. *European Journal of Gynaecological Oncology* 1, 198–200.

Aneiros, J., Garcia del Moral, R., Beltran, E. & Nogales, F.F. (1982) Epithelioid leiomyoma of the vulva. *Diagnostic Gynecology and Obstetrics* 4, 351–355.

Audet-Lapointe, P., Paquin, F., Guerard, M.J. *et al.* (1980) Leiomyosarcoma of the vulva. *Gynecologic Oncology* 10, 350–355.

Bagella, M.P., Fadda, G. & Cherchi, P.L. (1990) Non-Hodgkin's lymphoma: a rare primary vulvar localization. *European Journal of Gynaecologic Oncology* 11, 153–156.

Bai, P. & Sun, J. (1995) Primary malignant lymphoma of the female genital tract: clinical analysis of 15 cases. *Chinese Journal of Obstetrics and Gynecology* 30, 614–617.

Barnhill, D.R., Boling, R., Nobles, W., Crooks, L. & Burke, T. (1988) Vulvar dermatofibrosarcoma protruberans. *Gynecologic Oncology* 30, 149–152.

Bartels, U., Krauss, T., Sattler, B., Maghsudi, M. & Kuhn, W. (1995) Therapie eines ausgedehnten Lymphangiomes der Vulva. *Zentralblatt für Gynäkologie* 117, 220–223.

Begin, L.R., Clement, P.B., Kirk, M.E. *et al.* (1985) Aggressive angiomyxoma of pelvic soft parts: a clinicopathological study of nine cases. *Human Pathology* 16, 621–628.

Bianco, R. & Samuel, S. (1958) Neurilemmoma della vulva. *Tumori* 44, 326–336.

Birch, H.W. & Sondag, D.R. (1961) Granular cell myoblastoma of the vulva: report of five cases with special tissue stains in one. *Obstetrics and Gynecology* 18, 443–454.

Blair, C. (1970) Angiokeratoma of the vulva. *British Journal of Dermatology* 83, 409–411.

Bo, A.V., Bianchi, G., Kron, J.B. & Miglioli, P. (1976) Si un caso ad eccezionale sopravvenza di sarcoma della vulva. *Minerva Ginecologica* 28, 145–149.

Bock, J.E., Andreasson, B., Thorn, A. & Holck, S. (1985) Dermatofobrosarcoma protuberans of the vulva. *Gynecologic Oncology* 20, 129–135.

Bond, S.J., Seibel, N. & Kapur, S. (1994) Rhabdomyosarcoma of the clitoris. *Cancer* 73, 1884–1886.

Brooks, J.S.J. (1994) The spectrum of fibrohistiocytic tumours with special emphasis on malignant fibrous histiocytoma. *Current Diagnostic Pathology* 1, 3–12.

Brooks, J.S.J. & LiVolsi, V.A. (1987) Liposarcoma presenting on the vulva. *American Journal of Obstetrics and Gynecology* **156**, 73–75.

Brown. J.V. & Stenchever, M.A. (1989) Cavernous lymphangioma of the vulva. *Obstetrics and Gynecology* **73**, 877–879.

Bryan, W.E. (1955) Neurilemmoma of the vulva. *Journal of Obstetrics and Gynaecology of the British Empire* **62**, 949–950.

Buckingham J.C. & McClure, H.J. (1955) Reticulum cell sarcoma of the vulva: report of a case. *Obstetrics and Gynecology* **6**, 138–143.

Castaldo, T.W., Petrilli, E.S., Ballon, S.C. *et al.* (1980) Endodermal sinus tumor of the clitoris. *Gynecologic Oncology* **9**, 376–380.

Chalubinski, K., Breitenecker, G. & Tatra, G. (1992) Maligne Lymphome an Vulva und Vagina. *Geburtshilfe und Frauenheilkunde* **52**, 630–631.

Chambers, D.C. (1979) Granular cell myoblastoma of the vulva. *Journal of the National Medical Association* **71**, 1071–1073.

Cheah, P.L., Looi, L.M. & Sivanesaratnam, V. (1993) Aggressive angiomyxoma of the vulva with an unusual vascular finding. *Pathology* **25**, 250–252.

Clark, J.R. & Wheelock, J.R. (1988) Angiokeratoma of the vulva: a case report. *Journal of Reproductive Medicine* **33**, 473–474.

Coates, J.B. & Hales, J.S. (1973) Granular cell myoblastoma of the vulva. *Obstetrics and Gynecology* **41**, 796–799.

Cohen, P.R., Young, A.W. Jr. & Tovell, H.M. (1989) Angiokeratoma of the vulva: diagnosis and review of the literature. *Obstetrical and Gynecological Survey* **44**, 339–346.

Colgan, T.J., Dardick, I. & O'Connell, G. (1991) Paraganglioma of the vulva. *International Journal of Gynecological Pathology* **10**, 203–208.

Copeland, L.J., Sneige, N., Stringer, A. *et al.* (1985) Alveolar rhabdomyosarcoma of the female genitalia. *Cancer* **56**, 849–856.

Craighead, P.S. & du Toit, P.F. (1993) Endodermal sinus tumour of the vulva: an interesting clinico-pathological problem. *European Journal of Surgical Oncology* **19**, 203–205.

Craven, E.M. & Bresnahan, K. (1983) Neuroma of the clitoris. *Delaware Medical Journal* **55**, 341–342.

Curtin, J.P., Saigo, P., Slucher, B. *et al.* (1995) Soft-tissue sarcoma of the vagina and vulva: a clinicopathologic study. *Obstetrics and Gynecology* **86**, 269–272.

Darnalt-Restrepo, E. (1957) Hemangiomas de la vulva et de la vagina. *Revista Columniana de Obstetricia* **8**, 272–276.

Davos, I. & Abell, M.R. (1976) Soft tissue sarcomas of vulva. *Gynecologic Oncology* **4**, 70–86.

Degefu, S., Dhurandhar, H.N., O'Quinn, A.G. & Fuller, P.N. (1984) Granular cell tumor of the clitoris in pregnancy. *Gynecologic Oncology* **19**, 246–251.

deSousa, L.M. & Lash, A.F. (1959) Hemangiopericytoma of the vulva. *American Journal of Obstetrics and Gynecology* **78**, 295–298.

Dgani, R., Czernobilsky, B., Borenstein, R. & Lancet, M. (1978) Granular cell myoblastoma of the vulva: report of four cases. *Acta Obstetricia et Gynecologica Scandinavica* **57**, 385–387.

Dini, S. (1959) Rare osservazione di neurinoma del piccolo labbro vulvare. *Archivo de Becchi* **29**, 867–875.

DiSaia, P.J., Rutledge, F. & Smith, J.P. (1971) Sarcomas of the vulva: a report of 12 patients. *Obstetrics and Gynecology* **38**, 180–184.

Di Sant Agnese, P.A. & Knowles, D.M. (1980) Extracardiac rhabdomyoma: a clinicopathological study and review of the literature. *Cancer* **46**, 780–789.

Dotters, D.J., Fowler, W.C., Powers J.K. & McKune, B.K. (1986) Argon laser therapy of vulvar angiokeratoma. *Obstetrics and Gynecology* **68**, 56s–59s.

Doyle, W.F. & Hutchinson, J.R. (1968) Granular cell myoblastoma of the clitoris. *American Journal of Obstetrics and Gynecology* **100**, 589–590.

Dudley, A.G., Young, R.H., Lawrence, W.D. & Scully, R.E. (1983) Endodermal sinus tumor of the vulva in an infant. *Obstetrics and Gynecology* **61**, 76s–79s.

Egwuato, V.E., Ejeckam, G.C. & Okaro, J.M. (1980) Burkitt's lymphoma of the vulva: a case report. *British Journal of Obstetrics and Gynaecology* **87**, 827–830.

Elchalal, U., Dgani, R., Zosmer, A. *et al.* (1991) Malignant fibrous histiocytoma of the vagina and vulva successfully treated by combined chemotherapy and radiotherapy. *Gynecologic Oncology* **42**, 91–93.

Elchalal, U., Lifshitz-Mercer, B., Dgani, R. & Zalel, Y. (1992) Aggressive angiomyxoma of the vulva. *Gynecologic Oncology* **47**, 260–262.

Fetsch, J.F., Laskin, W.B., Lefkowitz, M., Kindblom, F.J. & Meis-Kindblom, J.M. (1996) Aggressive angiomyxoma: a clinicopathologic study of 29 female patients. *Cancer* **78**, 79–90.

Fletcher, C.D.M. (1994) Haemangiopericytoma—a dying breed? Reappraisal of an 'entity' and its variants: a hypothesis. *Current Diagnostic Pathology* **1**, 19–23.

Fletcher, C.D.M. (1995) Soft tissue tumors. In: *Diagnostic Histopathology of Tumors* (ed. C.D.M. Fletcher), pp. 1043–1096. Churchill Livingstone, Edinburgh.

Fletcher, C.D.M., Tsang, W.Y.W., Fisher, C., Lee, K.C. & Chan, J.K.C. (1992) Angiomyofibroblastoma of the vulva: a benign neoplasm distinct from aggressive angiomyxoma. *American Journal of Surgical Pathology* **16**, 373–382.

Friedrich, E.G. & Wilkinson, E.J. (1985) Vulvar surgery for neurofibromatosis. *Obstetrics and Gynecology* **65**, 135–138.

Fukaminzu, H., Matsumoto, K., Inoue, K. & Moriguchi, T. (1982) Large vulvar lipoma. *Archives of Dermatology* **118**, 447.

Gallup, D.G., Abell, M.R. & Morley, G.W. (1976) Epithelioid sarcoma of the vulva. *Obstetrics and Gynecology* **48**, 14s–17s.

Gardaise, J., Marie, M. & Bertrand, G. (1974) Chlorome à localizations génitales multiples. *Semaine des Hôpitaux de Paris* **51**, 609–616.

Genton, G.Y. & Maroni, E.S. (1987) Vulval liposarcoma. *Archives of Gynaecology* **240**, 63–66.

Gerbie, A.B., Hirsch, M.R. & Greene, R.R. (1955) Vascular tumors of the female genital tract. *Obstetrics and Gynecology* **6**, 499–507.

Gersell, D.J. & Fulling, K.H. (1989) Localized neurofibromatosis of the female genitourinary tract. *American Journal of Surgical Pathology* **13**, 873–878.

Giannone, R. & Avezzi, G. (1959) Emangioma cavernose della vulva. *Rivista Italiana de Ginecologia* **53**, 471–479.

Gifford, R. & Birch, H.W. (1973) Granular cell myoblastoma of multicentric origin involving the vulva: a case report. *American Journal of Obstetrics and Gynecology* **117**, 184–187.

Gomez-Bravo-Topete, E., Martinez-Martinez, M. & Hendrichs-Troeglen, B. (1993) Enfermedad von Recklinghausen con tumoracion a expensas de vulva: presentacion de una caso. *Ginecologica et Obstetricia Mexicana* **61**, 156–159.

Granter, S.R., Nucci, M.R. & Fletcher, C.D.M. (1997) Aggressive angiomyxoma: reappraisal of its relationship to angiomyofibroblastoma in a series of 16 cases. *Histopathology* **30**, 1–10.

Greer, D.M. & Pederson, W.C. (1981) Pseudo-masculinization of the clitoris. *Plastic and Reconstructive Surgery* **68**, 787–788.

Guenther, L. & Shum, D. (1993) Granular cell tumor of the vulva. *Pediatric Dermatology* **10**, 153–155.

Guercio, E., Siliquini, GP., Aimone, V. *et al.* (1982) Emangiopericytoma della vulva. *Minerva Ginecologica* **34**, 451–460.

Guidozzi, F., Sadan, U., Koller, A.B. & Marks, S.R. (1987) Combined chemotherapy and irradiation therapy after radical surgery for leiomyosarcoma of the vulva: a case report. *South African Medical Journal* **71**, 327–328.

Gulienetti, R. (1959) Haemangiomata of the external genitals. *British Journal of Plastic Surgery* **12**, 228–233.

Habeck, J.D. (1992) Aggressives Angiomyxome der Vulva und des Perineums. *Zentralblatt für Pathologie* **138**, 303–306.

Haddad, H.M. & Jones, W.H. (1960) Clitoral enlargement simulating pseudohermaphroditism. *American Journal of Diseases of Children* **99**, 282–287.

Hahn, G.A. (1958) Gynecologic considerations in malignant lymphoma. *American Journal of Obstetrics and Gynecology* **75**, 673–683.

Hall, D.J., Burns, J.C. & Goplerud, D.R. (1979) Kaposi's sarcoma of the vulva: a case report and brief review. *Obstetrics and Gynecology* **54**, 478–483.

Hall, D.J., Grimes, M.M. & Goplerud, D.R. (1980) Epithelioid sarcoma of the vulva. *Gynecologic Oncology* **9**, 237–246.

Hall, J.S.E. & Amin U.F. (1981) Fibrosarcoma of the vulva: case reports and discussion. *International Surgery* **86**, 185–187.

Harwood, C.A. & Mortimer, P.S. (1993) Acquired lymphangiomata mimicking genital warts. *British Journal of Dermatology* **129**, 334–336.

Hensley, G.T. & Friedrich, E.G. (1973) Malignant fibroxanthoma: a sarcoma of the vulva. *American Journal of Obstetrics and Gynecology* **116**, 289–291.

Hilgers, R.D., Pai, R., Barton, S.A., Aisenbrey, G. & Bowling, M.C. (1986) Aggressive angiomyxoma of the vulva. *Obstetrics and Gynecology* **68**, 60s–62s.

Hisaoka, M., Kouho, H., Aoki, T., Daimaru, Y. & Hashimoto, H. (1995) Angiomyofibroblastoma of the vulva: a clinicopathologic study of seven cases. *Pathology International* **45**, 487–492.

Hoffmann, J. (1962) Die Neurofibromatose der Vulva unter dem Erscheinunsbild eines Pseudohermaphroditismus. *Zentralblatt für Gynäkologie* **84**, 961–966.

Horowitz, I.R., Copas, P. & Majmudar, B. (1995) Granular cell tumors of the vulva. *American Journal of Obsterics and Gynecology* **173**, 1710–1713.

Htwe, M., Deppisch, L.M. & Saint Julien, J.S. (1995) Hormone-dependent aggressive angiomyxoma of the vulva. *Obstetrics and Gynecology* **86**, 697–699.

Iliya, F.A., Muggia, F.M., O'Leary, J.A. & King, T.M. (1968) Gynecologic manifestations of reticulum cell sarcoma. *Obstetrics and Gynecology* **31**, 266–269.

Imachi, M., Tsukamoto, N., Kamura, T. *et al.* (1991) Alveolar rhabdomyosarcoma of the vulva: report of two cases. *Acta Cytologica* **35**, 345–349.

Imperial, R. & Helwig, E.B. (1967) Angiokeratoma of the vulva. *Obstetrics and Gynecology* **29**, 307–312.

James, G.B., Guthrie, W. & Buchan, A. (1969) Embryonic sarcoma of the vulva in an infant. *Journal of Obstetrics and Gynaecology of the British Commonwealth* **76**, 458–461.

Johnson, T.L., Kennedy, A.W. & Segal, G.H. (1991) Lymphangioma circumscriptum of the vulva: a report of two cases. *Journal of Reproductive Medicine* **36**, 808–812.

Joswig, E.H. & Joswig-Priewe, H. (1974) Retikulumzellsarcom im Bereich der Vulva und Vagina. *Zentralblatt für Gynäkologie* **96**, 1040–1043.

Kaplan, E.G., Chadburn, A. & Caputo, T.A. (1996) HIV-related primary non-Hodgkin's lymphoma of the vulva. *Gynecologic Oncology* **61**, 131–138.

Kaplan, M.A., Jacobson, M.O., Ferry, J.A. & Harris, N.L. (1993) T-cell lymphoma of the vulva in a renal allograft recipient with associated hemophagocytosis. *American Journal of Surgical Pathology* **17**, 842–849.

Karlen, J.R., Johnson, K. & Kashkari, S. (1996) Dermatofibrosarcoma protuberans of the vulva: a case report. *Journal of Reproductive Medicine* **41**, 267–269.

Katenkamp, D. & Stiller, D. (1980) Unusual leiomyoma of the vulva with fibroma-like pattern and pseudoelastin formation. *Virchows Archiv. A, Pathological Anatomy and Histopathology (Berlin)* **388**, 361–368.

Katenkamp, D., Kosmehl, M., Mentzel, T. & Reinke, J. (1993) Das Angiomyofibroblastom (AMFB) der Vulva und Paravaginalregion—eine neue Entitat. *Pathologie* **14**, 131–137.

Katz, V.L., Askin, F.B. & Bosch, B.D. (1986) Glomus tumor of the vulva: a case report. *Obstetrics and Gynecology* **67**, 43s–45s.

Kauffmann-Friedman, K. (1978) Hemangioma of clitoris—confused with adreno-genital-syndrome: a case report. *Plastic and Reconstructive Surgery* **62**, 452–454.

Kaufman, R.H. & Gardner, H.L. (1965) Benign mesodermal tumors. *Clinical Obstetrics and Gynecology* **8**, 953–981.

Keller, J. (1951) Fibrosarcoma of labium vulvae. *Canadian Medical Association Journal* **64**, 574–576.

Kenny, F.M., Fetterman, G.H. & Preeyasombat, C. (1966) Neurofibromata simulating a penis and labioscrotal gonads in a girl with von Recklinghausen's disease. *Pediatrics* **37**, 956–959.

King, D.F., Bustillo, M., Broen, E.N. & Hirose, F.M. (1979) Granular cell tumors of the vulva: a report of three cases. *Journal of Dermatologic Surgery and Oncology* **5**, 794–797.

Klein, M., Heinz, R., Stierer, M., Kuhnel, E. & Beck, A. (1993) Die Erstemanifestation der Non-Hodgkins-Lymphom im Labium majus. *Zentralblatt für Gynäkologie* **115**, 131–132.

Kohorn, E.I., Merino, M.J. & Goldenhersh, M. (1986) Vulvar pain and dyspareunia due to glomus tumor. *Obstetrics and Gynecology* **67**, 41s–42s.

Kondratiev, L.N. & Kurillov, A.L. (1971) Soft tissue alveolar sarcoma of the vulva. *Arkhiv Patologii (Moscow)* **33**, 80–82.

Krag-Moller, L.B., Nygaard-Nielsen, M. & Trolle, C. (1990) Leiomyosarcoma vulvae. *Acta Obstetrica et Gynecologica Scandinavica* **68**, 187–189.

Krishnamurphy, S.C. & Sampat, M.B. (1981) Endodermal sinus (yolk sac) tumor of the vulva in a pregnant female. *Gynecologic Oncology* **11**, 379–382.

Kuller, J.A., Zucker, P.K. & Peng, T.C. (1990) Vulvar leiomyosarcoma in pregnancy. *American Journal of Obstetrics and Gynecology* **162**, 164–166.

Labardini, M.M., Kallet, H.A. & Cerny, J.C. (1968) Urogenital neurofibromatosis simulating an intersex problem. *Journal of Urology* **98**, 627–632.

Laricchia, R., Wierdis, T., Loiudice, L., Trisolini, A. & Riezzo, A. (1977) Neoformazione vulvare (mieloblastoma) come prima manifestazione di una leucemia acuta mieloblastica. *Minerva Ginecologica* **29**, 957–961.

Lawrence, W.D. & Shingleton, H.M. (1978) Malignant Schwannoma of the vulva: a light and electron microscopic study. *Gynecologic Oncology* **6**, 527–537.

Leake, J.F., Buscema, J., Cho, K.R. & Currie, J.L. (1991) Dermatofibrosarcoma protuberans of the vulva. *Gynecologic Oncology* **41**, 245–249.

Lenaz, M.P., Nguyen, T.C. & Hewett, W.J. (1987) Leiomyosarcoma of the vulva. *Connecticut Medicine* **51**, 705–706.

Lesoin, A., Destee, A., Lafitte, J.J. & Jmin, M. (1983) Myoblastoma à cellules granuleuses: revue de la litérature à propos 3 observations. *Larc Médicale* **3**, 232–235.

Lieb, S.M., Gallousis, S. & Freedman, H. (1979) Granular cell myoblastoma of the vulva. *Gynecologic Oncology* **8**, 12–20.

LiVolsi, V.A. & Brooks, J.J. (1987) Soft tissue tumors of the vulva. In: *Pathology of the Vulva and Vagina* (ed. E.J. Wilkinson), pp. 209–238. Churchill Livingstone, New York.

Lovelady, S.B., McDonald, J.R. & Waugh, J.M. (1941) Benign tumors of vulva. *American Journal of Obstetrics and Gynecology* **42**, 309–313.

Lupi, G., Jin, R. & Clemente, C. (1996) Malignant rhabdoid tumor of the vulva: a case report and review of the literature. *Tumori* **82**, 93–95.

Magori, A. & Szegvari, M. (1973) Rezidiverender und metastasieren der Abriskoff Tumor der Vulva. *Zentralblatt für Allgemeine Pathologie und Pathologischen Anatomie* **117**, 265–273.

Majmudar, B., Castellano, P.Z., Wilson, R.W. & Siegel, R.J. (1990) Granular cell tumors of the vulva. *Journal of Reproductive Medicine* **35**, 1008–1014.

Mandai, K., Moriwaki, S. & Motoi, M. (1990) Aggressive angiomyxoma of the vulva: report of a case. *Acta Pathologica Japonica* **40**, 927–934.

Marcos, C., Martinez, L., Esquivias, J.J. *et al.* (1992) Primary non-Hodgkin lymphoma of the vulva. *Acta Obstetricia et Gynecologica Scandinavica* **71**, 298–300.

Matias, C., Nunes, J.F., Vicente, L.F. & Almeida, M.O. (1990) Primary malignant rhabdoid tumour of the vulva. *Histopathology* **7**, 576–578.

Messina, A.M. & Strauss, R.G. (1976) Pelvic neurofibromatosis. *Obstetrics and Gynecology* **47**, 63s–66s.

Migliorini, A. & Amato, A. (1978) In tema de patologia neoplastica della vulva: rara caso di neurinoma del clitoride. *Minerva Ginecologica* **30**, 543–545.

Milia, S., Firinh, C. & Pirisi, G. (1982) Neurofibromatosi con localizzazione vulvare: a proposito di un caso. *Minerva Ginecologica* **34**, 1055–1058.

Miller, G.C. (1979) Neurofibromatosis affecting the vulva: case report. *Military Medicine* **144**, 542–543.

Mobius, W. & Krause, W. (1974) Das Vulvahanabguin beim Saugling und Kleinkind und seine Behandlung. *Zentralblatt für Gynäkologie* **96**, 280–286.

Morris, P.G. (1982) Granular cell myoblastoma of the vulva: report of two cases and review of the literature. *Journal of Obstetrics and Gynaecology* **2**, 178–180.

Muram, D. & Gold, S.S. (1993) Vulvar ulceration in girls with myelocytic leukemia. *Southern Medical Journal* **86**, 293–294.

Murugan, S., Srinivasan, G., Kaleelullah, M.C. & Rajkumar, L. (1992) A case report of lymphangioma circumscriptum of the vulva. *Genitourinary Medicine* **68**, 331.

Nam, J.H., Park, M.C., Lee, K.H. *et al.* (1992) Primary non-Hodgkin's malignant lymphoma of the vulva: a case report. *Journal of Korean Medical Science* **7**, 271–275.

Neri, A., Peled, Y. & Braslavski, D. (1993) Vulvar leiomyoma. *Acta Obstetricia et Gynecologica Scandinavica* **72**, 221–222.

Newman, P.L. & Fletcher, C.D.M. (1991) Smooth muscle tumours of the external genitalia: a clinicopathological analysis of a series. *Histopathology* **18**, 523–529.

Nielsen, G.P., Rosenberg, A.E., Koerner, F.C., Young, R.H. & Scully, R.E. (1996a) Smooth muscle tumors of the vulva: a clinicopathological study of 25 cases and review of the literature. *American Journal of Surgical Pathology* **20**, 779–793.

Nielsen, G.P., Rosenberg, A.E., Young, R.H. *et al.* (1996b) Angiomyofibroblastoma of the vulva and vagina. *Modern Pathology* **9**, 284–291.

Nirenberg, A., Ostor, A.G., Slavin, J., Riley, C.B. & Rome, R.M. (1995) Primary vulvar sarcomas. *International Journal of Gynecological Pathology* **14**, 55–62.

Novick, N.L. (1985) Angiokeratoma vulvae. *Journal of the American Academy of Dermatology* **12**, 561–563.

Nucci, M.R. & Fletcher, C.D.M. (1998) Liposarcoma (atypical lipomatous tumors) of the vulva: a clinicopathologic study of six cases. *International Journal of Gynecological Pathology* **17**, 17–23.

Palermino, D.A. (1964) Leiomyoma of the vulva: report of a case. *Obstetrics and Gynecology* **24**, 301–302.

Pandhi, R.K., Beci, T.R. & Dhawar, I.K. (1975) Leiomyosarcoma of the labium majus with extensive metastases. *Dermatologica* **150**, 70–74.

Panidis, D., Rousso, D., Achparaki, A., Georgiadis, H. & Viassis, G. (1993) Recurrence of dermatofibrosarcoma protuberans of the vulva: a clinical, histological and ultrastructural study. *European Journal of Gynaecological Oncology* **14**, 182–186.

Patel, S., Kapadia, A., Desai, A. & Dave, K.S. (1993) Leiomyosarcoma of the vulva. *European Journal of Gynaecologic Oncology* **14**, 406–407.

Penkar, S.J., Trani, S., Prabhu, V.L., Candes, F.P. & Nimbkar, S.A. (1992) Endodermal sinus tumor of the vulva (a case report). *Journal of Postgraduate Medicine* **38**, 44–45.

Perrone, T., Swanson, P.E., Twiggs, L., Ulbright, T.M. & Dehner, L.P. (1989) Malignant rhabdoid tumor of the vulva: is distinction from epithelioid sarcoma possible? A pathologic and immunohistochemical study. *American Journal of Surgical Pathology* **13**, 848–858.

Petsche, H. & Radinger, C. (1954) Ein Fall von Morbus Recklinghausen mit Ovarialplasie und Pseudohermaphroditismus masculinus externus. *Weiner Zeitschrift für Nervenheilkunde und deren Grenzgebiete* **10**, 252–259.

Piver, M.S., Tsukada, Y. & Barlow, J. (1972) Epithelioid sarcoma of the vulva. *Obstetrics and Gynecology* **40**, 839–842.

Powell, E.B. (1946) Granular cell myoblastoma. *Archives of Pathology* **42**, 517–524.

Radman, H.M. & Bhagavan, B.S. (1969) Granular cell myoblastoma of the vulva. *Obstetrics and Gynecology* **33**, 501–505.

Raju, G.C. & Naraysingh, V. (1987) Granular cell tumours of the vulva. *Australian and New Zealand Journal of Obstetrics and Gynaecology* **27**, 349–352.

Ramioul, H. (1952) Un nouveau cas de sarcoma vulvaire (réticulo-endothéliome malin). *Gynaecologia* **133**, 74–81.

Ravikumar, V.R. & Lakshmanan, D. (1983) A solitary neurofibroma of the clitoris masquerading as an intersex. *Journal of Pediatric Surgery* **18**, 617.

Reymond, R.D., Hazra, T.A., Edlow, D.W. & Bawab, M.S. (1972) Haemangiopericytoma of the vulva with metastasis to bone 14 years later. *British Journal of Radiology* **45**, 765–768.

Riedel, H. (1964) Zysten und Geschwulste der auseren Genitale und der Vagina. *Zentralblatt für Gynäkologie* **86**, 1479–1508.

Robertson, A.J., McIntosh, W., Lamont, P. & Guthrie, W. (1981) Malignant granular cell tumour (myoblastoma) of the vulva: a report of a case and review of the literature. *Histopathology* **5**, 69–79.

Salm, R. & Evans, D.J. (1985) Myxoid leiomyosarcoma. *Histopathology* **9**, 159–169.

Santala, M., Suonio, S., Syrjanen, K., Uronen, M.T. & Saarikoski, S. (1987) Malignant fibrous histiocytoma of the vulva. *Gynecologic Oncology* **27**, 121–126.

Schepel, S.J. & Tolhurst, D.E. (1981) Neurofibromata of clitoris and labium majus simulating a penis and testicle. *British Journal of Plastic Surgery* **34**, 221–223.

Schiller, H.M. & Madge, G.E. (1970) Reticulum cell sarcoma presenting as a vulvar lesion. *Southern Medical Journal* **63**, 471–472.

Shen, T.-J., D'Ablaing, G. & Morrow, C.P. (1982) Alveolar soft part sarcoma of the vulva: report of first case and review of literature. *Gynecologic Oncology* **13**, 120–128.

Siegle, J.C. & Cartmell, L. (1995) Vulvar leiomyoma associated with estrogen/progestin therapy: a case report. *Journal of Reproductive Medicine* **40**, 58–59.

Simo, M., Zapata, C., Esquius, J. & Domingo, J. (1992) Aggressive angiomyxoma of the female pelvis and perineum: report of two cases and review of the literature. *British Journal of Obstetrics and Gynaecology* **99**, 925–927.

Skalova, A., Michal, M., Husek, K., Zamecnik, M. & Leivo, I. (1993) Aggressive angiomyxoma of the pelvioperoneal region: immunohistological and ultrastructural study of seven cases. *American Journal of Dermatopathology* **15**, 446–451.

Smit, W.L.R., Knobel, J. & van der Merwe, J.V. (1984) Leiomioom en leiomiosarcoma van die vulva: gevalbeskry wings. *South African Medical Journal* **66**, 961–962.

Soltan, M.H. (1981) Dermatofibrosarcoma protuberans of the vulva. *British Journal of Obstetrics and Gynaecology* **88**, 203–205.

Sood, M., Mandal, A.K. & Ganesh, K. (1991) Lymphangioma cirumscriptum of the vulva. *Journal of the Indian Medical Association* **89**, 262–263.

Steeper, T. & Rosai, J. (1983) Aggressive angiomyxoma of the female pelvis and perineum. *American Journal of Surgical Pathology* **7**, 463–476.

Stenchever, M.A., McDivett, R.W. & Fisher, J.A. (1973) Leiomyoma of the clitoris. *Journal of Reproductive Medicine* **2**, 75–76.

Strayer, S.A., Yum, M.N. & Sutton, G.P. (1992) Epithelioid hemangioendothelioma of the clitoris: a case report with immunohistochemical and ultrastructural findings. *International Journal of Gynecological Pathology* **11**, 234–239.

Talerman, A. (1973) Sarcoma botyroides presenting as a polyp on the labium majus. *Cancer* **32**, 994–999.

Tan, G.W., Lim-Tan, S.K. & Salmon, Y.M. (1989) Epithelioid sarcoma of the vulva. *Singapore Medical Journal* **30**, 308–310.

Taussig, F.J. (1937) Sarcoma of the vulva. *American Journal of Obstetrics and Gynecology* **33**, 1017–1026.

Tavassoli, F.A. & Norris, H.J. (1979) Smooth muscle tumors of the vulva. *Obstetrics and Gynecology* **53**, 213–217.

Taylor, R.N., Bottles, K. & Miler, T.R. (1985) Malignant fibrous histiocytoma of the vulva. *Obstetrics and Gynecology* **66**, 145–148.

Terada, K.Y., Schmidt, R.W. & Roberts, J.A. (1988) Malignant Schwannoma of the vulva: a case report. *Journal of Reproductive Medicine* **33**, 969–972.

Toti, R., Danti, M. & Fruscella, L. (1995) Angiomiofibroblastoma della vulva: presentazione di un caso clinico. *Minerva Ginecologica* **47**, 51–53.

Uhlin, S.R. (1980) Angiokeratoma of the vulva. *Archives of Dermatology* **116**, 112–113.

Ulbright, T.M., Brokaw, S.A., Stehman, F.B. & Roth, L.M. (1983) Epithelioid sarcoma of the vulva: evidence suggesting a more aggressive behaviour than extra-genital epithelioid sarcoma. *Cancer* **52**, 1462–1469.

Ungerleider, R.S., Donaldson, S.S., Warnke, R.A. & Wilbur, J.R. (1978) Endodermal sinus tumor: the Stanford experience and the first reported case arising in the vulva. *Cancer* **41**, 1627–1634.

Venter, P.F., Rohm, G.F. & Slabber, C.F. (1981) Giant neurofibromas of the labia. *Obstetrics and Gynecology* **57**, 128–130.

Verbov, J.L. & Manglabruks, K. (1978) Angiokeratoma of vulva. *Dermatologica* **156**, 296–298.

Verhaegh, M., Clay, A., Demaille, M.C. & Caty, A. (1977) Les sarcomes vulvaires (à propos de 3 observations). *Lille Médicale* **22**, 675–677.

Void, I.N. & Jerve, F. (1984) Granular cell myoblastoma of the vulva: a report of three cases. *Annales Chirurgiae et Gynaecologicae Fenniae* **17**, 281–283.

Wesche, N.A., Fletcher, C.D.M., Dias, P. *et al.* (1995) Immunohistochemistry of MyoD1 in adult pleomorphic soft tissue sarcomas. *American Journal of Surgical Pathology* **19**, 261–269.

Wevers, A.C., Kroon, B.B., Albus-Lutter, C.E. & Gortzak, E. (1989) Epithelioid sarcoma. *European Journal of Surgical Oncology* **15**, 345–349.

Wishart, J. (1973) Reticulosarcoma of the vulva complicating azathioprine-treated dermatomyositis. *Archives of Dermatology* **108**, 563–564.

Wolber, R.A., Talerman, A., Wilkinson, E.J. & Clement, P.B. (1991) Vulvar granular cell tumors with pseudocarcinomatous hyperplasia: a comparative analysis with well-differentiated squamous carcinoma. *International Journal of Gynecological Pathology* **10**, 59–66.

Woodruff, J.D. & Brack, C.B. (1958) Unusual malignancies of the vulvo-urethral region: a report of twelve cases. *Obstetrics and Gynecology* **12**, 677–686.

Woodruff, J.M., Marshall, M.L., Godwin, T.A. *et al.* (1983) Plexiform (multinodular) Schwannoma: a tumor simulating the plexiform neurofibroma. *American Journal of Surgical Pathology* **7**, 691–697.

Yamashita, Y., Yamada, T., Ueki, K., Ueki, M. & Sugimoto, O. (1996) A case of vulvar schwannoma. *Journal of Obstetrics and Gynaecology* **22**, 31–34.

Yamazaki, M., Hiruma, M., Trie, H. & Ishibashi, A. (1992) Angiokeratoma of the clitoris: a subtype of angiokeratoma vulvae. *Journal of Dermatology* **19**, 553–555.

Yokoyama, R., Hashimoto, H., Daimaru, Y. & Enjoji, M. (1987) Superficial leiomyomas: a clinicopathologic study of 34 cases. *Acta Pathologica Japonica* **37**, 1415–1422.

Zakut, H., Lotan, M. & Lipnitzsky, M. (1985) Vulval haemangiopericytoma: a case report. *Acta Obstetrica et Gynecologica Scandinavica* **64**, 619–621.

Zenetta, G., Bellorini, R. & Berra, G. (1981) Il mioblastoma cellule granulose della vulva: presentazione di un caso. *Chirurgia Italiana* **33**, 616–619.

Chapter 10: Epithelial tumours of the vulva

H. Fox & C.H. Buckley

Benign epithelial tumours

Fibroepitheliomatous polyp (skin tag)

These common vulval lesions, which probably do not truly merit being classed as tumours, are usually solitary and appear as soft, sometimes wrinkled, polypoidal nodules (Fig. 10.1). Although usually small they can attain a striking size and become pendulous. The tags have a fibrovascular connective tissue core covered by squamous epithelium (Fig. 10.2), which may be atrophic or, more commonly, mildly acanthotic and hyperkeratotic. Cellular atypia is occasionally seen in the stromal cells of a fibroepitheliomatous polyp.

Squamous papilloma

These are solitary lesions of the middle aged and elderly, and macroscopically resemble fibroepitheliomatous polyps. They consist of a local papillomatous overgrowth of the epidermis: the stroma is formed of vascular fibrous tissue and the lesion differs from a skin tag only by having a higher epithelial/stromal ratio.

Basal cell papilloma

These lesions occur on the vulva, usually on the mons pubis or in the genitocrural folds, and are pigmented, warty and superficial. Histologically the lesion is somewhat papillary and lies superficial to the basal layer of the surrounding epidermis (Fig. 10.3); it is formed of sheets and cords of cells, which are small and regular and resemble those of the normal basal layer of the epidermis. Within the lesion there are usually keratin-containing cysts and there may be associated hyperkeratosis.

Keratoacanthoma

These occur rarely in the vulva, where they are most likely to be located on the outer surface of the labia majora (Rhatigan & Nuss 1985). The tumour is rapidly growing and within the course of a few weeks can develop into a hemispherical nodule with a central keratin-plugged crater 1–2 cm in diameter. Typically the lesion continues to grow for about 6 months and then involutes. Histologically (Fig. 10.4) there is a large central crater filled with keratin with the epidermis extending as a lip over the edge of the crater: the margins and base of the crater are formed by lobulated masses of squamous cells, each lobule having a peripheral layer of small, dark basal-like cells. There is little pleomorphism but mitotic figures, of normal form, may be numerous. This lesion can be mistaken for a squamous cell carcinoma but the short history, the absence of any associated vulval intraepithelial neoplasia (VIN) and the presence of the typical crater help in making a distinction.

Yell (1991) reported an example at the vulva of the rare generalized eruptive keratoacanthoma, described by Grzybowski.

Condylomata acuminata (genital warts) (see also Chapter 4)

These benign neoplasms are clearly of viral aetiology and are the result of infection by human papillomavirus (HPV) types 6 and 11 (Oriel & Almeida 1970, Woodruff *et al.* 1980, Kurman *et al.* 1981), which are usually transmitted by sexual contact; in young children the infection may be acquired by close non-sexual contact (Stumpf 1980).

Condylomas form multiple, sometimes confluent, papillary or verrucous lesions on the skin (Fig. 10.5) and mucous membrane of the vulva, perineum and perianal region, most frequently along the edges of the labia minora, in the interlabial sulcus or around the introitus. Flat (subclinical) condylomas also occur but are difficult or impossible to see without resort to colposcopy.

Histologically, the epithelium, which is flat or covers fine fibrovascular cores, is parakeratotic, or less commonly hyperkeratotic, and acanthotic (Fig. 10.6). Koilocytes are usually present in the upper layers of the epithelium and are regarded as being a hallmark of HPV infection (Fig. 10.7). To warrant recognition as a koilocyte the nucleus of the cell

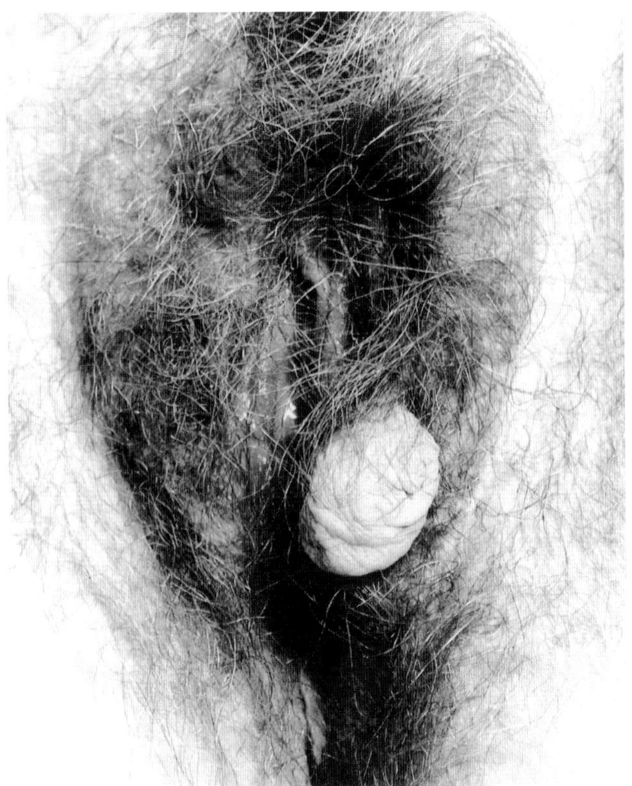

Fig. 10.1 A large fibroepithelial polyp of the vulva.

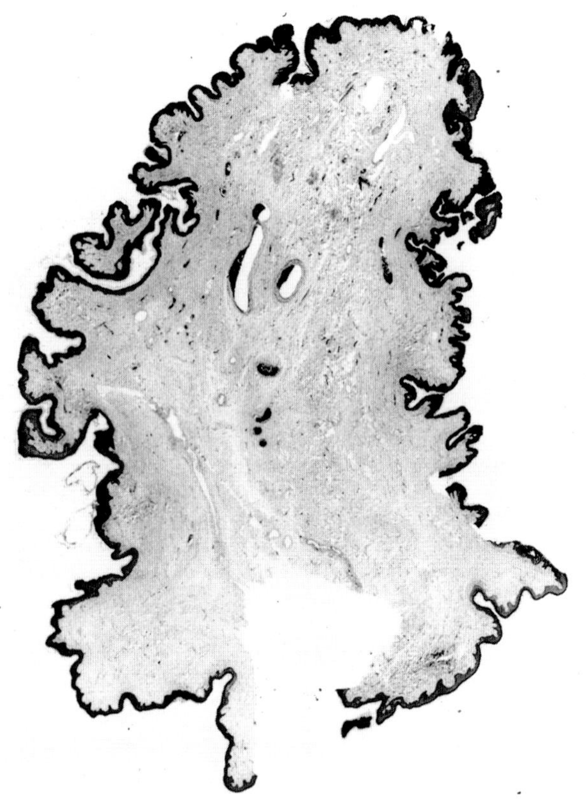

Fig. 10.2 Histological appearances of a vulval fibroepithelial polyp.

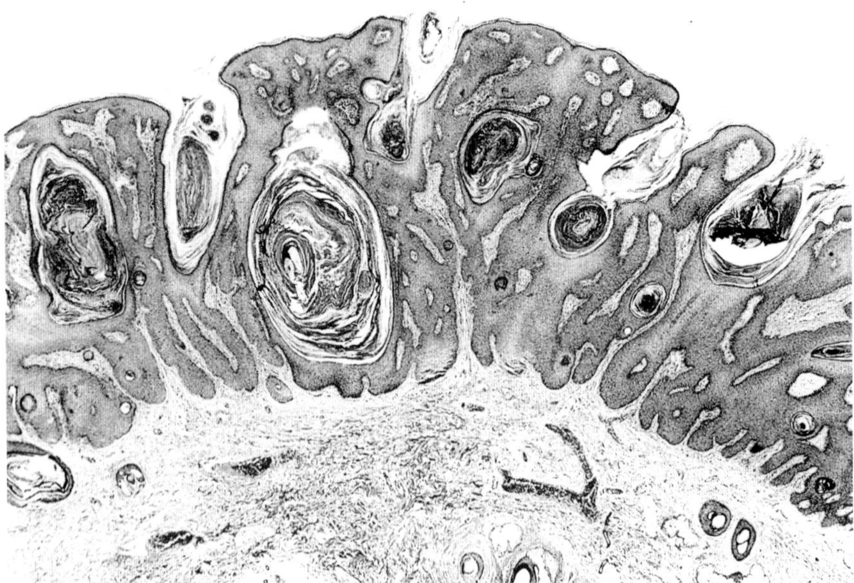

Fig. 10.3 A basal cell papilloma of the vulva.

should be enlarged and hyperchromatic and have a wrinkled outline, and there should be perinuclear cavitation of the cytoplasm; it is important to distinguish these from the clear glycogenated cells of the normal vestibular epithelium. Multinucleated cells and individual cell keratinization are typical features whilst occasional mitotic figures, of normal form, may be seen. The underlying stroma often shows a chronic inflammatory cell infiltrate.

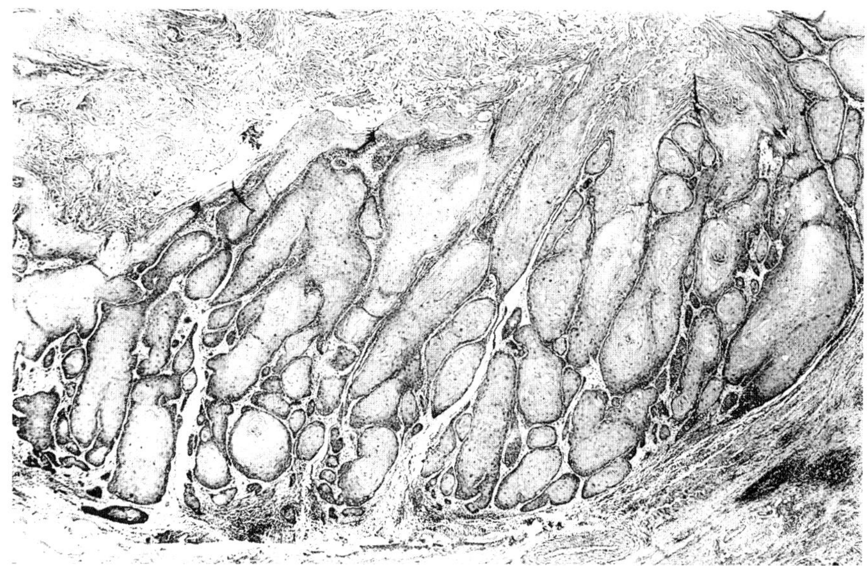

Fig. 10.4 A keratoacanthoma of the vulva: the wall of the lesion is formed by lobulated tongues of squamous epithelium and a keratin plug fills the crater.

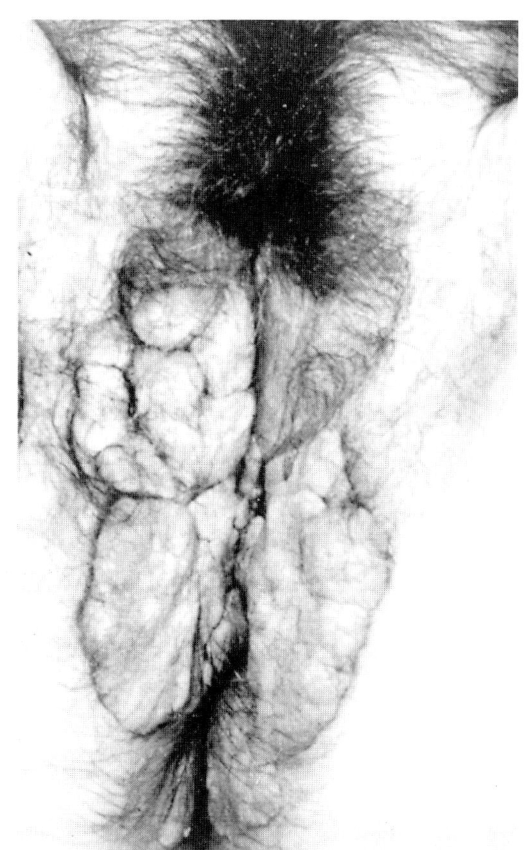

Fig. 10.5 Florid condylomata of the vulva.

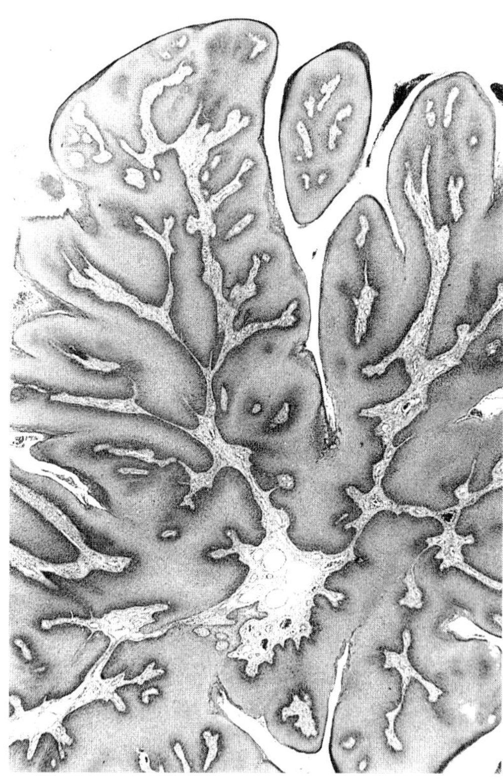

Fig. 10.6 Condyloma acuminatum: fine fibrovascular cores are covered by acanthotic squamous epithelium which is mildly hyperkeratotic.

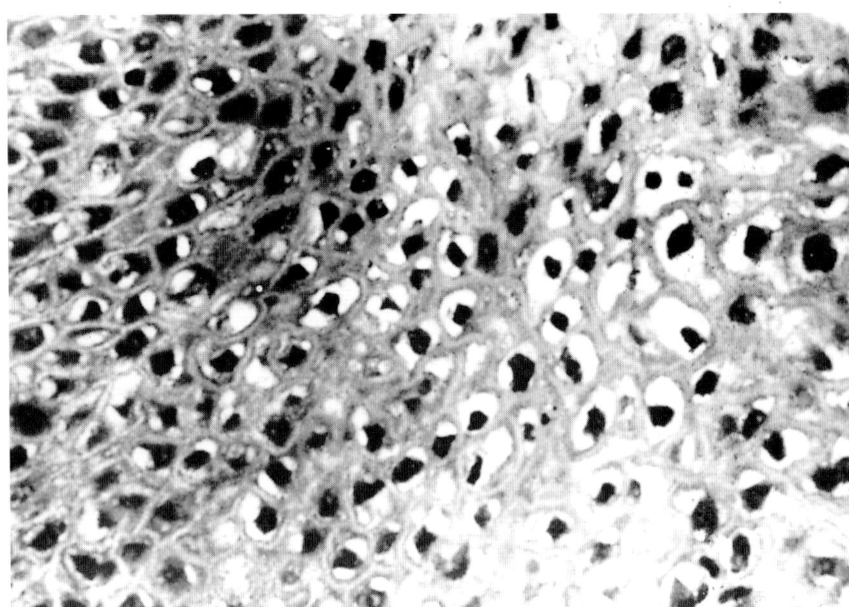

Fig. 10.7 High-power view of the epithelium in a condyloma acuminatum. Numerous koilocytes are present.

Biopsies from anogenital warts that have recently been treated with podophyllin may be difficult to evaluate, as there can be ballooning of the cells, vacuolation of the cytoplasm, nuclear enlargement and metaphase arrest (Pope *et al.* 1973) but a distinction can be drawn from VIN by the absence of abnormal mitotic figures and of any abnormality in chromatin pattern (Wade & Ackerman 1979).

Intraepithelial neoplastic disease

Paget's disease

Paget's disease of the vulva is a form of intraepithelial neoplasia characterized by the presence within the vulval epidermis and skin appendages of adenocarcinomatous cells. In approximately 20% of cases Paget's disease is associated with an underlying adenocarcinoma in the skin adnexae or Bartholin's gland and it is thought that under such circumstances the malignant Paget cells reach the epidermis by upward migration along the ducts (Koss *et al.* 1968, Tchange *et al.* 1973, Creasman *et al.* 1975, Hart & Millman 1977, Lee *et al.* 1977, Webb & Beswick 1983, Hastrup & Andersen 1988). In a further 10–20% of cases vulval Paget's disease is associated with a more distant neoplasm, most commonly in the breast and less frequently in such sites as the urinary tract, the anorectal area or elsewhere in the female genital tract (Helwig & Graham 1963, Fetherston & Friedrich 1972, Friedrich *et al.* 1975, Taylor *et al.* 1975, Lee *et al.* 1977, Breen *et al.* 1978, Jones *et al.* 1979, McKee & Hertogs 1980, Tuck & Williams 1985, Degefu *et al.* 1986, Baehrendtz *et al.* 1994, Fishman *et al.* 1995); the nature of this association is obscure for it is not thought that the Paget cells represent a metastatic lesion from a distant primary site.

In most patients with vulval Paget's disease neither a locally invasive nor a distant neoplasm is found and the neoplastic cells appear to have developed *in situ* from pluripotential germinative cells in the basal layer of the epidermis (Woodruff 1955, Medenica & Sahihi 1972, Salazar & Gonzalez-Angulo 1984, Guarner *et al.* 1989, Urabe *et al.* 1990). The Paget cells may also involve sweat gland ducts but whether the cells arise in the epidermis and migrate into the adnexae (Woodruff 1955), develop simultaneously in the epidermis and skin appendages (Fenn *et al.* 1971, Medenica & Sahihi 1972, Olson *et al.* 1991) or develop in sweat gland ducts and migrate to the dermis (Roth *et al.* 1977, Kariniemi *et al.* 1984, Mazoujian *et al.* 1984, Moll & Moll 1985) is a matter of debate. There is, however, an increasing acceptance that Paget cells are usually either of apocrine origin or are showing apocrine differentiation (Mazoujian *et al.* 1984, Merot *et al.* 1985, Moll & Moll 1985, Nagle *et al.* 1985).

Most patients with Paget's disease are elderly, the majority being above the age of 60, and their most common complaint is of pruritus for anything from a few months to 10 years, the average being about 2 years. Macroscopically, there are multiple, erythematous, eczematoid, moderately well-demarcated, scaly patches or plaques (Fig. 10.8): occasionally, the patches are hyperkeratotic and appear white. The lesions occur most commonly on the labia majora but they may also involve the perineum and perianal area.

Histologically, the Paget cells form clusters and nests (Fig. 10.9), with or without tubule formation, or lie singly in the epidermis (Fig. 10.10). The larger nests are in the basal and parabasal layers whilst small nests of cells and single cells tend to be in the more superficial parts of the epidermis. The cells are often seen in the outer root sheaths of hair follicles (Fig. 10.11) in eccrine and apocrine sweat gland ducts and in sebaceous glands. The Paget cells are large, oval and have abundant vacuolated cytoplasm and large, vesicular, pale, oval or round nuclei; some cells may have a signet ring appearance. The affected epidermis may be otherwise normal, acanthotic, hyperkeratotic or parakeratotic, and may contain atypical dyskeratotic cells; the underlying dermis usually shows a non-specific chronic inflammatory cell infiltrate.

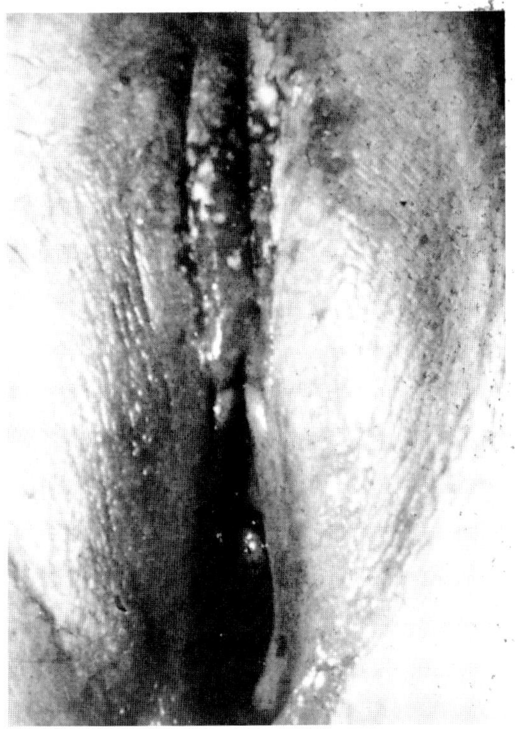

Fig. 10.8 Paget's disease of the vulva; extensive eroded erythema and whitish patches.

Paget cells stain positively with mucicarmine, aldehyde fuchsin (Helwig & Graham 1963) and periodic acid-Schiff stain (PAS)/Alcian blue after diastase digestion (Belcher 1972). Melanin is usually absent (Helwig & Graham 1963, Salazar & Gonzalez-Angulo 1984) but is occasionally present in patients whose skin is heavily pigmented (Medenica & Sahihi 1972, Jones *et al.* 1979); nevertheless the finding of intracellular melanin in large cells with clear cytoplasm should raise the possibility of superficial spreading melanoma, with which Paget's disease may be confused. The Paget cells stain positively for CEA (Kariniemi *et al.* 1984, Oji *et al.* 1984, Stapleton 1984, Nagle *et al.* 1985, Anthony *et al.* 1986, Mori *et al.* 1989, Olson *et al.* 1991), epithelial membrane antigen (Mori *et al.* 1989, Olson *et al.* 1991) and, in 60% of cases, for gross cystic disease protein (Mazoujian *et al.* 1984, Guarner *et al.* 1989, Olson *et al.* 1991). Their positive staining for 54-kDa cytokeratin contrasts with the negative reaction found in a superficial spreading melanoma (Shah *et al.* 1987); the cells also stain positively with Cam 5.2 (Helm *et al.* 1992) and with the monoclonal antibody B72.3, which is a marker for adenocarcinoma (Olson *et al.* 1991). They give a negative reaction for S-100.

The prognosis, in terms of survival, for patients with vulval Paget's disease and without an associated malignant neoplasm is generally very good. However, in some cases, the intraepithelial lesion gives rise to an adenocarcinoma, which invades the dermis, may metastasize to lymph nodes and can cause death (Creasman *et al.* 1975, Parmley *et al.* 1975, Hart & Millman 1977, Lee *et al.* 1977, Breen *et al.* 1978, Jones

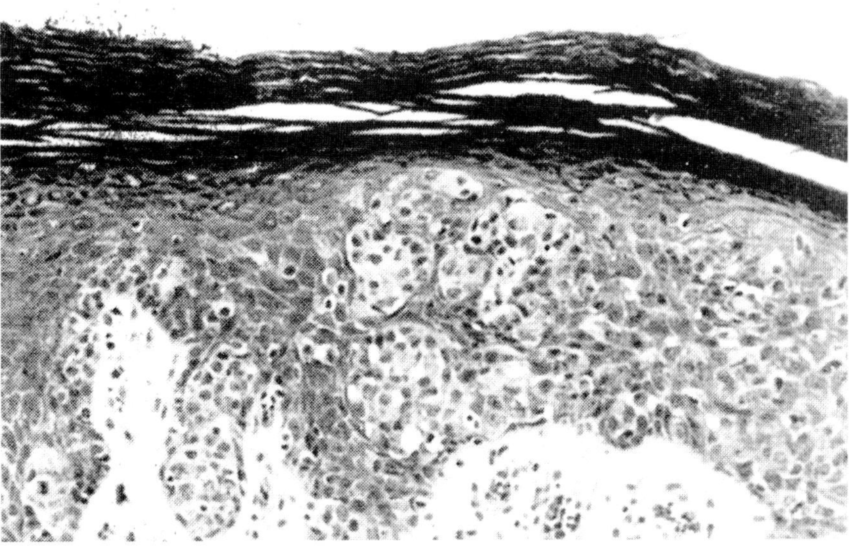

Fig. 10.9 Paget's disease of the vulva: large, pale-staining Paget cells form nests in the rete ridges and in the Malpighian layer of the epidermis.

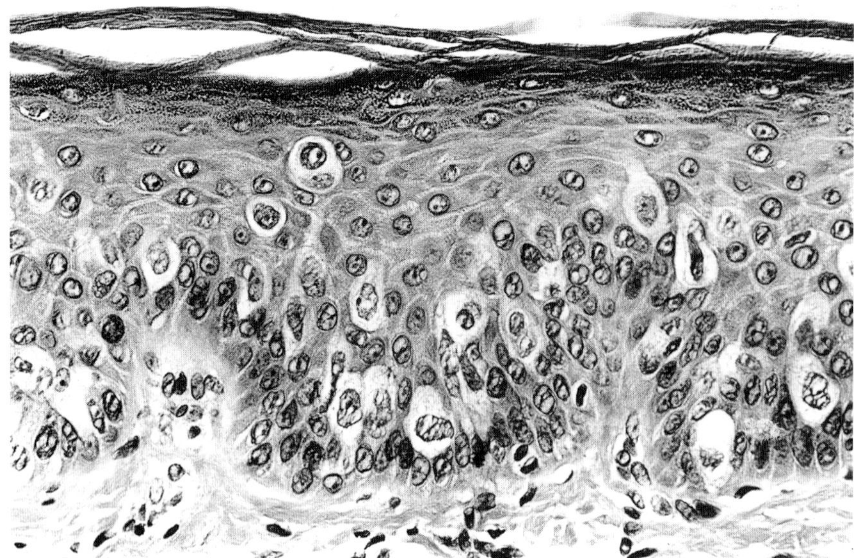

Fig. 10.10 Paget's disease of the vulva: large, round Paget cells are scattered in the epidermis.

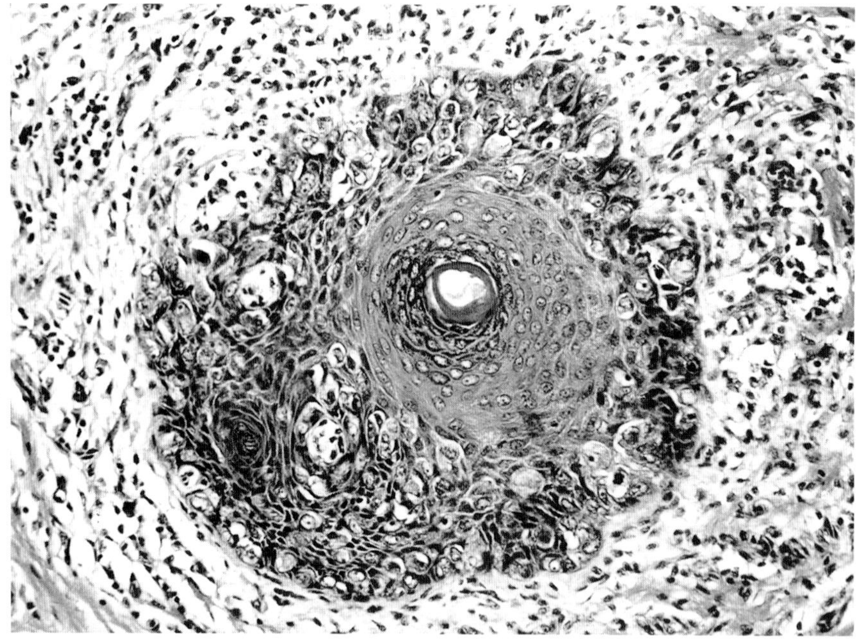

Fig. 10.11 Paget's disease: Paget cells are forming aggregates at the margin of this skin appendage.

et al. 1979, Feuer *et al.* 1990, Evans & Neven 1991, Hawley *et al.* 1991, Baehrendtz *et al.* 1994); extensive lymph node metasases have been noted in a patient in whom the dermal invasion was to a depth of only 1 mm (Fine *et al.* 1995).

Treatment of intraepithelial vulval Paget's disease is by surgical excision but recurrence occurs in nearly 40% of cases. This is due partly to the apparently multifocal nature of the disease and partly to the tendency of the lesion to extend beyond the clinically apparent margins (Gunn & Gallager 1980). It is generally thought useful to undertake frozen sections of resection margins to ensure adequate excision (Stacy *et al.* 1986, Curtin *et al.* 1990, Kodama *et al.* 1995) and whilst some have claimed that immunocytochemistry is superior to histology in assessing the resection margins (Bacchi *et al.* 1992) others have been unable to confirm this (Ganjei *et al.* 1990). Recurrence can, however, occur even when the resection margins have been free of Paget's cells (Bergen *et al.* 1989) and Fishman *et al.* (1995), who found no correlation between margin status and the risk of recurrence, suggest that intraoperative frozen sections should only be used in patients in whom there is concern with respect to an associated invasive carcinoma. It is of considerable practical and theoretical significance that recurrence can occur not only in residual skin but also in skin grafts taken from other parts of the body (de Jonge & Knobel 1988, Misas *et al.* 1990, DiSaia *et al.* 1995, Geisler *et al.* 1995). Recurrence can be both repetitive and extensive, often requiring repeated surgery and, in very exceptional cases, necessitating treatment as extreme as pelvic exenteration (Geisler *et al.* 1997). In patients with recurrent disease, other modalities of treatment include radiotherapy, carbon dioxide laser, topical 5-fluorouracil or bleomycin, and oral retinoids.

Vulval intraepithelial neoplasia

In this account the term vulval intraepithelial neoplasia (VIN) is restricted to intraepithelial squamous neoplasia and does not include Paget's disease or intraepithelial melanocytic lesions. The term does, however, encompass, and replace, those conditions previously known as Bowen's disease, Bowenoid papulosis, erythroplasia of Queyrat, squamous carcinoma-*in-situ* and dystrophy with atypia. VIN is characterized by disorientation and loss of squamous epithelial architecture and maturation together with a variable degree of cytological atypia; the lesion is graded into VIN 1, VIN 2 and VIN 3 but most accounts of the epidemiology, clinical features and natural history of the disease relate only to VIN 3 and not to the lesser grades of this condition.

Epidemiology

The incidence of VIN appears to have genuinely increased markedly during the last 25 years, particularly in younger woman, and the mean age at diagnosis has fallen progressively from 50 years in series reported before 1975 to, currently, about 33 years with a modal peak at 28 years (Ferenczy 1992, Sturgeon *et al.* 1992). There is a strong association with sexually transmitted diseases such as syphilis and gonorrhoea, their incidence in various series of women with VIN ranging from 22% to 60% (Collins *et al.* 1970, Forney *et al.* 1977, Friedrich *et al.* 1980). A history of herpes vulvitis is obtained in 10–12% of women with VIN whilst condylomata acuminata are present in between 15 and 30% (Abell 1965, Forney *et al.* 1977, Buscema *et al.* 1980a, Friedrich *et al.* 1980, Caglar *et al.* 1982, Bernstein *et al.* 1983a, Daling *et al.* 1984). A high proportion (variously estimated as between 11 and 80%) of patients with VIN have concurrent, past or subsequent cervical intraepithelial neoplasia (CIN) (Buscema *et al.* 1980a, Friedrich *et al.* 1980, Benedet & Murphy 1982, Caglar *et al.* 1982, DiPaola *et al.* 1982, Andreasson & Bock 1985, Bornstein *et al.* 1988, Ferenczy 1992). In view of the high incidence of associated CIN it is not suprising that many of the epidemiological factors operative for CIN, such as early onset of sexual activity, oral contraceptive use and multiple sexual partners, are also associated with VIN (Ferenczy 1992).

Aetiology

A clear association between VIN and HPV type 16 infection has been abundantly demonstrated (Pelisse *et al.* 1985, Obalek *et al.* 1986, Bergeron *et al.* 1987, Gupta *et al.* 1987, Reid *et al.* 1987, Beckmann *et al.* 1988, Bender *et al.* 1988, Buscema *et al.* 1988, Twiggs *et al.* 1988, Nuovo *et al.* 1990, Pilotti *et al.* 1990, Park *et al.* 1991, van Beurden *et al.* 1995), although in one study HPV 16 was found to be no more likely to be associated with VIN than HPV 6 or 11 (Cone *et al.* 1991). A significant proportion of cases of VIN are, however, negative when tested for HPV even by the most sophisticated techniques currently available and it is becoming increasingly clear that there are two distinct types of VIN: one associated with HPV infection and one not related to viral infection. The HPV-associated type of VIN occurs predominantly, but by no means solely, in younger patients and tends to be a multicentric and multifocal disease, whilst the non-HPV-associated form is usually found in older women and is commonly unifocal and unicentric (Haefner *et al.* 1995).

It has been suggested that herpes simplex virus type 2 (HSV 2) may play a role in the aetiology of VIN, possibly by acting synergistically with HPV (zur Hausen 1982), whilst there also appears to be a clear correlation between VIN and cigarette smoking (Wilkinson *et al.* 1988, Friedrich *et al.* 1992, Ferenczy 1992).

Clinical features

As already remarked, VIN in young women tends to be HPV associated, multifocal and often associated with lesions in the cervix, vagina and perineal skin, whilst in older patients intraepithelial disease is usually non-HPV associated, restricted to the vulva and unifocal (Crum *et al.* 1984, Twiggs *et al.* 1988, Husseinzadeh *et al.* 1989, Spitzer *et al.* 1989, Ferenczy 1992).

The most common presenting complaint of women with VIN 3 is pruritus, but about one-third will have noticed an abnormality of the vulval skin and a substantial proportion, ranging in different series from 18 to 46%, are asymptomatic (Buscema *et al.* 1980a, Friedrich *et al.* 1980, Caglar *et al.* 1982, DiPaola *et al.* 1982, Bernstein *et al.* 1983a, Andreasson & Bock 1985, Powell *et al.* 1986, Ragnarsson *et al.* 1987, Fiorica *et al.* 1988), the lesion being detected incidentally during the course of treatment of vulval condylomata or CIN.

VIN may be discrete and sharply localized but can involve the entire vulva; the most frequent site for a discrete lesion is on the posterior part of the labia minora. The gross appearances are extremely variable, as the lesions may be white, dull grey, red, brown, variegated red and white or darkly pigmented; they may be flat, granular or warty. The pigmented lesions have been segregated by some into a separate entity of 'Bowen's papulosis' (Wade *et al.* 1979); their histological features and natural history do not, however, differ in any respect from those of non-pigmented lesions (Obalek *et al.* 1986, Bergeron *et al.* 1987) and there is no justification for this separate categorization.

Histology

VIN may be undifferentiated or differentiated, the former tending to occur in younger women and being frequently associated with both HPV infection and smoking, and the latter occurring more commonly in older women and often not associated with HPV infection (Haefner *et al.* 1995, Kaufman 1995, Lininger & Tavassoli 1996). Two basic patterns of undifferentiated VIN are seen (Buscema *et al.* 1980a): one (Fig. 10.12) in which cells of basal or parabasal type extend into the upper layers of the epidermis—basaloid VIN—and the other (Fig. 10.13) in which premature cellular maturation occurs often in association with epithelial multinucleation, corps ronds and koilocytosis (Fig. 10.14)—Bowenoid or 'warty' VIN. Common to both forms is the presence of mitotic figures, often abnormal, above the basal layers of the epithelium (Fig. 10.15), cellular and nuclear pleomorphism, a high nuclear/cytoplasmic ratio, irregular clumping of nuclear chromatin and, in many cases, either parakeratosis or hyperkeratosis. It is not uncommon, in both forms of VIN, for pigmentary incontinence to occur and for the underlying dermis to contain

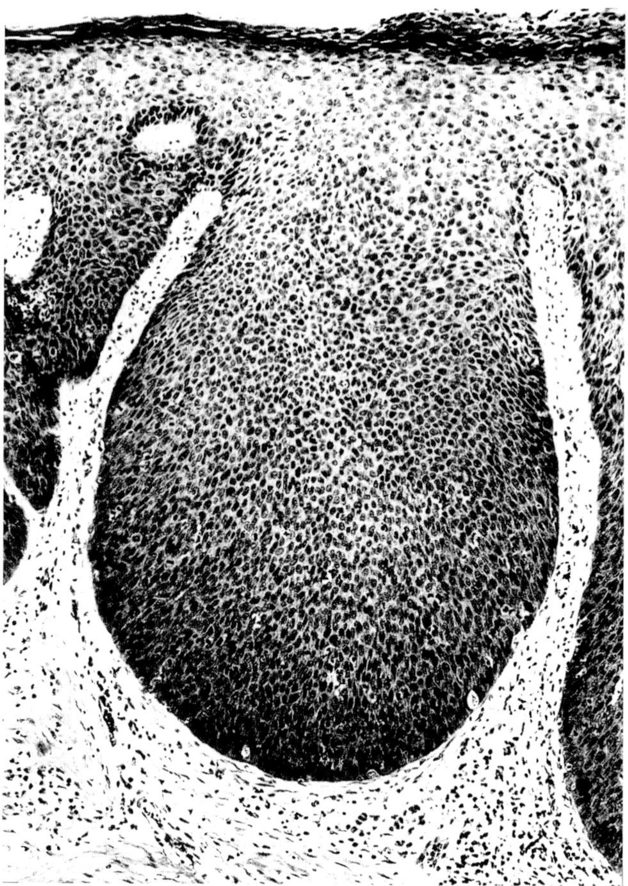

Fig. 10.12 Basaloid type of VIN 3: the epithelium is occupied throughout its depth by cells resembling those of the normal basal layer.

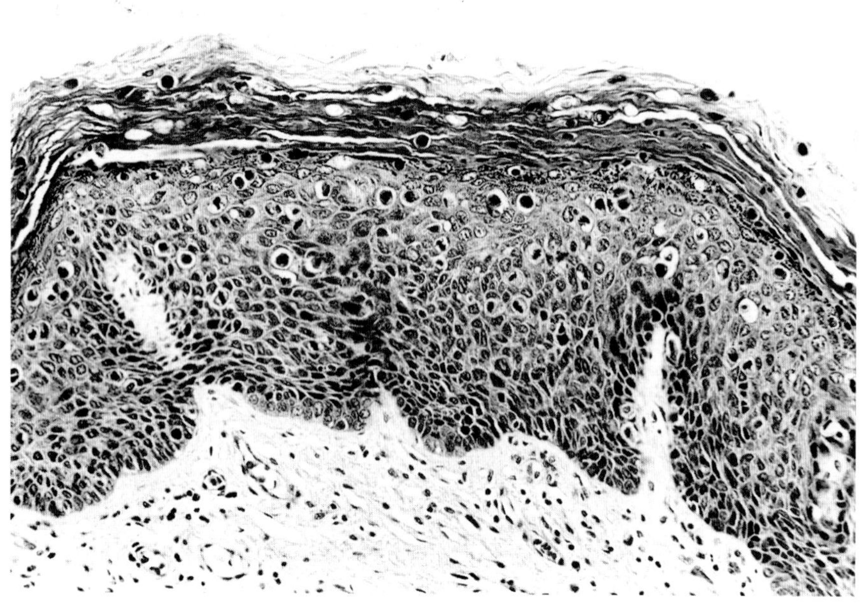

Fig. 10.13 Bowenoid VIN 3: the cellular atypia is characterized by the presence of koilocytes, corps ronds and frequent mitotic figures.

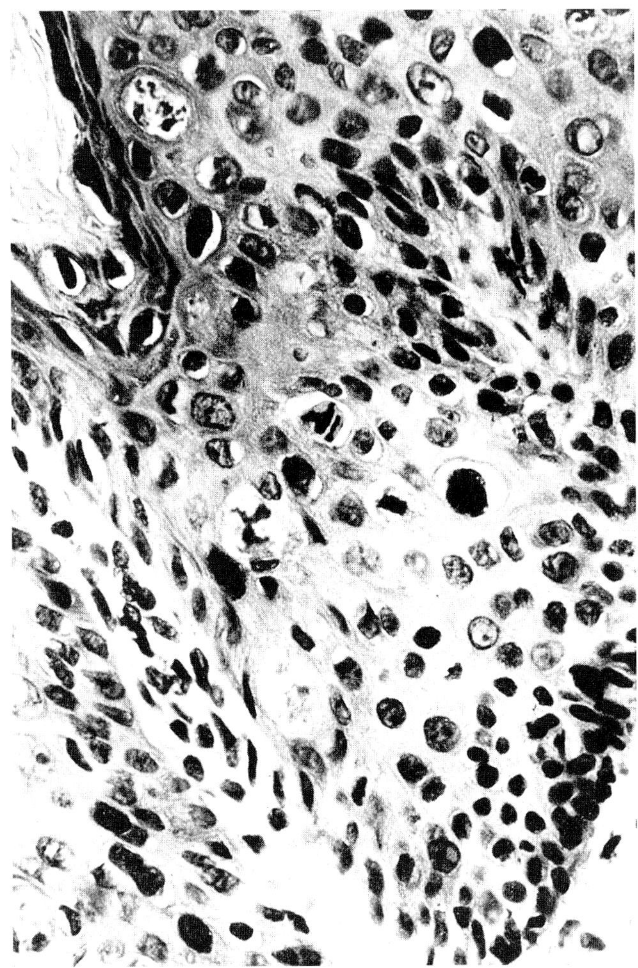

Fig. 10.14 High-power view of Bowenoid VIN 3.

large numbers of melanin-laden macrophages, these being responsible for the pigmentation which is sometimes macroscopically apparent. Either form of VIN may extend into pilosebaceous units or, less commonly, into sweat glands (Mene & Buckley 1985, Baggish *et al.* 1989, Shatz *et al.* 1989). The two forms of undifferentiated VIN not uncommonly exist together in the same patient and they are not mutually exclusive of each other.

A differentiated VIN is one in which the epithelium shows little or no atypia above the basal or parabasal layers but where large eosinophilic keratinocytes with abnormal nuclei are present in the basal layers and such cells, or intraepithelial pearls, are also present in the rete ridges (Fig. 10.16), the nuclei in these areas having coarse chromatin and prominent nucleoli (Buscema & Woodruff 1980, Wilkinson *et al.* 1986). This is a very uncommon form and is usually associated with lichen sclerosus.

It is usual to grade undifferentiated VIN, though the validity of such grading is open to debate. When cellular abnormalities and lack of both stratification and cytoplasmic differentiation are limited to the lower third of the epithelium the lesion is classed as VIN 1. Extension of the abnormal cells into the middle third of the epithelium puts the lesion into the category of VIN 2 whilst involvement of the upper third warrants a grading of VIN 3. Grading of a basaloid VIN is relatively easy but the grading of a Bowenoid VIN is often difficult and sometimes impossible. A differentiated VIN cannot be graded but should probably be regarded, for clinical purposes, as a VIN 3.

Natural history

Virtually nothing is known about the natural history of

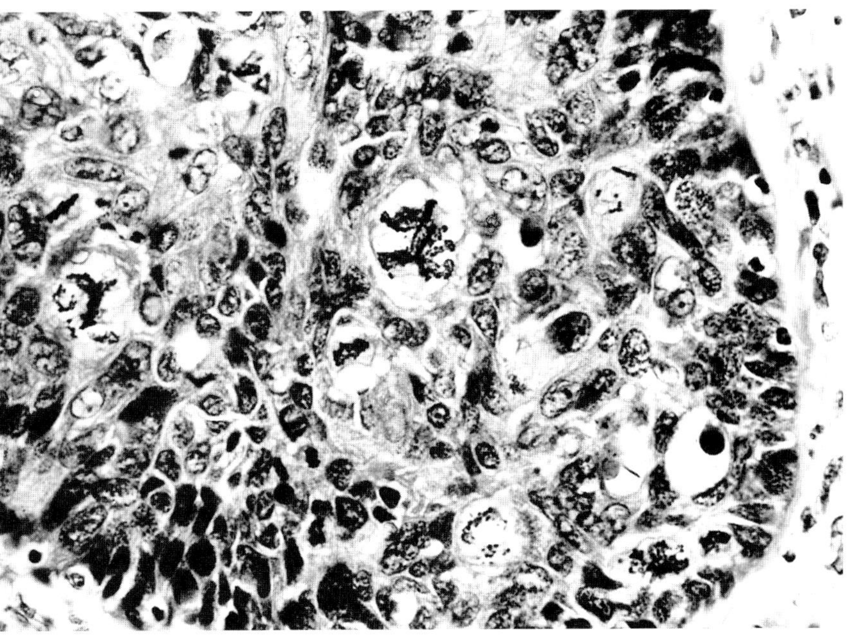

Fig. 10.15 VIN 3: abnormal mitotic figures are present.

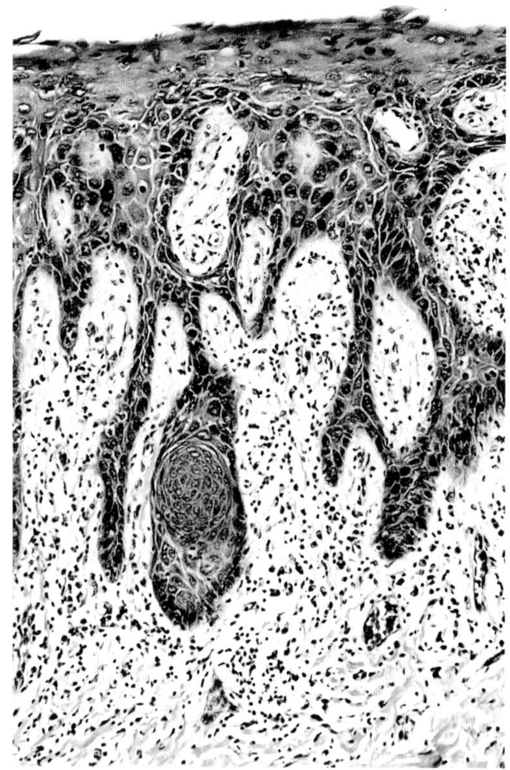

Fig. 10.16 Differentiated VIN. Within the epithelium there is relatively little atypia but there is a well-formed squamous pearl within an elongated rete ridge.

VIN 1 and 2 and the risk of such lesions evolving into an invasive carcinoma has not been determined: the risk is, however, almost certainly very low (Friedrich 1981).

There is no doubt that VIN 3 can progress to an invasive squamous cell carcinoma (Gardiner *et al.* 1953, Collins *et al.* 1970, Jones & Buntine 1978, Jones & McLean 1986) and, indeed, VIN 3 is present in the epithelium adjacent to an invasive vulval squamous cell carcinoma in 20–30% of cases (Buscema *et al.* 1980b, Zaino *et al.* 1982, Leibowitch *et al.* 1990). Nevertheless the potential for progression of VIN 3 to an invasive carcinoma, particularly the Bowenoid type in younger patients, has generally been thought to be low and usually estimated to be no more than 3–4% (Fiorica *et al.* 1988). The risk of invasion is not, however, consistently low and it is possible that it has been seriously underestimated in the past (Jones & Rowan 1994), particularly in elderly women, in whom progression to an invasive lesion can occur in up to 19% of cases of VIN (Crum 1992). Further, unexpected stromal invasion in cases of VIN 3 can easily be missed; Chafe *et al.* (1988) found unexpected stromal invasion in 20% of patients in whom the resected vulvar skin was subjected to serial blocking. Whilst in most cases this represented only very superficial stromal invasion, it has to be borne in mind that invasion of only the most minor degree is associated with a significant risk of progression to a frankly invasive carcinoma (Herod *et al.* 1996) and may, on occasion, be associated with metastatic disease (see later).

Untreated cases of VIN 3 may undergo spontaneous regression (Friedrich 1972, Skinner *et al.* 1973, Friedrich *et al.* 1980, Bernstein *et al.* 1983a), this being particularly the case for young woman with multifocal disease.

Management and prognosis

Because of the perceived low rate of progression of VIN the current tendency is to treat the lesion, especially in young patients, by the most conservative means consistent with complete eradication. Techniques such as laser vaporization, local surgical excision, loop electrosurgical excision or skinning vulvectomy are now widely employed (Ferenczy 1992, Ferenczy *et al.* 1994). Whichever of these techniques is employed the lesion will recur in about 10–12% of patients. In more elderly women a less conservative surgical approach may well be warranted.

Malignant epithelial neoplasms

Microinvasive squamous cell carcinoma of the vulva

Attempts have been made to define a vulval equivalent of the microinvasive carcinoma of the cervix. The theoretical definition of such an entity is straightforward for it means that a neoplasm has escaped from the confines of the epithelium but is invading the underlying stroma to such a limited extent that the risk of nodal metastasis is negligible. Achieving a practical definition of such an entity has, however, proved more difficult.

In 1974 Wharton *et al.* reported that none of 25 patients with carcinomas of 2 cm or less in diameter and invading to a depth of 5 mm or less suffered nodal metastases or recurrence, whilst of 20 women with tumours of similar diameter but invading to a depth of greater than 5 mm, five had lymph node spread and three died of their tumour. Largely as a result of this study a microinvasive carcinoma of the vulva was therefore defined as 'a squamous cell carcinoma 2 cm or less in diameter with no more than 5 mm stromal invasion; the presence of confluence, vascular channel permeation or cellular anaplasia does not exclude the case from this category'. It very rapidly became apparent, however, that approximately 15% of patients with a neoplasm meeting this definition had inguinal node metastases at the time of initial surgery (Barnes *et al.* 1980, Wilkinson *et al.* 1982, Hoffman *et al.* 1983, Boyce *et al.* 1984, Hacker *et al.* 1984, Wilkinson 1985, 1987, Sedlis *et al.* 1987). It was therefore suggested that a cut-off point of invasion to a depth of 3 mm should be used for defining a microinvasive

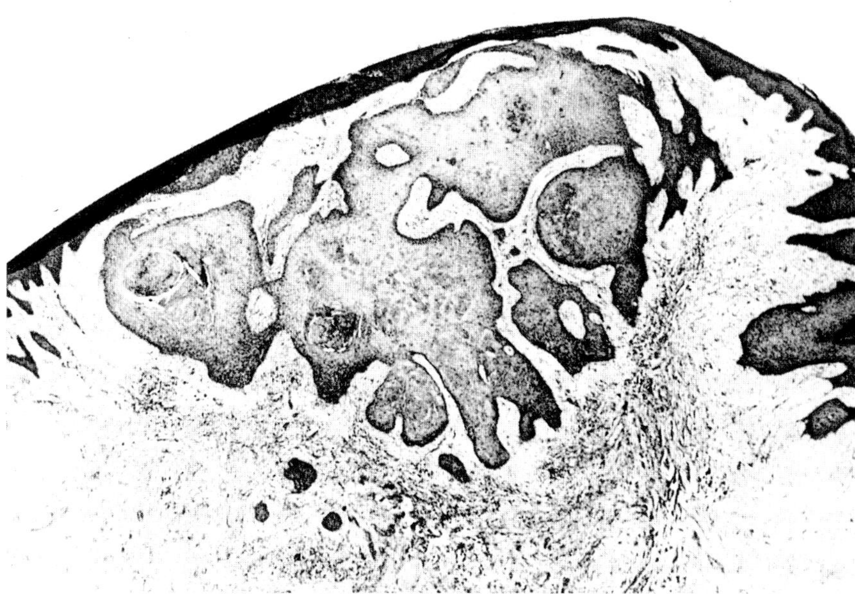

Fig. 10.17 A small squamous cell carcinoma of the vulva, which is invading to a depth of less than 3 mm from the surface epithelium.

carcinoma (Jafari & Cartnick 1976, Magrina *et al.* 1979, Chu *et al.* 1982, Hoffman *et al.* 1983) but even with invasion limited to this depth (Fig. 10.17) there is a nodal metastasis rate of 12% (Wilkinson 1987). There have also been reports of nodal metastases, and in some cases eventual death, in patients whose tumours invaded to a depth of between 1 and 2 mm (DiPaola *et al.* 1975, Parker *et al.* 1975, Yazigi *et al.* 1978, Magrina *et al.* 1979, Barnes *et al.* 1980, Kolstad *et al.* 1982, Hacker *et al.* 1983, 1984, Ross & Ehrmann 1987). It has thus become apparent that it is only those neoplasms that invade to a depth of 1 mm or less that are associated with a negligible risk of nodal spread (Kolstad *et al.* 1982, Hacker *et al.* 1983, 1984, Ross & Ehrmann 1987, Sedlis *et al.* 1987, Wilkinson 1987); it has to be stressed that the words 'negligible risk' are used rather than 'no risk', as of approximately 150 patients with tumours invading to a depth of less than 1 mm there has been one who suffered a groin recurrence (Atamtede & Hoogerland 1989) and one who developed groin metastases and eventually died of disseminated carcinoma (van der Velden *et al.* 1992).

It was consideration of the above findings that led the International Society for the Study of Vulvovaginal Disease to decide, in 1984, that the term 'microinvasive carcinoma of the vulva' was misleading and dangerous when taken with the definition current at that time and to recommend that its use be discontinued and that the designation stage 1a invasive carcinoma of the vulva be used to describe solitary lesions with a maximum diameter of 2 cm, and a maximum depth of invasion of 1 mm (Kneale 1984). This recommendation was clearly justified, although the term 'superficially invasive squamous cell carcinoma' is often used, rather unsatisfactorily, as a synonym for stage 1a carcinoma. It should be noted that the presence of vascular space invasion, very rarely seen in tumours invading to a depth of less than 1 mm, does not invalidate a diagnosis of stage 1a cancer, as this finding does not appear to be of any clinical significance in tumours of this size (Buscema *et al.* 1981, Hacker *et al.* 1983, Dvoretsky *et al.* 1984). Other possible prognostic factors, such as a confluent pattern of growth, a spray pattern of growth and tumour differentiation, do not appear to be of any importance when considering rigidly defined stage 1a lesions.

Two problems do, however, remain. The first is the point from which measurement of depth of invasion should be made. Measurements may be made from the epithelial-stromal junction of the most superficial dermal papillae adjacent to the tumour, from the granular layer, from the surface of the epithelium, from the tip of the rete ridge or from the tip of the rete ridge adjacent to the tumour (Wilkinson *et al.* 1982). Wilkinson (1987) recommends measurement from the epithelial-stromal junction of the nearest dermal papillae on the grounds that this measurement is not influenced by hyperkeratosis, tumour ulceration, epithelial hyperplasia or VIN. Wells and Jenkins (1994) suggest, however, that depth of invasion should be measured in a manner analagous to that in which early stromal invasion of the cervix is measured, i.e. from the point of origin of the invasive cells from the non-invasive epithelium; this seems an eminently sensible suggestion.

A second problem is the ability of the pathologist to distinguish between early invasion and tangential sectioning or involvement of skin appendages by VIN. Features suggestive of true invasion include an inflammatory infiltrate at the point of invasion, isolated squamous cells 'streaming' into the stroma, increased cytoplasmic eosinophilia of the invading cells, nuclear chromatin clearing and visible nucleoli in the invading cells, and a desmoplastic response at the site of invasion (Wilkinson 1987).

The reason for defining a group of vulval carcinomas with a very low risk of nodal metastases is that they can be treated by conservative measures and hence treatment of stage 1a invasive carcinoma is, in many centres, by wide local excision without groin node dissection (Kelley *et al.* 1992).

Invasive squamous cell carcinoma
(see also Chapter 5)

Squamous cell carcinoma accounts for between 80 and 90% of malignant vulval neoplasms and for about 3–4% of gynaecological cancers (Krupp 1992).

Epidemiology, aetiology and pathogenesis

It is becoming increasingly clear that there are, in epidemiological and aetiological terms, at least two quite different types of squamous cell carcinoma of the vulva (Crum 1992, Kurman *et al.* 1993, Hording *et al.* 1994, Trimble *et al.* 1996). The less common occurs in relatively young women, is usually preceded by VIN and is associated with HPV infection, particularly HPV types 16 and 18, whilst the more frequent form develops in elderly patients, is not commonly associated with VIN and is generally not linked to HPV infection (Andersen *et al.* 1991, Toki *et al.* 1991, Crum 1992, Messing & Gallup 1995). This recently defined heterogeneity makes it difficult to interpret many of the older epidemiological studies of vulval cancer, most of which have considered the disease as a single entity. Within these limitations, however, the incidence of vulval cancer appears to be highest in Latin America and the Caribbean and lowest in Asia. There was thought to be an inverse correlation with socioeconomic status but this disappears on multivariate analysis and earlier claims of an association with obesity, hypertension and diabetes mellitus have not withstood the tests of case control studies and multivariate analysis (Mabuchi *et al.* 1985, Brinton *et al.* 1990); likewise, menstrual and reproductive factors have not been linked to increased risk (Mack *et al.* 1992).

It is probable that younger patients with HPV-associated vulval carcinoma share many epidemiological features with those suffering from cervical carcinoma, such as an association with condylomas, multiple sexual partners and cigarette smoking (Mabuchi *et al.* 1985, Brinton *et al.* 1990, Andersen *et al.* 1991, Trimble *et al.* 1996); by contrast, none of these factors appears to be applicable to the non-HPV-associated carcinomas occurring in older women (Crum 1992).

An association of vulval cancer with syphilis and chronic granulomatous disease has been long documented in certain populations, such as Jamaicans and black Americans (Salzstein *et al.* 1956, Green *et al.* 1958, Hay & Cole 1970, Franklin & Rutledge 1972, Sengupta 1981). Vulval carcinomas related to these diseases occur, however, in women below the age of 60 years and it is almost certain that these infections are surrogates for sexual activity at a young age and for HPV infection (Crum 1992).

It seems highly probably that HPV infection is a carcinogenic factor, or cofactor, in the development of vulval cancer in younger patients but possible carcinogenic factors in non-HPV-associated vulval carcinoma in older women have not been defined. There is a historical association, clearly not valid today, between vulval carcinoma and industrial exposure to mineral oils in women working in the cotton industry (Gerrard 1932, Stacy 1939) whilst an association has also been noted with the use of hair dyes (Hennekens *et al.* 1979) and with coffee drinking (Mabuchi *et al.* 1985), neither of which appears to offer a very convincing aetiological hypothesis. *p53* mutation is relatively commonly detectable in older women with HPV-negative tumours (Pilotti *et al.* 1996, Lee *et al.* 1994) but the aetiological significance of such a mutation is still uncertain.

HPV-negative invasive squamous carcinoma in elderly women is often associated with either squamous hyperplasia or lichen sclerosus in the adjacent skin (Gomez-Rueda *et al.* 1994, Hording *et al.* 1994). That any associated squamous hyperplasia is, however, probably not the direct precursor of such invasive lesions is suggested by a study which found that, whilst the neoplasms were monoclonal and showed *p53* mutation, the hyperplastic skin was polyclonal and without evidence of *p53* mutation (Kim *et al.* 1996). The last word on this topic may not, however, have been written, as in a subsequent investigation some cases of squamous hyperplasia were found to be monoclonal (Crum *et al.* 1997). The relationship between lichen sclerosus and squamous carcinoma is a complex one: the vast majority of women with lichen sclerosus do not develop invasive carcinoma, but longitudinal analysis of a cohort of women with this condition has clearly shown them to be at increased risk (Carli *et al.* 1995). The carcinomas associated with lichen sclerosus may, however, be either HPV positive or HPV negative (Crum *et al.*).

Clinical features and gross pathology

Three-quarters of women with vulval squamous cell carcinoma are aged over 60 years (Green 1978, Benedet *et al.*

1979), the mean age at initial diagnosis being 66 years (Japaze *et al.* 1977). The common presenting complaints are of a vulval lump, pruritus, discharge, bleeding and pain.

The majority of squamous carcinomas (70%) develop on the labia, most commonly the labia majora (Fig. 10.18). The second commonest site, accounting for between 11 and 24% of cases, is the clitoris (Japaze *et al.* 1977, Benedet *et al.* 1979, Zaino 1987). In about 10% of cases the tumour is so large that its precise site of origin is uncertain. Multifocal disease is uncommon but 'kissing' tumours are sometimes seen on the adjacent surfaces of the labia. Over 50% of the tumours are ulcerated whilst about one-third are papillary and about 10% are plaque-like.

Spread

Squamous carcinomas spread directly to adjacent tissues, by the lymphatics to the inguinal, femoral and pelvic nodes, and, rarely, late in the course of the disease, via the bloodstream to the lungs, liver and bones. Nearly 30% of patients have inguinal nodal metastases at the time of initial diagnosis and 10–20% have pelvic node metastases. When the primary tumour is limited to one side, more than 80% of inguinal nodal metastases occur in the ipsilateral nodes (Krupp & Bohm 1978), 5–15% occur only in the contralateral nodes, and bilateral nodal involvement occurs in 15–30% (Way 1982). When the inguinal nodes are free from tumour the pelvic nodes are not usually affected (Curry *et al.* 1980, Podratz *et al.* 1983a, Shimm *et al.* 1986), although occasional exceptions to this general rule do occur (Krupp & Bohm 1978). Bilateral inguinal node metastases are present in nearly 40% of patients with clitoral tumours (Krupp 1992).

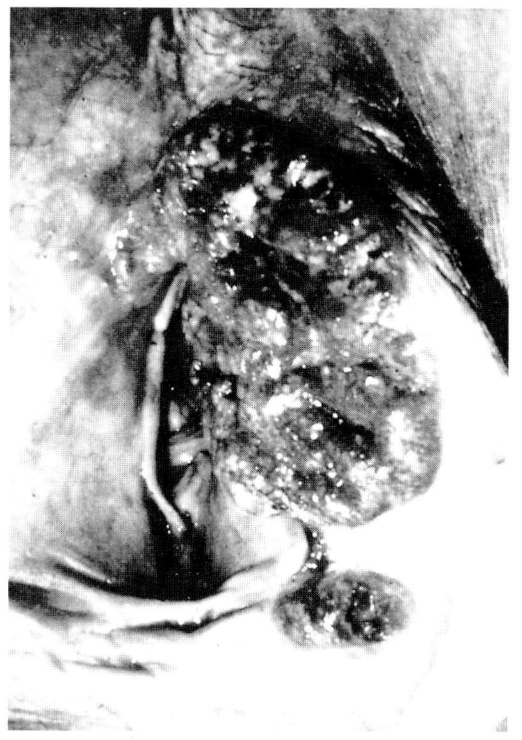

Fig. 10.18 An invasive squamous cell carcinoma of the vulva.

Staging

The FIGO clinical staging system that was in use until relatively recently was highly inaccurate, particularly in respect to the presence or absence of groin lymph node metastases, and has now been replaced by a combined clinical and surgical staging system (Shepherd 1995). This is detailed in Table 10.1 and it is seen that the presence of groin nodal metastases must be histopathologically confirmed.

Histopathology

Within recent years squamous cell carcinomas of the vulva have been subdivided into three separate categories, which differ from each other not only in their histological appearances but also in relationship to patient age, association with HPV infection and origin from pre-existing VIN (Toki *et al.* 1991, Kurman *et al.* 1993). These three categories are:

1 typical keratinizing squamous cell carcinoma;
2 basaloid carcinoma;
3 warty carcinoma.

Table 10.1 Combined Clinical and Pathological Staging of Vulvar Carcinoma (FIGO 1995).

Stage I	Tumour confined to the vulva, 2 cm or less in diameter, no metastases in the groin nodes
Stage Ia	Depth of invasion not exceeding 1 mm (calculated from the nearest dermal papilla)
Stage Ib	All others
Stage II	Tumour confined to the vulva, more than 2 cm in diameter, no metastases in the groin nodes
Stage III	Tumour of any size with adjacent spread to the vagina, urethra and/or perineum and/or anus and/or: unilateral pathologically confirmed groin lymph node metastases
Stage IVA	Tumour of any size infiltrating the bladder mucosa and/or rectal mucosa, including the upper part of the urethral mucosa, and/or fixed to the bone and/or: pathologically confirmed bilateral groin lymph node metastases
Stage IVB	Distant metastases and/or: pathologically confirmed pelvic lymph node metastases

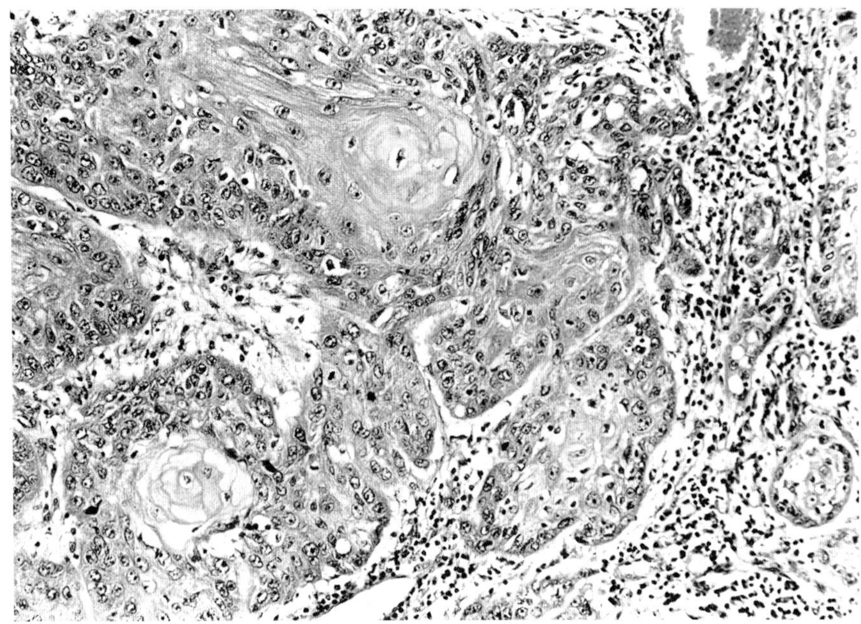

Fig. 10.19 A well-differentiated invasive squamous cell carcinoma of the vulva. The tumour is composed of nests of squamous cells showing differentiation towards their centre with the formation of epithelial pearls.

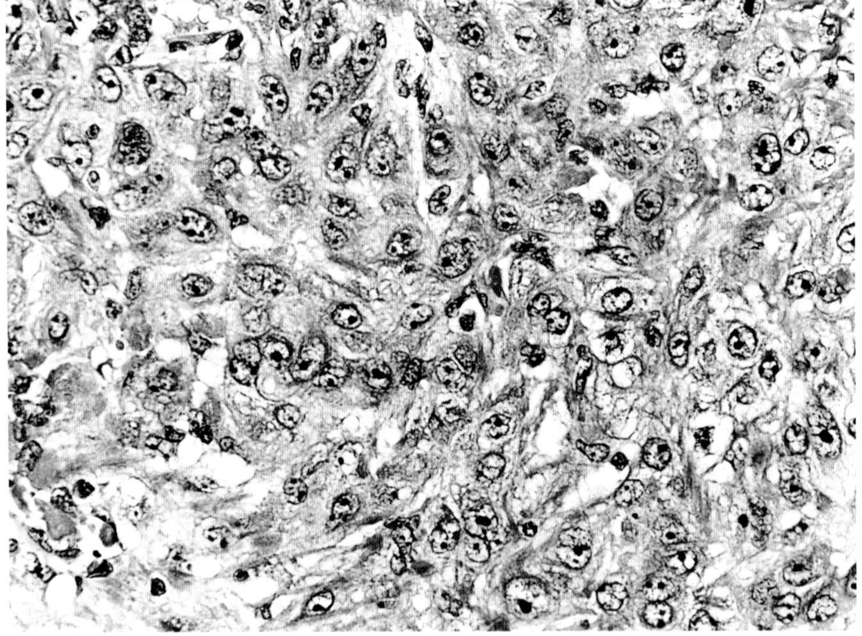

Fig. 10.20 A poorly differentiated squamous cell carcinoma of the vulva.

Typical keratinizing squamous cell carcinomas (Fig. 10.19) account for about 65% of cases, occur predominantly in women aged more than 65 years and are infrequently associated with HPV infection. The adjacent non-involved epithelium usually shows squamous hyperplasia or lichen sclerosus, and VIN is relatively rarely seen, when present tending to be of the differentiated type. Well-differentiated squamous cell carcinomas form rounded nests of mature squamous cells with keratin pearls in their centres, which may in some instances almost entirely replace the squamous cells. Desmosomes are evident, mitotic figures are sparse and found at the periphery of the nests and there is only slight nuclear atypia. Moderately differentiated squamous cell carcinomas show less keratinization within the cell nests and the squamous cells are less mature: there is a higher nuclear/cytoplasmic ratio, greater nuclear atypia and more marked mitotic activity with mitotic figures throughout the nests. In poorly differentiated squamous cell carcinomas (Fig. 10.20) the cells tend to be arranged in sheets, cords or small clusters; squamous pearls are still

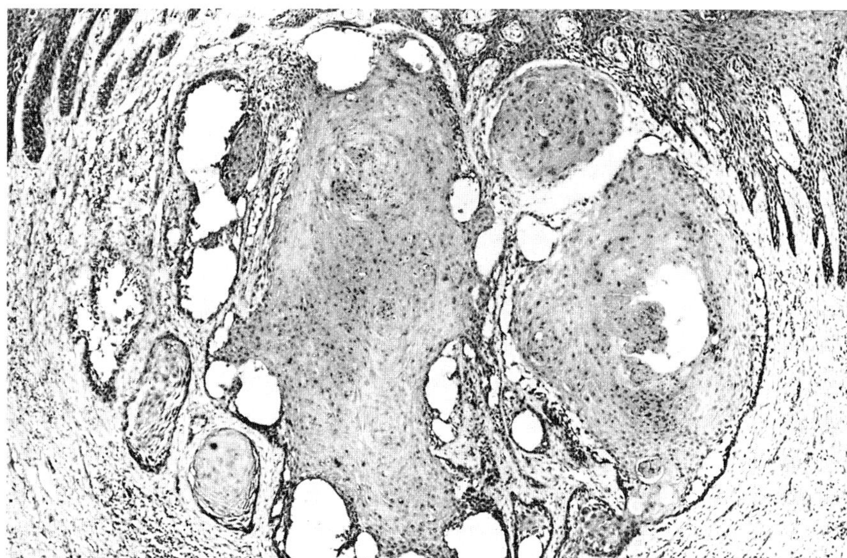

Fig. 10.21 An adenoid squamous cell carcinoma of the vulva. This has gland-like spaces, some of which contain acantholytic cells.

present but there is considerable nuclear atypia and pleomorphism, and marked mitotic activity.

Basaloid carcinomas form about 28% of invasive neoplasms, are frequently associated with HPV types 16 or 18 and occur in relatively young patients, i.e. below the age of 60 years. The adjacent non-involved epithelium commonly shows a basaloid type of VIN 3. The tumours are formed of masses, nests, clusters or cords of basal type cells with scanty cytoplasm and a high nuclear/cytoplasmic ratio. There may be some focal squamous maturation but keratin pearls are not present and desmosomes are not seen: there is moderate mitotic activity.

Warty carcinomas constitute approximately 7% of invasive carcinomas and these also occur in younger patients and are associated with HPV infection. The adjacent uninvolved epithelium usually shows a Bowenoid VIN 3. These neoplasms have an exophytic condylomatous appearance with rounded or spiky papillary projections that contain fibrovascular cores and are covered by hyperkeratotic squamous epithelium. At its base the tumour is formed of jagged or irregularly shaped nests of epithelium. Squamous pearls are present and there is a variable degree of nuclear pleomorphism and cytological atypia; multinucleated cells may be seen. Hyperchromatic nuclei with wrinkled membranes are seen in cells showing cytoplasmic vacuolization, i.e. koilocytic atypia.

It is clear that there are marked differences between typical squamous cell carcinoma and neoplasms associated with HPV infection, and it is probable that this histological subdivision is of prognostic importance in so far as HPV-negative tumours appear to have a worse prognosis than do those which are HPV positive (Ansink *et al.* 1994, Monk *et al.* 1995); it remains to be determined, however, whether the histological subdivision of the HPV-associated neoplasms into basal and warty types is of any real clinical significance.

An adenoid variant of squamous cell carcinoma (Fig. 10.21) has been described in which there is acantholysis in the centres of some or all of the infiltrating cell nests to produce cystic spaces lined by cubo-columnar cells (Lasser *et al.* 1974); the pesudoglands thus formed to not contain mucin, which distinguishes this variant from a true adenosquamous carcinoma.

A spindle-cell variant of squamous cell carcinoma is well recognized but occurs with great rarity at the vulva. Such a neoplasm can usually be distinguished from a sarcoma by its positive staining for cytokeratins and negative reaction for vimentin.

Prognosis

The overall 5-year survival rate for patients with vulval carcinoma is now about 75% (Andreasson *et al.* 1982, Podratz *et al.* 1983a, Krupp 1992). For patients with no nodal metastases the survival rate is between 90 and 100% whilst for those with inguinal spread the survival rate is between 30 and 70%, this falling to less than 25% if pelvic nodes are involved (Monaghan 1987, 1990, DiSaia & Creasman 1989). The most important factor governing prognosis is the absence or otherwise of nodal spread (Burger *et al.* 1995) and, whilst various tumour-associated factors are, on univariate analysis, of prognostic value, it is probable that these are largely indicative of the risk of, and are subordinate to, nodal metastasis (Lingard *et al.* 1992, Homesley *et al.* 1993). Thus, tumour diameter, tumour thickness, tumour differentiation, tumour grade, the presence of vascular space invasion and pattern of tumour growth all appear to be prognostic indicators (Franklin & Rutledge 1972, Krupp & Bohm 1978, Benedet *et al.* 1979, Andreasson *et al.* 1982, Podratz *et al.* 1983a, Hacker *et al.* 1984, Monaghan & Hammond 1984, Boyce *et al.* 1984, Shimm *et al.* 1986, Abroa *et al.* 1990, Heaps *et al.* 1990, Husseinzadah *et al.* 1990, Hopkins *et al.* 1991, Lingard *et al.* 1992, Onnis *et al.* 1992, Ayhan *et al.* 1993). Multiple regression analysis has, however, shown that only clinical stage and, within stage II, tumour thickness allow for a clear division into 'high-risk' and 'low-risk' cases (Bryson *et al.* 1991): low-risk cases are stage I patients, together with stage II patients with a tumour thickness of up to 5 mm thick, whilst stage II patients with a tumour more than 5 mm thick, together with stage III and IV patients, constitute the high-risk group.

In patients with nodal metastases the presence of extracapsular spread has indicated a particularly poor prognosis in most (Origoni *et al.* 1992, Paladina *et al.* 1994, van der Velden *et al.* 1995), but not all (Burger *et al.* 1995), studies.

Application of the newer techniques of tumour assessment to squamous cell carcinomas of the vulva has yielded rather inconsistent and inconclusive results. DNA ploidy has been found to be of considerable prognostic importance in some studies (Kaern *et al.* 1992) but not in others (Ballouk *et al.* 1993, Dolan *et al.* 1993) whilst morphometric studies have not yet yielded information of prognostic value (Bjerregaard *et al.* 1993). Immunohistochemical demonstration of p53 protein was found to be indicative of a poor prognosis in one study (Kohlberger *et al.* 1995) but was not of useful prognostic value in another (Kagie *et al.* 1997). Tumours with a diffuse pattern of staining for the cell proliferation market Ki67 were shown to be associated with a reduced patient survival by Hendricks *et al.* (1994) but this finding awaits further confirmation.

Verrucous carcinoma

Verrucous carcinomas of the vulva are distinctly uncommon (Japaze *et al.* 1982) but their true incidence is almost impossible to assess, largely because no definite criteria have been established to allow for a clear distinction to be drawn between this lesion and a giant condyloma of Buschke–Loewenstein. Indeed, there has been little agreement as to whether these are separate and distinct entities, arbitrarily defined morphological stages in a pathological continuum, or identical lesions. Some have felt that a clear clinical and histological distinction can be drawn between these two conditions (Partridge *et al.* 1980a,b) but others, an increasing majority, believe the two lesions to be a single entity and have recommended that the term 'giant condyloma of Buschke–Lowenstein' be abandoned (Gallousis 1972, Kluzak & Kraus 1987), a recommendation that will be followed in this account.

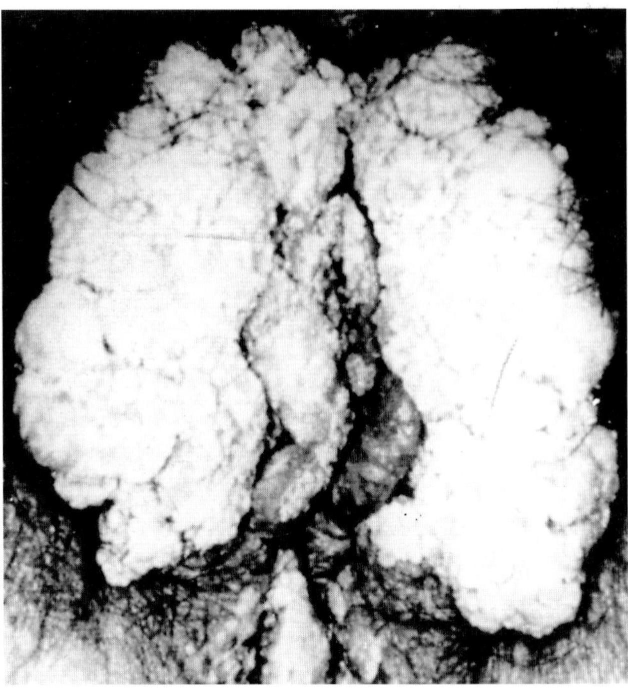

Fig. 10.22 A verrucous carcinoma of the vulva.

Verrucous carcinomas tend to occur at a generally older age than typical carcinomas, most patients being postmenopausal and a high proportion in their eighth or ninth decade. In one large series there was serological evidence of syphilis in 12.5% of cases (Japaze *et al.* 1982) whilst at least 50% of patients also have vulval condylomas. The clinical presentation may be very similar to that of a more conventinal squamous carcinoma but some grow very rapidly and can attain a huge size. The tumour (Fig. 10.22) classically appears as a warty or papillary, fungating, often ulcerated, 'cauliflower-like' mass, which may be pink, grey, yellowish or white. The most common site is the labium majus but not infrequently the neoplasm involves both labia and sometimes the entire vulva.

Histologically (Fig. 10.23), the tumour is composed of papillary fronds of mature stratified squamous epithelium with pushing, bulbous rete ridges. The broad rete ridges appear to be compressing and pushing against the underlying stroma rather than truly invading it and their basal margins are intact, smooth, regular and clearly defined. Hyperkeratosis is usually marked whilst acanthosis is often of a striking degree. There is a virtually total lack of cellular atypia, and delay in maturation is not a feature, basal type cells being seen only in the two or three layers immediately abutting on the basal membrane. Mitotic figures, if present, are confined to the basal layers and are of

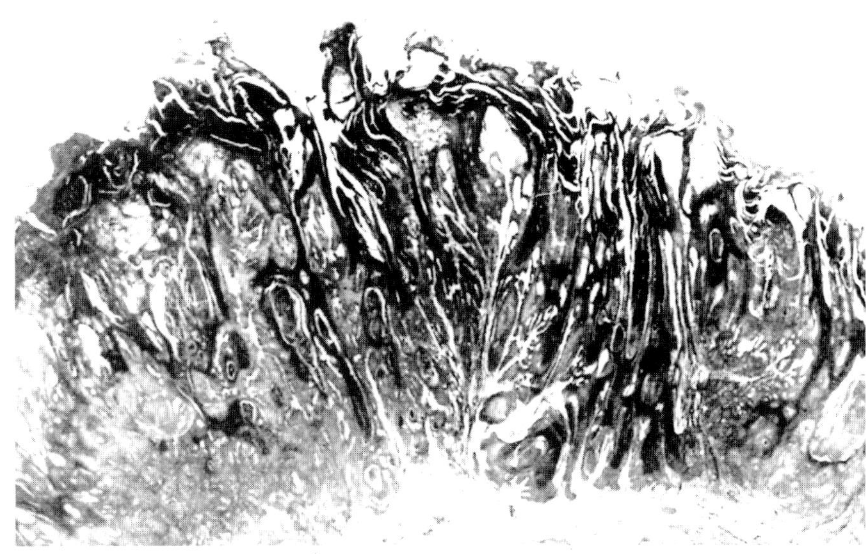

Fig. 10.23 A verrucous carcinoma of the vulva showing extensive warty-like growth with accumulated surface keratin.

normal form. Koilocytes are almost invariably present and this is in accord with the frequent, although far from invariable, presence of HPV 6 or 11 in these lesions (Rando *et al.* 1986, Crowther *et al.* 1988). There is always a well-marked, non-specific chronic inflammatory cell infiltrate adjacent to the base of the tumour. Verrucous carcinomas show a very homogeneous staining pattern for keratins, which contrasts with the disorganized and patchy staining reaction seen in typical squamous cell carcinomas (Brisigotti *et al.* 1989).

In view of the bland histological appearances of a verrucous carcinoma, it is hardly surprising that the pathologist, especially one who is not fully aware of the clinical details, will often report a biopsy from such a neoplasm as being histologically benign, a diagnosis of a condyloma or squamous papilloma often being proffered. Not uncommonly it is only when the neoplasm recurs or continues to show rapid growth and relentless invasive tendencies that the contrast between the aggressive nature of the tumour and its paradoxically innocuous histology raises the possibility of a verrucous carcinoma.

The natural history of a verrucous carcinoma is towards recurrence and local invasion (Lucas *et al.* 1974). If primary removal is incomplete, as is often the case, recurrence is inevitable and does, in fact, occur in about one-third of cases. Although recurrences are usually typical of verrucous carcinoma, they can, very occasionally, take the form of a typical squamous carcinoma (Levitan *et al.* 1992). The neoplasm tends to invade adjacent structures and can sometimes encircle, without actually invading, lymph nodes. True lymphatic spread to nodes can occur (Vayrynen *et al.* 1981) but is most exceptional, as are distant metastases (Stehman *et al.* 1980).

Treatment is by wide local excision (Lucas *et al.* 1974, Isaacs 1976, Partridge *et al.* 1980a, Stehman *et al.* 1980, Japaze *et al.* 1982, Andersen & Sorensen 1988, Gadducci *et al.* 1989). Lymphadenectomy has its advocates (Gallousis 1972, Selium & Lankeroni 1979) but in view of the extremely low incidence of nodal metastases this is an unnecessarily radical procedure (Isaacs 1976, Powell *et al.* 1978). The 5-year survival rate following surgery is 80% but it is only 46% for patients treated with a combination of surgery and radiotherapy, this being because irradiation can induce an anaplastic transformation of the neoplasm (Kraus & Perez-Mesa 1966).

Basal cell carcinoma

Basal cell carcinomas of the vulva are thought to be rare, accounting for only 2–4% of malignant vulval neoplasms (Copas *et al.* 1996). This may well be true amongst cases referred to a gynaecological oncologist but in non-referral hospitals their incidence is much higher, as high as 28% in a Dutch population (van der Velden 1995). Virtually nothing is known about aetiological factors, as, rather obviously, the vulva is not an area commonly exposed to sunlight; a few patients have had previous radiotherapy to the vulval area (Breen *et al.* 1975) but this is a far from common antecedent factor.

Women with these tumours are usually white and elderly (Palladino *et al.* 1969, Breen *et al.* 1975, Cruz-Jimenez & Abell 1975, Zerner 1975), although occasional examples are encountered in younger women (Ambrosini *et al.* 1980). Patients present with a history, of extremely variable length, of pruritus, bleeding or awareness of a mass, which may be ulcerated. Most basal cell carcinomas are confined to the anterior part of the labia majora, although they may also develop around the clitoris, mons, urethra or fourchette (Schueller 1965, Palladino *et al.* 1969, Deppisch 1978). They are usually between 1 and 7 cm in diameter but can occasionally attain a diameter as great as 10 cm (Dudzinski *et al.* 1984). The tumours may form a nodule (Fig. 10.24), with or without ulceration, an exophytic lesion or an excoriated area; they may also be erythematous, polypoidal, papillomatous, cystic or plaque-like (Bean & Becker 1968, Breen *et al.* 1975, Goldstein & Kent 1975, Deppisch 1978, Merino *et al.* 1982) whilst pigmentation is common.

Histologically (Figs 10.25 & 10.26), the appearances of a vulval basal cell carcinoma are identical to those occurring elsewhere in the skin, and the patterns seen most commonly in vulval lesions are the superficial, solid, morphoea-like (or sclerosing) and keratotic (Siegler & Greene 1951, Ackles & Pratt 1956, Marcus 1960, Schueller 1965, Bean & Becker 1968, Cruz-Jimenez & Abell 1975, Goldstein & Kent 1975, Dudzinski *et al.* 1984). A pure adenoid pattern (Fig. 10.27) is rather uncommon, although adenoid foci are not infrequently present in predominantly solid neoplasms (Goldstein & Kent 1975, Sworn *et al.* 1979, Merino *et al.* 1982); focal sebaceous differentiation is occasionally seen.

There have been seven cases of vulval basal cell carcinoma that have metastasized to inguinal or subcutaneous lymph nodes (Jimenez *et al.* 1975, Sworn *et al.* 1979, Perrone *et al.* 1987, Hoffman *et al.* 1988, Winkelmann & Llorens 1990, Gleeson *et al.* 1994, Mizushima & Ohara 1995) and it has been suggested that features such as bleeding, tumour thickness of greater than 1 cm, invasion of subcutaneous fat and a morphoea-like pattern of growth characterize those vulval basal cell carcinomas likely to metastasize (Perrone *et al.* 1987). This type of behaviour is, however, so unusual that it does not detract from the general principle that the treatment of vulval basal cell carcinomas is by wide local excision; inadequate primary excision is responsible for a recurrence rate of about 20% (Palladino *et al.* 1969) but there have been no recorded deaths from this neoplasm.

Adenocarcinoma

Primary adenocarcinomas of the vulva, arising in continuity with the epidermis and unrelated to underlying glandular structures or to endometriosis, are extremely rare. Tiltman

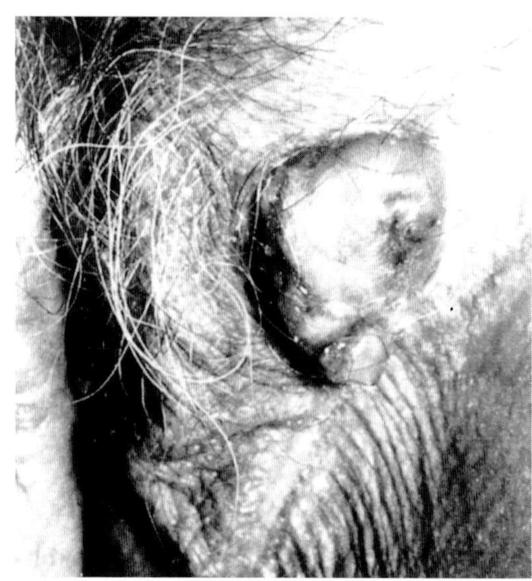

Fig. 10.24 A basal cell carcinoma of the vulva.

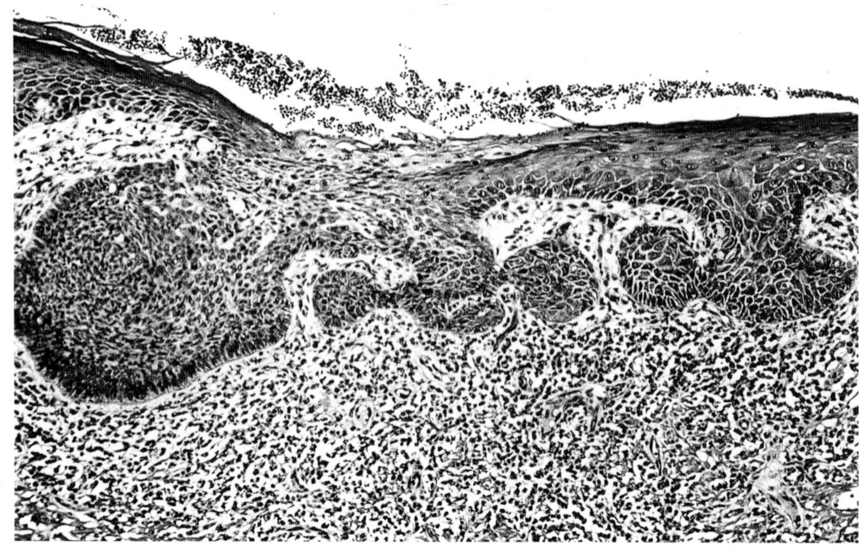

Fig. 10.25 Basal cell carcinoma of the vulva: superficial pattern. Several irregular tumour buds descend from the basal layer of the epidermis into the dermis; the peripheral layer of cells forms a palisade.

and Knutzen (1978) described a mucus-secreting adenocarcinoma that contained goblet cells and Paneth cells and bore a close resemblance to a large intestinal adenocarcinoma. Kennedy and Majmudar (1993) reported two adenocarcinomas that clearly arose in direct continuity with the epidermis, and these were also similar to an enteric adenocarcinoma, although neither contained goblet or Paneth cells and the one tumour tested was negative for CEA. Ghamande *et al.* (1995) described a colonic-type mucinous adenocarcinoma in the posterior fourchette that was CEA positive. It has been suggested that these neoplasms are of possible cloacogenic origin but those described by Tiltman and Knutzen and Ghamande *et al.* clearly arose in what was either a focus of gastrointestinal metaplasia or heterotopic intestinal tissue, this latter entity having been described as a cause of vulvar ulceration (Yeoh *et al.* 1987).

Adenosquamous carcinoma

Tumours of this type have been descibed in the vulva

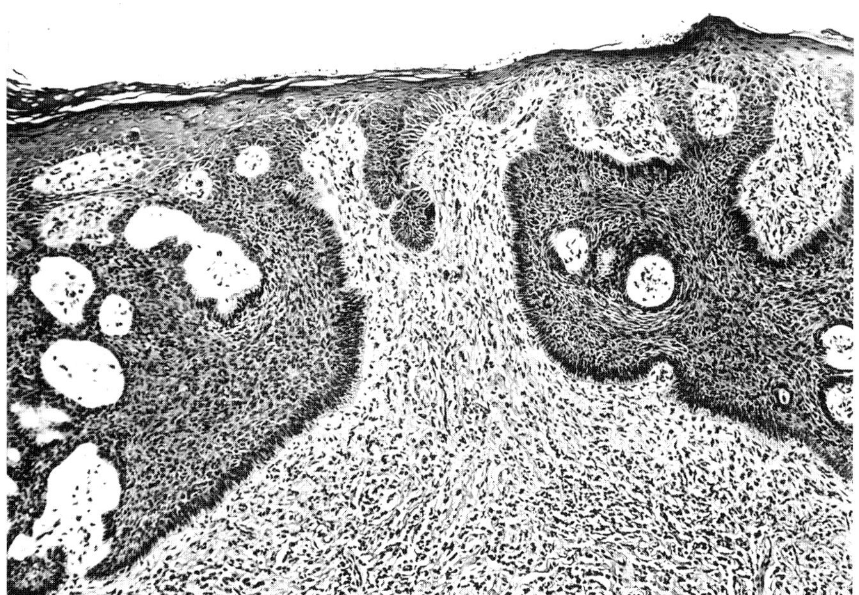

Fig. 10.26 Basal cell carcinoma of the vulva: solid pattern.

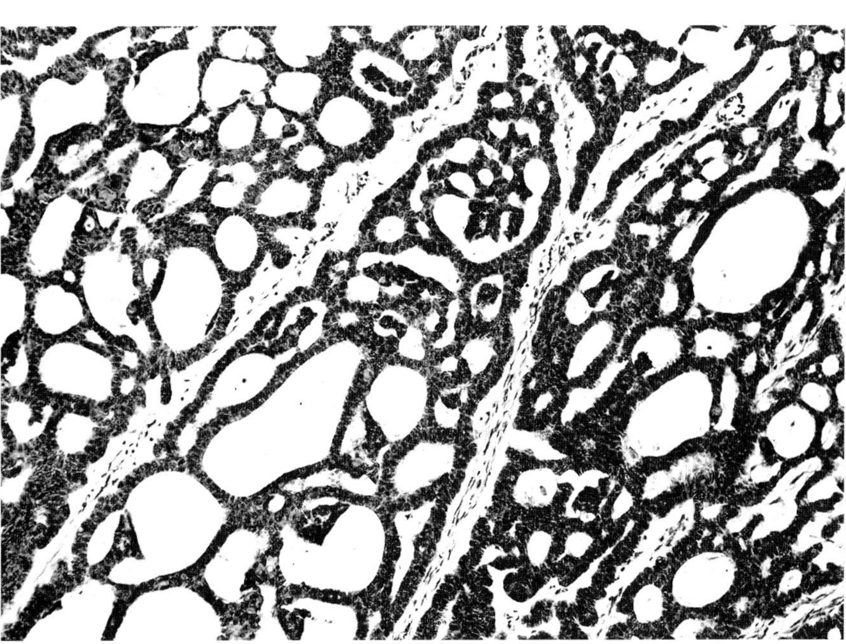

Fig. 10.27 Basal cell carcinoma of the vulva: adenoid pattern. Fine cords and trabeculae of tumour cells form a cribiform pattern.

(Underwood *et al.* 1978) but it is probable that they are derived from skin adnexae or Bartholin's gland.

Neuroendocrine tumours of the vulva

Merkel cell tumour

Merkel cell tumours are primary, small-cell, malignant neoplasms of the skin; they are usually classed as neuroendocrine neoplasms but proof that they are of neural crest origin is lacking. They are composed of fairly uniform cells with ill-defined margins and large, round, vesicular nuclei in which there are several nucleoli. They have scanty ambophilic cytoplasm and are round or spindled. The cells form solid sheets, compact nests, cords or trabeculae and occasional rosettes may be present. The tumours may show focal squamous differentiation and, at the vulva, are often associated with VIN 3. The tumours stain positively for neurone-specific enolase and about 50% of these neoplasms are Grimelius positive; electron microscopy reveals the presence of neurosecretory granules.

Only a few cases of vulval Merkel cell tumour have been recorded (Tang *et al.* 1982, Bottles *et al.* 1984, Copeland *et al.* 1985, Husseinzadah *et al.* 1988, Chandeying *et al.* 1989, Cliby *et al.* 1991, Loret-de-Mola *et al.* 1993, Scurry *et al.* 1996), one of which showed, focally, both squamous and glandular differentiation (Scurry *et al.* 1996). These are aggressive neoplasms that spread at an early stage to regional nodes and distant sites. The prognosis has been generally poor but some improvement has been achieved by supplementing surgery with chemotherapy.

Amphicrine tumour

Hidvegi *et al.* (1988) have described an amphicrine (adenocarcinoid) tumour of the vulva; this presented as an ulcerated vulval mass, present for 5 years and measuring 12 cm in diameter, in a 75-year-old woman.

Melanocytic lesions and neoplasms

Lentigo simplex, melanocytic naevi

The term 'melanosis', when applied to the vulva, is often used to describe both patchy or diffuse hyperpigmentation and lentigo simplex. Idiopathic vulvar melanosis is characterized by increased basal layer melanin pigmentation and deposition of melanin in dermal macrophages and is discussed in Chapter 5. When this change is associated with elongation of the rete pegs the lesion is classed as lentigo simplex (Fig. 10.28). Lentigines are the most common pigmented lesion of the vulva and occur as smooth, dark-brown spots measuring 1–5 mm in diameter on the labia minora and around the introitus.

Vulval naevi have been found in 2.3% of women (Rock *et al.* 1990). Intradermal, compound and junctional naevi occur at this site and although it has been claimed that the junctional type predominates (Friedrich 1976) this has not always been the case (Christensen *et al.* 1987, Rollason 1992). Juvenile (Spitz) naevi have also been described (Hulagu & Erez 1973).

A small proportion of vulval naevi in premenopausal women show atypical features (Friedman & Ackerman

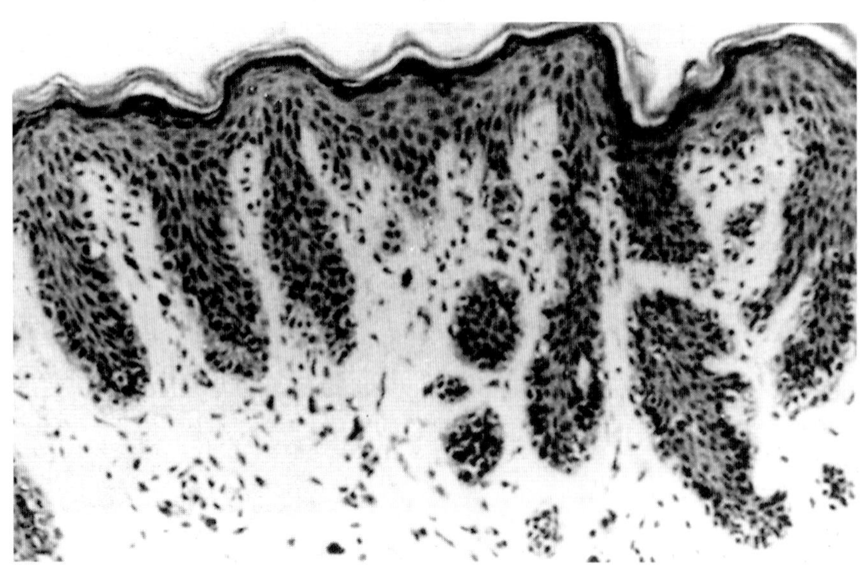

Fig. 10.28 A lentigo of the vulva.

1981). These include the presence of large pleomorphic epithelioid (or sometimes spindled) intraepidermal melanocytes with abundant eosinophilic cytoplasm and prominent nucleoli, variably sized intradermal melanocytic nests and confluence of intraepithelial melanocyte clusters; hair shafts and sweat gland ducts are commonly involved. In these lesions there is, however, an overall symmetry with cellular maturation in the deep dermis and no single-cell migration of melanocytes into the upper epidermis. Whether such lesions merit being classed as a variant of the so-called 'dysplastic' naevus is a moot and unresolved point (Christensen *et al.* 1987, Pierson 1987, Rollason 1992). There has, in fact, been only one report of a typical 'dysplastic' naevus of the vulva (Christensen *et al.* 1987).

Malignant melanoma

Malignant melanomas of the vulva constitute between 2 and 4% of all melanomas in females and have been variously estimated to account for between 3.6 and 10% of malignant vulvar neoplasms (Morrow & Rutledge 1972, Chung *et al.* 1975, Morrow & DiSaia 1976, Silvers & Halperin 1978, Pierson 1987, Bradgate *et al.* 1990, Rollason 1992). It is thought that about 10% arise in pre-existing vulval naevi (Curtin & Morrow 1992).

Vulval malignant melanoma does not occur in prepubertal girls but thereafter its incidence rises steadily to reach a peak in the sixth and seventh decades. Patients usually present with a relatively short history of, most commonly, a lump, although there may also be complaints of bleeding or itching. In some series the tumours have been predominantly central, i.e. involving the labia minora or the clitoris (Morrow & Rutledge 1972, Podratz *et al.* 1983b), but others have found an equal incidence of lateral (i.e. involving labia majora) and central neoplasms (Phillips *et al.* 1982, Jaramillo *et al.* 1985). The melanoma (Fig. 10.29) may be flat, elevated, nodular or polypoid and is often ulcerated; the colour ranges from brown to bluish-black but a small minority in this site are amelanotic and bear a close macroscopic resemblance to a squamous cell carcinoma. In some series most vulval melanomas have been of the superficial spreading variety (Fig. 10.30) but in others the nodular type (Fig. 10.31) has predominated (Bouma *et al.* 1982, Landthaler *et al.* 1985, Itala *et al.* 1986, Johnson *et al.* 1986) whilst both the mucosal lentiginous and neurotropic forms have been prominent in yet others (Benda *et al.* 1986, Blessing *et al.* 1991).

The 5-year survival rate for patients with a malignant melanoma of the vulva has ranged from 13 to 54% with a mean of about 30–35% (Symmonds *et al.* 1960, Janovski *et al.* 1962, Pack & Oropeza 1967, Yackel *et al.* 1970, Morrow & Rutledge 1972, Fenn & Abell 1973, Bozzetti *et al.* 1975, Chung *et al.* 1975, Karlen *et al.* 1975, Cleophax *et al.* 1977, Ragni & Tobon 1974, Edington & Monaghan 1980, Bouma *et al.* 1982, Phillips *et al.* 1982, Podratz *et al.* 1983b, Jaramillo *et al.* 1985, Landthaler *et al.* 1985, Benda *et al.* 1986, Itala *et al.* 1986, Woolcot *et al.* 1988, Bradgate *et al.* 1990, Blessing *et al.* 1991, Piura *et al.* 1992, Ragnarsson-Olding *et al.* 1993, Scheistroen *et al.* 1995). It should be noted, however, that 5-year survival is not synonymous with cure, for recurrences, and metastases can occur at any time up to 13 years after primary treatment (Bouma *et al.* 1982, Podratz *et al.* 1983b) and the 10-year survival rate is significantly lower than that noted at 5 years (Bradgate *et al.* 1990).

Melanomas of the vulva are staged in the same way as are squamous cell carcinomas at this site but the prognostic value of clinical stage in malignant melanoma is still open to debate. There seems little difference in survival rates between stage I and stage II cases (5-year survival 60–70%) and the outlook is agreed to be universally gloomy for patients with stage IV disease; some have also found stage III tumours to be associated with a very poor progno-

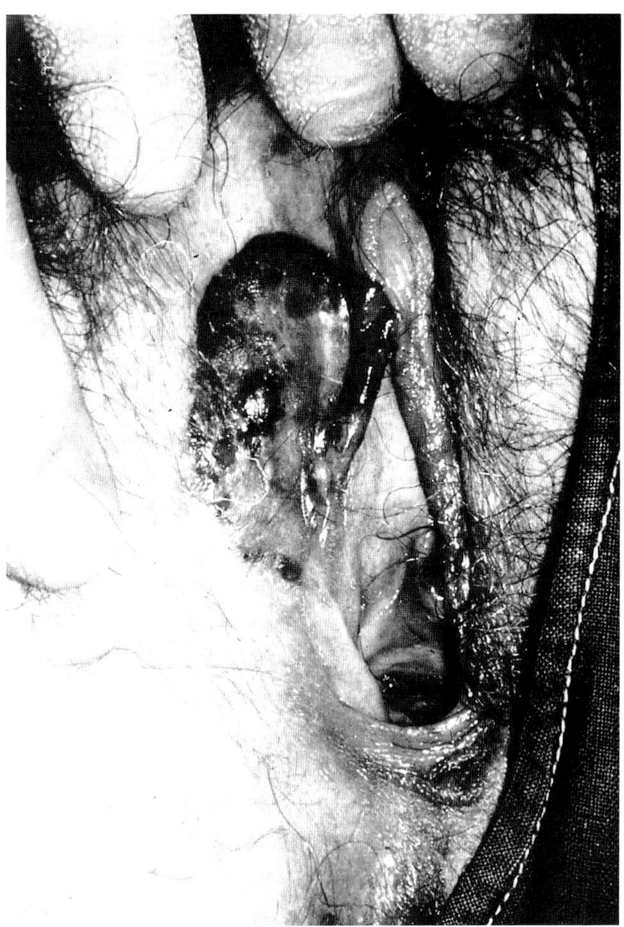

Fig. 10.29 A malignant melanoma of the vulva.

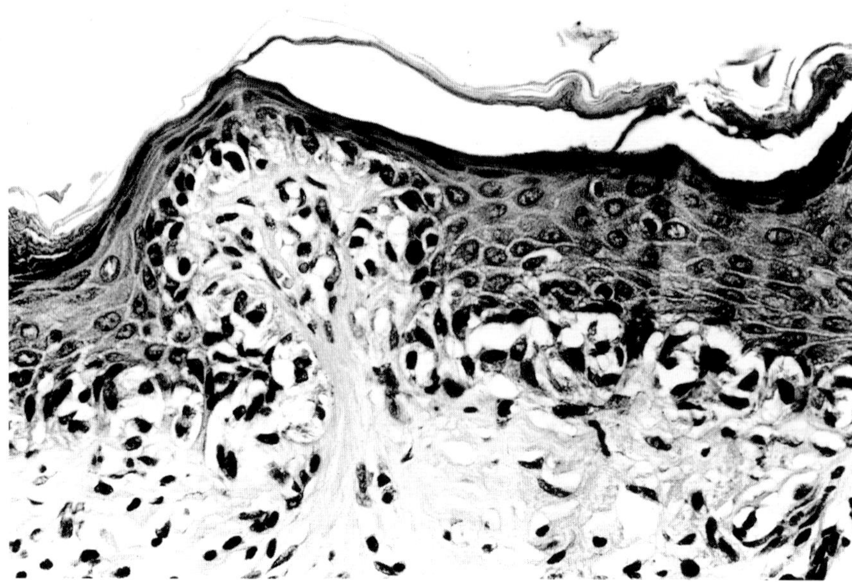

Fig. 10.30 Superficial spreading melanoma of the vulva. Pagetoid melanotic cells are invading the epidermis and spreading laterally within it.

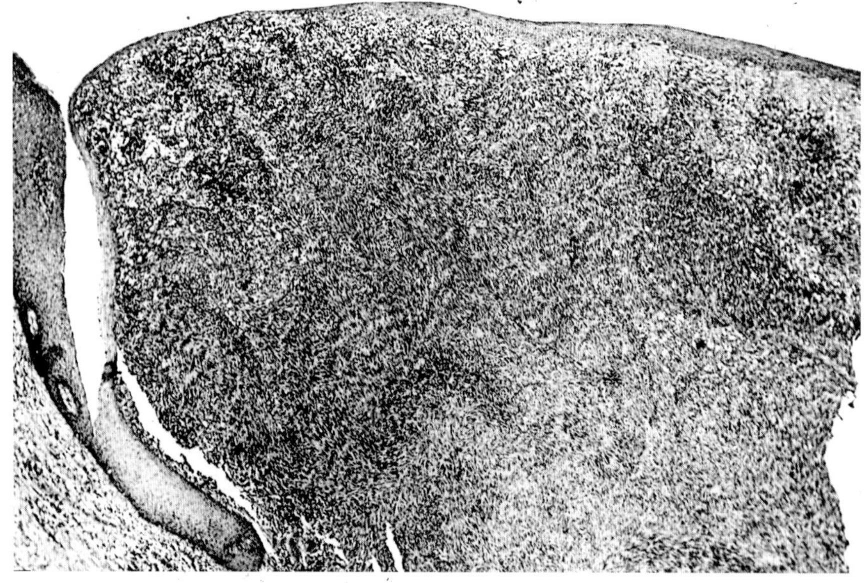

Fig. 10.31 A nodular malignant melanoma of the vulva.

sis (Morrow 1981, Jaramillo *et al.* 1985, Bradgate *et al.* 1990) whilst others have been unable to show that the prognosis for such neoplasms is any worse than is that for tumours in earlier stages (Phillips *et al.* 1982, Podratz *et al.* 1983b).

The diameter of a melanoma appears to be of little prognostic importance but it has been maintained that laterally sited tumours have a better prognosis than those which are centrally placed (Podratz *et al.* 1983b, Johnson *et al.* 1986), although it has been suggested that this is only true if the central neoplasms involve the urethra or vagina (Morrow 1981). Localization of the tumour to the clitoris has been noted as having a poor prognosis (Scheistroen *et al.* 1995). The traditional belief that superficial spreading melanomas have a better prognosis than their nodular counterparts has been upheld in some series (Podratz *et al.* 1983b, Itala *et al.* 1986, Johnson *et al.* 1986) but not in others (Chung *et al.* 1975, Bradgate *et al.* 1990). Other histological features, such as cell type, degree of atypia and number of mitotic figures, are not generally thought to be of prognostic value, although Bradgate *et al.* (1990) found that tumours containing epithelioid-type cells were associated with an

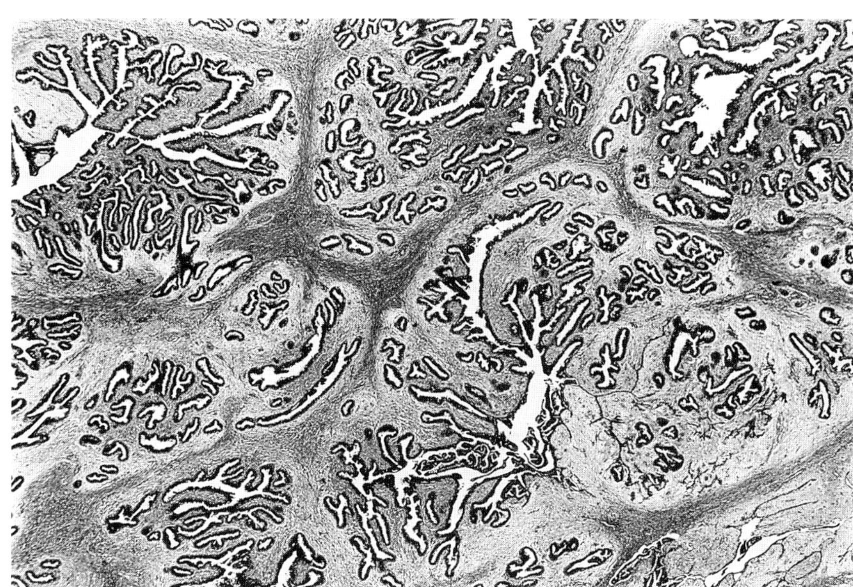

Fig. 10.32 A fibroadenoma of the vulva that is morphologically identical to a mammary fibroadenoma.

unusually poor outlook. DNA non-diploidy emerged as a major prognostic indicator of poor survival in women with vulvar melanomas who were studied by Scheistroen *et al.* (1995, 1996).

For melanomas confined to the vulva, histological microstaging is thought to be prognostically important (Dunton *et al.* 1995). Some have found Clark's levels, which define depth of tumour invasion in terms of dermal planes (Clark *et al.* 1969), to be of considerable prognostic significance (Phillips *et al.* 1982, Podratz *et al.* 1983b), but the value of this technique is limited by the fact that most vulval melanomas are already level IV, or worse, at presentation (Rollason 1992). Chung's modification of Clark's levels (Chung *et al.* 1975) suffers from the same disadvantage (Blessing *et al.* 1991). The Breslow technique measures tumour thickness (Breslow 1970) and there has been quite widespread, although not universal, agreement that tumour thickness is a dominant prognostic factor, melanomas less than 0.76 mm in thickness having an excellent prognosis and subsequent survival rates beyond this plummeting with increasing thickness (Phillips *et al.* 1982, Podratz *et al.* 1983a, Jaramillo *et al.* 1985); the value of Breslow microstaging has, however, not been confirmed in every study (Piura *et al.* 1992, Scheistroen *et al.* 1996).

Malignant melanoma has traditionally been treated by radical vulvectomy and node dissection but it has not been shown that the results following radical surgery are any better than those achieved by wide local excision (Davidson *et al.* 1987, Rose *et al.* 1988, Bradgate *et al.* 1990); there is therefore an increasing move towards purely local surgery, certainly for thin lesions (Tasseron *et al.* 1992, Trimble *et al.* 1992, Look *et al.* 1993, Dunton *et al.* 1995).

Tumours arising from ectopic tissues

Tumours of ectopic breast tissue

Neoplasms of this type are controversial: firstly, there is, as discussed in Chapter 8, some doubt as to whether ectopic breast tissue truly occurs in the vulva and, secondly, it is virtually impossible to distinguish between a mammary neoplasm in this site and a tumour of apocrine sweat gland origin.

Within the obvious limitations imposed by these two factors a number of fibroadenomas of the vulva (Fig. 10.32) have been described that were morphologically identical to those which commonly occur in normally sited mammary tissue (Friedel 1932, Roth 1936, Fisher 1947, Siegler & Gordon 1951, Burger & Marcuse 1954, Foushee & Pruitt 1967, Hassim 1969, Prasad *et al.* 1995); in none of these cases, however, was there clear evidence of derivation from non-neoplastic mammary tissue. Bilateral phyllodes tumours, which appeared to be associated with breast tissue, have been described (Tbakhi *et al.* 1993). An intraduct papilloma arising in vulval breast tissue has also been reported (Rickert 1980) but the distinction between such a neoplasm and a papillary hidradenoma is virtually impossible.

A small number of mammary-type adenocarcinomas of the vulva, thought to have originated in accessory breast tissue, have been documented (Green 1936, Hendrix & Behrman 1956, Guerry & Pratt-Thomas 1976, Guercio *et al.* 1984, Cho *et al.* 1985, Rose *et al.* 1990, Di Bonito *et al.* 1992, Bailey *et al.* 1993, Levin *et al.* 1995) but in very few of these neoplasms was a reasonably definite derivation from breast tissue established, the origin in most cases being only presumptive. Two of the reported neoplasms contained oestrogen receptors (Cho *et al.* 1985, Rose *et al.* 1990) but this finding is far from specific for tumours of mammary origin.

A single case of a neoplasm thought to be an intraductal carcinoma of mammary type arising within a papillary hidradenoma of the vulva has been recorded (Pelosi *et al.* 1991); the tumour reacted positively for apocrine cell markers and contained both oestrogen and progesterone receptors. The histogenetic ramifications of this case are, to say the least, complex.

Tumours arising in endometriosis

A single example of a clear-cell adenocarcinoma arising in vulval endometriosis has been recorded (Mesko *et al.* 1988); this arose in the canal of Nuck at the superior aspect of the labium majus.

Benign skin adnexal tumours

Syringoma (see also Chapter 5)

This is considered to be an adenoma of the intraepidermal eccrine sweat gland ducts, which occurs only rarely at the vulva (Brown & Freeman 1971, Carneiro *et al.* 1971, 1972, Isaacson & Turner 1979, Thomas *et al.* 1979, Young *et al.* 1980, Ghirardini 1982, Panizzon *et al.* 1987, Aquila-Martinez *et al.* 1989, Blazejak & Plewig 1989, Siemund 1989, Carter & Elliott 1990, Turan *et al.* 1996). The vulval lesions may occur in isolation or can be associated with similar lesions elsewhere on the body. The neoplasms can develop at any age but most occur in adolescents and young women.

Vulval syringomas are occasionally solitary but are usually multiple and are bilaterally symmetrical. They occur principally on the labia and are seen as small (1–4 mm in diameter), firm or fleshy, dome-shaped nodules. Histologically, a syringoma occurs in the dermis, is ill defined and appears as a proliferation of small ducts embedded in fibrous tissue (Fig. 10.33); comma-like tails extending from the ducts is a characteristic feature (Fig. 10.34). The ducts are lined by two rows of cells that are often focally flattened due to pressure. The duct lumina contain amorphous material that is diastase resistant and PAS positive. The ducts may become cystically dilated and can rupture with the elicitation of a foreign-body reaction (Thomas *et al.* 1979). One unusual case has been reported in which a vulval syringoma was admixed with pilosebaceous elements (Guindi *et al.* 1974).

Treatment is usually unnecessary except for cosmetic reasons. In occasional cases, however, the lesions may cause severe vulvar pruritus (Carter & Elliott 1990).

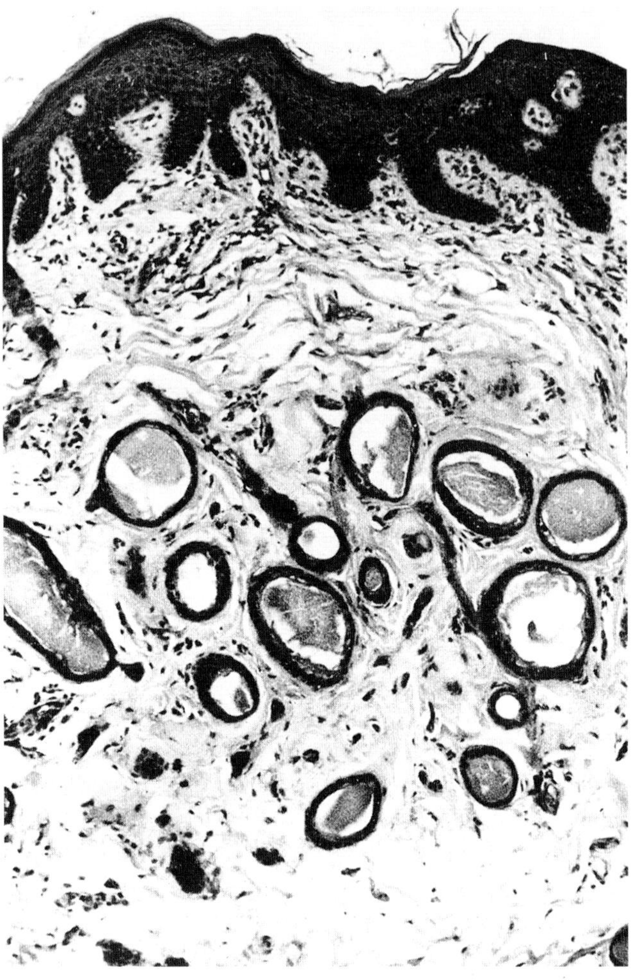

Fig. 10.33 A syringoma of the vulva.

Clear-cell hidradenoma

This is a rare eccrine sweat gland tumour, which is multinodular and composed of lobular masses of fusiform epidermoid and large clear cells, together with ducts, separated by fine fibrous tissue bands. It occurs with extreme rarity in the vulva, only one case having been reported, and not in great detail, at this site (Lever & Castleman 1952).

Papillary hidradenoma

This is a sweat gland adenoma showing apocrine differentiation and occurs almost exclusively in the anogenital region of middle-aged white women (Meeker *et al.* 1962, Nielson 1973, Donna *et al.* 1978). Van der Putte (1991) found a

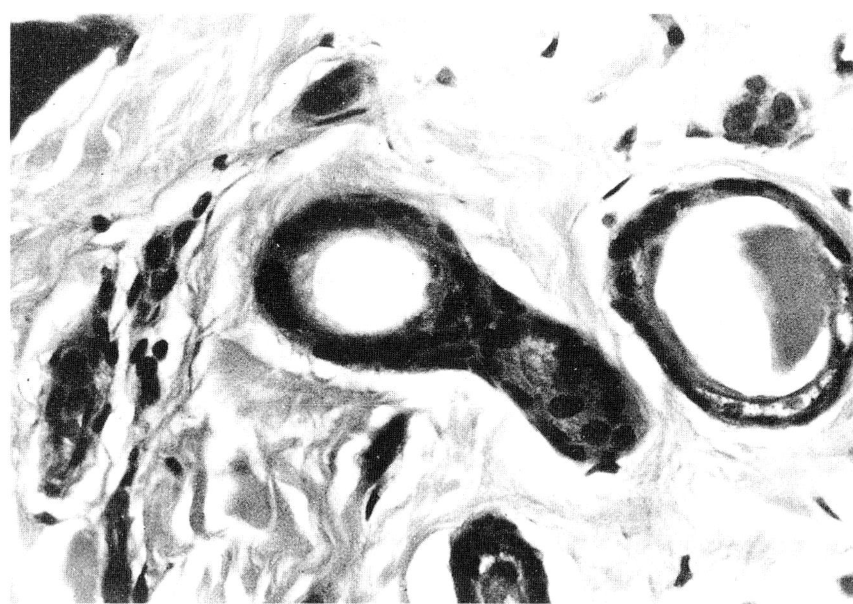

Fig. 10.34 A high-power view of a vulval syringoma showing an eccrine duct-like structure with a typical 'comma' appearance.

close association with anogenital glands in four out of five cases.

Papillary hidradenomas form firm, often asymptomatic but occasionally painful nodules, which whilst usually less than 2 cm in diameter can attain a considerable size (Kaufmann *et al.* 1987, Veraldi *et al.* 1990). They occur most commonly in the labia majora, interlabial sulcus, lateral surfaces of the labia minora or perineal region (Tappeiner & Wolff 1968, Lever & Schaumburg-Lever 1975, Basta & Madej 1990) and although usually single are occasionally multiple (Meeker *et al.* 1962, Woodworth *et al.* 1971). Curiously, when they are multiple all the lesions tend to develop on one side of the vulva (Hobbs 1965) (Fig. 10.35). In most patients the covering epidermis remains intact but in a proportion the elevated epithelium may become ulcerated (Donna *et al.* 1978) and the red, fleshy, adenomatous tissue protrudes through the cutaneous defect: such lesions may bleed on contact and may be mistaken clinically for a carcinoma (Basta & Madej 1990).

The tumours lie deep in the dermis, have no connection with the epidermis and are often clearly delineated from the surrounding tissues by a layer of compressed fibrous tissue. The neoplasm has a complex pattern of glandular acini, tubules and small cysts into which project papillae (Fig. 10.36). The epithelial component of the neoplasm is, for the most part, double layered (Fig. 10.37). The outer, or luminal, layer is formed of cuboidal or columnar cells with oval, pale-staining, basal nuclei and faintly eosinophilic, PAS-positive, diastase-resistant cytoplasm, which may show apocrine features as manifest by active decapitation

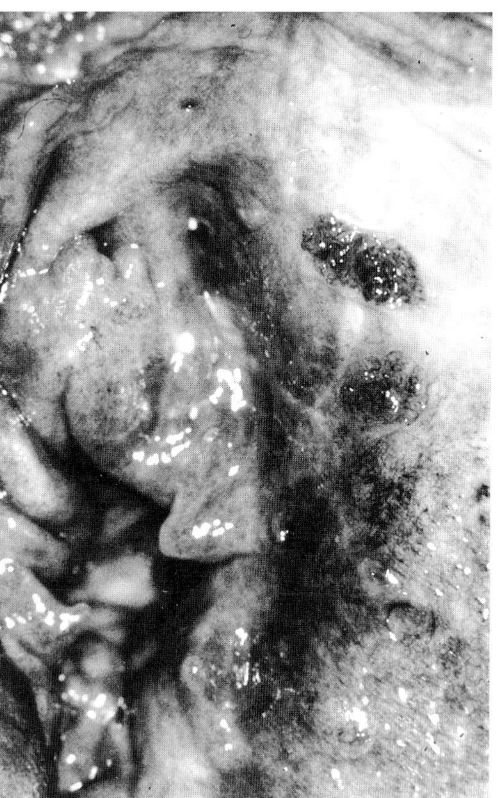

Fig. 10.35 Two hidradenomas on the left labium majus: erythematous and glistening appearance.

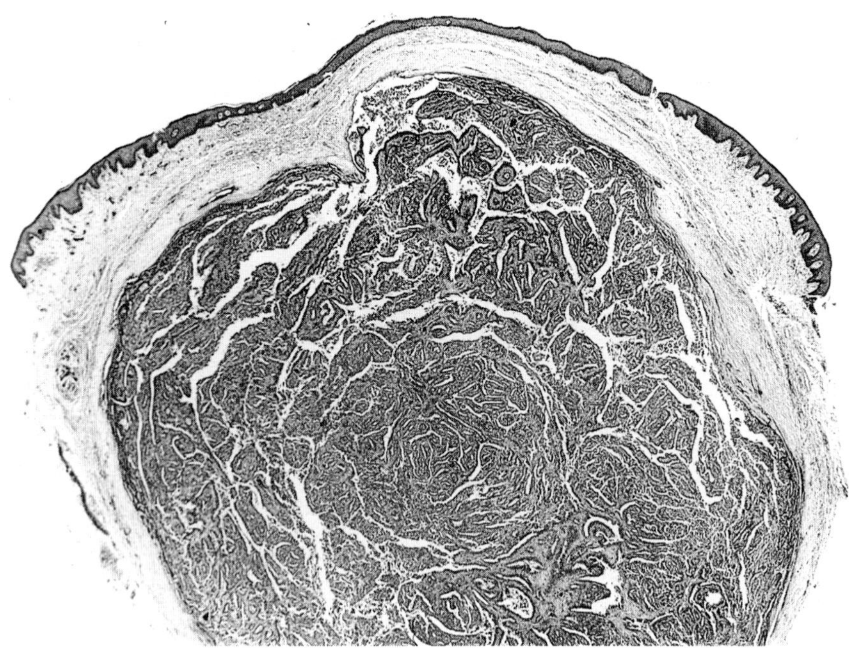

Fig. 10.36 A papillary hidradenoma of the vulva.

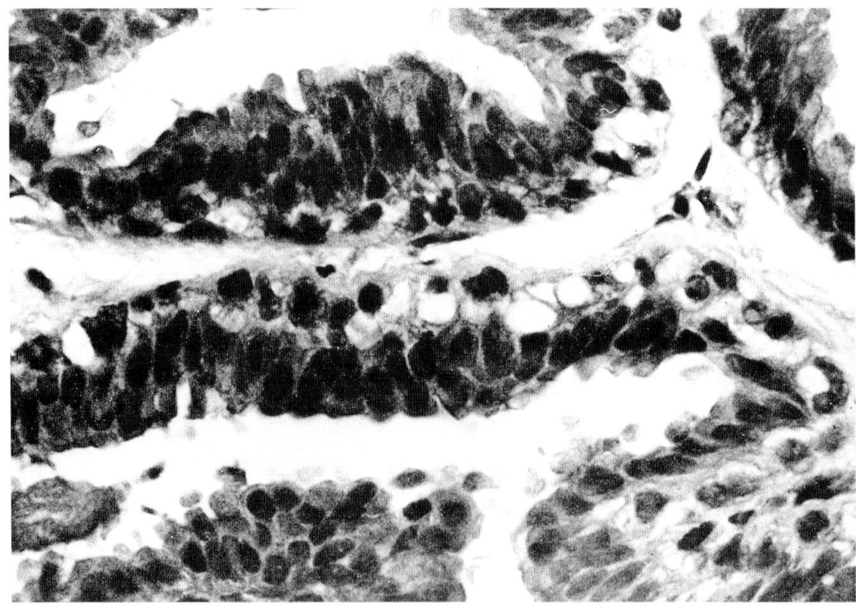

Fig. 10.37 Vulval papillary hidradenoma: high-power view showing double layer of cells.

secretion (Lever & Schaumburg-Lever 1975). The deeper layer is composed of smaller, more darkly staining cuboidal or spindle-shaped myoepithelial cells (Tappeiner & Wolff 1968, Hashimoto 1973).

Treatment of this benign lesion is by local excision (Woodworth *et al.* 1971, Lomeo *et al.* 1992). There have been two reasonably convincing examples of malignant change within a papillary hidradenoma: one was an apocrine carcinoma and was cured by wide local excision (Pelosi *et al.* 1991) whilst the other was an adenosquamous carcinoma, which proved rapidly fatal (Bannatyne *et al.* 1989).

Pilar tumour

This neoplasm, also known as a proliferating trichilemmal tumour, is thought to develop from the outer hair root sheath and usually occurs in the scalp. Very rarely, however,

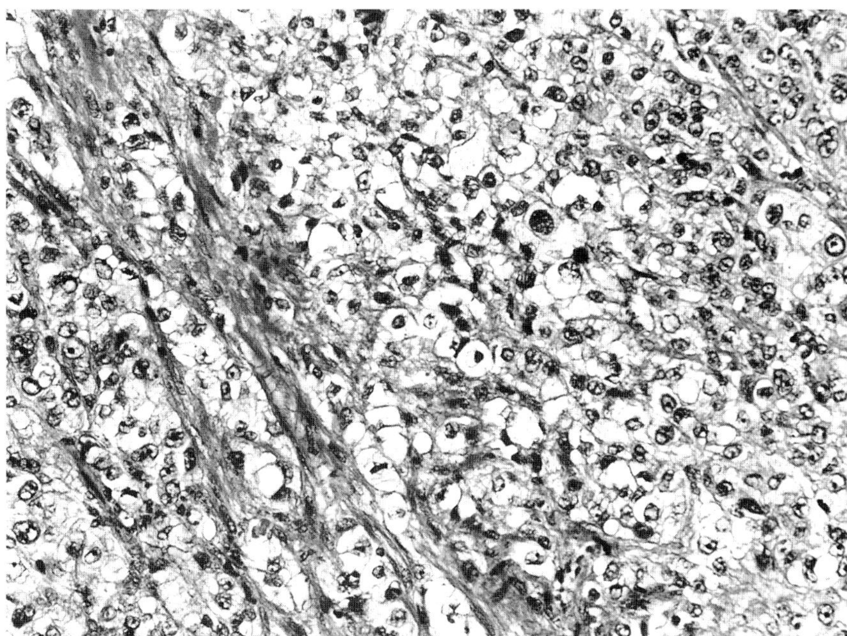

Fig. 10.38 A poorly differentiated sweat gland adenocarcinoma of the vulva.

this neoplasm arises at the vulva (Buchler *et al.* 1978, Avinoach *et al.* 1989), where it assumes some considerable importance because of the ease with which it can be misdiagnosed as a squamous cell carcinoma.

The tumour starts as a subcutaneous nodule, which may become elevated, ulcerate and discharge serosanguineous fluid. Histologically, the neoplasm shows no connection with the epidermis and is composed of strands and, more typically, lobules of squamous epithelium, which undergo a rather abrupt change in their centres to eosinophilic amorphous keratin, which may be focally calcified. The neoplasm is differentiated from a squamous cell carcinoma by its sharp demarcation from the surrounding stroma and abrupt transition to keratin without a granular layer. Treatment is by local excision.

Trichoepithelioma

These benign neoplasms of hair follicle origin can, extremely rarely, occur as a solitary vulval nodular lesion (Cho & Woodruff 1988). Histologically, they are distinct from the epidermis and are formed of irregular masses of small dark cells, which are very similar to those seen in a basal cell carcinoma. These cells surround keratin-filled horn cysts whilst structures resembling abortive hair follicles may be present.

A desmoplastic variant of the trichoepithelioma is recognized and whether this is a distinct entity from the trichoblastic fibroma, one example of which has been recorded as occuring in the vulva (Gilks *et al.* 1989), is a moot point.

Tumours with sebaceous differentiation

Sebaceous adenomas have been described in the vulva (Janovski & Douglas 1972, Novak & Woodruff 1979) but it appears likely that these were in fact examples of sebaceous gland hyperplasia (Rocamora *et al.* 1986).

Malignant skin adnexal tumours

Sweat gland carcinomas

These are rare, usually develop in postmenopausal women and occur most frequently on the labia majora and interlabial sulcus (Boehm & Morris 1971, Lee *et al.* 1977, Webb & Beswick 1983, Wick *et al.* 1985); many are associated with Paget's disease in the overlying dermis. They most commonly present as painless, or only mildly tender, firm, non-ulcerated dermal nodules, which may or may not be fixed to the underlying tissues; the tumours range in size from 0.5 to 10 cm.

The majority of vulval sweat gland carcinomas cannot be further histologically classified, as they lack features of either apocrine or eccrine differentiation (Fig. 10.38). They consist of infiltrating nests and cords of cells showing intercellular or intracellular lumina: stains for mucus are usually, although not invariably, positive. The tumours have infiltrating margins, and show nuclear pleomorphism, coarse clumping of nuclear chromatin, much mitotic activity, an increased nuclear/cytoplasmic ratio and, often, areas of necrosis.

In some cases vulval sweat gland carcinomas have shown

features of apocrine differentiation (Eichenberg 1934, Plachta & Speer 1954, Rosser & Hamlin 1957, Lee *et al.* 1977, Roth *et al.* 1977, Nazario *et al.* 1989). These neoplasms are characterized by a glandular pattern with papillary formations whilst their lining epithelial cells have abundant eosinophilic cytoplasm with diastase-resistant, PAS-positive granules and show decapitation secretion. Neoplasms of this type bear a marked resemblance to a ductal carcinoma of the breast and, in the vulva, distinction of apocrine sweat gland carcinoma from carcinoma arising in heterotopic breast tissue may be impossible unless an origin can be demonstrated from non-neoplastic tissue.

Some neoplasms have shown eccrine differentiation with the features of an eccrine porocarcinoma (Fig. 10.39), a syringoid eccrine carcinoma, a mucinous eccrine carcinoma or a clear-cell eccrine carcinoma (Wilner *et al.* 1976, Webb & Beswick 1983, Gartmann 1985, Wick *et al.* 1985, Fukuma *et al.* 1986, Messing *et al.* 1993, Ghamande *et al.* 1995, Rahilly *et al.* 1995, Massad *et al.* 1996).

It is difficult to glean from the literature any firm data about the natural history of vulval sweat gland carcinomas. There is certainly a quite high incidence of local recurrence and there may be distant metastases but the frequency with which local and distant spread occurs is impossible to assess; experience with sweat gland carcinomas elsewhere in the body does, however, suggest that they should be regarded as aggressive neoplasms (Fu & Reagan 1989). Treatment is surgical, although the radicality of surgical approach required is open to debate, and the tumours are insensitive to radiotherapy.

Sebaceous carcinomas

Only one convincing example of a sebaceous carcinoma of the vulva has been recorded (Jacobs *et al.* 1986); this was in continuity with the overlying epidermis, which showed Bowenoid VIN 3. Other sebaceous neoplasms recorded at this site appear to have been basal cell or squamous cell carcinomas showing sebaceous differentiation (Rulon & Helwig 1974).

Benign tumours of Bartholin's gland

Adenoma

Adenomas of Bartholin's gland are extremely rare (Foushee *et al.* 1968, Honore & O'Hara 1978). They present as a persistent or intermittent swelling of the posterolateral part of the vulva that is clinically indistinguishable from a cyst or abscess. Histologically, the tumour has pushing margins and is formed of closely packed secretory alveoli, which show a variable degree of branching and are lined by a tall, pale, mucus-secreting epithelium with small basal nuclei. There has been some debate, still unresolved, as to whether these lesions are really benign neoplasms or whether they should, more correctly, be regarded as focal hyperplasias or hamartomas.

Similar lesions have also been reported in small, unnamed, minor vestibular glands (Axe *et al.* 1986).

Mucinous cystadenoma

A single mucinous cystadenoma of Bartholin's gland has been reported (Chapman *et al.* 1987). This was a small vulval mass, which was formed of multiple branching, focally dilated mucus-secreting glands set in dense fibrous tissue. The term 'cystadenoma' hardly seems justified for this lesion and 'benign mucinous tumour' would be preferable.

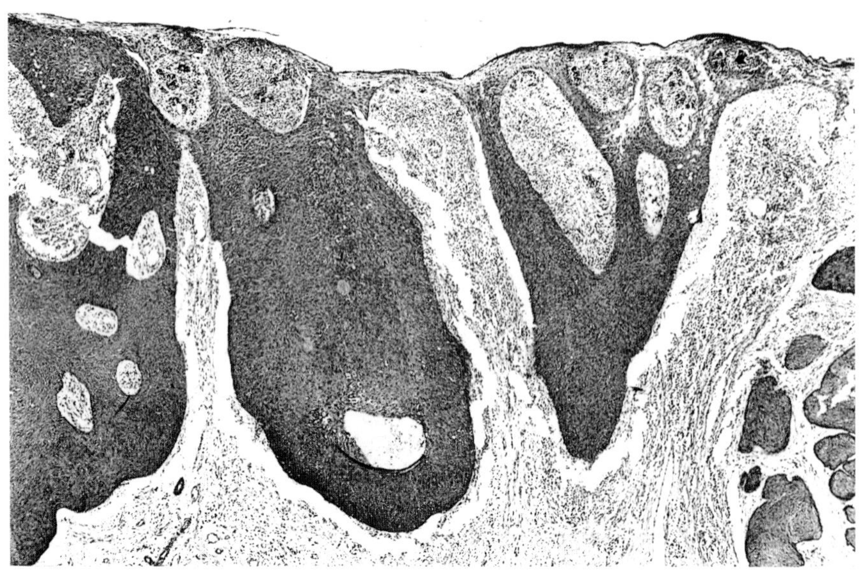

Fig. 10.39 A malignant eccrine poroma of the vulva.

Papilloma

A papilloma arising within a Bartholin's duct cyst has been described (Enghardt *et al.* 1993). The tumour was lined by an epithelium that consisted of columnar and stratified polygonal cells resembling squamous and transitional epithelium.

Malignant neoplasms of Bartholin's gland

Various types of carcinoma occur in Bartholin's gland and these are usually considered together. However, the adenoid cystic carcinoma of Bartholin's gland appears to be a distinctive clinicopathological entity which merits, and will receive here, separate consideration.

Carcinoma

Carcinoma of Bartholin's gland has been variously estimated as accounting for between 2 and 7% of malignant vulvar neoplasms (Wharton & Everett 1951, Masterson & Goss 1954, Barclay *et al.* 1964, Chamlian & Taylor 1972, Wahlstrom *et al.* 1978, Leuchter *et al.* 1982). It is of considerable interest to note that HPV 16 has been found, when looked for, in a high proportion of Bartholin's gland carcinomas (Scinicariello *et al.* 1992, Felix *et al.* 1993, Dancoisne *et al.* 1995).

The mean age at presentation is about 49–55 years (Barclay *et al.* 1964, Leuchter *et al.* 1982) but the age range is wide; a case was reported in a 14-year-old girl (Addison 1977) and a 91-year-old woman (Dennis *et al.* 1955). Cases have been reported in pregnancy (Dennis *et al.* 1955, Chamlian & Taylor 1972).

Bartholin's gland carcinoma most commonly presents as a vulval mass deep in the posterior part of the labium majus, often with pain or irritation and occasionally accompanied by vaginal discharge and bleeding. The tumour is only rarely associated with vulval Paget's disease (Hastrup & Andersen 1988). In a very high proportion of cases the initial clinical diagnosis is of a cyst or abscess; an abscess is, in fact, not uncommonly present and it is only when this fails to respond to conventional measures that the possibility of an underlying neoplasm is considered.

Bartholin's gland carcinoma is almost invariably unilateral, only very exceptional cases having been bilateral (Purola & Widholm 1966, Schweppe & Schlake 1980). The tumours are usually between 1 and 6 cm in diameter, although very much larger neoplasms occasionally occur (Lulenski & Naji 1964, Purola & Widholm 1966), and are generally solid and grey-white on section, often with foci of haemorrhage and necrosis.

Histologically, carcinomas of Bartholin's gland display no specific features and the criteria to be met for recognition that a carcinoma has arisen in a Bartholin's gland are that there should be Bartholin's gland elements adjacent to the tumour, that areas of transition from normal to neoplastic gland elements should be seen, that the tumour involves the site of Bartholin's gland and should be histologically compatible with an origin from the gland, and that no other concurrent primary tumour is present (Chamlian & Taylor 1972).

If adenoid cystic carcinomas are excluded then squamous carcinomas and adenocarcinomas, in approximately equal proportions, make up about 85% of Bartholin's gland carcinomas, the remainder being transitional carcinomas, adenosquamous carcinomas and anaplastic carcinomas (Barclay *et al.* 1964, Dodson *et al.* 1970, Trelford & Doks 1976, Leuchter *et al.* 1982). Squamous cell carcinomas have been thought to arise from metaplastic epithelium in the duct or acini (Chamlian & Taylor 1972, Copeland *et al.* 1986a) but a recent immunohistological study suggests that both they and adenocarcinomas arise from the transitional area of the duct (Felix *et al.* 1993). The squamous carcinomas are of varying degrees of differentiation and may contain well-formed epithelial pearls. Adenocarcinomas may be well or poorly differentiated (Tchang *et al.* 1973, Advani *et al.* 1978, Wahlstrom *et al.* 1978, Kuzuya *et al.* 1981). The well-differentiated adenocarcinomas may have a papillary, tubular or cribiform pattern and mucin secretion may be scanty or copious (Lulenski & Naji 1964); cells resembling those of the acini or ducts are often present and may be admixed with cuboidal cells of eccrine sweat gland type (Kuzuya *et al.* 1981). Poorly differentiated adenocarcinomas may resemble a ductal carcinoma of the breast or grow in sheets. Bland squamous metaplasia can occur in adenocarcinomas whilst adenosquamous carcinomas are occasionally encountered (Van Nagell *et al.* 1969, Dennefors & Bergman 1980, Wheelock *et al.* 1984). Transitional cell carcinomas are rare (Dodson *et al.* 1970, Wahlstrom 1978) and appear to arise from the duct (Wheelock *et al.* 1984); these resemble transitional cell cloacagenic carcinomas of the anal ducts and may show focal glandular or squamous differentiation. Two small-cell neuroendocrine carcinomas of Bartholin's gland have been reported (Jones *et al.* 1990, Philippe *et al.* 1990).

Treatment of a Bartholin's gland carcinoma is by surgery, usually radical vulvectomy and inguinofemoral lymphadenectomy, with adjuvant radiotherapy, and the overall 5-year survival rate is now between 60 and 80% (Copeland *et al.* 1986a, Heine & Vahrson 1987). At the time of treatment between 37 and 55% of patients will have inguinofemoral nodal metastases and of these about 18% will also have pelvic node metatases (Leuchter *et al.* 1982, Wheelock *et al.* 1984). The 5-year survival rate is probably only about 40% for patients with nodal spread; if more than two nodes contain tumour only 18% of patients survive for 5 years (Leuchter *et al.* 1982).

Adenoid cystic carcinoma

Neoplasms of this type comprise about 10% of malignant Bartholin's gland tumours (Copeland *et al.* 1986b) and are distinctive in both their histological appearance and their behaviour.

The tumour is composed of small, angular or oval cells with oval hyperchromatic nuclei and scanty cytoplasm, which resemble the luminal cells of the ductal epithelium, and modified myoepithelial cells, which have large angular nuclei without nucleoli. The cells form single or anastomosing strands, trabeculae and well-circumscribed nests with a cribriform growth pattern within which there are lumina and pseudolumina containing basophilic, PAS-positive after diastase digestion, amorphous material. The latter is a combination of reduplicated basal lamina material and proteoglycans (Orenstein *et al.* 1985). The cell nests are set in a fibrous stroma.

The histogenesis of an adenoid cystic carcinoma in this site is uncertain; Addison & Parker (1977) proposed an origin either from ductal epithelium or from vascular myoepithelial cells, whilst a more recent study has suggested that they are derived from reserve cells in the intercalated small ducts of the gland that have the capacity to differentiate into luminal epithelial cells or into myoepithelial cells (Tsukahara *et al.* 1991). Cytogenetic study of one neoplasm showed complex chromosomal changes involving chromosomes 1, 4, 6, 11, 22 and 14 (Kieche Schwartz *et al.* 1992) but whether this is a consistent pattern of abnormalities in these tumours remains to be determined.

Adenoid cystic carcinoma characteristically invades and spreads via the perineural spaces and is associated with a high incidence of local recurrence (Sayre 1949, Dennis *et al.* 1955, Murphy *et al.* 1962, Abell 1963, Eichner 1963, Dodson *et al.* 1978, Bernstein *et al.* 1983b, Copeland *et al.* 1986b, Rosenberg *et al.* 1989). The tumour pursues, however, an indolent and prolonged course with the mean time interval between primary treatment and recurrence being about 8 years (Copeland *et al.* 1986b, Lelle *et al.* 1994). Spread to regional lymph nodes does occur but is uncommon, whilst eventual haematogenous spread is to the lung, skeleton and liver (Abroa *et al.* 1985, Chapman *et al.* 1985, Copeland *et al.* 1986b, Rose *et al.* 1991), patients sometimes succumbing to their disease as long as 27 or 31 years after initial treatment (Sayre 1949, Lelle *et al.* 1994). The 5- and 10-year survival rates have been reported as 71 and 59%, respectively (Copeland *et al.* 1986b) but in a recent series of 11 patients all three deaths occurred more than 10 years after initial surgical treatment (Lelle *et al.* 1994). It has been suggested that adjuvant radiotherapy may be of value in those cases in which tumour involves the surgical resection margin (Depasquale *et al.* 1996).

Mixed tumours of the vulval region

The origin of mixed tumours of the vulval region is obscure but they probably arise from either Bartholin's gland or from sweat glands.

Benign mixed tumours

These contain both an epithelial and a mesenchymal component, both benign, and occur very infrequently at the vulva (Janovski & Douglas 1972, Wilson & Woodger 1974, Ordonez *et al.* 1981, Rorat & Wallach 1984). The neoplasms present, usually in women aged over 60 years, as a painless lump that has frequently been present for years rather than months and is commonly in the labium majus. The neoplasms are mobile, measure less that 2.5 cm in diameter, have a bosselated surface and on section may appear firm, cartilaginous or mucoid. Histologically, these tumours have an appearance identical to that of a pleomorphic adenoma of the salivary glands, an epithelial component forming tubules, cysts, cords, nest or sheets being set in a chrondromyxoid stroma in which mature cartilage is often present. Wide local excision appears to be curative.

Malignant mixed tumours

Only one malignant mixed tumour of the vulva has been recorded (Ordonez *et al.* 1981), this being an adenoid cystic carcinoma that had arisen in an otherwise typical benign mixed tumour (carcinoma *ex* mixed tumour), which gave rise to pulmonary metastases.

Benign tumours of the urethra

Nephrogenic adenoma

These are small polypoid or papillary lesions composed of a series of small tubules or glandular spaces of varying size and shape, some of which are cystically dilated (Fig. 10.40). The glandular spaces are lined by cuboidal or flattened cells with eosinophilic granular cytoplasm; their nuclei vary in size and may be hyperchromatic. The tubules may be in closely packed clusters or loosely scattered in the stroma.

Nephrogenic adenomas can occur in the urethral epithelium or in a urethral diverticulum (Peterson & Matsumoto 1978, Bhagavan *et al.* 1981, Summitt *et al.* 1994) and it is uncertain whether they are metaplastic, hamartomatous or neoplastic in nature.

Transitional cell papilloma

These have been described in the urethra (Roberts &

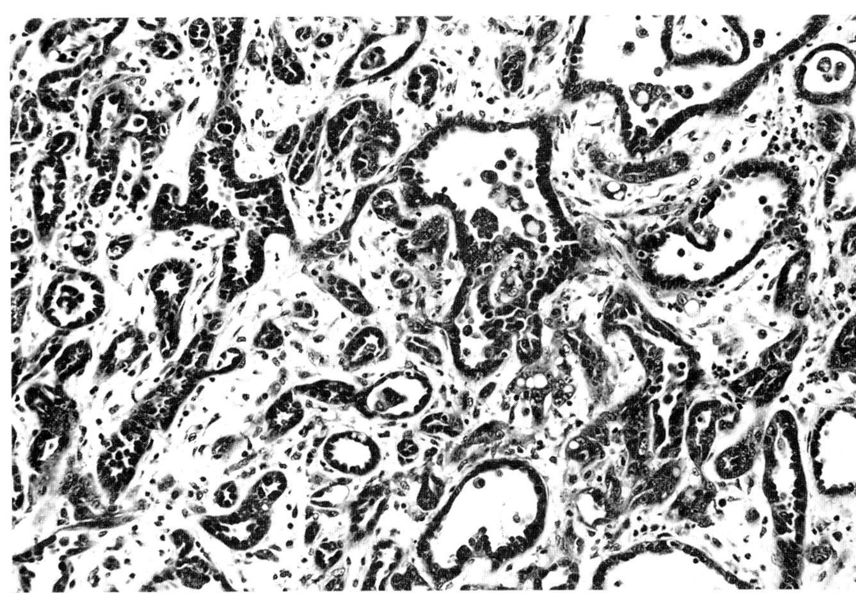

Fig. 10.40 A nephrogenic adenoma of the urethra. This contains glandular spaces of vaying size and shape, which are lined by cuboidal cells.

Melicow 1977) but are better considered as low-grade transitional cell carcinomas.

Villous adenoma

A papillary neoplasm resembling a villous adenoma of the large intestine may develop in the urethra (Howells *et al.* 1985), this presumably arising in a focus of intestinal metaplasia.

Malignant neoplasms of the urethra

Carcinoma

Carcinoma of the urethra is more common in females than in males, but nevertheless is rare, accounting for less than 1% of malignant disease of the female genital tract (Prempree *et al.* 1978, 1984). The peak incidence is between the fifth and seventh decades, the mean age at initial diagnosis being 63 years (Desai *et al.* 1973, Roberts & Melicow 1977, Bolduan & Farah 1981, Prempree *et al.* 1984).

Patients may present with haematuria, urethral or vaginal bleeding, with a wide variety of urinary symptoms or with a protruding meatal mass (Desai *et al.* 1973, Levine 1980).

About 70% of urethral carcinomas are either purely squamous or contain a mixture of malignant squamous and transitional epithelium (Levine 1980, Hopkins *et al.* 1983, Ampil 1985) whilst 10–20% are adenocarcinomas, which are thought to arise from the paraurethral glands, Skene's gland (Knoblick 1960, Grabstald 1973, Prempree *et al.* 1984) or foci of glandular metaplasia within the urethra (Ebel & Klinger, 1991). Pure transitional cell carcinomas account for the remainder (Bracken *et al.* 1976, Elkon *et al.* 1980). The squamous and transitional cell tumours may be papillary or solid whilst the adenocarcinomas may resemble a prostatic adenocarcinoma (Svanholm *et al.* 1987), be mucus-secreting (Ney *et al.* 1971), have a signet ring pattern (Klotz 1974) or be of clear-cell type (Murayama *et al.* 1978, Peven & Hidvegi 1985, Young & Scully 1985), these last resembling clear-cell adenocarcinomas of the vagina or ovary and being of unknown origin.

Urethral carcinoma spreads directly to local tissues such as the vagina, labia and bladder neck, and via the lymphatics to the inguinal, iliac, obturator and pre-sacral nodes, Distant metastasis is usually a very late phenomenon.

The 5-year survival rate for women with a urethral carcinoma is usually quoted as being between 20 and 30% (Bracken *et al.* 1976) with the outlook being particularly poor for patients with tumours involving the proximal urethra, with neoplasms more than 3 cm in diameter and for those with extraurethral spread (Rogers & Burns 1969, Levine 1980, Pempree *et al.* 1984, Ali *et al.* 1988), the histological type probably not being of prognostic importance (Bracken *et al.* 1976). Currently, however, treatment by radiotherapy, after excision or biopsy of the lesion, is achieving a 5-year survival rate of 41% (Garden *et al.* 1993).

Malignant melanoma

This is an extremely rare neoplasm of the urethra. Melanomas develop most commonly in the distal urethra, may be melanotic or amelanotic, can form a haemorrhagic or pigmented polyp, a black ulcerated area or a papillary mass, and are associated with an extremely poor prognosis

(Das Gupta & Grabstald 1965, Block & Hotchkiss 1971, Katz & Grabstald 1976, Godec *et al.* 1981, Robutti 1986, Sanz-Velez *et al.* 1989, Thum *et al.* 1990).

References

Abell, M.R. (1963) Adenocystic (pseudoadenomatous) basal cell carcinoma of vestibular glands of vulva. *American Journal of Obstetrics and Gynecology* **86**, 470–482.

Abell, M.R. (1965) Intraepithelial carcinomas of epidermis and squamous mucosa of vulva and perineum. *Surgical Clinics of North America* **46**, 1179–1198.

Abroa, F.S., Marques, A.F., Marziona, F. *et al.* (1985) Adenoid cystic carcinoma of Bartholin's gland: review of the literature and report of two cases. *Journal of Surgical Oncology* **30**, 132–137.

Abroa, F.S., Baracat, E.C., Marques, A.F. *et al.* (1990) Carcinoma of the vulva: clinicopathologic factors involved in inguinal and pelvic lymph node metastasis. *Journal of Reproductive Medicine* **35**, 1113–1116.

Ackles, R.C. & Pratt, J.P. (1956) Basal cell carcinoma of the vulva. *American Journal of Obstetrics and Gynecology* **72**, 1124–1126.

Addison, A. (1977) Adenocarcinoma of Bartholin's gland in a 14 year old girl: report of a case. *American Journal of Obstetrics and Gynecology* **127**, 214–215.

Addison, A. & Parker, R.T. (1977) Adenoid cystic carcinoma of the Bartholin's gland: a review of the literature and report of a patient. *Gynecologic Oncology* **5**, 196–201.

Advani, H., Waldo, E.D. & Bigelow, B. (1978) Bartholin's gland carcinoma: an ultrastructural study. *American Journal of Obstetrics and Gynecology* **130**, 362–364.

Ali, M.M., Klein, F.A. & Hazra, T.A. (1988) Primary female urethral carcinoma: a retrospective comparison of different treatment techniques. *Cancer* **62**, 54–57.

Ambrosini, L., Becagli, L. & Resta, P. (1980) Basal cell carcinoma of vulva. *European Journal of Gynaecological Oncology* **1**, 126–128.

Ampil, F.L. (1985) Primary malignant neoplasms of the female urethra. *Obstetrics and Gynecology* **66**, 799–804.

Andersen, E.S. & Sorensen, I.M. (1988) Verrucous carcinoma of the female genital tract: report of a case and review of the literature. *Gynecologic Oncology* **30**, 427–434.

Andersen, W.A., Franquemont, D.W., Williams, J., Tayor, P.T. & Crum, C.P. (1991) Vulvar squamous cell carcinoma and papillomavirus: two separate entities? *American Journal of Obstetric and Gynecology* **165**, 329–336.

Andreasson, B. & Bock, J.E. (1985) Intraepithelial neoplasia in the vulvar region. *Gynecologic Oncology* **21**, 300–305.

Andreasson, B., Bock, J.E. & Wisberg, E. (1982) Invasive cancer in the vulvar region. *Acta Obstetricia et Gynecologica Scandinavica* **61**, 113–119.

Ansink, A.C., Krul, M.R.M., de Weger, R.A. *et al.* (1994) Human papillomavirus, lichen sclerosus and squamous cell carcinoma of the vulva: detection and prognostic significance. *Gynecologic Oncology* **52**, 180–184.

Anthony, P.P., Freeman, K. & Warin, A.P. (1986) Case reports: extrammamary Paget's disease. *Clinical and Experimental Dermatology* **11**, 387–395.

Aquila-Martinez, A., Requena-Caballero, L., Ambrojo-Antunez, P. & Sanchez-Yus, E. (1989) Syringome de la vulva au-dessous d'une verrue séborrhéique. *Annales de Dermatologie et Vénéréologie* **116**, 323–324.

Atamtede, F. & Hoogerland, D. (1989) Regional lymph node recurrence following local excision for microinvasive vulvar carcinoma. *Gynecologic Oncology* **34**, 125–128.

Avinoach, H., Zirkin, H.J. & Glezerman, M. (1989) Proliferating trichilemmal tumor of the vulva: case report and review of the literature. *International Journal of Gynecological Pathology* **8**, 163–168.

Axe, S., Parmley, T., Woodruff, J.D. & Hlopak, B. (1986) Adenomas in minor vestibular glands. *Obstetrics and Gynecology* **68**, 16–18.

Ayhan, A., Tuncer, R., Tuncer, Z.S. *et al.* (1993) Risk factors for groin node metastasis in squamous carcinoma of the vulva: a multivariate analysis of 39 cases. *European Journal of Gynaecology Obstetrics and Reproductive Biology* **48**, 33–36.

Bacchi, C.E., Goldfogel, G.A., Greer, B.E. & Gown, A.M. (1992) Paget's disease and melanoma of the vulva: use of a panel of monoclonal antibodies to identify cell type and to microscopically define adequacy of surgical margins. *Gynecologic Oncology* **46**, 216–221.

Baehrendtz, H., Einhorn, N., Pettersson, F. & Silfversward, C. (1994) Paget's disease of the vulva: the Radiumhemmet series 1975–1990. *International Journal of Gynecological Cancer* **4**, 1–6.

Baggish, M.S., Sze, E.H., Adelson, M.D., Cohn, G. & Oates, R.P. (1989) Quantitative evaluation of the skin and accessory appendages in vulvar carcinoma *in situ*. *Obstetrics and Gynecology* **74**, 169–174.

Bailey, C.L., Sankey, H.Z., Donovan, J.T. *et al.* (1993) Primary breast cancer of the vulva. *Gynecologic Oncology* **50**, 379–383.

Ballouk, F., Ambros, R.A., Malfetano, J.H. & Ross, J.S. (1993) Evaluation of prognostic indicators in squamous carcinoma of the vulva including nuclear DNA content. *Modern Pathology* **6**, 371–375.

Bannatyne, P., Elliott, P. & Russell, P. (1989) Vulvar adenosquamous carcinoma arising in a hidradenoma papilliferum with rapidly fatal outcome: a case report. *Gynecologic Oncology* **35**, 395–398.

Barclay, D.L., Collins, C.G. & Macey, H.B. (1964) Cancer of the Bartholin's gland: a review and report of eight cases. *Obstetrics and Gynecology* **24**, 329–336.

Barnes, A.E., Crissman, J.D., Schellhas, H.F. & Azoury, R.S. (1980) Microinvasive carcinoma of the vulva: a clinicopathologic evaluation. *Obstetrics and Gynecology* **56**, 234–238.

Basta, A. & Madej, J.G. (1990) Hydradenoma of the vulva: incidence and clinical observations. *European Journal of Gynaecological Oncology* **11**, 185–189.

Bean, S.F. & Becker, F.T. (1968) Basal cell carcinoma of the vulva: a case report and review of the literature. *Archives of Dermatology* **98**, 284–286.

Beckmann, A.A., Kiviat, N.B., Daling, J.R., Sherman, K.J. & McDougall, J.K. (1988) Human papillomavirus type 16 in multifocal neoplasia of the female genital tract. *International Journal of Gynecological Pathology* **7**, 39–47.

Benda, J.A., Platz, C.E. & Anderson, B. (1986) Malignant melanoma of the vulva: a clinical-pathologic review of the 16 cases. *International Journal of Gynecological Pathology* **5**, 202–216.

Bender, H.G., Degen, K.W. & Beck, L. (1988) Human papilloma virus findings in the perimeter of vulvo-vaginal malignancies. *European Journal of Gynaecological Oncology* **9**, 287–290.

Benedet, J.L. & Murphy, K.J. (1982) Squamous carcinoma *in situ* of the vulva. *Gynecologic Oncology* **13**, 213–219.

Benedet, J.L., Turko, M., Fairey, R.N. & Boyes, D.A. (1979) Squamous carcinoma of the vulva: results of treatment 1938–1976. *American Journal of Obstetrics and Gynecology* **134**, 201–207.

Bergen, S., DiSaia, S., Liao, S.Y. & Berman, M.I. (1989) Conservative management of extramammary Paget' disease of the vulva. *Gynecologic Oncology* **33**, 151–156.

Bergeron, C., Naghashfar, Z., Canaan, C. *et al.* (1987) Human papillomavirus type 16 in intraepithelial neoplasia (Bowenoid papulosis) and coexistent invasive carcinoma of the vulva. *International Journal of Gynecological Pathology* **6**, 1–11.

Bernstein, S.G., Kovacs, B.R., Townsend, D.E. & Morrow, C.P. (1983a) Vulvar carcinoma *in situ*. *Obstetrics and Gynecology* **61**, 304–307.

Bernstein, S.G., Voet, R.L., Lifshitz, S. & Buchsbaum, H.J. (1983b) Adenoid cystic carcinoma of Bartholin's gland: case report and review of the literature. *American Journal of Obstetrics and Gynecology* **147**, 385–390.

Bhagavan, B., Tiasmson, E.M. & Wenk, R.E. (1981) Nephrogenic adenoma of the urinary bladder and urethra. *Human Pathology* **12**, 907–916.

Bjerregaard, B., Andreasson, B., Visfeldt, J. & Bock, J.E. (1993) The significance of histology and morphometry in predicting lymph node metastases in patients with squamous cell carcinoma of the vulva. *Gynecologic Oncology* **50**, 323–329.

Blazejak, T. & Plewig, G. (1989) Lokalisierte Syringome der Vulva. *Geburtshilfe und Frauenheilkunde* **49**, 1083–1084.

Blessing, K., Kernohan, N.M., Miller, I.D. & Al Nafussi, A.L. (1991) Malignant melanoma of the vulva; clinicopathological features. *International Journal of Gynecological Cancer* **1**, 81–87.

Block, N.L. & Hotchkiss, R.S. (1971) Malignant melanoma of the female urethra: report of a case with 5 year survival and review of the literature. *Journal of Urology* **105**, 251–255.

Boehm, B. & Morris, J.McL. (1971) Paget's disease and apocrine gland carcinoma of the vulva. *Obstetrics and Gynecology* **38**, 185–192.

Bolduan, J.P. & Farah, R.N. (1981) Primary urethral neoplasms: review of 30 cases. *Journal of Urology* **125**, 192–200.

Bornstein, J., Kaufman, R.H., Adam, E. & Adler-Storthz, K. (1988) Multicentric intraepithelial neoplasia involving the vulva: clinical features and association with human papillomavirus and herpes simplex virus. *Cancer* **62**, 1601–1604.

Bottles, K., Lacey, C.G., Goldberg, J. *et al.* (1984) Merkel cell carcinoma of the vulva. *Obstetrics and Gynecology* **63**, 61s–65s.

Bouma, J., Weening, J.J. & Elders, A. (1982) Malignant melanoma of the vulva: report of 18 cases. *European Journal of Obstetrics and Gynecology and Reproductive Biology* **13**, 237–251.

Boyce, J., Fruchtèr, R.G., Kasambilides, E. *et al.* (1984) Prognostic factors in carcinoma of the vulva. *Gynecologic Oncology* **20**, 364–377.

Bozzetti, F., Cascinelli, N., Cataldo, I. & Lupi, G. (1975) Prognosi del melanoma della vulva. *Tumori* **61**, 393–399.

Bracken, R.B., Johnson, D.E., Miller, L.S. *et al.* (1976) Primary carcinoma of the female urethra. *Journal of Urology* **116**, 188–192.

Bradgate, M.G., Rollason, T.P., McConkey, C. & Powell, J. (1990) Malignant melanoma of the vulva: a clinico-pathological study of 30 women. *British Journal of Obstetrics and Gynaecology* **97**, 124–133.

Breen, J.L., Neubecker, R.D., Greenwald, E. & Gregori, C.A. (1975) Basal cell carcinoma of the vulva. *Obstetrics and Gynecology* **46**, 122–129.

Breen, J.L., Smith, H. & Gregori, C.A. (1978) Extramammary Paget's disease. *Clinical Obstetrics and Gynecology* **21**, 1107–1115.

Breslow, A. (1970) Thickness, cross sectional areas and depth of invasion in the prognosis of malignant melanoma. *Annals of Surgery* **172**, 902–908.

Brinton, L.A., Nasca, P.C., Mallin, K. *et al.* (1990) Case control study of cancer of the vulva. *Obstetrics and Gynecology* **75**, 859–866.

Brisigotti, M., Moreno, A., Murcia, C., Matias-Guiu, X. & Prat, J. (1989) Verrucous cancinoma of the vulva: a clinicopathologic and immunohistochemical study of five cases. *International Journal of Gynecological Pathology* **8**, 1–7.

Brown, S.M. & Freeman, R.G. (1971) Syringoma limited to the vulva. *Archives of Dermatology* **104**, 331.

Bryson, S.C.P., Dembo, A.J., Colgan, T.J. *et al.* (1991) Invasive squamous cell carcinoma of the vulva: defining low and high risk groups for recurrence. *International Journal of Gynecological Cancer* **1**, 25–31.

Buchler, D.A., Sun, F. & Chuprevich, T. (1978) A pilar tumor of the vulva. *Gynecologic Oncology* **6**, 479–486.

Burger, M.P.M., Hollema, H., Emanuels, A.G. *et al.* (1995) The importance of the groin node status for the survival of T1 and T2 vulval carcinoma patients. *Gynecologic Oncology* **57**, 327–334.

Burger, R.A. & Marcuse, P.M. (1954) Fibroadenoma of vulva. *American Journal of Clinical Pathology* **24**, 965–968.

Buscema, J. & Woodruff, J.D. (1980) Progressive histobiologic alterations in the development of vulvar cancer: report of five cases. *American Journal of Obstetrics and Gynecology* **138**, 146–150.

Buscema, J., Woodruff, J.D., Parmely, T.H. & Genadry, R. (1980a) Carcinoma *in situ* of the vulva. *Obstetrics and Gynecology* **55**, 225–230.

Buscema, J., Stern, J. & Woodruff, J.D. (1980b) The significance of the histologic alterations adjacent to invasive vulvar carcinoma. *American Journal of Obstetrics and Gynecology* **137**, 902–909.

Buscema, J., Stern, J.L. & Woodruff, J.D. (1981) Early invasive carcinoma of the vulva. *American Journal of Obstetrics and Gynecology* **140**, 563–569.

Buscema, J., Naghashfar, Z. & Sawada, E. (1988) The predominance of human papillomavirus type 16 in vulvar neoplasia. *Obstetrics and Gynecology* **71**, 601–606.

Caglar, H., Tamer, S. & Hreshchyshn, M.M. (1982) Vulvar intraepithelial neoplasia. *Obstetrics and Gynecology* **60**, 346–349.

Carli, P., Catteneo, A., De Magnis, A. *et al.* (1995) Squamous cell carcinoma arising in vulval lichen sclerosus: a longitudinal cohort study. *European Journal of Cancer Prevention* **4**, 491–495.

Carneiro, S.J.C., Gardner, H.L. & Knox, J.W. (1971) Syringoma of the vulva. *Archives of Dermatology* **103**, 494–496.

Carneiro, S.J.C., Gardner, H.L. & Knox, J.M. (1972) Syringoma: three cases with vulvar involvement. *Obstetrics and Gynecology* **39**, 95–99.

Carter, J. & Elliott, P. (1990) Syringoma—an unusual cause of pruritus vulvae. *Australian and New Zealand Journal of Obstetrics and Gynecology* **30**, 382–383.

Chafe, W., Richards, A., Morgan, L. & Wilkinson, E.J. (1988) Unrecognized invasive carcinoma in vulvar intraepithelial neoplasia (VIN). *Gynecologic Oncology* **31**, 154–165.

Chamlian, D.L. & Taylor, H.B. (1972) Primary carcinoma of Bartholin's gland: a report of 24 patients. *Obstetrics and Gynecology* **38**, 489–494.

Chandeying, V., Sutthijumroon, S. & Tungphaisal, S. (1989) Merkel cell carcinoma of the vulva: a case report. *Asia Oceania Journal of Obstetrics and Gynaecology* **15**, 261–265.

Chapman, G.W., Benda, J.B. & Lifshitz, S. (1985) Adenoid cystic carcinoma of the vulva with lung metastases: a case report. *Journal of Reproductive Medicine* **30**, 217–220.

Chapman, G.W., Hassan, N., Page, D. *et al.* (1987) Mucinous cystadenoma of Bartholin's gland: a case report. *Journal of Reproductive Medicine* **32**, 939–941.

Cho, D. & Woodruff, J.D. (1988) Trichepithelioma of the vulva: report of two cases. *Journal of Reproductive Medicine* **33**, 317–319.

Cho, D., Buscema, J., Rosenhein, N.B. & Woodruff, J.D. (1985) Primary breast cancer of the vulva. *Obstetrics and Gynecology* **66**, 79s–81s.

Christensen, W.N., Friedman, K.J., Woodruff, J.D. & Hood, A.F. (1987) Histological characteristics of vulvar nevocellular nevi. *Journal of Cutaneous Pathology* **14**, 87–91.

Chu, J., Tamimi, H.K., Ek, M. & Figge, D.C. (1982) Stage I vulvar cancer: criteria for microinvasion. *Obstetrics and Gynecology* **59**, 716–719.

Chung, A.F., Woodruff, J.M. & Lewis, J.L. (1975) Malignant melanoma of the vulva: a report of 44 cases. *Obstetrics and Gynecology* **45**, 638–646.

Clark, W.H. Jr., From, L., Bernadino, E.A. & Mihm, M.C. (1969) Histogenesis and biologic behaviour of primary human malignant melanoma of the skin. *Cancer Research* **29**, 705–727.

Cleophax, J.P., Pelleron, J.P., Durand, J.C. & Lourant, M. (1977) Le mélanome de la vulva. *Gynécologie* **27**, 333–339.

Cliby, W., Soisson, A.P., Berchuck, A. & Clarke-Pearson, D.I. (1991) Stage 1 small cell carcinoma of the vulva treated with vulvectomy, lymphadenectomy, and adjuvant chemotherapy. *Cancer* **67**, 2415–2417.

Collins, C.G., Roman-Lopez, J.J. & Lee, F.Y.L. (1970) Intraepithelial carcinoma of the vulva. *American Journal of Obstetrics and Gynecology* **108**, 1187–1191.

Cone, R., Beckmann, A., Aho, M. *et al.* (1991) Subclinical manifestations of vulvar human papillomavirus infection. *International Journal of Gynecological Pathology* **10**, 26–35.

Copas, P.R., Spann, C.O. Jr., Majmudar, B. & Horowitz, I.R. (1996) Basal cell carcinoma of the vulva: a report of four cases. *Journal of Reproductive Medicine* **41**, 283–286.

Copeland, L.J., Cleary, K., Sneige, N. & Edwards, C.L. (1985) Neuroendocrine (Merkel cell) carcinoma of the vulva: a case report and review of the literature. *Gynecologic Oncology* **22**, 367–378.

Copeland, L.J., Sneige, N., Gershenson, D.M. *et al.* (1986a) Bartholin gland carcinoma. *Obstetrics and Gynecology* **67**, 794–801.

Copeland, L.J., Sneige, N., Gershenson, D.M. *et al.* (1986b) Adenoid cystic carcinoma of the Bartholin gland. *Obstetrics and Gynecology* **67**, 115–120.

Creasman, W.G., Gallager, H.S. & Rutledge, F. (1975) Paget's disease of the vulva. *Gynecologic Oncology* **3**, 133–148.

Crowther, M.E., Shepherd, J.H. & Fisher, C. (1988) Verrucous carcinoma of the vulva containing human papillomavirus-11: case report. *British Journal of Obstetrics and Gynaecology* **95**, 414–418.

Crum, C.P. (1992) Carcinoma of the vulva: epidemiology and pathogenesis. *Obstetrics and Gynecology* **79**, 448–458.

Crum, C.P., Liskow, A., Petras, P., Keng, W.C. & Frick, H.C. (1984) Vulvar intraepithelial neoplasia (severe atypia and carcinoma *in situ*). *Cancer* **54**, 1429–1434.

Crum, C.P., McLachlin, C.M., Tate, J.E. & Mutter, G. (1997) Pathobiology of vulvar squamous neoplasia. *Current Opinion in Obstetrics and Gynecology* **9**, 63–69.

Cruz-Jimenez, P.R. & Abell, M.R. (1975) Cutaneous basal cell carcinoma of the vulva. *Cancer* **36**, 1860–1868.

Curry, S.L., Wharton, J.T. & Rutledge, F.D. (1980) Positive lymph nodes in vulvar squamous carcinoma. *Gynecologic Oncology* **9**, 63–67.

Curtin, J.P. & Morrow, C.P. (1992) Melanoma of lower female genital tract. In: *Gynecologic Oncology*, 2nd edn (ed. M. Coppleson), pp. 1059–1068. Churchill Livingstone, Edinburgh.

Curtin, J.P., Rubin, S.C., Jones, W.B., Hoskins, W.J. & Lewis, J.L. Jr. (1990) Paget's disease of the vulva. *Gynecologic Oncology* **39**, 574–577.

Daling, J.R., Chu, J., Weiss, N.S., Emel, L. & Tamini, H.K. (1984) The association of condylomata acuminata and squamous carcinoma of the vulva. *British Journal of Cancer* **50**, 533–535.

Dancoisne, P., Riviere, J.P., Abossolo, T. *et al.* (1995) Cancer primitif de la glande de Bartholin et role étiopathogénétique du papillomavirus humain: rapport d'un nouveau cas. *Revue Française de Gynécologie et de l'Obstétrique* **90**, 220–221.

Das Gupta, T. & Grabstald, H. (1965) Melanoma of the genitourinary tract. *Journal of Urology* **93**, 607–614.

Davidson, T., Kissin, M. & Westbury, G. (1987) Vulvo-vaginal melanoma—should radical surgery be abandoned? *British Journal of Obstetrics and Gynaecology* **94**, 473–476.

Degefu, S., O'Quinn, A.G. & Dhurandhar, H.N. (1986) Paget's disease of vulva and urogenital malignancies: a case report and review of the literature. *Gynecologic Oncology* **25**, 347–354.

de Jonge, E.T. & Knobel, J. (1988) Recurrent Paget's disease after simple vulvectomy and skin grafting: a case report. *South African Medical Journal* **9**, 46–47.

Dennefors, B. & Bergman, B. (1980) Primary carcinoma of the Bartholin gland. *Acta Obstetricia et Gynecologica Scandinavica* **59**, 95–96.

Dennis, E.J., Hester, L.L. Jr. & Wilson, L.A. (1955) Primary carcinoma of Bartholin's glands: review; report of a case. *Obstetrics and Gynecology* **6**, 291–296.

Depasquale, S.E., McGuiness, T.B., Mangan, C.E., Husson, M. & Woodland, M.B. (1996) Adenoid cystic carcinoma of Bartholin's gland: a review of the literature and report of a patient. *Gynecologic Oncology* **61**, 122–125.

Deppisch, L.M. (1978) Basal cell carcinoma of the vulva. *Mt Sinai Journal of Medicine* **45**, 406–410.

Desai, S., Libertino, J.A. & Zinman, I. (1973) Primary carcinoma of the female urethra. *Journal of Urology* **110**, 693–695.

Di Bonito, L., Patriaca, S. & Falconieri, G. (1992) Aggressive 'breast-like' adenocarcinoma of vulva. *Pathology Research and Practice* **188**, 211–214.

DiPaola, G.R., Gomez-Rueda, N. & Arrhigi, L. (1975) Relevance of microinvasion in carcinoma of the vulva. *Obstetrics and Gynecology* **45**, 647–649.

DiPaola, G.R., Rueda-Leverone, N.G., Becardi, M.G. & Vighi, S. (1982) Vulvar carcinoma *in situ*: a report of 28 cases. *Gynecologic Oncology* **14**, 236–242.

DiSaia, P.J. & Creasman, W.T. (1989) *Clinical Gynecologic Oncology*, 3rd edn. Mosby, St Louis.

DiSaia, P.J., Dorian, G.E., Cappucchini, F. & Carpenter, P.M. (1995) A report of two cases of recurrent Paget's disease of the vulva in a split-thickness graft and its possible pathogenesis—labelled "retrodissemination". *Gynecologic Oncology* **57**, 109–112.

Dodson, M.G., O'Leary, J.A. & Averette, H.E. (1970) Primary carcinoma of Bartholin's gland. *Obstetrics and Gynecology* **35**, 578–584.

Dodson, M.G., O'Leary, J.A. & Averette, H.E. (1978) Adenoid cystic carcinoma of the vulva: malignant cylindroma. *Obstetrics and Gynecology* **51**, 26s–29s.

Dolan, J.R., McCall, A.R., Gooneratne, S., Walter, S. & Lansky, D.M. (1993) DNA ploidy, proliferation index, grade, and stage as prognostic factors for vulvar squamous cell carcinomas. *Gynecologic Oncology* **48**, 232–235.

Donna, A., Torchio, B. & Lampertico, P. (1978) L'idroadenoma papillifero della vulva: contributo casistico e revisione della letteratura. *Pathologica* **70**, 359–375.

Dudzinski, M.R., Askin, F.B. & Fowler, W.C. (1984) Giant basal cell carcinoma of the vulva. *Obstetrics and Gynecology* **63**, 57s–60s.

Dunton, C.J., Kautzy, M. & Hanau, C. (1995) Malignant melanoma of the vulva: a review. *Obstetrical and Gynecological Survey* **50**, 739–746.

Dvoretsky, P.M., Bonfiglio, T., Helmkamp. F. *et al.* (1984) The pathology of superficially invasive, thin vulvar squamous cell carcinoma. *International Journal of Gynecological Pathology* **3**, 331–342.

Ebel, K. & Klinger, D. (1991) Glandulare Metaplasie und primares Adenokarzinom der Urethra. *Urologe* **30**, 147–149.

Edington, P.T. & Monaghan, J.M. (1980) Malignant melanoma of the vulva and vagina. *British Journal of Obstetrics and Gynaecology* **87**, 422–424.

Eichenberg, H.E. (1934) Hidradenoma vulvae. *Zeitschrift für Gynäkologie und Geburtshilfe* **109**, 358–375.

Eichner, E. (1963) Adenoid cystic carcinoma of Bartholin's gland: review of the literature and report of a case. *Obstetrics and Gynecology* **21**, 608–613.

Elkon, D., Kim, J.A., Huddleston, A.L. *et al.* (1980) Primary carcinoma of female urethra. *Southern Medical Journal* **73**, 1439–1442.

Enghardt, M.H., Valente, P.T. & Day, D.H. (1993) Papilloma of Bartholin's gland duct cyst: first report of a case. *International Journal of Gynecological Pathology* **12**, 86–92.

Evans, A.T. & Neven, P. (1991) Invasive adenocarcinoma arising in extramammary Paget's disese of the vulva. *Histopathology* **18**, 355–360.

Felix, J.C., Cote, R.J., Kramer, E.E., Saigo, P. & Goldman, G.H. (1993) Carcinomas of Bartholin's gland: histogenesis and the etiological role of human papillomavirus. *American Journal of Pathology* **142**, 925–933.

Fenn, M.E. & Abell, M.R. (1973) Melanoma of vulva and vagina. *Obstetrics and Gynecology* **41**, 902–911.

Fenn, M.E., Morley, G.W. & Abell, M.R. (1971) Paget's disease of the vulva. *Obstetrics and Gynecology* **38**, 660–670.

Ferenczy, A. (1992) Intraepithelial neoplasia of the vulva. In: *Gynecologic Oncology*, 2nd edn (ed. M. Coppleson), pp. 443–463. Churchill Livingstone, Edinburgh.

Ferenczy, A., Wright, J.R. & Richart, R.M. (1994) Comparison of CO_2 laser surgery and loop electrosurgical excision/fulguration procedure (LEEP) for the treatment of vulvar intraepithelial neoplasia (VIN). *International Journal of Gynecological Cancer* **4**, 22–28.

Fetherston, W.C. & Friedrich, E.G. (1972) The origin and significance of vulvar Paget's disease. *Obstetrics and Gynecology* **49**, 735–744.

Feuer, G.A., Shevchuk, M. & Calanog, A. (1990) Vulvar Paget's disease: the need to exclude an invasive lesion. *Gynecologic Oncology* **38**, 81–89.

Fine, B.A., Fowler, L.J., Valente, P.T. & Gaudet, T. (1995) Minimally invasive Paget's disease of the vulva with extensive lymph node metastases. *Gynecologic Oncology* **57**, 262–265.

Fiorica, J.V., Cavanagh, D., Marsden, D.E. *et al.* (1988) Carcinoma *in situ* of the vulva: 24 years experience in southwest Florida. *Southern Medical Journal* **81**, 589–593.

Fisher, J.H. (1947) Fibroadenoma of supernumary mammary gland tissue in vulva. *American Journal of Obstetrics and Gynecology* **53**, 335–337.

Fishman, D., Chambers, S., Schwartz, P. & Kohorne, E. (1995) Extramammary Paget's disease of the vulva. *Gynecologic Oncology* **56**, 266–270.

Forney, J.P., Morrow, C.P., Townsend, D.E. & DiSaia, J.P. (1977) Management of carcinoma *in situ* of the vulva. *American Journal of Obstetrics and Gynecology* **127**, 801–806.

Foushee, J.H.S. & Pruitt, A.B. (1967) Vulvar fibroadenoma from aberrant breast tissue. *Obstetrics and Gynecology* **29**, 819–823.

Foushee, J.H.S., Reeves, W.J.U. & McCool, J.A. (1968) Benign masses of Bartholin's gland: solid adenomas, adenomas with cyst, and Bartholin's gland with varices or thrombosis or cavernous hemangioma. *Obstetrics and Gynecology* **31**, 695–701.

Franklin, E.W. & Rutledge, F.D. (1972) Epidemiology of epidermoid carcinoma of the vulva. *Obstetrics and Gynecology* **39**, 165–172.

Friedel, R. (1932) Ein Fibroadenoma einer Nebenbrustdruse in rechten labium majus. *Virchows Archiv* **286**, 62–69.

Friedman, R.J. & Ackerman, A.B. (1981) Difficulties in the histological diagnosis of melanocytic nevi on the vulvae of premenopausal women. In: *Pathology of Malignant Melanoma* (ed. A.B. Ackerman), pp. 119–127. Masson, New York.

Friedrich, E.G. (1972) Reversible vulvar atypia: a case report. *Obstetrics and Gynecology* **39**, 173–181.

Friedrich, E.G. (1976) *Vulvar Disease.* Saunders, Philadelphia.

Friedrich, E.G. (1981) Intraepithelial neoplasia of the vulva. In: *Gynecologic Oncology* (ed. M. Coppleson), pp. 303–319. Churchill Livingstone, Edinburgh.

Friedrich, E.G., Wilkinson, E.J., Steingraeber, P.H. & Lewis, J.D. (1975) Paget's disease of the vulva and carcinoma of the breast. *Obstetrics and Gynecology* **46**, 130–134.

Friedrich, E.G., Wilkinson, E.J. & Fu, Y.S. (1980) Carcinoma *in situ* of the vulva: a continuing challenge. *American Journal of Obstetrics and Gynecology* **136**, 830–843.

Fu, Y.S. & Reagan, J.W. (1989) *Pathology of the Uterine Cervix, Vagina, and Vulva.* Saunders, Philadelphia.

Fukuma, K., Inoue, S., Tamaka, N. *et al.* (1986) Eccrine adenocarcinoma of the vulva producing isolated alpha-subunit of glycoprotein hormones. *Obstetrics and Gynecology* **67**, 293–296.

Gadducci, A., De Punzio, C., Facchini, V., Rispoli, G. & Fioretti, P. (1989) The therapy of verrucous carcinoma of the vulva. *European Journal of Gynaecological Oncology* **10**, 284–287.

Gallousis, S. (1972) Verrucous carcinoma: report of three vulvar cases and review of the literature. *Obstetrics and Gynecology* **40**, 502–507.

Ganjei, P., Giraldo, K.A., Lampe, B. & Nadji, M. (1990) Vulvar Paget's disease: is immunocytochemistry helpful in assessing the surgical margins? *Journal of Reproductive Medicine* **35**, 1002–1004.

Garden, A.S., Zagars, G.K. & Delclos, L. (1993) Primary carcinoma of the female urethra: results of radiation therapy. *Cancer* **71**, 3102–3108.

Gardiner, S.H., Stout, F.E., Argobast, J.L. & Huber, C.P. (1953) Intraepithelial carcinoma of the vulva. *American Journal of Obstetrics and Gynecology* **63**, 539–549.

Gartmann, H. (1985) Eccrine porocarcinoma. *Zietschrift für Hauptkrankenheiten* **1**, 555–562.

Geisler, J.P., Stowell, M.J., Melton, M.E., Maloney, C.D. & Geisler, H.E. (1995) Extramammary Paget's disease of the vulva recurring in a skin graft. *Gynecologic Oncology* **56**, 446–447.

Geisler, J.P., Gates, R.W., Shirrell, W. *et al.* (1997) Extramammary Paget's disease with diffuse involvement of the lower female genito-urinary system. *International Journal of Gynecological Cancer* **7**, 84–87.

Gerrard, E.A. (1932) Epithelioma vulvae as an occupational disease among cotton operatives. *Transactions of the North of England Obstetrical and Gynaecological Society* 65–74.

Ghamande, S.A., Kasznica, J., Griffiths, C.T., Finkler, N.J. & Hamid, A.M. (1995) Mucinous adenocarcinomas of the vulva. *Gynecologic Oncology* **57**, 117–120.

Ghirardini, G. (1982) Syringoma limited to the vulva. *Diagnostic Gynecology and Obstetrics* **4**, 325–326.

Gilks, C.B., Clement, P.B. & Wood, W.S. (1989) Trichoblastic fibroma: a clinicopathologic study of three cases. *American Journal of Dermatopathology* **11**, 397–402.

Gissman, L., de Villiers, E.-M. & zur Hausen, H. (1982) Analysis of human genital warts (condylomata acuminata) and other genital tumours for HPC type 6 DNA. *International Journal of Cancer* **29**, 143–146.

Gleeson N.C., Ruffolo, E.M., Hoffman, M.S. & Cavanagh, D. (1994) Basal cell carcinoma of the vulva with groin node metastasis. *Gynecologic Oncology* **53**, 266–268.

Godec, C.J., Cass, A.S., Hitchcock, R. *et al.* (1981) Melanoma of the female urethra. *Journal of Urology* **126**, 553–555.

Goldstein, A.I. & Kent, D.R. (1975) All vulvar lesions should be biopsied: basal cell carcinoma—an example of the futility of diagnosis by gross appearance. *American Journal of Obstetrics and Gynecology* **121**, 173–174.

Gomez-Rueda, N., Garcia, A., Vighi, S. *et al.* (1994) Epithelial alterations adjacent to invasive squamous carcinoma of the vulva. *Journal of Reproductive Medicine* **39**, 526–530.

Grabstald, H. (1973) Tumors of the urethra in men and women. *Cancer* **32**, 1236–1255.

Green, H.J. (1936) Adenocarcinoma of supernumary breasts of the labia majora in a case of epidermoid carcinoma of the vulva. *American Journal of Obstetrics and Gynecology* **31**, 660–663.

Green, T.H. (1978) Carcinoma of the vulva: a reassessment. *Obstetrics and Gynecology* **52**, 462–469.

Green, T.H., Ulfelder, H. & Meigs, J.V. (1958) Epidermoid carcinoma of the vulva: an analysis of 238 cases. *American Journal of Obstetrics and Gynecology* **75**, 834–847.

Guarner, J., Cohen, C. & DeRose, P.B. (1989) Histogenesis of extramammary and mammary Paget cells: an immunohistochemical study. *American Journal of Dermatopathology* **11**, 313–318.

Guercio, F., Cesone, P., Saracino, A. *et al.* (1984) Adenocarcinoma in soto su glandola mammaria aberrente in sede vulvare. *Minerva Ginecologica* **36**, 315–319.

Guerry, R.L. & Pratt-Thomas, H.R. (1976) Carcinoma of supernumary breast of vulva with bilateral mammary cancer. *Cancer* **38**, 2570–2574.

Guindi, S.F., Silverberg, B.K. & Evans, T.L. (1974) Multifocal mixed adenoid tumors of the vulva. *International Journal of Gynaecology and Obstetrics* **12**, 138–140.

Gunn, R.A. & Gallager, H.S. (1980) Vulvar Paget's disease: a topographic study. *Cancer* **46**, 590–594.

Gupta, J., Pilotti, S., Shah, K.V., De Palo, G. & Rilke, F. (1987) Human papillomavirus-associated early vulvar neoplasia investigated by *in situ* hybridization. *American Journal of Surgical Pathology* **11**, 430–434.

Hacker, N.F., Nieberg, R.K., Berek, J.S. *et al.* (1983) Superficially invasive vulvar cancer with nodal metastases. *Gynecologic Oncology* **15**, 65–77.

Hacker, N.F., Berek, J.S., Lagasse, L.D., Nieberg, R.K. & Leuchter, R.S. (1984) Individualization of treatment for Stage I squamous cell vulvar carcinoma. *Obstetrics and Gynecology* **63**, 155–162.

Haefner, H., Tate, J., McLachlin, C. & Crum, C. (1995) Vulvar intraepithelial neoplasia: age, morphological phenotype, papillomavirus DNA, and coexisting invasive carcinooma. *Human Pathology* **26**, 147–154.

Hart, W.R. & Millman, J.B. (1977) Progression of intraepithelial Paget's disease of the vulva to invasive carcinoma. *Cancer* **40**, 233–237.

Hashimoto, K. (1973) Hidradenoma papilliferum: an electron microscopic study. *Acta Dermato-venereologica (Stockholm)* **53**, 22–30.

Hassim, A.M. (1969) Bilateral fibroadenoma in supernumary breasts of the vulva. *Journal of Obstetrics and Gynaecology of the British Commonwealth* **76**, 275–277.

Hastrup, N. & Andersen, F. (1988) Adenocarcinoma of Bartholin's gland associated with extramammary Paget's disease of the vulva. *Acta Obstetricia et Gynecologica Scandinavica* **67**, 375–377.

Hawley, I.C., Husain, F. & Pryse-Davies, J. (1991) Extramammary Pagets's disease of the vulva with dermal invasion and vulval intraepithelial neoplasia. *Histopathology* **18**, 374–376.

Hay, D.M. & Cole, F.M. (1970) Postgranulomatous epidermoid carcinoma of the vulva. *American Journal of Obstetrics and Gynecology* **108**, 479–484.

Heaps, J.M., Fu, Y.S., Montz, F.J., Hacker, N.F. & Berek, J.S. (1990) Surgical–pathologic variables predictive of local recurrence in squamous cell carcinoma of the vulva. *Gynecologic Oncology* **38**, 309–314.

Heine, O. & Vahrson, H. (1987) Das primare Karzinom der Bartholinischen Druse. *Geburtshilfe und Frauenheilkunde* **47**, 35–40.

Helm, K.F., Goellner, J.R. & Peters, M.S. (1992) Immunohistochemical stains in extramammary Paget's disease. *American Journal of Dermatopathology* **14**, 402–407.

Helwig, E.B. & Graham, J.H. (1963) Anogenital (extramammary) Paget's disease. *Cancer* **16**, 387–403.

Hendricks, J.B., Wilkinson, E.J., Kubilis, P. *et al.* (1994) Ki-67 expression in vulvar carcinoma. *International Journal of Gynecological Pathology* **13**, 205–210.

Hendrix, R.C. & Behrman, S.J. (1956) Adenocarcinoma arising in a supernumerary mammary gland in the vulva. *Obstetrics and Gynecology* **8**, 238–241.

Hennekens, C.H., Speizer, F.E., Rosner, B. *et al.* (1979) Use of permanent hair dyes and cancer amongst registered nurses. *Lancet* ii, 1390–1393.

Herod, J.J., Shafi, M.I., Rollason, T.P., Jordan, J.A. & Luesley, D.M. (1996) Vulvar intraepithelial neoplasia with superficially invasive carcinoma of the vulva. *British Journal of Obstetrics and Gynaecology* **103**, 453–456.

Hidvegi, J., Zsolnai, B. & Szinay, G. (1988) Amphicrine tumor of the vulva. *Pathology Research and Practice* **183**, 505–508.

Hobbs, J.E. (1965) Sweat gland tumors. *Clinical Obstetrics and Gynecology* **8**, 946–951.

Hoffman, J.S., Kumar, N.B. & Morley, G.W. (1983) Microinvasive squamous cell carcinoma of the vulva: search for a definition. *Obstetrics and Gynecology* **61**, 615–618.

Hoffman, M.S., Roberts, W.S. & Ruffolo, E.H. (1988) Basal cell carcinoma of the vulva with inguinal lymph node metastases. *Gynecologic Oncology* **29**, 113–119.

Homesley, M.D., Bundy, B.N., Sedlis, A. *et al.* (1993) Prognostic factors for groin node metastasis in squamous cell carcinoma of the vulva: a Gynecologic Oncology Group study. *Gynecologic Oncology* **49**, 279–283.

Honore, L.H. & O'Hara, K.E. (1978) Adenomas of the Bartholin's gland: report of three cases. *European Journal of Obstetrics, Gynecology and Reproductive Biology* **8**, 335–340.

Hopkins, M.P., Reid, G.C., Vettrano, I. & Morley, G.W. (1991) Squamous cell carcinoma of the vulva: prognostic factors influencing survival. *Gynecologic Oncology* **43**, 113–117.

Hopkins, S.C., Vider, M., Nag, S.K. *et al.* (1983) Carcinoma of the female urethra: reassessment of modes of therapy. *Journal of Urology* **129**, 958–961.

Hording, U., Junge, J., Daugaard, S. *et al.* (1994) Vulvar squamous cell carcinoma and papillomaviruses: indications for two different etiologies. *Gynecologic Oncology* **52**, 241–246.

Howells, M.R., Baylis, M.S. & Howell, S. (1995) Benign urethral villous papilloma. *British Journal of Obstetrics and Gynaecology* **92**, 1070–1071.

Hulagu, C. & Erez, S. (1973) Juvenile melanoma of the clitoris. *Journal of Obstetrics and Gynaecology of the British Commonwealth* **80**, 89–91.

Husseinzadeh, N., Wesseler, T., Newman, N., Shbaro, I. & Ho, P. (1988) Neuroendocrine (Merkel cell) carcinoma of the vulva. *Gynecologic Oncology* **29**, 105–112.

Husseinzadeh, N., Newman, N.J. & Wesseler, T.A. (1989) Vulvar intraepithelial neoplasia: a clinicopathological study of carcinoma *in situ* of the vulva. *Gynecologic Oncology* **33**, 157–163.

Husseinzadeh, N., Wesseler, T., Schneider, D., Schellhas, H. & Nahhas, W. (1990) Prognostic factors and the significance of cytologic grading in invasive squamous cell carcinoma of the vulva: a clinicopathologic study. *Gynecologic Oncology* **36**, 192–199.

Isaacs. J.H. (1976) Verrucous carcinoma of the female genital tract. *Gynecologic Oncology* **4**, 259–263.

Isaacson, D. & Turner, M.L. (1979) Localized vulvar syringomas. *Journal of the American Academy of Dermatology* **1**, 352–356.

Itala, J., DiPaola, G.R., Gomez-Rueda, N., Perez-Lloret, I. & Buquet, R. (1986) Melanoma of the vulva: the experience at Buenos Aires University. *Journal of Reproductive Medicine* **31**, 836–838.

Jacobs, D.M., Sandles, L.G. & Leboit, P.E. (1986) Sebaceous carcinoma arising from Bowen's disease of the vulva. *Archives of Dermatology* **122**, 1191–1192.

Jafari, K. & Cartnick, F.N. (1976) Microinvasive squamous cell carcinoma of the vulva. *Gynecologic Oncology* **4**, 158–166.

Janovski, N.A. & Douglas, C.P. (1972) *Diseases of the Vulva.* Harper & Row, Hagerstown, MD.

Janovski, N.A., Marshall, D. & Taki, A. (1962) Malignant melanoma of the vulva. *American Journal of Obstetrics and Gynecology* **84**, 523–536.

Japaze, H., Garcia-Bunuel, R. & Woodruff, J.D. (1977) Primary vulvar neoplasia: a review of *in-situ* and invasive carcinoma, 1935–1972. *Obstetrics and Gynecology* **49**, 401–411.

Japaze, H., Dinh, T.V. & Woodruff, J.D. (1982) Verrucous carcinoma of the vulva: study of 24 cases. *Obstetrics and Gynecology* **60**, 462–466.

Jaramillo, B.A., Gansel, P., Averette, H.E., Sevin, B.L. & Lovecchio, J.L. (1985) Malignant melanoma of the vulva. *Obstetrics and Gynecology* **66**, 398–401.

Jimenez, H.T., Fenoglio, C.M. & Richart, R.M. (1975) Vulvar basal cell carcinoma with metastasis: a case report. *American Journal of Obstetrics and Gynecology* **121**, 285–286.

Johnson, T.L., Kumar, N.B., White, C.D. & Morley, G.W. (1986) Prognostic features of vulvar melanoma: a clinicopathologic analysis. *International Journal of Gynecological Pathology* **5**, 110–118.

Jones, I. & Buntine, D. (1978) Progression of vulval carcinoma *in situ*. *Australian and New Zealand Journal of Obstetrics and Gynaecology* **18**, 274–276.

Jones, M.A., Mann, E.W., Caldwell, C.L. *et al.* (1990) Small cell neuroendocrine carcinoma of Bartholin's gland. *American Journal of Clinical Patholgy* **94**, 439–442.

Jones, R.E. Jr., Austin, C. & Ackerman, A.B. (1979) Extramammary Paget's disease: a critical re-examination. *American Journal of Dermatopathology* **1**, 101–132.

Jones, R.W. & McClean, M.R. (1986) Carcinoma *in situ* of the vulva: a review of 31 treated and five untreated cases. *Obstetrics and Gynecology* **68**, 499–503.

Jones, R.W. & Rowan, D. (1994) Vulvar intraepithelial neoplasia III: a clinical study of the outcome in 113 cases with relation to the later development of invasive vulvar carcinoma. *Obstetrics and Gynecology* **84**, 741–745.

Kaern, J., Iversen, T., Trope, C., Pettersen, E.O. & Nesland, J.M. (1992) Flow cytometric DNA measurements in squamous cell carcinoma of the vulva: an important prognostic method. *International Journal of Gynecological Cancer* **2**, 169–174.

Kagie, M.J., Kenter, G.G., Tollenaar, R.A.E.M. *et al.* (1997) p53 protein overexpression, a frequent observation in squamous cell carcinoma of the vulva and in various synchronous vulva epithelia, has no value as a prognostic parameter. *International Journal of Gynecological Pathology* **16**, 124–130.

Kariniemi, A.L., Forsman, L., Wahlstrom, T., Vesterinen, E. & Andersson, L. (1984) Expression of differentiation antigens in mammary and extramammary Paget's disease. *British Journal of Dermatology* **110**, 203–210.

Karlen, J.R., Pivers, M.S. & Barlow, J.J. (1975) Melanoma of the vulva. *Obstetrics and Gynecology* **45**, 181–185.

Katz, J.I. & Grabstald, H. (1976) Primary malignant melanoma of the female urethra. *Journal of Urology* **116**, 454–457.

Kaufman, R. (1995) Intraepithelial neoplasia of the vulva. *Gynecologic Oncology* **56**, 8–21.

Kaufmann, T., Pawl, N.O., Soifer, I., Greston, W.M. & Kleiner, G.J. (1987) Cystic papillary hidradenoma of the vulva: case report and review of the literature. *Gynecologic Oncology* **26**, 240–245.

Kelley, J.L., Burke, T.W., Tornos, C. *et al.* (1992) Minimally invasive vulvar carcinoma: an indication for conservative surgical therapy. *Gynecologic Oncology* **44**, 240–244.

Kennedy, J.C. & Majmudar, B. (1993) Primary adenocarcinoma of the vulva, possibly cloacogenic: a report of two cases. *Journal of Reproductive Medicine* **38**, 113–116.

Kieche-Schwartz, M., Kommoss, F., Schmidt, J. *et al.* (1992) Cytogenetic analysis of an adenoid cystic carcinoma of the Bartholin's gland: a rare, semimalignant tumor of the female genitourinary tract. *Cancer Genetics and Cytogenetics* **61**, 26–30.

Kim, Y.T., Thomas, N.F., Kessis, T.D. *et al.* (1996) p53 mutations and clonality in vulvar carcinomas and squamous hyperplasia: evidence suggesting that squamous hyperplasia do not serve as direct precursors of human papillomavirus-negative vulvar carcinomas. *Human Pathology* **27**, 389–395.

Klotz, P.G. (1974) Carcinoma of Skene's gland associated with urethral diverticulum: a case report. *Journal of Urology* **112**, 487–488.

Kluzak, T.R. & Kraus, F.T. (1987) Condylomata, papillomas, and verrucous carcinoma of the vulva and vagina. In: *Pathology of the Vulva and Vagina* (ed. E.J. Wilkinson), pp. 49–77. Churchill Livingstone, New York.

Kneale, B.L.G. (1984) Report of the ISSVD Task Force. *Journal of Reproductive Medicine* **29**, 454–456.

Knoblick, R. (1960) Primary adenocarcinoma of the female urethra: a review and report of 3 cases. *American Journal of Obstetrics and Gynecology* **80**, 353–364.

Kodama, S., Kaneko, T., Saito, M. *et al.* (1995) A clinicopathologic study of 30 patients with Paget's disease of the vulva. *Gynecologic Oncology* **56**, 63–70.

Kohlberger, P., Kainz, C., Breitenecker, G. *et al.* (1995) Prognostic value of immunohistochemically detected p53 expression in vulvar carcinoma. *Cancer* **76**, 1786–1789.

Kolstad, P., Iversen, T., Abeler, V. & Adlders, J. (1982) Microinvasive carcinoma of the vulva—definition and treatment problems. *Clinical Oncology* **1**, 355–362.

Koss, L.G., Ladinsky, S. & Brockunier, A. (1968) Paget's disease of the vulva. *Obstetrics and Gynecology* **31**, 513–525.

Kraus, F.T. & Perez-Mesa, C. (1966) Verrucous carcinoma: clinical and pathologic study of 105 cases including oral cavity, larynx and genitalia. *Cancer* **19**, 26–38.

Krupp, P.J. (1992) Invasive tumors of vulva: clinical features, staging and management. In: *Gynecologic Oncology*, 2nd edn (ed. M. Coppleson), pp. 479–491. Churchill Livingstone, Edinburgh.

Krupp, P.J. & Bohm, J.W. (1978) Lymph gland metastases in invasive squamous cell cancer of the vulva. *American Journal of Obstetrics and Gynecology* **130**, 943–952.

Kurman, R.J., Shaw, K.V., Lancaster, W.D. & Jenson, A.B. (1981) Immunoperoxidase localization of papillomavirus antigens in cervical dysplasia and vulvar condylomata. *American Journal of Obstetrics and Gynecology* **140**, 931–935.

Kurman, R.J., Toki, T. & Schiffman, M.H. (1993) Basaloid and warty carcinomas of the vulva: distinctive types of squamous cell carcinoma frequently associated with human papillomaviruses. *American Journal of Surgical Pathology* **17**, 133–145.

Kuzuya, K., Matsutama, M., Nishi, Y., Chihara, T. & Suchi, T. (1981) Ultrastructure of adenocarcinoma of Bartholin's gland. *Cancer* **48**, 1392–1398.

Landthaler, M., Braun-Falco, D., Richter, K., Baltzer, J. & Zander, J. (1985) Maligne Melanoma der Vulva. *Deutsche Medizinische Wochenschrift* **110**, 789–794.

Lasser, A., Cornog, J.L. & Morris, J.McL. (1974) Adenoid squamous cell carcinoma of the vulva. *Cancer* **33**, 224–227.

Lee, S.C., Roth, L.M., Ehrlich, C. & Hall, J.A. (1977) Extramammary Paget's disease of the vulva. *Cancer* **39**, 2540–2549.

Lee, Y.Y., Wilczynski, S.P., Chumakov, A., Chih, D. & Koeffler, H.P. (1994) Carcinoma of the vulva: HPV and p53 mutations. *Oncogene* **9**, 1655–1659.

Leibowitch, M., Neill, S., Pelisse, M. & Moyal-Barracco, M. (1990) The epithelial changes associated with squamous cell carcinoma of the vulva: a review of the clinical, histological and viral findings in 78 women. *British Journal of Obstetrics and Gyneaecology* **97**, 1135–1139.

Lelle, R.J., Davis, K.P. & Roberts, J.A. (1994) Adenoid cystic carcinoma of the Bartholin's gland: the University of Michigan experience. *International Journal of Gynecological Cancer* **4**, 145–149.

Leuchter, R.S., Hacker, N.F., Voet, R.L. *et al.* (1982) Primary carcinoma of Bartholin's gland: a report of 14 cases and review of the literature. *Obstetrics and Gynecology* **60**, 361–367.

Lever, W.F. & Castleman, B. (1952) Clear cell myoepithelioma of the skin: report of ten cases. *American Journal of Pathology* **28**, 691–699.

Lever, W.F. & Schaumberg-Lever, G. (1975) *Histopathology of the Skin*, 5th edn. Lippincott, Philadelphia.

Levin, M., Pakarakas, R.M., Chang, H.A., Maiman, M. & Goldberg, S.L. (1995) Primary breast carcinoma of the vulva: a case report and review of the literature. *Gynecologic Oncology* **56**, 448–451.

Levine, R.L. (1980) Urethral cancer. *Cancer* **45**, 1965–1972.

Levitan, Z., Kaplan, A.L. & Kaufman, R.H. (1992) Advanced squamous cell carcinoma of the vulva after treatment for verrucous carcinoma: case report. *Journal of Reproductive Medicine* **37**, 889–892.

Lingard, D., Free, K., Wright, R.G. & Battistutta, D. (1992) Invasive squamous cell carcinoma of the vulva; behaviour and results in the light of changing management regiments: a review of clinicopathological features predictive of regional lymph node involvement and local recurrence. *Australian and New Zealand Journal of Obstetrics and Gynaecology* **32**, 137–145.

Lininger, R.A. & Tavassoli, F.A. (1996) The pathology of vulvar neoplasia. *Current Opinion in Obstetrics and Gynecology* **8**, 63–68.

Lomeo, A.M., Manzione, L., Martoccia, G. *et al.* (1992) Idrocistoadenoma papillifero della vulva; descrizione di un caso. *Minerva Ginecologica* **44**, 126–127.

Look, K.Y., Roth, L.M. & Sutton, G.P. (1993) Vulvar melanoma reconsidered. *Cancer* **72**, 143–146.

Loret-de-Mola, J.H., Hudock, P.A., Steinetz, C. *et al.* (1993) Merkel cell carcinoma of the vulva. *Gynecologic Oncology* **51**, 272–276.

Lucas, W.E., Benirschke, K. & Lebhertz, T.B. (1974) Verrucous carcinoma of the female genital tract. *American Journal of Obstetrics and Gynecology* **119**, 435–440.

Lulenski, C.R. & Naji, A.F. (1964) Mucin secreting adenocarcinoma of Bartholin's gland. *Obstetrics and Gynecology* **24**, 542–544.

Mabuchi, K., Bross, D.S. & Kessler, I.I. (1985) Epidemiology of cancer of the vulva: a case control study. *Cancer* **55**, 1843–1848.

Mack, T.M., Cozen, W. & Quinn, M.A. (1992) Epidemiology of cancer of the endometrium, ovary, vulva and vagina. In: *Gynecologic Oncology*, 2nd edn (ed. M. Coppleston), pp. 31–54. Churchill Livingstone, Edinburgh.

McKee, P.H. & Hertogs, K.T. (1980) Endocervical adenocarcinoma and vulval Paget's disease: a significant association. *British Journal of Dermatology* **103**, 443–448.

Magrina, J.F., Webb, M.J., Gaffey, T.A. & Symmonds, R.E. (1979) Stage I squamous cell cancer of the vulva. *American Journal of Obstetrics and Gynecology* **134**, 453–459.

Marcus, S.L. (1960) Basal cell and basal–squamous cell carcinoma of the vulva. *American Journal of Obstetrics and Gynecology* **79**, 461–469.

Massad, L.S., Bitterman, P. & Clarke-Pearson, D.L. (1996) Metastatic clear cell eccrine hidradenocarcinoma of the vulva: survival after primary surgical resection. *Gynecologic Oncology* **61**, 287–290.

Masterson, J.G. & Goss, A.S. (1954) Carcinoma of Bartholin's gland: review of the literature and report of a new case in an elderly patient treated by radical operation. *American Journal of Obstetrics and Gynecology* **69**, 1323–1332.

Mazoujian, G., Pinkus, G.S. & Haagensen, D.E. Jr. (1984) Extramammary Paget's disease—evidence for an apocrine origin: an immnunoperoxidase study of gross cystic disease fluid protein-15, carcino-embryonic antigen, and keratin proteins. *American Journal of Surgical Pathology* **8**, 43–50.

Medenica, M. & Sahihi, T. (1972) Ultrastructural study of a case of extramammary Paget's disease of the vulva. *Archives of Dermatology* **105**, 236–243.

Meeker, J.H., Neubecker, R.D. & Helwig, E.B. (1962) Hidradenoma papilliferum. *American Journal of Clinical Pathology* **37**, 182–195.

Mene, A. & Buckley, C.H. (1985) Involvement of the vulval skin appendages by intraepithelial neoplasia. *British Journal of Obstetrics and Gynecology* **92**, 634–638.

Merino, M.J., LiVolsi, V.A., Schwartz, P.E. & Rudnicki, J. (1982) Adenoid basal cell carcinoma of the vulva. *International Journal of Gynecological Pathology* **1**, 299–306.

Merot, Y., Mazoujian, G., Pinkus, G., Momtaz, T.K. & Murphy, G.F. (1985) Extramammary Paget's disease of the perianal and perineal regions: evidence of apocrine derivation. *Archives of Dermatology* **121**, 750–752.

Mesko, J.D., Gates, H., McDonald, T.W., Youmans, R. & Lewis, J. (1988) Clear cell (mesonephroid) adenocarcinoma of the vulva arising in endometriosis: a case report. *Gynecologic Oncology* **29**, 385–391.

Messing, M.J. & Gallup, O.G. (1995) Carcinoma of the vulva in young women. *Obstetrics and Gynecology* **86**, 51–54.

Messing, M.J., Richardson, M.S., Smith, M.T., King, L. & Gallup, O.G. (1993) Metastatic clear cell hydradenocarcinoma of the vulva. *Gynecologic Oncology* **48**, 264–268.

Misas, J.E., Larson, J.E., Podczaski, E., Manetta, A. & Mortel, R. (1990) Recurrent Paget disease of the vulva in a split-thickness graft. *Obstetrics and Gynecology* **76**, 543–544.

Mizushima, J. & Ohara, K. (1995) Basal cell carcinoma of the vulva with lymph node and skin metastasis—report of a case and review of 20 Japanese cases. *Journal of Dermatology* **22**, 36–42.

Moll, I. & Moll, R. (1985) Cells of extramammary Paget's disease express cytokeratins different from those of epidermal cells. *Dermatology* **84**, 3–8.

Monaghan, J.M. (1987) Vulvar carcinoma: the case for individualization of treatment. *Baillière's Clinical Obstetrics and Gynaecology* **1**, 263–276.

Monaghan, J.M. (1990) The management of carcinoma of the vulva. In: *Clinical Gynaecological Oncology*, 2nd edn (eds J.H. Shepherd & J.M. Monaghan), pp. 140–167. Blackwell Scientific Publications, Oxford.

Monaghan, J.M. & Hammond, I.G. (1984) Pelvic node dissection in the treatment of vulval carcinoma—is it necessary? *British Journal of Obstetrics and Gynaecology* **91**, 270–274.

Monk, B., Burger, R., Lin, F. *et al.* (1995) Prognostic significance of human papillomavirus DNA in vulvar carcinoma. *Obstetrics and Gynecology* **85**, 709–715.

Mori, O., Hachisuka, H. & Sasai, Y. (1989) Immunohistochemical demonstration of epithelial membrane antigen (EMA), carcinoembryonic antigen (CEA), and keratin on mammary and extramammary Paget's disease. *Acta Histochemica* **85**, 93–100.

Morrow, C.P. (1981) Melanoma of the female genital tract. In: *Gynaecologic Oncology*, 1st edn (ed. M. Coppleston), pp. 784–793. Churchill Livingstone, Edinburgh.

Morrow, C.P. & DiSaia, P.J. (1976) Malignant melanoma of the female genitalia: a clinical analysis. *Obstetrical and Gynecological Survey* **31**, 233–271.

Morrow, C.P. & Rutledge, F.N. (1972) Melanoma of the vulva. *Obstetrics and Gynecology* **39**, 745–752.

Murayama, T., Komatsu, H., Asano, M., Tahara, M. & Nakamura, T. (1978) Mesonephric adenocarcinoma of the urethra in a woman: report of a case. *Journal of Urology* **120**, 500–501.

Murphy, J., Wilson, J.M. & Bickel, D.A. (1962) Adenoid cystic carcinoma of the Bartholin gland and pregnancy. *American Journal of Obstetrics and Gynecology* **83**, 612–614.

Nagle, R.B., Lucas, D.O., McDaniel, K.M., Clark, V.A. & Schmalzel, G.M. (1985) New evidence linking mammary and extramammary Paget cells to a common cell phenotype. *American Journal of Clinical Pathology* **83**, 431–438.

Nazario, A.C., Noronha, P. de A., Salomao, C. & de Lima, G.R. (1989) Carcinoma de celulas apocrinas de vulva: relato de um caso. *Revista Paulista da Medicina* **107**, 122–124.

Ney, C., Miler, H.L. & Ochs, D. (1971) Adenocarcinoma in a diverticulum of the female urethra: a case report of mucinous adenocarcinoma with a summary of the literature. *Journal of Urology* **106**, 874–877.

Nielson, N.C. (1973) Hidradenoma of the vulva. *Acta Obstetricia et Gynecologica Scandinavica* **52**, 387–389.

Novak, E.R. & Woodruff, J.D. (1979) *Novak's Gynecologic and Obstetric Pathology*, 8th edn. Saunders, Philadelphia.

Nuovo, G.J., Friedman, D. & Richart, R.M. (1990) *In situ* hybridization analysis of human papillomavirus DNA segregation patterns in lesions of the female genital tract. *Gynecologic Oncology* **36**, 256–262.

Obalek, S., Jablonska, S., Beaudenon, S., Walczak, L. & Orth, G. (1986) Bowenoid papulosis of the male and female genitalia: risk of cervical neoplasia. *Journal of the American Academy of Dermatology* **14**, 433–444.

Oji, M., Furue, M. & Tamaki, K. (1984) Serum carcinoembryonic antigen level in Paget's disease. *British Journal of Dermatology* **110**, 211–213.

Olson, D.J., Fujimura, M., Swanson, P. & Okagaki, T. (1991) Immunohistochemical features of Paget's disease of the vulva with and without adenocarcinoma. *International Journal of Gynecological Pathology* **10**, 285–295.

Ordonez, N.G., Manning, J.T. & Luna, M.A. (1981) Mixed tumors of the vulva: a report of two cases probably arising in Bartholin's gland. *Cancer* **48**, 181–185.

Orenstein, J.M., Dardick, I. & van Nostrand, A.W.P. (1985) Ultrastructural similarities of adenoid cystic carcinoma and pleomorphiadenoma. *Histopathology* **9**, 623–638.

Oriel, J.D. & Almeida, J.D. (1970) Demonstration of virus particles in human genital warts. *British Journal of Venereal Diseases* **47**, 1–13.

Origoni, M., Sideri, M., Garsia, S., Cannelli, S.G. & Ferrari, A.G. (1992) Prognostic value of pathological patterns of lymph node positivity in squamous cell carcinoma of the vulva stage III and IVa FIGO. *Gynecologic Oncology* **45**, 313–316.

Pack, G.T. & Oropeza, R.A. (1967) A comparative study of melanoma and epidermoid carcinoma of the vulva: a review of 44 melanomas and 58 epidermoid carcinomas (1930–1965). *Reviews in Surgery* **24**, 305–324.

Paladina, D., Cross, P., Lopes, A. & Monaghan, J.M. (1994) Prognostic significance of lymph node variables in squamous cell carcinoma of the vulva. *Cancer* **74**, 2491–2496.

Palladino, V.S., Duffy, J.L. & Bures, G.J. (1969) Basal cell carcinoma of the vulva. *Cancer* **24**, 460–470.

Panizzon, R., Mitsuhashi, Y. & Schnyder, U.W. (1987) Das Syringom der Vulva. *Hautarzt* **38**, 607–609.

Park, J.S., Jones, R.W., McLean, M.R. *et al.* (1991) Possible etiologic heterogeneity of vulvar intraepithelial neoplasia: a correlation of pathologic characteristics with human papillomavirus detection by *in situ* hybridization and polymerase chain reaction. *Cancer* **67**, 1599–1607.

Parker, R.T., Duncan, I., Rampone, J. & Creasman, W. (1975) Operating management of early invasive epidermoid carcinoma of the vulva. *American Journal of Obstetrics and Gynecology* **123**, 349–354.

Parmley, T.H., Woodruff, J.D. & Julian, C.G. (1975) Invasive vulvar Paget's disease. *Obstetrics and Gynecology* **46**, 341–346.

Partridge, E.E., Murad, T., Shingleton, H.M., Austin, J.M. & Hatch, K.D. (1980a) Verrucous lesions of the female genitalia. I. Giant condylomata. *American Journal of Obstetrics and Gynecology* **137**, 412–418.

Partridge, E.E., Murad, T., Shingleton, H.M., Austin, J.M. & Hatch, K.D. (1980b) Verrucous lesions of the female genitalia. II. Verrucous carcinoma. *American Journal of Obstetrics and Gynecology* **137**, 419–424.

Pelisse, M., Orth, G., Croissant, O. *et al.* (1985) Données anatomocliniques et virologiques dans vingt cas de maladie de Bowen vulvaire. *Annales de Dermatologie et de Vénéréologie* **112**, 749–750.

Pelosi, G., Martignoni, G. & Bonetti, F. (1991) Intraductal carcinoma of mammary-type apocrine epithelium arising within a papillary hydradenoma of the vulva: report of a case and review of the literature. *Archives of Pathology and Laboratory Medicine* **115**, 1249–1254.

Perrone, T., Twiggs, L.B., Adcock, L.I. & Dehner, L.P. (1987) Vulvar basal cell carcinoma: an infrequently metastasizing neoplasm. *International Journal of Gynecological Pathology* **6**, 152–165.

Peterson, L.J. & Matsumoto, L.M. (1978) Nephrogenic adenoma in urethral diverticulum. *Urology* **11**, 193–195.

Peven, D.R. & Hidvegi, D.F. (1985) Clear-cell adenocarcinoma of the female urethra. *Acta Cytologica* **29**, 142–146.

Philippe, E., Vetter, J.M., Dellenbach, P. & Petit, J.C. (1990) Carcinome neuro-endocrine d'une glande de Bartholin. *Journal de Gynécologie, Obstétrique et Biologie de la Reproduction, Paris* **19**, 717–719.

Phillips, G.L., Twiggs, L.B. & Okagaki, T. (1982) Vulvar melanoma: a microstaging study. *Gynecological Oncology* **14**, 80–88.

Pierson, K.K. (1987) Malignant melanomas and pigmented lesions of the vulva. In: *Pathology of the Vulva and Vagina* (ed. E.J. Wilkinson), pp. 155–179. Churchill Livingstone, New York.

Pilotti, S., Rotola, A., D'Amato, L. *et al.* (1990) Vulvar carcinomas: search for sequences homologous to human papillomavirus and herpes simplex virus DNA. *Modern Pathology* **3**, 442–448.

Pilotti, S., Dhongi, R., D'Amato, L. *et al.* (1996) Papillomavirus, p 53 alteration and primary carcinoma of the vulva. *European Journal of Cancer* **29**, 924–925.

Piura, B., Egan, M., Lopes, A. & Monaghan, J.M. (1992) Malignant melanoma of the vulva: a clinicopathologic study of 18 cases. *Journal of Surical Oncology* **50**, 234–240.

Plachta, A. & Speer, F.D. (1954) Apocrine gland adenocarcinoma and extramammary Paget's disease of the vulva: review of the literature and report of a case. *Cancer* **7**, 910–919.

Podratz, K.C., Symmonds, R.E., Taylor, W.F. & Williams, T.J. (1983a) Carcinoma of the vulva: analysis of treatment and survival. *Obstetrics and Gynecology* **61**, 63–74.

Podratz, K.C., Gaffey, T.A., Symmonds, R.E., Johansen, K.L. & O'Brien, P.C. (1983b) Melanoma of the vulva: an update. *Gynecologic Oncology* **16**, 153–168.

Pope, C., Ingella, H.P. & Strecker, H. (1973) Light and electron microscopic observations following repeated podophyllin benzoin therapy of condyloma acuminata. *Archives of Gynecology* **215**, 417–425.

Powell, J.L., Franklin, E.W., Nickerson, J.F. & Burrell, M.O. (1978) Verrucous carcinoma of the female genital tract. *Gynecologic Oncology* **6**, 565–573.

Powell, L.C. Jr., Dinh, T.V., Rajaraman, E.V. *et al.* (1986) Carcinoma *in situ* of the vulva: a clinicopathologic study of 50 cases. *Journal of Reproductive Medicine* **31**, 808–813.

Prasad, K.R., Kumari, G.S., Aruna, C.A., Durga, K. & Kameswari, V.R. (1995) Fibroadenoma of ectopic breast tissue in the vulva: a case report. *Acta Cytologica* **39**, 791–792.

Prempree, T., Wizenberg, M.J. & Scott, R.M. (1978) Radiation treatment of primary carcinoma of the female urethra. *Cancer* **42**, 1177–1184.

Prempree, T., Amornmarn, R. & Patanaphan, V. (1984) Radiation therapy in primary carcinoma of the female urethra. II. An update on results. *Cancer* **52**, 729–733.

Purola, E. & Widholm, O. (1966) Primary carcinoma of Bartholin's gland. *Acta Obstetricia et Gynecologica Scandinavica* **45**, 205–210.

Ragnarsson, B., Raabe, N., Willems, J. & Pettersson, F. (1987) Carcinoma *in situ* of the vulva. *Acta Oncologica* **26**, 277–280.

Ragnarsson-Olding, B., Johansson, H., Rutqvist, L.E. & Ringborg, U. (1993) Malignant melanoma of the vulva and vagina: trends in incidence and distribution, and long term survival among 245 consecutive cases in Sweden 1960–1984. *Cancer* **71**, 1893–1897.

Ragni, M.V. & Tobon, H. (1974) Primary malignant melanoma of the vagina and vulva. *Obstetrics and Gynecology* **43**, 658–664.

Rahilly, M.A., Beattie, G.J. & Lessells, A.M. (1995) Mucinous eccrine carcinoma of the vulva with neuroendocrine differentiation. *Histopathology* **27**, 82–86.

Rando, R.F., Selacek, T.V., Hunt, J. *et al.* (1986) Verrucous carcinoma of the vulva associated with an unusual Type 6 human papilloma virus. *Obstetrics and Gynecology* **67**, 70s–75s.

Reid, R., Greenberg, M., Jenson, A.B. *et al.* (1987) Sexually transmitted papillomaviral infections. I. The anatomic distribution and pathologic grade of neoplastic lesions associated with different viral types. *American Journal of Obstetrics and Gynecology* **156**, 212–222.

Rhatigan, R.M. & Nuss, C.R. (1985) Keratoacanthoma of the vulva. *Gynecologic Oncology* **21**, 118–123.

Rickert, R.R. (1980) Intraductal papilloma arising in supernumerary vulvar breast tissue. *Obstetrics and Gynecology* **55**, 84s–85s.

Roberts, T.W. & Melicow, M.M. (1977) Pathology and natural history of urethral tumors in females: review of 65 cases. *Urology* **10**, 583–589.

Robutti, F. (1986) Primary malignant melanoma of the female urethra. *European Urology* **12**, 62–63.

Rocamora, A., Santonja, C., Vives, E. & Varona, C. (1986) Sebaceous gland hyperplasia of the vulva: a case report. *Obstetrics and Gynecology* **68**, 63s–65s.

Rock, B., Hood, A.F. & Rock, J.A. (1990) Prospective study of vulvar nevi. *Journal of the American Academy of Dermatology* **22**, 104–106.

Rogers, R.E. & Burns, B. (1969) Carcinoma of the female urethra. *Obstetrics and Gynecology* **33**, 54–57.

Rollason, T.P. (1992) Malignant melanoma and related lesions of the lower female genital tract. In: *Advances in Gynaecological Pathology* (ed. D. Lowe & H. Fox), pp. 119–143. Churchill Livingstone, Edinburgh.

Rorat, E. & Wallach, R.E. (1984) Mixed tumors of the vulva: clinical outcome and pathology. *International Journal of Gynecolgical Pathology* **3**, 323–328.

Rose, P.G., Piver, M.S., Tsukada, Y. & Lau, T. (1988) Conservative therapy for melanoma of the vulva. *American Journal of Obstetrics and Gynecology* **159**, 52–55.

Rose, P.G., Roman, L.D., Reale, F.R., Tak, W.K. & Hunter, R.E. (1990) Primary adenocarcinoma of the breast arising in the vulva. *Obstetrics and Gynecology* **76**, 537–539.

Rose, P.G., Tak, W.K., Reale, F.R. & Hunter, R.E. (1991) Adenoid cystic carcinoma of the vulva: a radiosensitive tumor. *Gynecologic Oncology* **43**, 81–83.

Rosenberg, P., Simonsen, E. & Risberg, B. (1989) Adenoid cystic carcinoma of Bartholin's gland: a report of five cases treated with surgery and radiotherapy. *Gynecologic Oncology* **34**, 145–147.

Ross, M.J. & Ehrmann, R.I. (1987) Histologic pronostications in Stage I squamous cell carcinoma of the vulva. *Obstetrics and Gynecology* **70**, 774–784.

Rosser, E.I. & Hamlin, I.M.E. (1957) Paget's disease of the vulva. *Journal of Obstetrics and Gynaecology of the British Empire* **64**, 127–130.

Roth, L.M., Lees, S.C. & Ehrlich, C.E. (1977) Paget's disease of the vulva: a histogenetic study of five cases including ultrastructural observations and review of the literature. *American Journal of Surgical Pathology* **1**, 193–206.

Roth, V. (1936) Zystichen Adenofibrom und der Basis einer persistierenden Brustdrusenanlage in der linken grossen Schamlippe. *Zeitschrift für Geburtshilfe* **112**, 245–251.

Rulon, D.B. & Helwig, E.B. (1974) Cutaneous sebaceous neoplasms. *Cancer* **33**, 82–102.

Salazar, H. & Gonzalez-Angulo, A. (1984) Ultrastructural diagnosis in gynaecological pathology. *Clinics in Obstetrics and Gynaecology* **11**, 25–77.

Salzstein, S.L., Woodruff, J.D. & Novak, E.R. (1956) Postgranulomatous carcinoma of the vulva. *Obstetrics and Gynecology* **7**, 80–90.

Sanz-Valez, J.I., Esclarin-Duny, M.A., Abad-Roger, J., Abascal-Agorreta, M. & Vera-Alvarez, J. (1989) Melanoma de uretra distal femenina: a proposito de un caso. *Actas Urologica Espagnol* **13**, 63–64.

Sayre, G.P. (1949) Cylindroma ofthe vulva: adenocarcinoma, cylindroma type, of the vulva: report of a case of twenty seven years duration. *Mayo Clinic Proceedings* **24**, 224–233.

Scheistroen, M., Trope, C., Kaern, J., Pettersen, E.O., Abeler, V.M. & Kristensen, G.B. (1995) Malignant melanoma of the vulva: evaluation of prognostic factors with emphasis on DNA plody in 75 patients. *Cancer* **75**, 72–80.

Scheistroen, M., Trope, C., Kaern, J. *et al.* (1996) Malignant melanoma of the vulva FIGO stage I: evaluation of prognostic factors in 43 patients with emphasis on DNA ploidy and surgical treatment. *Gynecologic Oncology* **61**, 253–258.

Schueller, E.F. (1965) Basal cell cancer of the vulva. *American Journal of Obstetrics and Gynecology* **93**, 199–208.

Schweppe, K.W. & Schlake, W. (1980) Adenocarzinom der Bartholinschen Druse. *Geburtshilfe und Frauenheilkunde* **40**, 437–443.

Scinicariello, F., Rady, P., Hannigna, E., Dinh, T.V. & Tyring, S.K. (1992) Human papillomavirus type 16 found in primary transitional cell carcinoma of the Bartholin's gland and in a lymph node metastasis. *Gynecologic Oncology* **47**, 263–266.

Scurry, J., Brand, A., Planner, Dowling, J. & Rode, J. (1996) Vulvar Merkel cell tumor with glandular and squamous differentiation. *Gynecologic Oncology* **62**, 292–297.

Sedlis, A., Homesley, H., Bundy, B.N. *et al.* (1987) Positive groin lymph nodes in superficial squamous cell vulvar cancer: a Gynecologic Oncology Group study. *American Journal of Obstetrics and Gynecology* **156**, 1159–1164.

Selium, M.A. & Lankeroni, M.R. (1979) Verrucous carcinomas of the vulva. *Journal of Reproductive Medicine* **22**, 92–96.

Sengupta, B.S. (1981) Carcinoma of the vulva in Jamaican women. *Acta Obstetricia et Gynecologica Scandinavica* **60**, 537–544.

Shah, K.D., Tabibzadeh, S.S. & Gerber, M.A. (1987) Immunohistochemical distinction of Paget's disease from Bowen's disease and superficial spreading melanoma with the use of monoclonal cytokeratin antibodies. *American Journal of Pathology* **88**, 689–695.

Shatz, P., Bergeron, C., Wilkinson, E.J., Arseneau, J. & Ferenczy, A. (1989) Vulvar intraepithelial neoplasia and skin appendage involvement. *Obstetrics and Gynecology* **74**, 769–774.

Shepherd, J.H. (1995) Staging announcement, FIGO staging of gynecologic cancers: cervical and vulva. *International Journal of Gynecological Cancer* **5**, 319.

Shimm, D.S., Fuller, A.F., Orlow, E.L., Dosoretz, D.E. & Aristizibal, S.A. (1986) Prognostic variables in the treatment of squamous cell carcinoma of the vulva. *Gynecologic Oncology* **24**, 343–358.

Siegler, A.M. & Greene, H.J. (1951) Basal cell carcinoma of the vulva: a report of 5 cases and review of the literature. *American Journal of Obstetrics and Gynecology* **62**, 1219–1224.

Siegler, M. & Gordon, R. (1951) Fibroadenoma in a supernumerary breast of the vulva. *American Journal of Obstetrics and Gynecology* **62**, 1367–1369.

Siemund, J. (1989) Syringome an der Vulva. *Zentralblatt für Gynäkologie* **111**, 1517–1520.

Silvers, D.H. & Halperin, A.J. (1978) Cutaneous and vulvar melanoma: an update. *Clinical Obstetrics and Gynecology* **21**, 1117–1118.

Skinner, M.S., Sternberg, W.H., Ichinose, H. & Collins, J. (1973) Spontaneous regression of Bowenoid atypia of the vulva. *Obstetrics and Gynecology* **42**, 40–46.

Spitzer, M., Krumbolz, B.A. & Seltzer, V. (1989) The multicentric nature of disease related to human papillomavirus infection of the female genital tract. *Obstetrics and Gynecology* **73**, 303–307.

Stacy, J.E. (1939) Epithelioma of the vulva. *Proceedings of the Royal Society of Medicine* **32**, 304–308.

Stacy, D., Burrell, M.O. & Franklin, E.W. (1986) Extramammary Paget's disease of the vulva and anus: use of intraoperative frozen-section margins. *American Journal of Obstetrics and Gynecology* **155**, 519–523.

Stapleton, J.J. (1984) Extramammary Paget's disease in a young black woman: a case report with histogenic confirmation by immunostaining. *Journal of Reproductive Medicine* **29**, 444–446.

Stehman, F.B., Castaloo, T.W., Charles, E.H. & Lagasse, L. (1980) Verrucous carcinoma of the vulva. *International Journal of Obstetrics and Gynaecology* **17**, 523–525.

Stumpf, P.G. (1980) Increasing occurrence of condylomata acuminata in premenarchal children. *Obstetrics and Gynecology* **56**, 262–264.

Sturgeon, S.R., Brinton, L.A., Devesa, S.S. & Kurman, R.J. (1992) *In situ* and invasive vulvar cancer incidence trends (1973 to 1987). *American Journal of Obstetrics and Gynecology* **166**, 1482–1485.

Summitt, R.L., Murrmann, S.C. & Flax, S.D. (1994) Nephrogenic adenoma in a urethral diverticulum: a case report. *Journal of Reproductive Medicine* **39**, 473–476.

Svanholm, H., Andersen, O.P. & Rohl, H. (1987) Tumour of female paraurethral duct: immunohistochemical similarity with prostatic carcinoma. *Virchows Archiv. A, Pathological, Anatomy and Histopathology (Berlin)* **411**, 395–398.

Sworn, M.J., Hammond, G.T. & Buchanan, R. (1979) Metastatic basal cell carcinoma of the vulva: case report. *British Journal of Obstetrics and Gynaecology* **86**, 332–334.

Symmonds, R.E., Pratt, J.H. & Dockerty, M.D. (1960) Melanoma of the vulva. *Obstetrics and Gynecology* **15**, 543–553.

Tang, C-K., Nedwich, A., Toker, C. & Zaman, A.N.F. (1982) Unusual cutaneous carcinoma with features of small cell (oat cell-like) and squamous cell carcinoma: a variant of malignant Merkel cell neoplasm. *American Journal of Dermatopathology* **4**, 537–548.

Tappeiner, J. & Wolff, K. (1968) Hidradenoma papilliferum: eine enzymehistochemische und elektronmikroskopische Studie. *Hautarzt* **19**, 101–109.

Tasseron, E.W., van der Esch, E.P., Hart, A.A., Brutel de la Riviere, G. & Aartsen, E.J. (1992) A clinicopathological study of 30 melanomas of the vulva. *Gynecologic Oncology* **46**, 170–175.

Taylor, P.T., Stenwig, J.T. & Klausen, H. (1975) Paget's disease of the vulva: a report of 18 cases. *Gynecologic Oncology* **3**, 46–60.

Tbakhi, A., Cowan, D.F., Kumar, D. & Kyle, D. (1993) Recurring phyllodes tumor in aberrant breast tissue of the vulva. *American Journal of Surgical Pathology* **17**, 946–950.

Tchang, F., Okagaki, T. & Richart, R.M. (1973) Adenocarcinoma of Bartholin's gland associated with Paget's disease of vulvar area. *Cancer* **31**, 221–225.

Thomas, J., Majmudar, B. & Gorelkin, I. (1979) Syringoma localized to the vulva. *Archives of Dermatology* **115**, 95–96.

Thum, G., Wechsel, H.W. & Merkel, K.H. (1990) Das primare maligne Melanom des distalen Urogenitaltraktes: Fallbericht und Literaturubersicht. *Urologe* **29**, 158–160.

Tiltman, A.J. & Knutzen, V.K. (1978) Primary adenocarcinoma of the vulva originating in misplaced cloacal tissue. *Obstetrics and Gynecology* **51**, 30s–33s.

Toki, T., Kurman, R.J., Park, J.S. *et al.* (1991) Probable nonpapillomavirus etiology of squamous cell carcinoma of the vulva in older women: a clinicopathologic study using *in situ* hybridization and polymerase chain reaction. *International Journal of Gynecological Pathology* **10**, 107–125.

Trelford, J.D. & Does, P.H. (1976) Bartholin's gland carcinomas: five cases. *Gynecologic Oncology* **4**, 212–221.

Trimble, C.L., Hildesheim, A., Brinton, L.A., Shah, K.V. & Kurman, R.J. (1996) Heterogenous etiology of squamous carcinoma of the vulva. *Obstetrics and Gynecology* **87**, 59–64.

Trimble, E.L., Lewis, J.L. Jr., Williams, E.L. *et al.* (1992) Management of vulvar melanomas. *Gynecologic Oncology* **45**, 254–258.

Tsukahara, Y., Mori, A., Fukuta, I., Katsuyama, T. & Yamagami, O. (1991) Adenoid cystic carcinoma of Bartholin's gland: a clinical, immunohistochemical and ultrastructural study of a case with regard to its histogenesis. *Gynecological and Obstetrical Investigation* **31**, 110–113.

Tuck, S.M. & Williams, A. (1985) Paget's disease of the vulva complicated by bladder carcinoma: case report. *British Journal of Obstetrics and Gynaecology* **92**, 416–418.

Turan, C., Ugur, M., Kutluay, L. *et al.* (1996) Vulval syringoma exacerbated during pregnancy. *European Journal of Obstetrics, Gynecology and Reproductive Biology* **64**, 141–142.

Twiggs, L.B., Okagaki, T., Clark, B. *et al.* (1988) A clinical, histopathologic, and molecular biologic investigation of vulvar intraepithelial neoplasia. *International Journal of Gynecological Pathology* **7**, 48–55.

Underwood, J.W., Adcock, L.L. & Okagaki, T. (1978) Adenosquamous carcinoma of skin appendage (adenoid squamous cell carcinoma, pseudoglandular squamous cell carcinoma, adenoacanthoma of sweat gland of Lever) of the vulva. *Cancer* **42**, 1851–1855.

Urabe, A., Matsukuma, A., Shimizu, N. *et al.* (1990) Extramammary Paget's disease: comparative histopathologic studies of intraductal carcinoma of the breast and apocrine adenocarcinoma. *Journal of Cutaneous Pathology* **17**, 257–265.

van Beurden, M., ten Kate, F.J., Smits, H.L. *et al.* (1995) Multifocal VIN III and multicentric lower genital tract neoplasia is associated with transcriptionally active HPV. *Cancer* **75**, 2879–2884.

van der Putte, S.C.J. (1991) Anogenital 'sweat' glands: histology and pathology of a gland that may mimic mammary glands. *American Journal of Dermatopathology* **13**, 557–565.

van der Velden, J. (1996) Some aspects of the management of squamous cell carcinoma of the vulva. Thesis, University of Utrecht.

van der Velden, J., Kooyman, C.D., van Lindert, A.C.M. & Heintz, A.P.M. (1992) A stage 1a vulvar carcinoma with an inguinal lymph node recurrence after local excision: a case report and literature review. *International Journal of Gynecological Cancer* **2**, 157–159.

van der Velden, J., van Lindert, A.C.M., Lammes, F.B. *et al.* (1995) Extracapsular growth of lymph node metastases in squamous cell carcinoma of the vulva, the impact on recurrence and survival. *Cancer* **75**, 2885–2890.

Van Nagell, J.R. Jr., Tweeddale, D.W. & Roddick, J.W. Jr. (1969) Primary adenoacanthoma of the Bartholin's gland: report of a case. *Obstetrics and Gynecology* **34**, 87–90.

Vayrynen, M., Romppanen, T., Koskela, E., Castren, A.O. & Syrjanen, K. (1981) Verrucous squamous cell carcinoma of the female genital tract: report of three cases and survey of the literature. *International Journal of Obstetrics and Gynaecology* **19**, 351–356.

Veraldi, S., Schianchi-Veraldi, R. & Marini, D. (1990) Hidradenoma papilliferum of the vulva: report of a case characterized by unusual clinical behaviour. *Journal of Dermatological Surgery and Oncology* **16**, 674–676.

Wade, T.R. & Ackerman, A.B. (1979) The effects of podophyllin resin on condyloma acuminata. *Archives of Dermatology* **115**, 1349.

Wade, T.R., Kopf, A.W. & Ackerman, A.B. (1979) Bowenoid papulosis of the genitalia. *Archives of Dermatology* **115**, 306–308.

Wahlstrom, T., Vesterinen, E. & Saksela, E. (1978) Primary carcinoma of Bartholin's glands: a morphological and clinical study of six cases including a transitional cell carcinoma. *Gynaecologic Oncology* **6**, 354–362.

Way, S. (1982) *Malignant Disease of the Vulva*. Churchill Livingstone, Edinburgh.

Webb, J.B. & Beswick, I.P. (1983) Eccrine hidradenocarcinoma of the vulva with Paget's disease: case report and review of the literature. *British Journal of Obstetrics and Gynaecology* **90**, 90–95.

Wells, M. & Jenkins, M. (1994) Selected topics in the histopathology of the vulva. *Current Diagnostic Pathology* **1**, 41–47.

Wharton, J.T., Gallager, S. & Routledge, F.N. (1974) Microinvasive carcinoma of the vulva. *American Journal of Obstetrics and Gynecology* **111**, 159–162.

Wharton, L.R. Jr. & Everett, H.S. (1951) Primary malignant Bartholin's gland tumors. *Obstetrical and Gynecological Survey* **6**, 1–8.

Wheelock, J.B., Gopelrud, D.R., Dunn, L.T. & Oates, J.F. (1984) Primary carcinoma of the Bartholin gland: a report of ten cases. *Obstetrics and Gynecology* **63**, 820–824.

Wick, M.R., Goellner, J.R., Wolfe, J.T. & Su, W.P.D. (1985) Vulvar sweat gland carcinomas. *Archives of Pathology and Laboratory Medicine* **109**, 43–47.

Wilkinson, E.J. (1985) Superficial invasive carcinoma of the vulva. *Clinical Obstetrics and Gynecology* **28**, 188–195.

Wilkinson, E.J. (1987) Superficially invasive carcinoma of the vulva. In: *Pathology of the Vulva and Vagina* (ed. E.J. Wilkinson) pp. 103–117. Churchill Livingstone, New York.

Wilkinson, E.J., Rico, M.J. & Pierson, K.K. (1982) Microinvasive carcinoma of the vulva. *International Journal of Gynecological Pathology* **1**, 29–39.

Wilkinson, E.J., Cook, J.C., Friedrich, E.G. & Massey, J.K. (1988) Vulvar intraepithelial neoplasia: association with cigarette smoking. *Colposcopic Gynecology and Laser Surgery* **4**, 153–159.

Wilner, R.B., Greenwald, M. & Wendelken, H. (1976) Eccrine carcinoma of the vulva: report of a case. *Journal of the American Osteopathic Assosociation* **76**, 282–285.

Wilson, D. & Woodger, B.A. (1974) Pleomorphic adenoma of the vulva. *Journal of Obstetrics and Gynaecology of the British Commonwealth* **81**, 1000–1002.

Winkelmann, S.E. & Llorens, A.S. (1990) Metastatic basal cell carcinoma of the vulva. *Gynecologic Oncology* **38**, 138–140.

Woodruff, J.D. (1955) Paget's disease of the vulva. *Obstetrics and Gynecology* **10**, 10–16.

Woodruff, J.D., Braun, L., Calvieri, R. *et al.* (1980) Immunologic identification of papillomavirus antigen in condylomatous tissue from the female genital tract. *Obstetrics and Gynecology* **56**, 727–732.

Woodworth, H., Dockerty, M.B., Wilson, R.B. & Pratt, J.H. (1971) Papillary hidradenoma of the vulva: a clinicopathologic study of 69 cases. *American Journal of Obstetrics and Gynecology* **110**, 501–508.

Woolcot, R.J., Henry, R.J.W. & Houghton, C.R.S. (1988) Malignant melanoma of the vulva: Australian experience. *Journal of Reproductive Medicine* **33**, 699–702.

Yackel, D.B., Symmonds, R.E. & Kempers, R.D. (1970) Melanoma of the vulva. *Obstetrics and Gynecology* **35**, 23–29.

Yazigi, R., Piver, M.S. & Tsukada, Y. (1978) Microinvasive carcinoma of the vulva. *Obstetrics and Gynecology* **35**, 625–631.

Yell, J.A. (1991) Grzybowski's generalized eruptive keratoacanthoma. *Journal of the Royal Society of Medicine* **84**, 170–171.

Yeoh, G., Bannatyne, P., Kossard, S. *et al.* (1987) Intestinal heterotopia: an unusual cause of vulval ulceration: a case report. *British Journal of Obstetrics and Gynaecology* **94**, 600–602.

Young, A.W. Jr., Herman, E.W. & Tovell, H.M.M. (1980) Syringoma of the vulva; incidence, diagnosis and cause of pruritis. *Obstetrics and Gynecology* **55**, 515–518.

Young, R.H. & Scully, R.E. (1985) Clear cell adenocarcinoma of the bladder and urethra: a report of three cases and review of the literature. *American Journal of Surgical Pathology* **9**, 816–826.

Zaino, R.J. (1987) Carcinoma of the vulva, urethra, and Bartholin's glands. In: *Pathology of the Vulva and Vagina* (ed. E.J. Wilkinson), pp. 119–153. Churchill Livingstone, New York.

Zaino, R.J., Husseinzadeh, N., Nahas, W. & Mortel, R. (1982) Epithelial alterations in proximity to invasive squamous carcinoma of the vulva. *International Journal of Gynecological Pathology* **1**, 173–184.

Zerner, J. (1975) Basal cell carcinoma of the vulva: a report of six cases and review of the literature. *Journal of the Maine Medical Association* **65**, 127–129.

zur Havsen, H. (1982) Human genital cancer: synergism between two virus infections and initiating events. *Lancet* **ii**, 1370–1372.

Chapter 11: Surgical procedures in benign vulval disease

B.J. Paniel

Ambiguous external genitalia

Female pseudohermaphroditism

The commonest cause of female pseudohermaphroditism is congenital adrenal hyperplasia. These children should always be reared as a female because if the uterus, tubes and ovaries are present they can become fertile women and bear children later in life.

The operation is performed in two stages. The first stage is a perineoplasty, which is done to open up the vulva and vagina. The simplest perineotomy consists of separating the adherent labia majora in the midline. This operation is suitable for Prader stages II and III (Prader 1954), where the urogenital sinus is close to the perineal skin (Fig. 11.1a–c). Normal childbirth may be possible later. A V–Y plastic operation (Fortunoff *et al.* 1964) can be used for Prader stages III and IV where the urogenital sinus is situated deep inside. An inverted U-shaped incision is made as shown in Fig. 11.2a (see p. 279), which is then undermined to free a flap (Fig. 11.2b). A perineotomy is extended as a midline incision to the posterior vaginal wall. The flap that is created is then used to fill the defect (Fig. 11.2c). Normal vaginal delivery in the future may be possible, but a caesarean section is often preferred so that the good cosmetic result of the procedure can be preserved. A transperineal operation has been described by Hendren (1977), which is done to bring the vagina down. It is reserved for those rare cases that are highly masculinized and where the vagina opens into the urethra.

The second stage is the reduction of the clitoral hypertrophy. There are numerous procedures that have been described including excision, embedding, or excision with a ventral or a dorsal flap. The most satisfactory procedure (Ferry *et al.* 1977) consists of freeing the clitoris from its dorsal and ventral attachments and then resecting the inferior two-thirds of the corpora cavernosa preserving the dorsal vasculoneural bundle. The cavernosa arteries are clamped and sutured; after a cuneiform resection, the glans clitoris is attached to the symphysis pubis and the preserved clitoral hood is lowered and used to cover the raw surfaces and to refashion the labia minora. A medial incision is made 1 month later to divide the large clitoral hood into two labia minora.

Male pseudohermaphroditism

In the case of male pseudohermaphroditism when the sex assignment is going to be female, the feminizing genitoplasty is similar to that described for female pseudohermaphroditism, but in addition an artificial vagina has to be constructed either by instrumental dilatation of the vaginal dimple according to Frank's method (Frank 1938) or by surgical means. The testes need to be removed because of the risk of malignant changes later in life. This is done by a Pfannenstiel incision or at the time of the clitoridoplasty (Strafford & Cleary 1976).

Bladder exstrophy

This condition occurs predominantly in females. The vulva has a characteristic appearance where the mons pubis is flattened or depressed, both the labia minora and majora diverge, and the clitoris is bifid. At puberty the growth of pubic hair is split into two halves which extend out towards the inguinal area. A medial perineotomy is done to widen the narrowed introitus. This correction will allow future sexual intercourse. Unfortunately the procedure may be complicated by genital prolapse. A simple clitoridoplasty brings together the divided clitoris. A double Z-plasty (Erich 1959), however, gives a result that looks more like a normal vulva. In this procedure (Fig. 11.3a–d, see p. 280) two inguinal triangular flaps covered with hair are exchanged with two medial hairless triangular flaps; the hair-bearing mons pubis is thus reconstructed and the vulva closed.

Labia minora hypertrophy

Hypertrophy of the labia minora is not a congenital malformation but a developmental anomaly. It is never seen in prepubertal girls where the labia minora are tiny or not

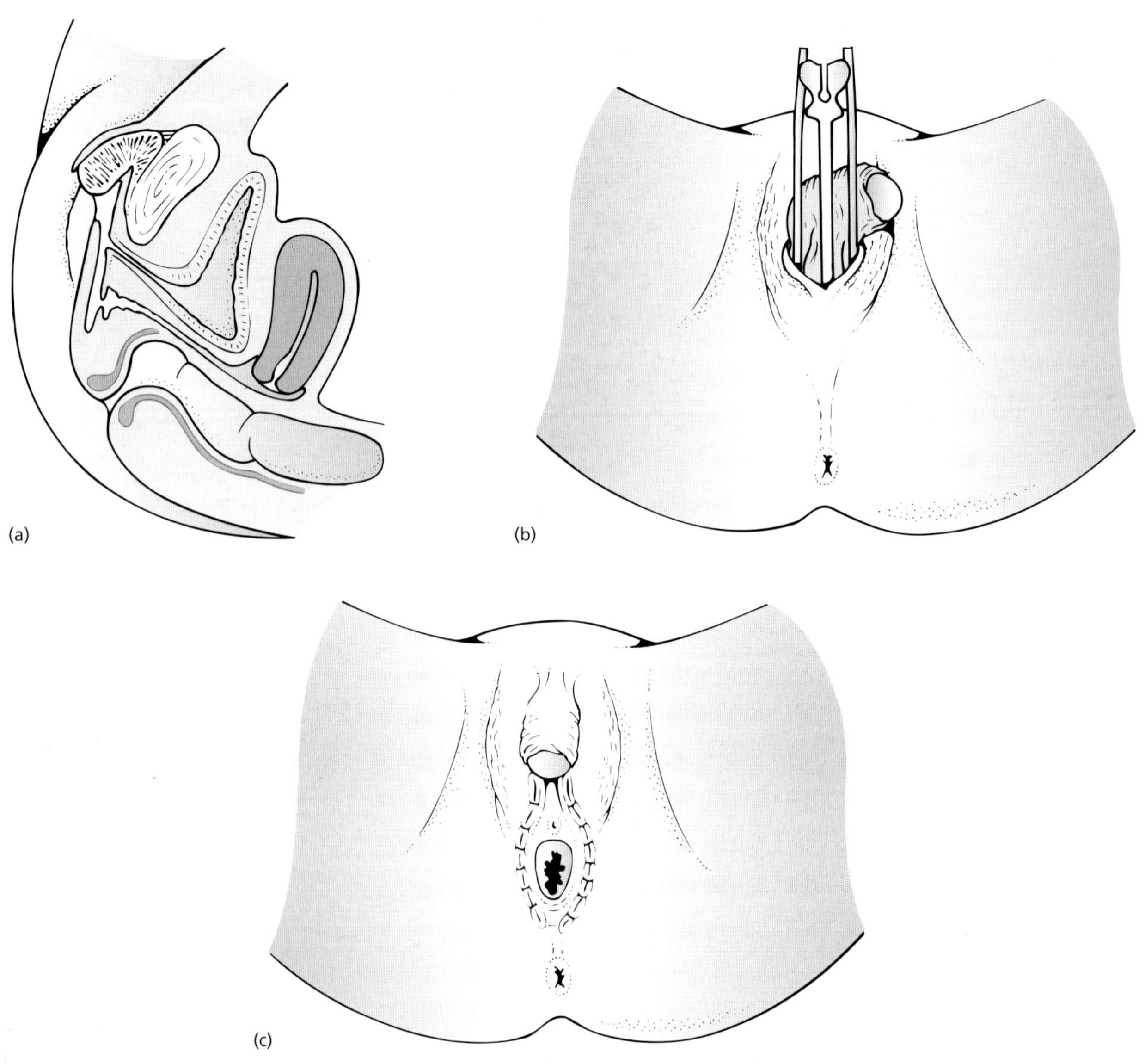

Fig. 11.1 Perineotomy. (a) Sagittal section showing the urogenital sinus close to the perineal skin. (b) A median incision is made to open up the sinus. (c) Mucocutaneous suture after sinus has been opened.

developed. The abnormality may be uni- or bilateral, symmetrical or asymmetrical and of varying degrees. It is usually asymptomatic but sometimes there is a complaint of irritation particularly with exercise and later in life the enlargement may interfere with sexual intercourse. However, the majority of patients complained for cosmetic reasons, feeling that the excessive, pendulous skin makes them less feminine. In such cases reduction can be achieved by one of three procedures as outlined below.

Complete nymphectomy

The labia minora are spread out but not stretched. An incision is made on the outer surface from the point where the labium minus divides to encircle the clitoris. The line of the incision runs along the interlabial sulcus and ends where the labium minus merges into the inner aspect of the labium majus ending before the posterior lateral labial commissure. The incision on the inner aspect of the labium minus matches that already made on the outside border and is down to the level of Hart's line or slightly higher than the level on the opposite edge to enable eversion of the final suture. The labium minus is then amputated by joining the two incisions and cutting across the vascular fibroelastic body of the labium minus (Fig. 11.4, see p. 281). The incision is completed either with a scalpel or scissors.

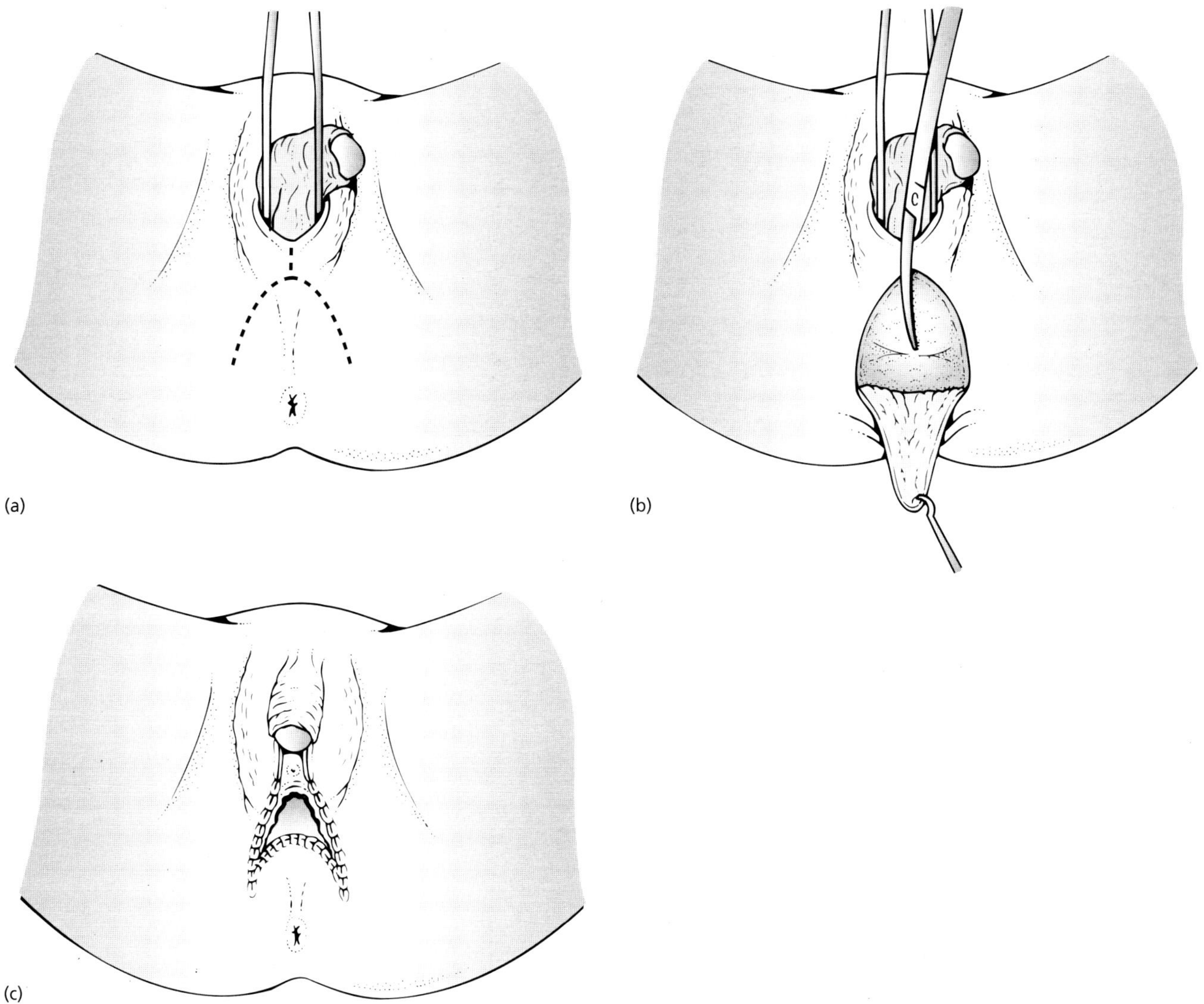

Fig. 11.2 Posterior cutaneous flap. (a) Urogenital sinus deeply situated: inverted U-shaped incision. Apex near the orifice of the urogenital sinus base near the anal margin. (b) Dissection of the perineal cutaneous flap followed by a median perineotomy. (c) The flap is used to fill the triangular defect.

Haemostasis is achieved with clips or Vicryl Rapide 4.0 to avoid a haematoma. The free edges are sutured with 3.0 or 4.0 absorbable suture with interrupted or running stitches. Any remaining stitches are removed 15 days later and the patients are warned that initially they will experience strange, transitory sensations produced by the inner surface of the labia majora rubbing against each other.

Subtotal nymphectomy

This procedure was first described by Hodgkinson and Hait (1984). The incision starts at the glans clitoris just below where the labia minora divide and finishes where the labia minora merge into the tissue a little way from the fourchette. This curved incision leaves a labium minus that has a maximum breadth of 1 cm, and a free edge that is pink and not pigmented. However, in normal women with small labia minora the free borders of the labia are very often not pigmented. The labia are sutured with interrupted stitches or by oversewing with colourless absorbable thread 4.0. There is no special postoperative care required.

Reduction nymphoplasty

This procedure results in the most natural-looking labia minora in that the resulting free edges of the labia minora are pigmented which more closely resembles the normal. In addition there is preservation of the two main functions of

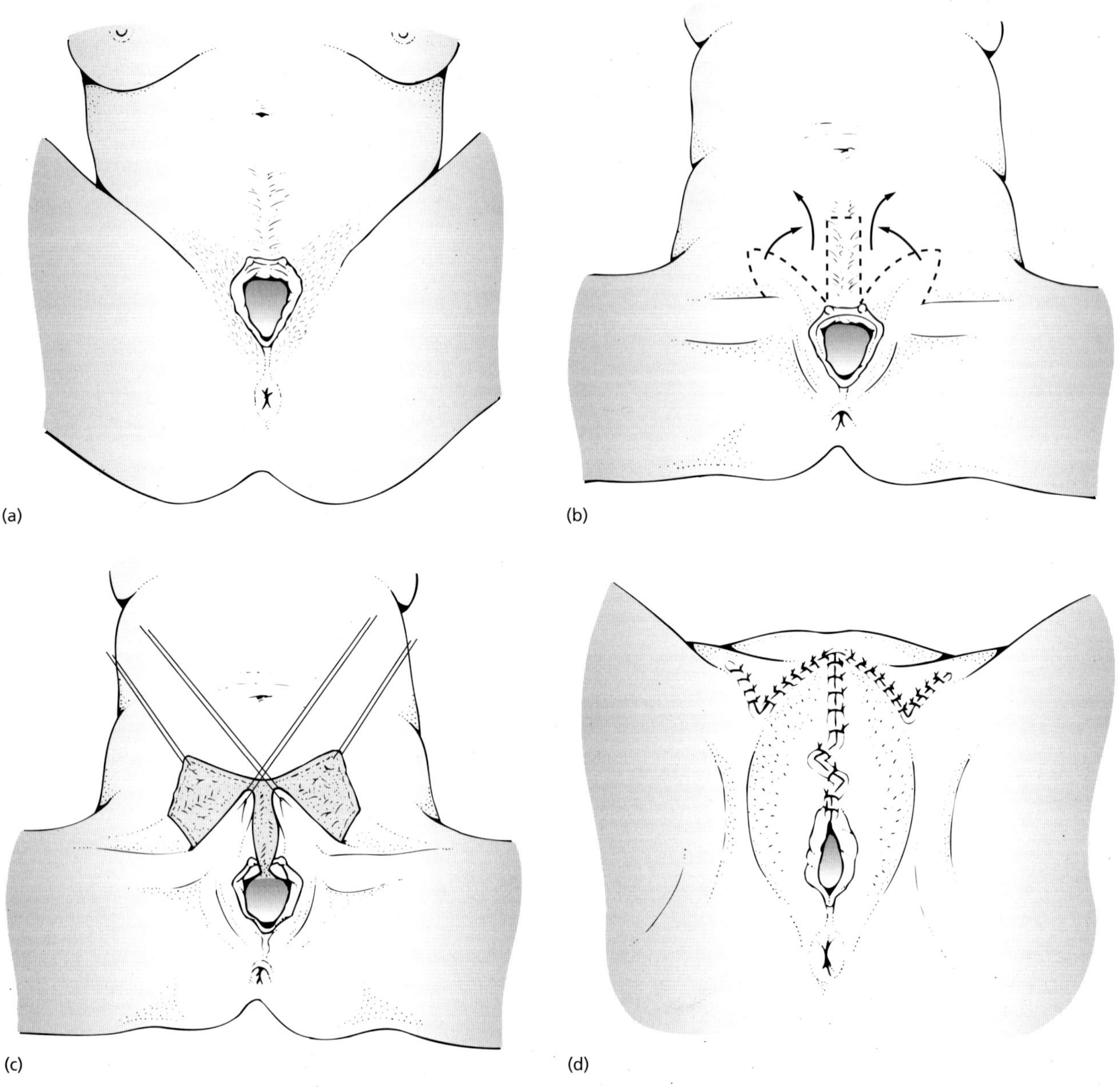

Fig. 11.3 Double Z-plasty.

the labia minora, i.e. firstly to provide a lubricated smooth surface to facilitate intercourse and secondly to protect the inner aspects of the vulva by virtue of their natural apposition (Paniel *et al.* 1985).

Each labium minus is laid out but not stretched and a pair of Kocher forceps is placed along the length and the base of the labium minus near the interlabial sulcus. Another pair is placed at an angle of approximately 90° to the first pair, demarcating two labial segments, which should be of identical dimensions in order to avoid any asymmetry (Fig. 11.5a, see p. 282). Each labial segment may have a base smaller than its length because of its rich blood supply. After incising along the forceps with the scalpel haemostasis is achieved using coagulating forceps (Fig. 11.5b). The superior labial segment is gently spread out and the edges are joined by one or two stitches at exactly the same levels, without trying to cover the entire raw edge, in order to avoid unwanted tension. The segments are sutured in three planes by fine stitches using 4.0 thread (Fig. 11.5c). A buried running stitch joins the fibroelastic body of the minora. A running suture or separate sutures ensure approximation of the outer and inner edges. Inevitably

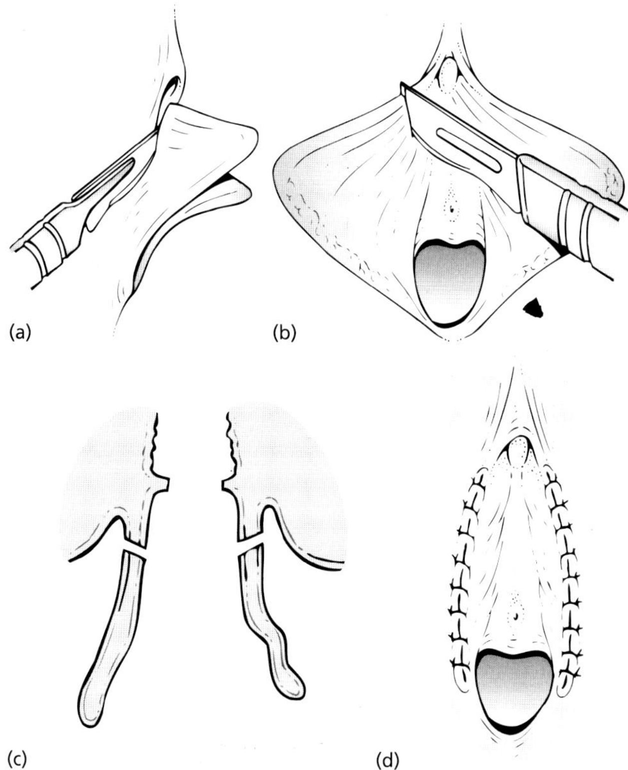

Fig. 11.4 Complete nymphectomy. (a) Incision on the outer surface; (b) incision on the inner aspect; (c) incision is slightly higher than the level on the opposite edge to enable eversion of the primal suture; (d) suturing of edges.

there is a formation of dog-ears, which can be resected or may be left to flatten out with time.

Postoperative care consists of simple cleansing twice daily. Any residual stitches are removed 3 weeks later, under local anaesthetic if necessary.

Vulval trauma

There are various causes of vulval trauma.

Obstetric trauma

This is not infrequent and occurs on the vulva or perineum during delivery.

VULVAL TEARS

These may be anterior around the meatus or clitoris and are usually unilateral. They frequently bleed and may need pressure or suturing to achieve haemostasis. Lateral tears of the labia minora are simple grazes, which cause pain only when urine is passed. Usually they heal spontaneously but sometimes the healing of a torn mucosa may lead to subsequent formation of mucous cysts. Radial tears (Fig. 11.6, see p. 282), labia minora perforations (Fig. 11.7, see p. 283) and labial detachment (Fig. 11.8, see p. 283) are also possible complications and can be easily repaired by excision and suturing in the three planes as already described above.

Surgical trauma

POST-PROLAPSE REPAIR

Not infrequently a surgical procedure undertaken to correct one problem gives rise to another. A good example of this is the vaginal narrowing that can occur after a prolapse repair. This occurs after a posterior colpoperineorraphy has been carried out and the vagina is thought to be sufficiently adequate at the time, as it often is. However, it may become narrow later because of the atresia that develops at the time of the menopause when oestrogen diminishes. There may be eventual stenosis of the vaginal opening that may give rise to dyspareunia or even apareunia.

Treatment is straightforward and involves a median perineotomy, i.e. Fenton's operation, which can be done under local anaesthesia, epidural or general anaesthetic (Fig. 11.9, see p. 284).

A median incision is made using either a scalpel or a pair of scissors running from the hymenal ring to the perineal body, simultaneously cutting through the vestibule. The perineal area is opened up and it is now important to free the vaginal wall and perineal skin by undermining on either side of the incision with a pair of blunt, curved dissecting scissors, particularly at each extremity to enable mobilization of the tissues without tension. If the perineal body has become fibrosed because of previous surgery it is important to free the right and left sides with a cuneiform incision in order to make it more supple and facilitate suturing. Good haemostasis is essential to prevent haematoma formation. The longitudinal incision is then sutured transversely. A tacking stitch is placed centrally. The edges may develop dog-ears, which can be easily resected. Suturing is done with absorbable thread 3.0 and gradually the areas are sewn together, working from the ends towards the centre.

There is very little postoperative discomfort. Sometimes a slight dehiscence occurs; this means longer healing but fortunately does not affect the long-term results. Any residual sutures are removed 3–4 weeks later. Sexual intercourse can then be resumed but postmenopausal women are advised to use oestrogen therapy. The outcome of this operation is usually very satisfactory.

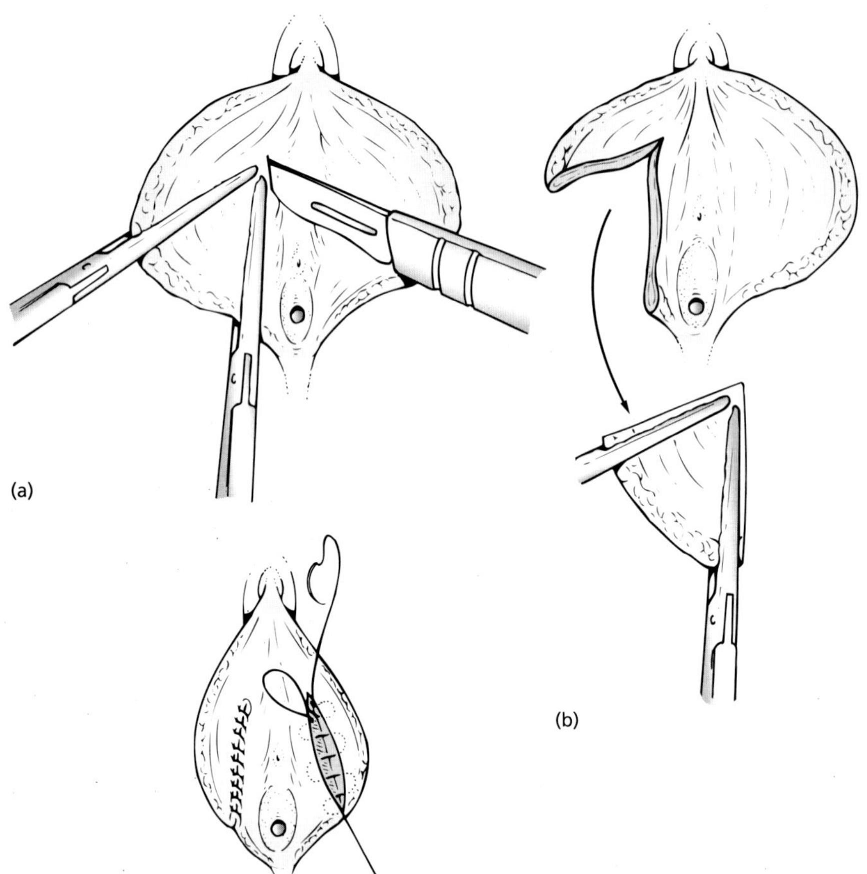

Fig. 11.5 Reduction nymphoplasty. (a) Two pairs of Kocher forceps are placed demarcating the labial segment to be excised. (b) Excision of the large inferior segment. (c) Suture of the smaller anterior segment in three planes.

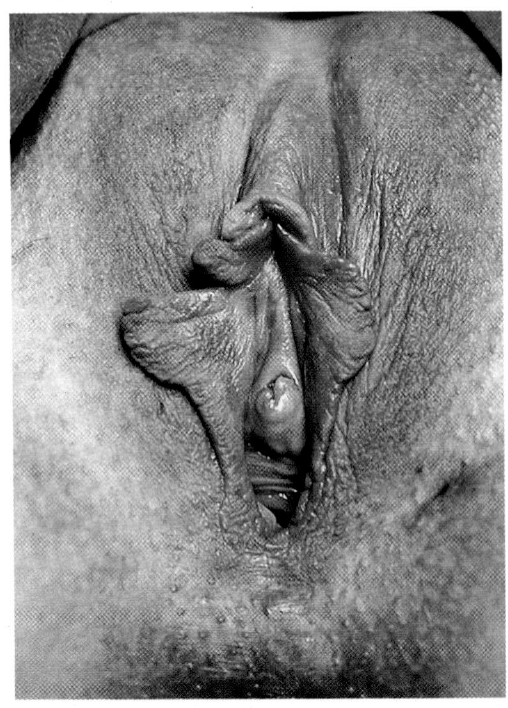

Fig. 11.6 Radial tear.

POST-VULVECTOMY

There are several surgical procedures available to correct the introital stenosis that may follow either simple or radical vulvectomy.

The Z-plasty is frequently used to correct post-operative scarring and the results are usually good. The annular constriction of the vaginal opening is eliminated and the gusset effect gives it a certain elasticity (Fig. 11.10, see p. 285).

In cases of introital stenosis following vulvectomy, a Z-plasty (Scott *et al.* 1963, Wilkinson 1971) is performed on one side. An incision is made into the introital opening measuring approximately 2.5 cm. The other two incisions of identical length form 60° angles, one of the incisions running into the introital opening and the other into the perineal skin. The pieces defined in this way are dissected with skin hooks to prevent crushing. They are then switched and stitched together. A mirror-image Z-plasty is made on the opposite side. An in-dwelling bladder catheter is inserted and a vaginal tampon is left in place 24–48 hours.

A unilateral or bilateral transposition flap taken from the labium majorus is suitable for stenosis of the vaginal

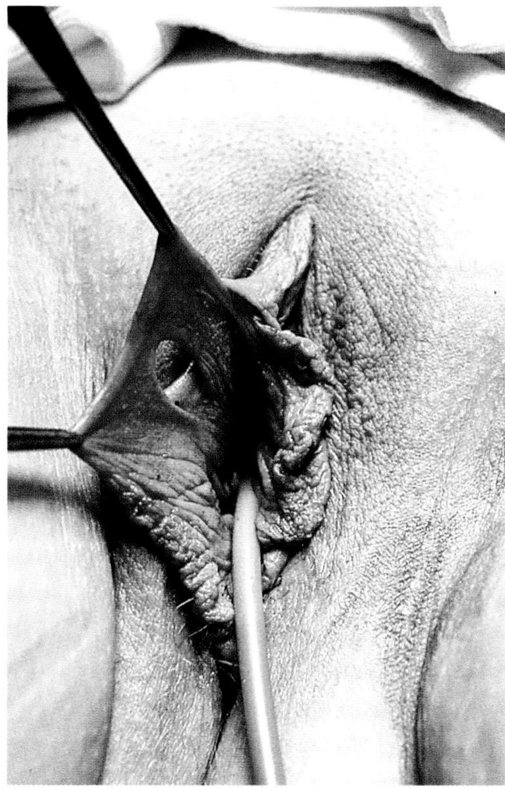

Fig. 11.7 Labium minus perforation.

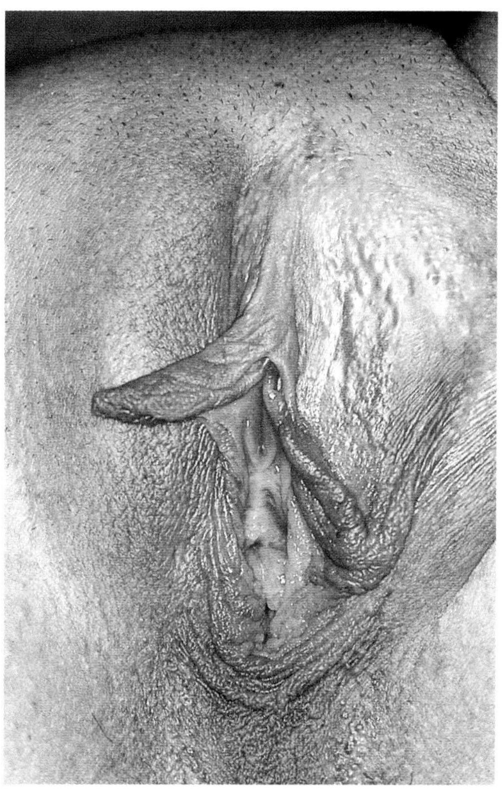

Fig. 11.8 Labial detachment.

opening and of the lower end of the vagina (Patterson & Rhodes 1958). The operation starts with a lateral or posterolateral incision resembling an extended episiotomy, which creates a triangular defect. A cutaneous full-thickness triangular flap is then drawn out on the labium majorus to cover the defect (Fig. 11.11, see p. 286).

The cutaneous and the mucosal edges are then carefully sutured. The non-dissected angle separating the flaps from the raw surfaces stays in place. It inevitably raises itself in a dog-ear, which usually flattens with time because of the elasticity of the surrounding skin. The edges of the donor site are closed by simple approximation after having undermined the edges. If the correction of the stenosis is insufficient the procedure should be repeated on the opposite side at the same time as the operation or it can be done later. Postoperatively a suitable vaginal tampon is left in place for 24–48 hours to apply a light compression on the flap in its new position to avoid the development of a haematoma. The completed skin graft has a very small risk of retraction but in such a case the aesthetic considerations should yield precedence to the functional result and the patient should be warned about this.

AFTER INCISION AND DRAINAGE OF BARTHOLIN'S ABSCESS

The incision and drainage of a Bartholin's abscess through the interlabial sulcus can result in either partial detachment of a labium minus, or the development of a fistulous track, which oozes mucus. The treatment consists of removal of Bartholin's duct and gland and then resuturing the labium minus. To avoid this complication it is preferable to make the incision in the nymphohymenal sulcus.

AFTER LASER THERAPY

The complications following carbon dioxide ablation of vulval intraepithelial neoplasia (VIN) 3 include synechiae formation of the labia minora and vestibule. These secondary adhesions are very common after lasering of lesions in the fourchette, fossa navicularis and vestibule. The partly fused labia tear apart during sexual intercourse causing dyspareunia. To avoid this complication it is recommended that in the case of bilateral lesions only one side is treated at a time. If the fourchette or fossa navicularis are involved with VIN 3 it is preferable to deal with the problem surgically followed by reconstruction using the posterior vaginal wall.

(a)

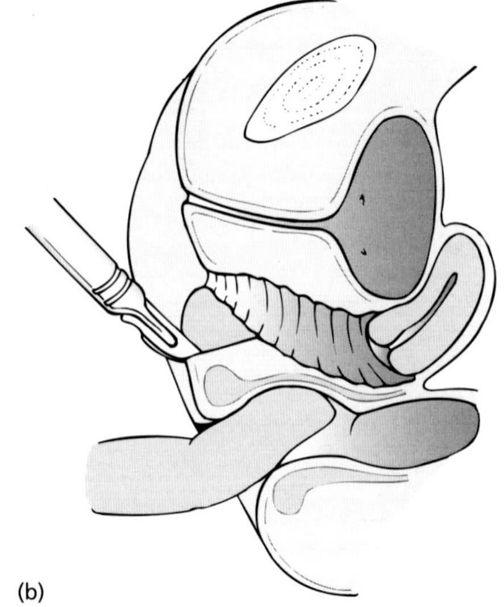

(b)

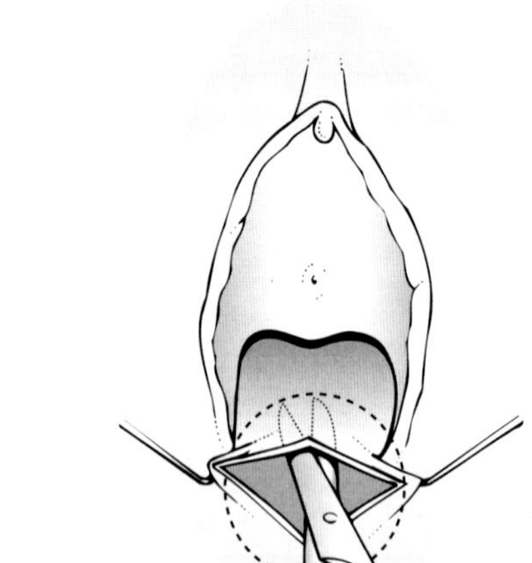

(c)

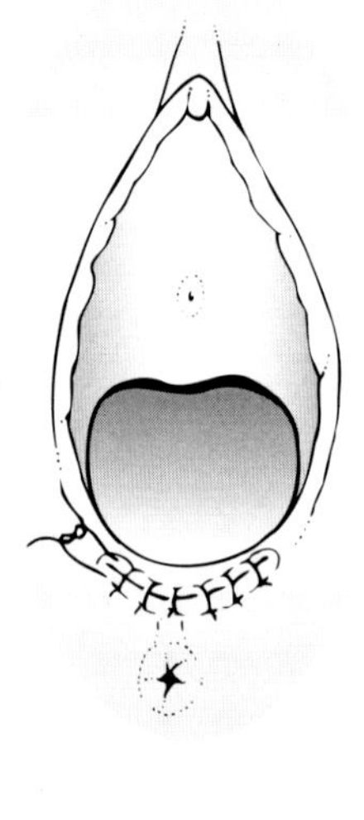

(d)

Fig. 11.9 Median perineotomy (Fenton's operation). (a) and (b) Longitudinal incision running from the hymenal ring to the perineal skin and cutting into the perineal body; (c) undermining vaginal wall and perineal skin; (d) transverse suturing. (Paniel *et al.* 1985.)

Post-coital fissures

HYMENAL FISSURES

These occur in young nulliparous women and are one cause of superficial dyspareunia (Michlewitz 1986, Moyal-Barracco *et al.* 1998). Post-coital bleeding and precise site of pain correspond to the areas of the hymenal tears of first intercourse and serve to make the diagnosis. The areas of scarring can fissure during vaginal examination particularly if there is any tension on the hymenal ring (i.e. opening a vaginal speculum to take a cervical smear) or during sexual intercourse particularly with a change of partner.

These fissures are arranged in a radial fashion around the hymenal ring usually between 3 and 4 and 8 and 9 o'clock. (Fig. 11.12, see p. 287). They may be uni- or bilateral and look like linear erosions. They can extend from the hymenal ring into the vagina or nymphohymenal sulcus. They may go unnoticed and it is important to try to display the hymen well and this is done by grasping the labia between the thumb and index finger and stretching them gently out and down.

The fissures heal rapidly in a few days after intercourse, leaving behind a pale scarred site, which refissures at each intercourse. Avoiding intercourse even for long periods does not prevent recurrence. Spontaneous cure does occur but may take a long time.

The treatment entails the excision of the fissures sagittally and resuturing the edges of the vestibular and vaginal mucosa transversely. The procedure is most suitable for removing the scarred area, which is particularly vulnerable to the tension that is exerted at the time of sexual intercourse. The radial incisions are made with a scalpel blade or a pair of scissors each at 60° cutting lightly into the mucosa

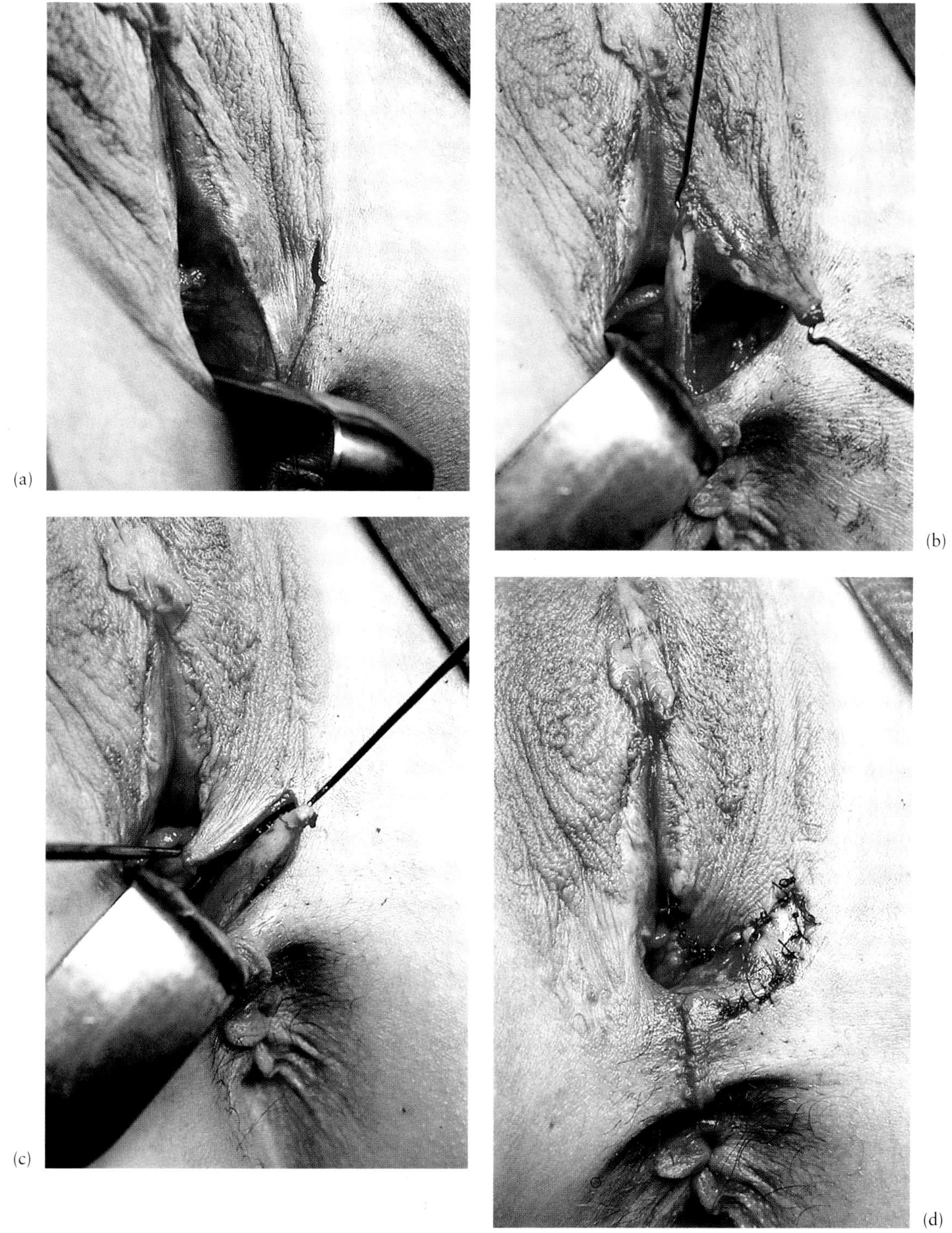

Fig. 11.10 (a) Lines of the incision; (b) raising a flap; (c) transposition of flaps; (d) final suturing.

above and below and deeply into the base of the fibrous insertion of the hymen. At 5 and 7 o'clock, care is taken to avoid the excretory ducts of the Bartholin's glands. At 11 and 1 o'clock near the urethral meatus, the incisions are made deeper to ensure dissociation of the meatus from the hymen and avoid the development of post-coital recurrent cystitis. Interrupted stitches are made using fine absorbable thread, and are placed transversely to achieve haemostasis.

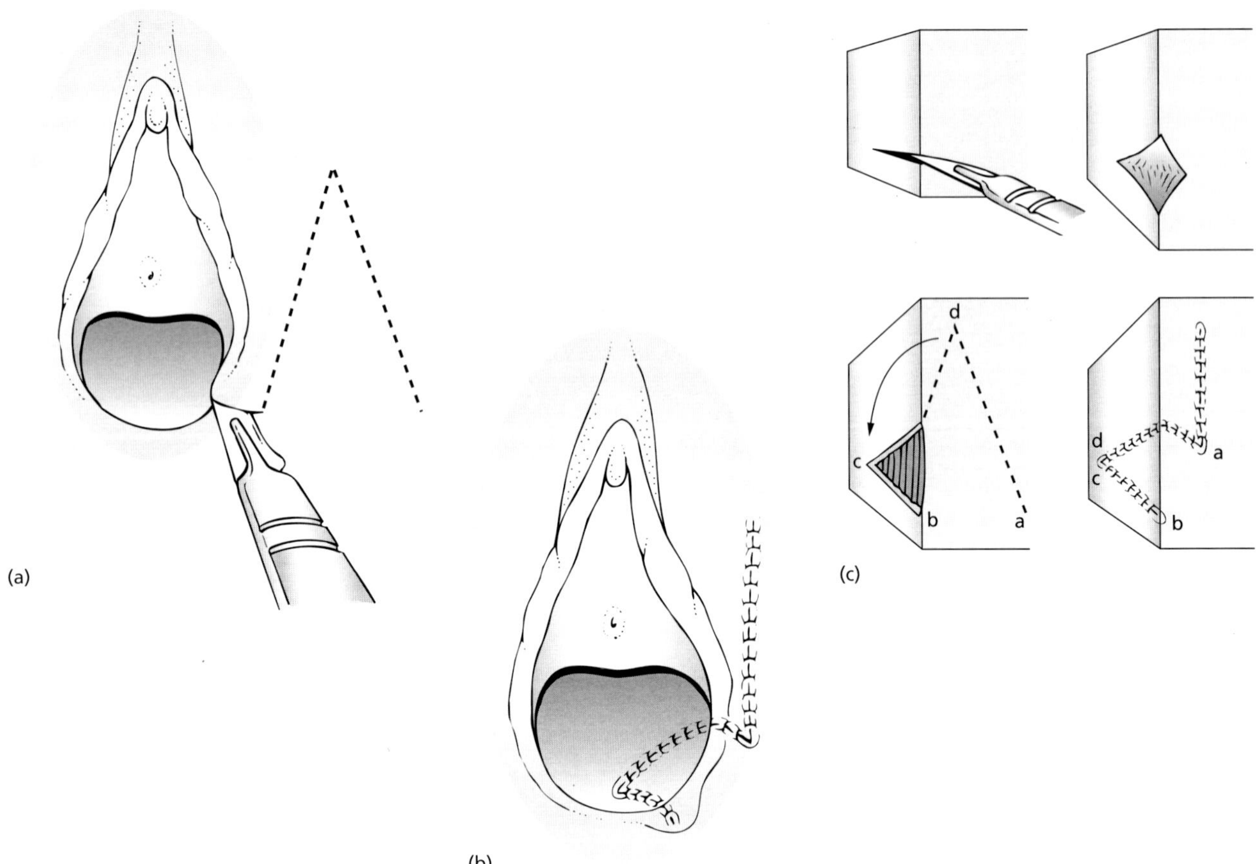

Fig. 11.11 Transposition flap. (a) Incision to make a triangular flap. (b) Positioning and suturing. (c) Diagram to show procedure in three dimensions.

Sexual intercourse can be resumed a month postoperatively when healing is complete. It is important to reassure the patient beforehand to lessen her apprehension.

FOSSA NAVICULARIS FISSURES

These fissures are a cause of secondary superficial dyspareunia (Michlewitz 1986, Berville-Levy *et al.* 1998, Moyal-Barracco *et al.* 1998). Following penetration the patient senses vulval tearing, sometimes accompanied by bleeding and this may be followed for several days by spontaneous localized burning of the vulva, often triggered by micturition. These symptoms return with each intercourse and understandably lead to difficulties with sexual relations; the patient eventually dreads and avoids intercourse. On gently examining the vulva the fissure can be seen the length of the posterior vestibule in the midline (Fig. 11.13, see p. 287) running from the hymen to the fourchette. Sometimes after intercourse there will be a very fine white scar, which may only be faintly visible but with a more thorough examination it may readily split open. There is no evidence of lichen sclerosus or lichen planus but in some cases the delicate epithelium of the fossa navicularis has been damaged following previous treatment of lesions in this area with carbon dioxide laser, liquid nitrogen or electrocoagulation. Reducing the frequency of sexual intercourse and the use of bland emollients may help, but if these measures fail, surgical treatment has to be considered. Quadrilateral excision of the vestibular mucosa including the fissure with dissection and cleavage of the posterior vaginal wall for 2–3 cm is required. This provides a flap of vaginal wall, which can be used to fill in the defect, and the tissue can be sutured without tension.

HYMENORRAPHY

It is technically feasible to repair the hymen after forced or consensual sexual activity. This is done using a vaginal flap, or by suture in three planes, after excision of the membrane from 2 o'clock to 10 o'clock.

Female sexual mutilation

After clitoridectomy no worthwhile reconstruction is pos-

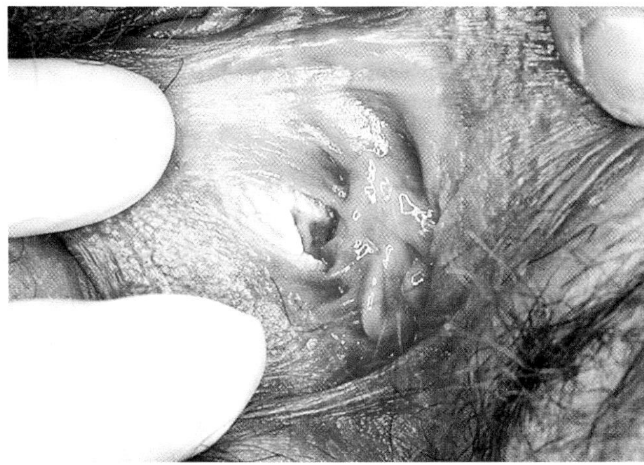

Fig. 11.12 Hymenal fissure (courtesy of M. Moyal-Barracco).

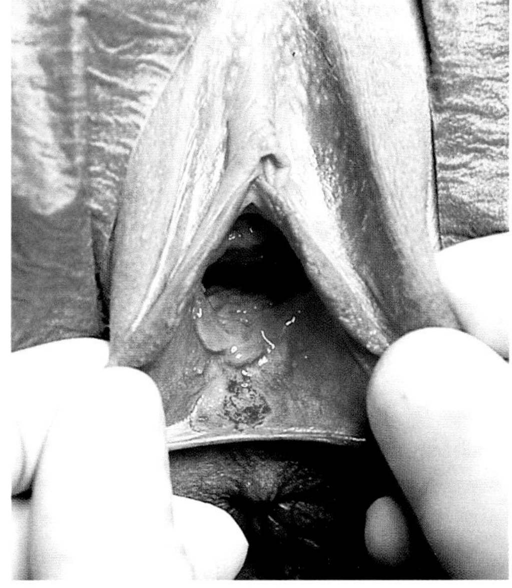

Fig. 11.13 Fossa navicularis fissure (courtesy of S. Berville).

sible. Infibulation or pharaonic circumcision as practised in Mali, Sudan and the Horn of Africa consists of removal of the labia minora and suturing with acacia spines after freshening of the edges, with or without a clitoridectomy. A little hole that is made by leaving a small stick of wood in place while suturing remains open in front of the posterior commissure to allow urine and menstrual blood to flow out. Surgical correction consists of separating the labia minora along the midline and then suturing their free borders so that a nearly normal appearance can be obtained. This will allow normal sexual function and vaginal delivery later in life.

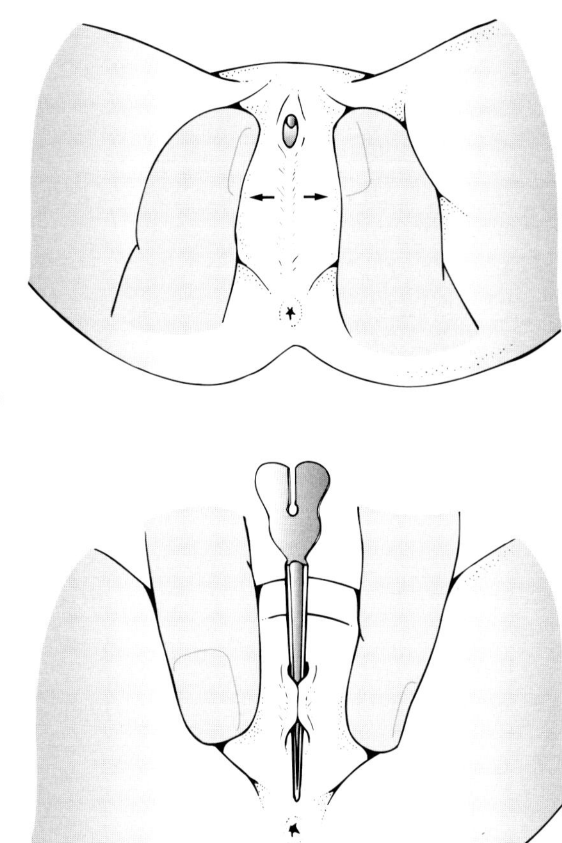

Fig. 11.14 Labial adhesions. (a) Digital separation; (b) instrumental separation.

Labial adhesions

Labial adhesions are relatively common and they are acquired and not congenital (Guillarme *et al.* 1995). The condition is usually asymptomatic but there is often parental concern. If the children are symptomatic they present with dysuria, urinary tract infections and vulval irritation. On inspection and parting of the labia majora the vulva appears flat as the free edges of the inner aspects of the vulva are adherent one upon the other. This join is seen as a fine line running anteroposteriorly and the adherence may be complete or partial. There is always a small opening at the level of the urethral meatus. Medical management includes the use of bland emollients and topical oestrogen.

It is particularly important to reassure the parents that labial adhesions are a common and harmless phenomenon that usually resolves spontaneously. This strong reassurance may well diffuse their anxiety and avoid surgical intervention in those asymptomatic children where the abnormality has been noted by chance.

For a long time it was a not uncommon practice to separate the adhesions either manually or instrumentally after cleansing the skin. The former technique involved placing a thumb on each labium majus and quicky splitting the adhesion by applying firm but gentle pressure in an outward and downward direction (Fig. 11.14a). The second technique involved passing either a lubricated hollow sound or forceps into the opening of the adhesion (Fig. 11.14b). The adhesion is then broken down. These manoeuvres leave torn edges on either side of the vulva with little or no bleeding. The frequent applications of an emollient often help healing and prevent resealing. If there is any suggestion of secondary infection a topical antibiotic should be used. The separation of the labia by these techniques is very effective but further adhesions are common. Even with local anaesthesia this digital and instrumental separation is quite brutal and painful, resulting in a tearful and distressed child. The memory of these traumatic events leaves the child fearful of further gynaecological examination and may in later life lead to psychosexual problems. Furthermore the child's mother is usually present during the procedure and she is often appalled by the distress caused to her child.

Surgical division of the adhesion under a general anaesthetic is done only under exceptional circumstances. It is a procedure reserved for those cases where resealing has occurred after several previous divisions. The free edges are sutured to help prevent resealing. The two main reasons for intervention are symptomatic children and parental pressure. The pressure usually comes from the mother who is anxious that her daughter may have sexual problems later in life.

Lichen sclerosus

Surgical intervention in lichen sclerosus is indicated only for the post-inflammatory sequelae of the disease.

Introital stenosis

VULVOPERINEOPLASTY

Vulvoperineoplasty is indicated on the rare occasions where there is introital stenosis following lichen sclerosus (Paniel 1984, Paniel *et al.* 1984). Patients present with either dyspareunia or apareunia. The procedure involves:

1 wide dissection and mobilization of the posterior wall of the vagina;

2 reduction of the height of the perineal body;

3 advancement and eversion of the posterior vaginal wall (Fig. 11.15).

The patient is placed in the lithotomy position and under general anaesthetic or epidural the procedure begins as for a posterior colpoperineorrhaphy. A marker thread is passed through the posterior extremity of each labium minus. By lifting and stretching out the two threads the mucocutaneous junction can be seen and the initial incision is made along this line. A triangular flap of perineal skin that has often been involved in the disease process is excised together with the subcutaneous tissue. The base of the triangle is represented by a border of tissue made by the initial vulval incision. The summit of the triangle is always situated closely to the anal margin.

The edge of the vestibular mucosa is lifted by a pair of dissecting forceps stretching out the tissue so that the blade can delicately undermine the area. Ring forceps then replace the dissecting forceps and are held in the left hand between the thumb and index while the extended third and fourth fingers of this hand are placed under the vaginal wall to facilitate the dissection. The dissection is done freely and widely with the blade or scissors without ever losing contact with the lower vaginal wall. In this way, the rectovaginal plane of cleavage is reached. The division is done digitally for 6–7 cm just to the vicinity of the pouch of Douglas. The fibrous perineal body now exposed is incised medially just near the anal sphincter. If the vaginal opening is not sufficiently wide, two paramedian incisions are made. The completion of the radial incisions is effected by digital dissection. The height of fibrous perineal body is thus reduced.

A posterior vaginal flap is then made and brought down. The posterior vaginal wall is incised longitudinally on both sides of the ring forceps at the level of the lateral gutters of the vagina for 3–4 cm, taking care to avoid the ductal openings of the Bartholin's glands. The lower extremity of the vaginal flap, which was grasped and damaged by the pressure of the ring forceps, is then excised. The thin vaginal epithelium, which is supple and well vascularized, is then easily drawn down to the exterior, making a perfect cover for the perineal defect. A small median sagittal incision is made on the inferior edge of the flap to improve the laxity on either side. The suturing must be done without tension and the best way to achieve this is by using interrupted absorbable sutures 3.0. This leaves a widened introitus that will eventually be able to withstand the trauma of coitus. Both sides of the flap as well as the mucocutaneous edges are brought together by interrupted sutures. There are small lateral vestibular defects, which are left to heal spontaneously.

An appropriately sized tampon wrapped in paraffin gauze is left in place for 24 hours together with an indwelling urinary catheter. The pressure exerted by the tampon prevents haematoma formation under the flap.

The procedure takes a trained surgeon 25–45 minutes. Healing is usually straightforward and the patient may be discharged 24–48 hours later once the local discomfort is controlled. Any sutures that have not dissolved sponta-

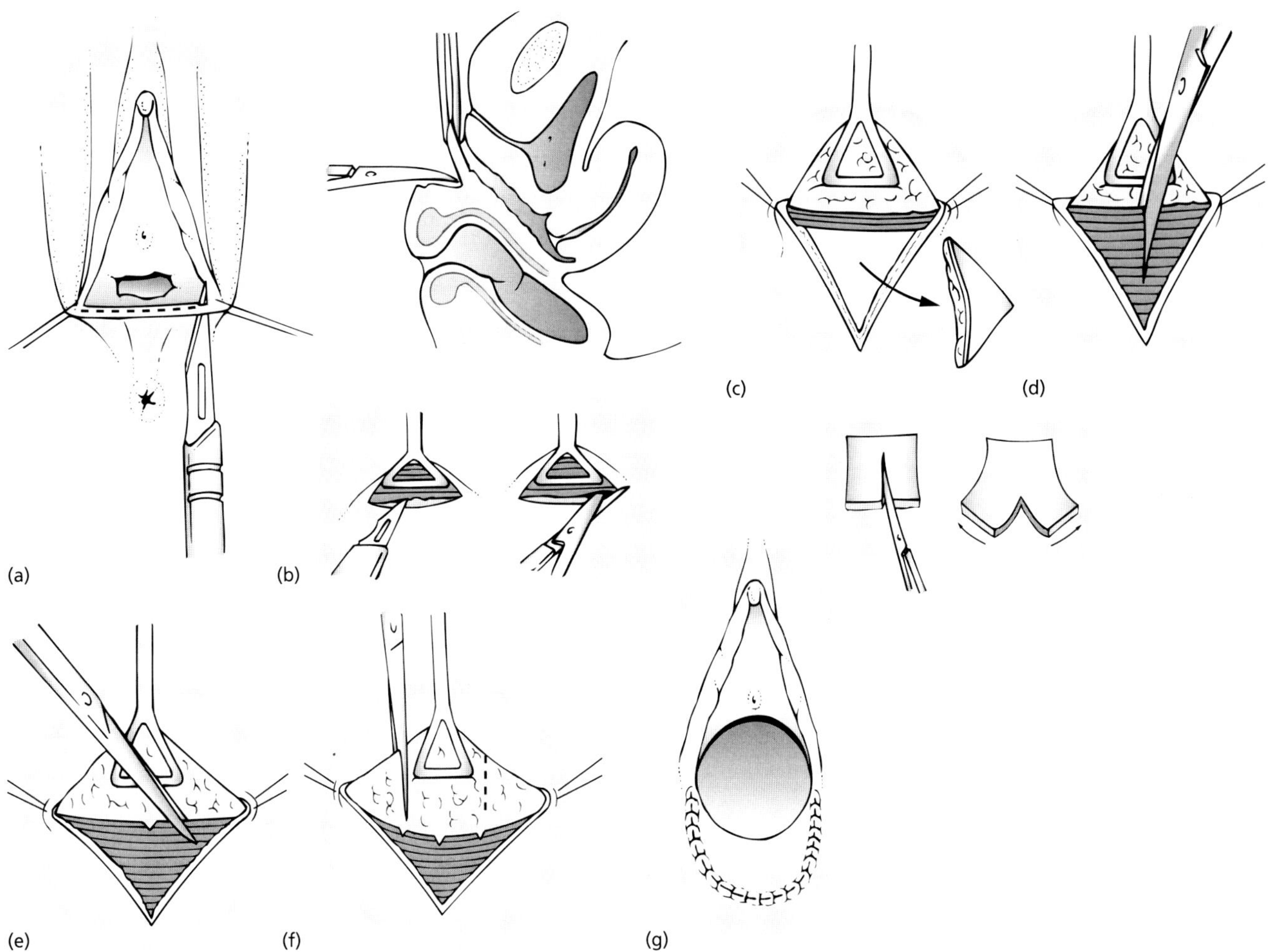

Fig. 11.15 Vulvoperineoplasty. (a) Mucocutaneous incision; (b) dissection of the posterior vaginal wall; (c) excision of a triangular patch of perineal skin; (d, e), radial incision of the fibrous perineal body to reduce its height; (f) individualization of a vaginal flap; (g) the vaginal flap is drawn down, making a cover for the perineal defect, and sutured.

neously are removed 2–3 weeks postoperatively. The operation not only successfully restores the introitus to an adequate size but also leaves an area that is not attacked later by lichen sclerosus. The vaginal epithelium that now covers this site seems to remain unaffected, as has been shown by biopsies carried out up to 15 years later. The patient should not discontinue the use of the topical steroids.

Adhesions

Adhesions due to epithelial atrophy with lichen sclerosus are usually localized to the fourchette, labia minora or clitoral prepuce.

FOURCHETTE ADHESIONS

These usually consist of synechiae, which tear during sexual intercourse or on clinical examination. There may be light bleeding when they are disrupted and patients often complain of dyspareunia. The adhesions reform after healing and tear again with further disturbance. The treatment is simple, consisting of a median perineotomy, i.e. Fenton's operation. This is done under local or general anaesthesia by incising the adhesion, perineal skin, vestibular mucous membrane and the summit of the perineal body. The mucosal edges are undermined and sutured transversely using interrupted stitches of 3.0 Vicryl.

LABIA MINORA ADHESIONS

Extensive labial synechiae or a fused vulva is a rare finding, usually occurring in postmenopausal women. The appearance is similar to that seen after ritual infibulation where there is only a small orifice posteriorly. The synechiae are freed and the edges are sutured with fine absorbable thread.

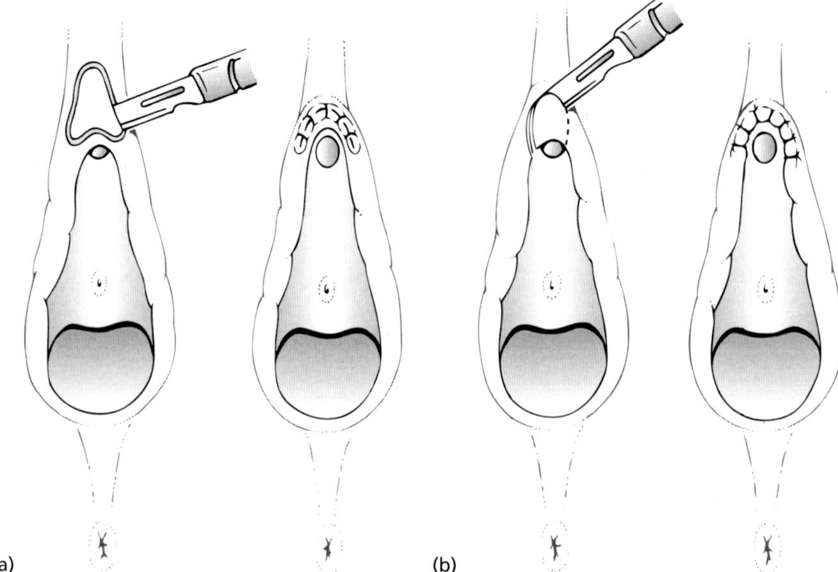

Fig. 11.16 Prevention of re-adhesion. (a) Resection of a segment of the clitoral hood in the shape of a tricorn. (b) Circumcision.

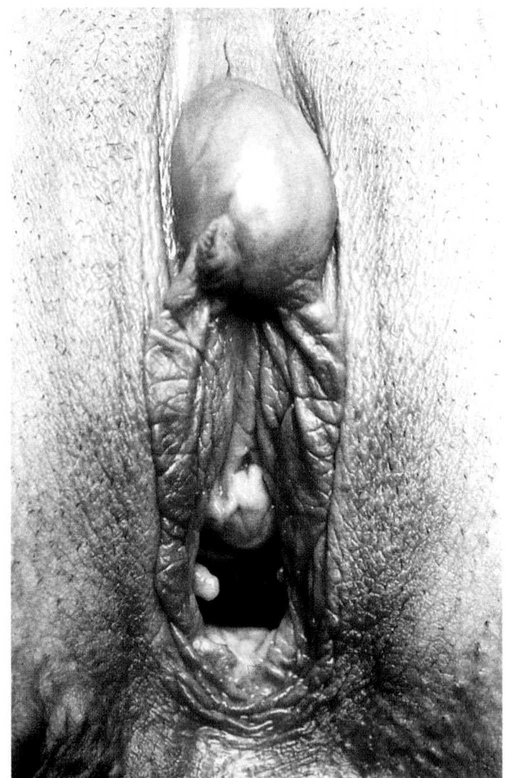

Fig. 11.17 Clitoral pseudocyst.

CLITORAL ADHESIONS

The clitoris is frequently buried in lichen sclerosus and although this is often symptomless many patients prefer the area to be freed for aesthetic reasons. The adhesions are delicately incised and then, using a probe, the hood is freed from the glans.

Prevention of readhesion is achieved either by resection of a fragment of the clitoral hood in the shape of a tricorn hat, which everts the free edge (Fig. 11.16a), or by excision of the clitoral hood, which is the equivalent to a circumcision (Fig. 11.16b).

Sometimes periclitoral adhesion results in a pseudocyst containing smegma, which can lead to a misdiagnosis of a tumour or cyst (Fig. 11.17). It may be complicated by secondary infection with fistula formation. The only treatment that can be offered is subtotal or total circumcision.

Lichen planus and other bullous and erosive diseases

Vulvovaginal adhesions

Vulvovaginal adhesions are associated with several erosive mucosal diseases, which result in scarring and adhesion of the vagina, vestibule or labia minora. These erosive diseases include lichen planus, cicatricial pemphigoid, toxic epidermal necrolysis and Stevens–Johnson syndrome.

The active inflammatory dermatosis is treated medically. Surgery is only required for post-inflammatory adhesions. In the vulva the localized scarring results in burying of the clitoris, labial adhesions or introital stenosis. The buried glans clitoris is freed surgically and then circumcision can

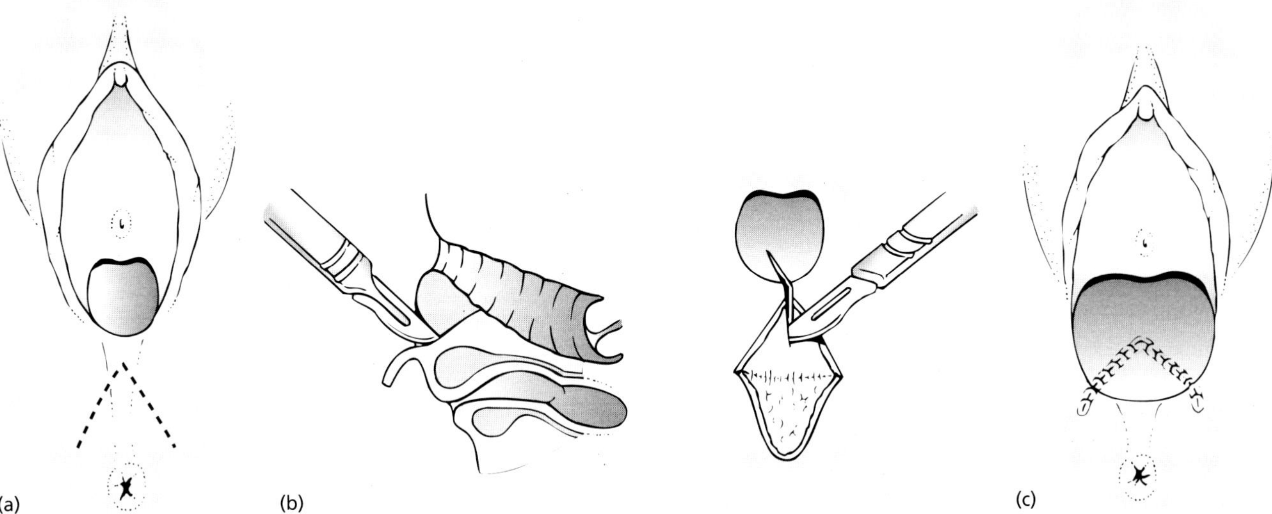

Fig. 11.18 Posterior perineal cutaneous flap. (a) A V-shaped flap is made on the perineal skin. (b) The perineal body is reduced by radial incisions and digital dissection. (c) The perineal flap covers the triangular defect and is sutured with 3.0 or 4.0 Vicryl.

be done to prevent recurrence. Anterior and lateral fusion are divided by sagittal incisions followed by transverse suturing. The adhesions of the fourchette can be corrected by a procedure similar to a median perineotomy.

If there is vestibular stenosis without vaginal wall involvement a perineoplasty may be performed. In those cases with associated vulvovaginal involvement, the healthy surrounding skin of the perineal area is used for reconstruction by carrying out an inverse V–Y plasty. This procedure is identical to that used by Fortunoff to open the urogenital sinus in cases of sexual ambiguity. A V-shaped flap is made on the perineal skin. The apex is at the top of the fourchette and the base lies flush with the anal margin. It is advisable to ensure that the length of the base is equal to the length of the flap so as not to compromise the vascularization. The flap is then dissected from the apex to the base, taking care to preserve a suitable thickness and fatty support. The perineal body is reduced by radial incisions and by digital dissection. The posterior wall of the vagina is then incised along the median line. The gaping sides of the incision allow the recovery of a normal calibre for the introitus and lower vagina. After haemostasis the cutaneous flap is pulled up into the interior of the vaginal conduit to fit into the triangular defect caused by the perineotomy, and the tissue is then sutured with Vicryl 3.0 or 4.0 (Fig. 11.18). A tampon for haemostasis is left in place for 24 hours.

Vaginal adhesions alone have various clinical aspects but the problem most frequently encountered is partial fusion of the anterior and posterior walls of the vagina along the lateral edges. This produces a concentric narrowing of the vagina. Sometimes a small speculum can be passed but otherwise the adhesions may result in the appearance of a funnel-shaped narrowing with a small opening at its apex through which the secretions and menstrual blood can flow out. Rarely a complete adhesion may cause retention of the menstrual flow. The first stage of the procedure is removal of the adhesion with a blade or a blunt instrument, following the line of the fusion, keeping a finger in the rectum and an in-dwelling catheter in the urethra. The areas underlying the adhesions are haemorrhagic with little or no mucosal covering. The second stage involves the prevention of refusion by placing in the vagina a prosthetic device identical to that used after the surgical treatment of vaginal aplasia. The device is changed every 8–10 days and then daily for 4–8 weeks. As epithelialization is progressing the device is worn only at night and when epithelialization is nearly complete frequent sexual intercourse or the use of a 35-mm vaginal dilator several times daily is encouraged. To prevent further adhesions the device or dilator can be coated in a topical corticosteroid. The patient should nevertheless be made aware of the risk of recurrence.

References

Berville-Levy, S., Moyal-Barracco, M. & Paniel, B.J. (1997) Fissures of the fossa navicularis: 20 cases treated by vulvo perineoplasty. In: *XIVth International Congress of the I.S.S.V.D.* Baveno, Italy, 14–18 September.

Erich, J.B. (1959) Plastic repairs of the female perineum in a case of exstrophy of the bladder. *Mayo Clinic Proceedings* 34, 235–237.

Ferry, C., Sgro, J.C. & Solente, J.J. (1977) Résection de l'organe péno-clitoridien conservant le gland avec son innervation, chez les interseés à vocation féminine—Bases anatomiques et technique opératoire. *Revue Française d'Endocrinologie Clinique, Nutrition et Métabolisme* **18**, 247–254.

Fortunoff, S.J., Lattimer, J.K. & Edson, M. (1964) Vaginoplastic technique for female pseudohermaphrodites. *Surgery, Gynecology and Obstetrics* **118**, 545–548.

Frank, R.T. (1938) Formation of an artificial vagina without operation. *American Journal of Obstetrics and Gynecology* **35**, 1053–1055.

Guillarme, P., Haddad, B., Touboul, C. & Paniel, B.J. (1995) Coalescence des petites lèvres. *Références en Gynécologie Obstétrique* 3, 245–250.

Hendren, W.H. (1977) Surgical management of urogenital sinus abnormalities. *Journal of Pediatric Surgery* **12**, 339–357.

Hodgkinson, D.J. & Hait, G. (1984) Aesthetic vaginal labioplasty. *Plastic and Reconstructive Surgery* **74**, 414–416.

Michlewitz, H. (1986) Laser ablation of hymeneal fissures. *Journal of Reproductive Medicine* **31**, 63–64.

Moyal-Barracco, M., Berville-Levy, S. & Paniel, B.J. (1997) Mechanical hymeneal fissures: 18 cases. In: *XIVth International Congress of the I.S.S.V.D.* Baveno, Italy, 14–18 September.

Paniel, B.J., Berville-Levy, S. & Moyal-Barracco, M. (1984) La vulvopérinéoplastie. *Journal de Gynécologie Obstétrique et Biologie de la Réproduction* **31**, 91–99.

Paniel, B.J. Truc, J.B., Robichez, B. & Poitout, P. (1984) Vulvo-perinéoplastie. *Presse Médicale* **13**, 1895–1898.

Paniel, B.J., Truc, J.B., Robichez, B., Malouf, A. & Poitout, P. (1985) Chirurgie des lésions bénignes de la vulve. *Encyclopédie Medicochirurgicale.* Techniques Chirurgicales Gynocologie. Elsevier, Paris, France. No. 41885.6.85.

Paniel, B.J., Haddad, B. & Meneux, E. (1996) Malformations vaginales. *Encyclopédie Medicochirurgicale.* Techniques Chirurgicales Gynocologie. Elsevier, Paris, France. No. 41855.A.

Patterson, T.J.S. & Rhodes, P. (1958) Treatment of stenosis of the vagina by a thigh flap. *Journal of Obstetrics and Gynaecology of the British Empire* **65**, 481–482.

Prader, A. (1954) Der genitalbefund beim Pseudohermaphroditismus des kongenitalen adrenogenital syndroms. Morphologie, Haüfigkeit, Entwicklung und Vererbung der verschiedenen genital formen. *Helvetica Paediatrica Acta* **9**, 231.

Scott, J.W., Gilpin, C.R. & Vence, C.A. (1963) Vulvectomy, introital stenosis and Z plasty. *American Journal of Obstetrics and Gynecology* **85**, 132–133.

Strafford, J.C. & Cleary, R.E. (1976) A simplified surgical approach to the incomplete form of testicular feminization. *Obstetrics and Gynecology* **48**, 244–245.

Wilkinson, E.J. (1971) Introital stenosis and Z plasty. *Obstetrics and Gynecology* 38, 638–640.

Chapter 12: Surgical procedures in malignant vulval disease

J.M. Monaghan

Knowledge of the malignant potential of both vulval dermatoses and vulval intraepithelial lesions has been unclear so that most surgeons have tended to use an aggressive, radical approach to surgical treatment, often resulting in unnecessary damage to the vulval architecture, which has led to significant physical and psychosexual morbidity. In recent times better categorization of vulval cancer has resulted in a more individualized approach in which the surgical treatment is more closely suited to the malignant potential of the lesion.

Consent

As with all major vulval procedures there is a possibility of mutilation. It is therefore vital that the patient and her partner fully understand the nature of the condition and the impact and extent of any treatment. The need for surveillance and possibly further treatment has to be stressed, with emphasis on the increased risk of recurrence when more conservative techniques are used.

Delineation of vulval lesions

It is important to record the skin changes graphically in the patient's records. A simple line drawing remains an excellent way of recording changes, although there are now very sophisticated techniques available, including computerized images and digital camera systems. Whatever the method, a graphic record is vital as the disease is a chronic management problem with multiple visits and treatments being the norm.

Extramammary Paget's disease

Initially, local excision with the aim of achieving disease-free margins is the usual procedure. The margins may, however, be difficult to identify because of the way in which the disease tends to extend under the epithelial surface; a margin wider than that suggested clinically will often be required to achieve a clear histological border. This problem is further discussed elsewhere (see Chapter 10). Should an underlying adenocarcinoma be found, bilateral lymphadenectomy is indicated. In the absence of such a lesion, recurrences are common but appear to be superficial, and they may be dealt with by local excisions or by non-surgical means such as topical 5-fluorouracil or bleomycin, the carbon dioxide laser or oral retinoids. In those who are unfit for surgery, radiotherapy has as role for the primary as well as for recurrent disease (Burrows *et al.* 1995).

The association with carcinomas elsewhere should be remembered, and appropriate screening procedures carried out.

Vulval intraepithelial neoplasia

Treatment options

NON-SURGICAL TECHNIQUES

Attempts to treat vulval intraepithelial neoplasia with topical cytotoxic agents and with immunotherapy, for example interferon, have been disappointing.

SURGICAL TECHNIQUES

During the last 15 years surgical treatment options have evolved as more information has become available. Initially surgical excision was the most commonly used modality. There was a vogue for laser vaporization during the 1980s; this technique was used extensively. However, it became increasingly clear that there was a significant risk of missing invasive disease as there is no final specimen for assessment of pathology. A shift back to excisional techniques has taken place, using either the knife excision or the laser as a cutting tool. In more recent times the loop diathermy has also been used to obtain excisional specimens.

Laser excision

The patient is put into the colposcopic examination position and the lesion identified and mapped. If the lesion is small it is possible to remove it in the colposcopy clinic under local anaesthesia. However, in the vast majority of cases it is more practicable to perform the procedure under general anaesthesia in a day-care unit. It is important not to drape the patient fully or to use any alcohol-based skin preparation as the fire risk is high when an open laser is employed. The carbon dioxide laser is the ideal instrument for this procedure, the smallest spot size at high power being used. In this mode the cutting ability of the laser is superb, giving a clean cut with reduced edge char and cleanly dividing vessels so as to allow them to retract and seal.

The previous mapping is checked and confirmed with a fresh application of 5% acetic acid (Fig. 12.1a). It is important to outline the lesion at this point before the acetic acid changes decline. Although a plastic surgery ink-marker may be used, the lesion is better outlined with the laser. The outline should include a margin of at least 3 mm; this is easily seen as two to three times the laser burn width (Fig. 12.1b). Once the lesion is outlined the depth of the cut can be increased, beginning at the lower margin of the lesion. As the cut is deepened the specimen edge is picked up with a skin hook or forceps (Fig. 12.2a), thus placing the subcutaneous tissues on tension and allowing the laser beam to cut rapidly through. The entire specimen is thus stripped off with considerable control of small vessel bleeding (Fig. 12.2b).

The defect that is left can then be sutured together if small (Fig. 12.3) or skin grafted as a primary step; or if it is in a difficult area, for example, round the anus, it can be left to granulate with surprisingly good results. Postoperative care consists of meticulous local cleansing (carried out by the patient) and analgesia when necessary. There is surprising variability in the amount of pain experienced.

For widespread lesions of vulval intraepithelial neoplasia, surgical management involving removal of the entire vulval skin has been devised, i.e. simple vulvectomy or skinning vulvectomy. These procedures are now rarely performed.

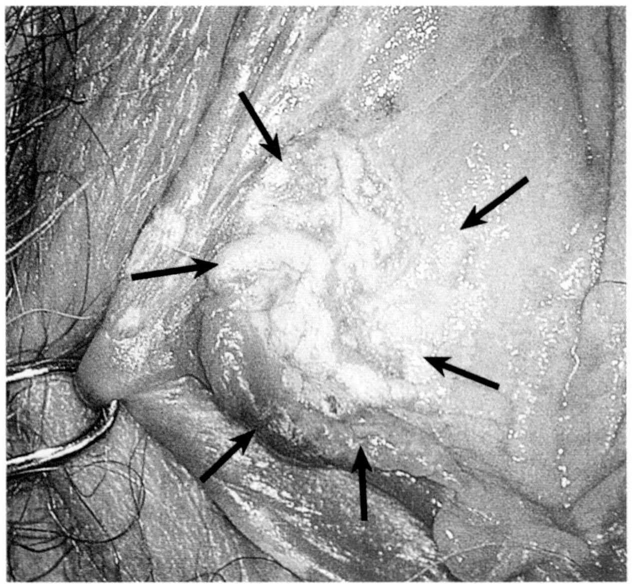

(a)

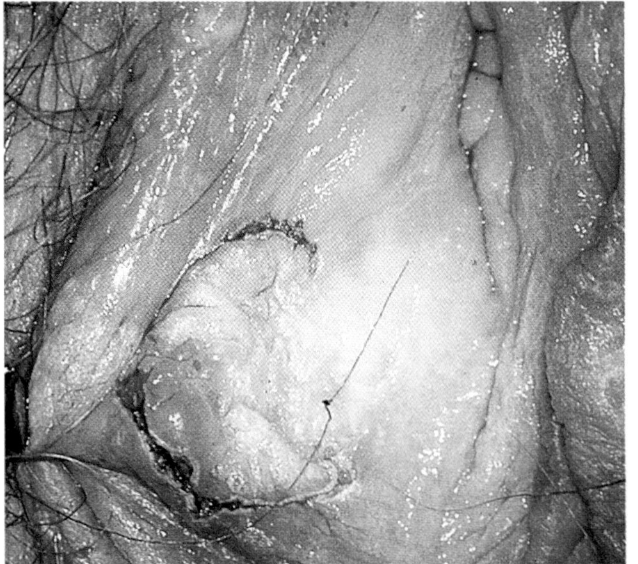

(b)

Fig. 12.1(a,b) Excision of VIN by the cutting of CO_2 laser. The technique involves the initial delineation of the affected area (see arrows).

Simple vulvectomy

The procedure is normally carried out under general anaesthesia. The patient is placed in the lithotomy position and the lesions to be removed are carefully mapped and compared with any previous mapping.

Two oval incisions are made to include the mapped area of abnormality (Fig. 12.4) but not so deep as to reach the perineal fascia. A margin of normal tissue of approximately 1 cm is necessary around the lesion. The specimen is elevated with tissue forceps and by playing the knife across the deep surface the entire skin block is removed.

Bleeding tends to occur from three main points: the clitoral area and the posterolateral parts of the vulva over the pudendal vessels. These vessels are picked up and tied or can be oversewn with a 3.0 Vicryl suture (Fig. 12.5). Good haemostasis over the whole area is important. All that is now required is for the defect to be closed using a series of interrupted 3.0 Vicryl sutures (Fig. 12.6). It is important not to hood the urethra or to generate too much tension. Usually when the patient is taken down from the lithotomy position there is little tension in the wound. Catheterization of the bladder is maintained for the first 3 days postopera-

(a)
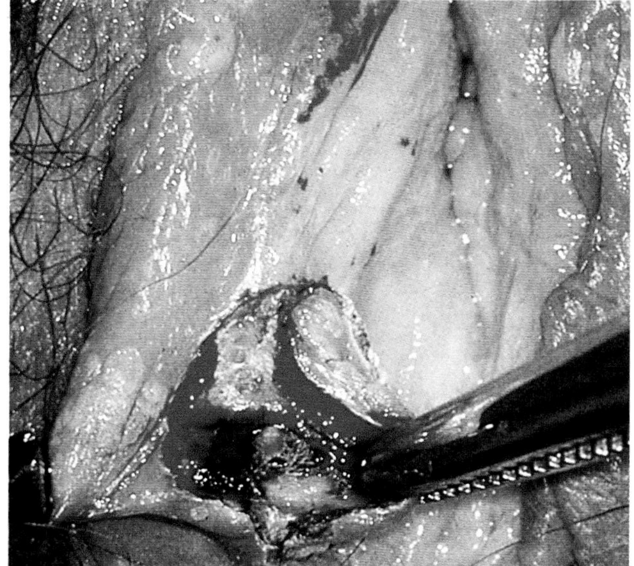

(b)
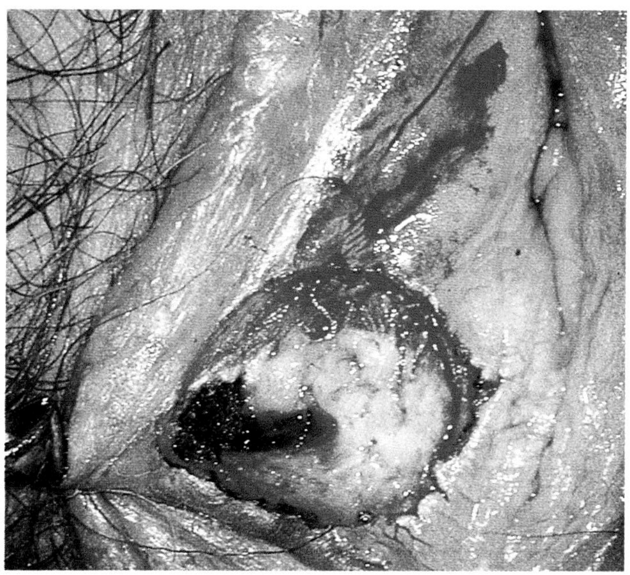

Fig. 12.2(a,b) The incision is then deepened to about 2.5 mm to allow the epidermis and dermis to be undercut.

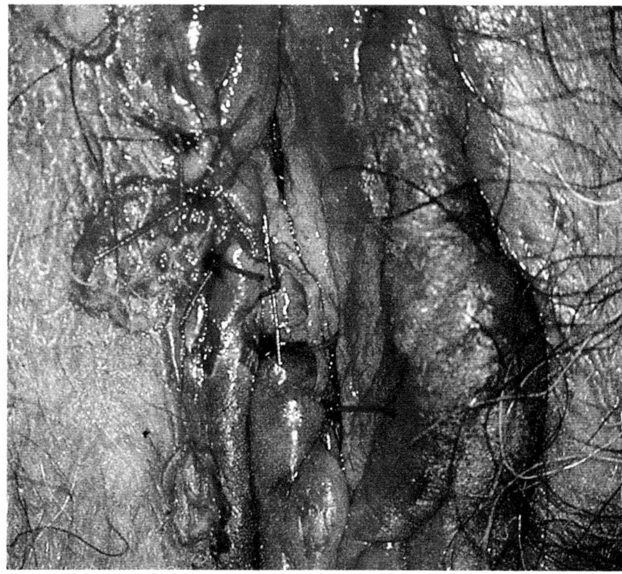

Fig. 12.3 The undercutting process shown has resulted in the small area of VIN being removed, and the edges of the wound can be approximated with fine, absorbable sutures.

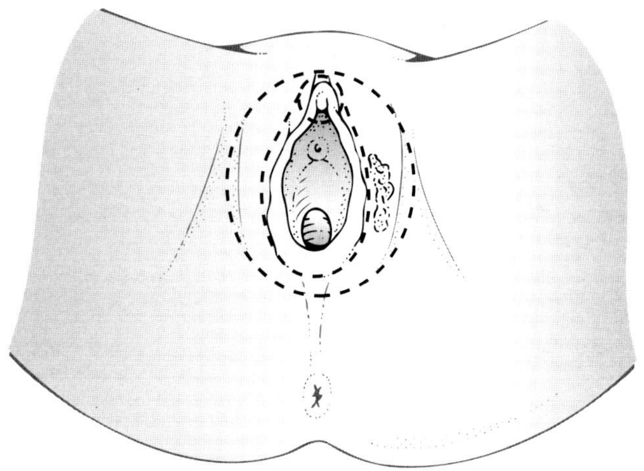

Fig. 12.4 Simple vulvectomy. Two oval incisions are made preserving the clitoris where possible.

tively so as to keep the area clean and dry. Healing is remarkably rapid with an excellent cosmetic result.

Skinning vulvectomy

This procedure will allow maintenance of some vulval structures and facilitates preservation of the clitoris when this is indicated. The procedure is similar to simple vulvectomy apart from the fact that only the skin is removed (Fig. 12.7). The defect can be filled with a skin graft from the thigh or buttock (Fig. 12.8). Although this procedure appears attractive, the author's experience is that the skin quality is poor and there may be recurrence of the disease in the graft (Cox *et al.* 1986).

Local surgical excision

A small lesion can be removed using simple knife surgical excision with little tissue loss. The skin on the vulva is commonly loose and easily moved to repair small defects. Multiple small excisions are feasible, and preferable to vulvectomy in young women.

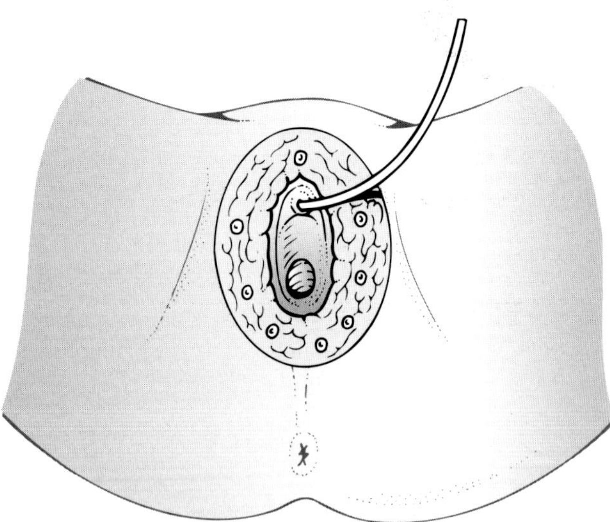

Fig. 12.5 Simple vulvectomy. Vessels being oversewn with a 3.0 Vicryl suture.

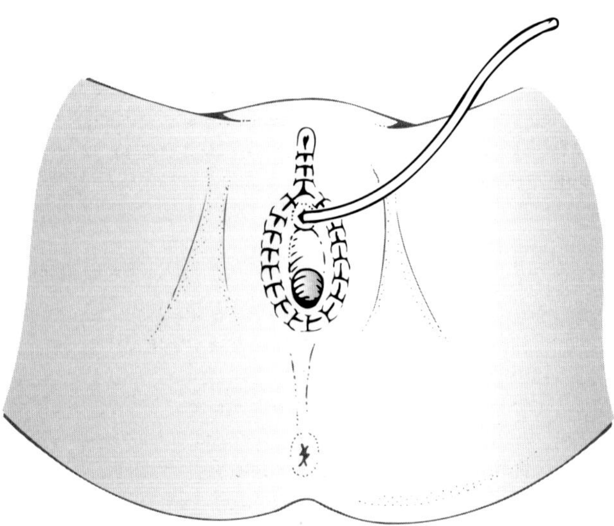

Fig. 12.6 Simple vulvectomy. Series of interrupted 3.00 Vicryl sutures.

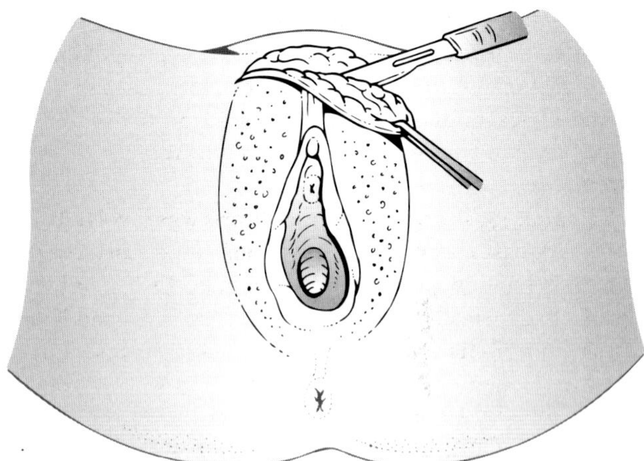

Fig. 12.7 Skinning vulvectomy. Removal of skin.

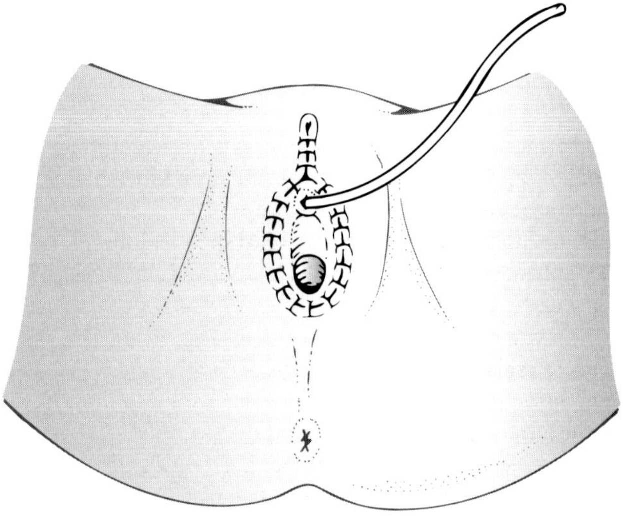

Fig. 12.8 Skinning vulvectomy. The defect can be filled with a skin graft from the thigh or buttocks.

Squamous cell carcinoma

Vulval carcinoma is rare, representing 4–5% of genital cancers. It is a problem mainly affecting the elderly, the average age at presentation being in the late seventh decade; however, the age range is wide and it can be seen at a much earlier time of life.

Surgical anatomy and routes of spread

SITE OF TUMOUR AND LYMPHATIC DRAINAGE

Most carcinomas of the vulva affect the labia majora and minora, on the left side slightly more often than the right; and the second commonest single site is the clitoris.

The clitoris

It has been thought that carcinomas affecting the clitoris require more aggressive management. Its lymphatics were said to communicate directly with the pelvic lymphatics (Parry-Jones 1963) but this direct communication has never been satisfactorily demonstrated. Iversen and Aas (1983) did not find any evidence of such communication. They demonstrated the frequent bilateral flow of the clitoral lymphatics and evidence of contralateral flow alone from laterally placed injection of radionucleide (technetium) in the labia (in 28 of 42 or 67% of cases). They did not demonstrate higher lymph flow rates from any particular part of the vulva. However, care must be used in interpreting this work as they studied patients suffering from carcinoma of the cervix and no allowance could be made for any disturbance of lymphatic drainage in the presence of vulval carcinoma.

In the author's earlier series the clitoris was involved in 54 out of 200 cases, 47 of whom had nodal dissection. Twenty-five (53%) had metastases to the groin nodes but only two (4.2%) had metastases to the pelvic nodes. Piver and Xynos (1983) in a similarly sized series came to the same conclusion. Andreasson and Nyboe (1985) consider that the clitoris is a high-risk site, giving a poorer overall prognosis, but the author feels that the pelvic nodes should not be routinely dissected simply because the clitoris or any other particular site on the vulva is involved.

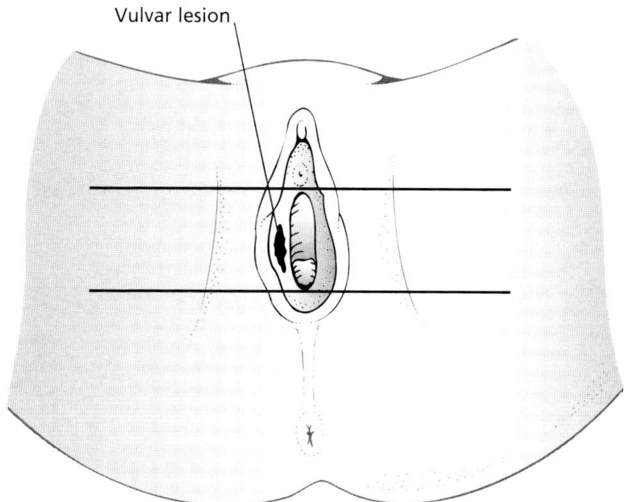

Fig. 12.9 A simple technique for defining lateral lesions.

Laterality

It has been proposed that, when stage Ib vulval carcinoma (see Table 10.1, p. 245) affects the labia alone, and does not impinge on the clitoris, urethra, vagina, fourchette or perianal region, it may be reasonable to carry out a local excision or vulvectomy plus an ipsilateral groin node dissection, the contralateral nodes being preserved. This proposal is based on the belief that contralateral spread alone and bilateral spread from a laterally placed tumour is extremely rare. Hacker *et al.* (1984) had never seen positive contralateral nodes with negative ipsilateral nodes. They also argued that if ipsilateral nodes are found to be negative then a contralateral dissection is unnecessary. In an analysis of 296 patients in the author's series it was found that, of 71 stage Ib carcinomas where the groin nodes had been dissected, in the 40 patients where the tumour was laterally placed, only six (14%) patients had positive nodes. Five of the six patients had positive nodes that were on the same side as the carcinoma. Thus, this particular group may well benefit from a more limited approach. It is of interest that contralateral spread alone, and bilateral spread, did occur in those carcinomas which affected midline structures and in stage II and III disease, as was found by Hoffman *et al.* (1985).

Definition of lateral tumours. It may be difficult for the clinician to be certain of identifying a tumour that is truly lateral and can therefore be treated using the more conservative approach mentioned above. The author would recommend the following simple technique, which can be used for all patients. If a horizontal line is drawn through the lower border of the urethra and through the upper border of the fourchette then any tumour lying between these two lines can be regarded as 'lateral' and treated more conservatively (Fig. 12.9).

If the vulva is extensively involved by vulval intraepithelial neoplasia a limited resection would clearly have a high risk of recurrence, so when using more conservative incisions due attention must be paid to the remaining vulval skin with appropriate biopsies being taken. Normally a margin of 1 cm is acceptable for preinvasive disease.

Lymph node metastases

The main cause of failure of treatment of cancer of the vulva is inability to control lymphatic and distant metastases. Control of local disease is relatively simple. Detailed knowledge of the lymphatic drainage and anatomy of the regional lymph nodes is essential if the diagnosis and treatment of vulval carcinoma are to be improved (Fig. 12.10).

Most cancers of the vulva are well-differentiated squamous tumours with a slow growth pattern, local invasion and superficial spread being common. Lymphatic spread occurs in approximately 30–40% of patients and is primarily to the inguinal lymphatics and then sequentially to the pelvic lymphatics. Blood-borne spread is extremely rare. It is almost superfluous to spend time identifying nodal metastases preoperatively as with very few exceptions the nodes must be removed as an integral part of treatment. Gross involvement can be identified but micrometastases are undiagnosable preoperatively and if not removed are potentially lethal.

PREOPERATIVE IDENTIFICATION OF LYMPHATIC SPREAD AND NODAL INVOLVEMENT

The techniques available to the clinician for preoperatively diagnosing metastatic disease include the following.

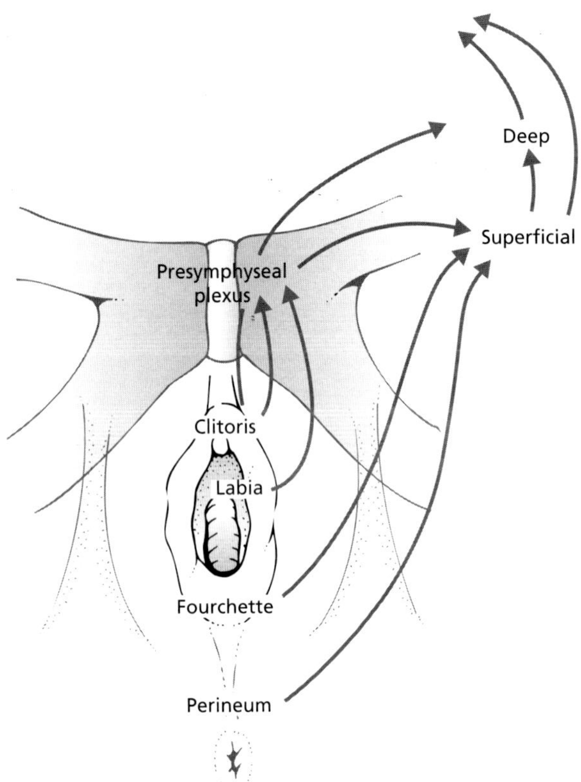

Fig. 12.10 General schematic representation of the major drainage channels of the vulva. Lymphatics and regional nodes of perineum, fourchette and labia are located within the subcutaneous fatty tissue of the vulva, mons veneris and femoral triangle.

Palpation

This method of assessment is notoriously inaccurate, with error rates of 13 to 39% (Benedet *et al.* 1979, Monaghan 1985).

Computed axial tomography scan

This non-invasive technique has a relatively high false-positive and false-negative rate plus an unacceptably high limit of resolution. The method is reasonably accurate in the para-aortic region but is unacceptably inaccurate in the pelvis and groin.

Magnetic resonance imaging

This technique, again non-invasive, has a possible place in diagnosis, as recently modifications using tissue subtraction techniques have shown great promise in being able to differentiate cancer tissue from normal, opening the way to identifying metastatic cancer at an early stage. Unfortunately the facility is not widely available because of its high capital cost.

Ultrasound

The effectiveness of groin ultrasound in both identifying nodes and differentiating between positive and negative nodes has been demonstrated and is currently being explored in trials.

Lymphangiography

Many authorities have shown the value of this technique. However, an equal number have highlighted the pitfalls of the method, which can include the difficulties of identifying micrometastases, and the equivocal value of the lymphogram because of fatty infiltration and hyperplasia. Very high levels of skill and experience are required to make this technique of value to the clinician.

Fine needle aspiration

Fine needle aspiration of lymph nodes or suspicious areas is a frequently used technique, often saving major operative procedures or biopsies and commonly modifying management (McDonald *et al.* 1983, Fortier *et al.* 1985). The morbidity is low even in potentially dangerous areas such as the posterior thorax. False positives are virtually nil. The specificity of the investigation is close to 100% and the sensitivity may reach 90%. Open biopsy can now be restricted to those patients with negative or unsatisfactory results.

Thus, preoperative assessment of groin node status remains unsatisfactory, and at present it is recommended that a complete groin node dissection should be performed for all invasive disease except in the case of an International Society for the Study of Vulvovaginal Disease (ISSVD) stage Ia lesion (see Table 10.1, p. 245). This has been defined by the ISSVD and accepted by FIGO as a lesion of the vulva measuring less than 2 cm in diameter with a depth of invasion of less than 1 mm (see Chapter 10). Multiple sites are excluded from this definition. The general consensus is that wide local excision is satisfactory in this category.

Intraoperative sampling of lymph nodes has been used to determine whether to proceed to removal of deep inguinal nodes, or to carry out pelvic node dissection. Curry *et al.* (1980) stated that where four or more nodes were involved in the groin then pelvic node dissection should be carried out. DiSaia *et al.* (1979) have recommended dissection of the superficial nodes initially, removing a sentinel node and performing frozen sections. If the node demonstrates metastases then the remainder of the groin dissection should be performed. More recently Levenback *et al.* (1994) have shown a neat technique for identification of the 'sentinel' node using an injection of vital blue dye into the leading edge of the tumour. Dissection of the groin then allows identification of the 'blue' node and a decision as to the extent of surgery can be made on the basis of frozen section examination of this node. A preliminary experience with this method has shown it to be of considerable interest, although there are circumstances where the node is not readily identified, for example where an excision biopsy has been performed prior to definitive surgery. In an extended experience the same group, has indicated that the 'blue' node can be found in a wide variety of sites including the deep inguinal region (Levenback *et al.* 1995). The degree of involvement of the groin nodes by metastases will determine further action.

Plan of management

From the information now available it is clear that a high degree of individualization of management can be achieved for patients with carcinoma of the vulva. The most important principle to be followed is to apply the *principle of adequate margins*, which must include not only the lateral margins but also the medial margins, particularly where the cancer arises close to the urethra, vagina or anus. The author proposes the following methods of management.

Patients with stage Ia carcinoma (see above) may be treated with wide local excision alone. For those with a stage Ib tumour, a radical vulvectomy with bilateral groin node dissection may be performed through separate incisions. Where the tumour is laterally placed and there is no significant pre-invasive skin change a wide local excision of the tumour on the vulva combined with an ipsilateral groin node dissection is appropriate. The margins should be as close to 2 cm as possible.

For later-stage disease with carcinomas up to 4 cm in diameter, a radical vulvectomy and bilateral groin node dissection through either separate incisions or a 'butterfly' incision should be carried out, making certain that the cancer is completely encompassed with a 2-cm-wide margin of the normal tissue. For carcinomas greater than 4 cm in diameter or where there are clinically involved groin nodes, a pelvic node dissection may be added to the groin node dissection and the groins should be dissected *en bloc* in direct continuity with the radical vulvectomy, emptying a 'butterfly' incision. Radiotherapy to the groin and pelvic nodal areas following radical vulvectomy and groin dissection may be used as an alternative to pelvic node dissection where three or more groin nodes are involved.

Where the cancer extends to involve the anus or lower rectum an anovulvectomy with colostomy or a posterior exenteration should be performed together with groin and pelvic node dissection (Grimshaw *et al.* 1991).

The radical surgical management of cancer of the vulva should be carried out in centres with considerable surgical, anaesthetic and nursing experience of the disease. This multidisciplinary approach will result in high feasibility of operation (96.8% of patients in the author's series, personal series), and excellent long-term survivals. In a series of 575 cases the author had an overall actuarial five-year survival of 72%, with an operative mortality of 2%. When the groin nodes were negative this increased to 94.7%; it fell to 62% when they were positive, with an operative mortality of 2%.

Patient preparation

The patient should be admitted 1–2 days prior to surgery depending on the size of the tumour for optimal preparation of the site. A longer preoperative period increases the risk of developing thromboembolic disease.

Thromboembolic prophylaxis

These patients are at a very high risk of developing thromboembolic disease, as they are often old, obese and may have degenerative diseases of the cardiovascular, respiratory and joint systems; they often already have major difficulties in mobility. The author chooses low-dose subcutaneous heparin (5000 units twice a day). The modern fractionated heparin used as a single daily dose has proved of great value in high-risk patients. Antithromboembolic stockings and intraoperative muscle pumps are of value. However, early mobilization following the operation remains the cornerstone of efforts to reduce thromboembolic risks.

Prophylactic antibiotics

In general, wound infections can be reduced for all surgery if intraoperative prophylactic antibiotics are used. Any allergies should be noted and an appropriate antibiotic regimen employed. A single intravenous dose of a broad-spectrum antibiotic may be given during the induction of anaesthesia.

It is helpful to the surgeon if radical surgery is performed under either a spinal or an epidural anaesthetic. The advantages are twofold. Firstly, small-vessel oozing is reduced with a concomitant reduction in intraoperative blood loss. Secondly, the patient requires either minimal general anaesthesia or none, which is of particular benefit when the patient is frail. However, some anaesthetists prefer to use hypotensive techniques, which are also acceptable.

Lymphadenectomy

The patient is positioned lying supine with the feet approximately 25 cm apart and supported by an ankle rest to elevate the calves from the table. Some authorities recommend the 'ski' position (Symmonds & Webb 1981) so that two and even three teams can operate simultaneously; in the author's view this is a recipe for confusion and does not significantly speed up the operation. A partial Trendelenburg position is sometimes necessary to facilitate access to the groins, especially if the patient is overweight.

THE SKIN INCISION

Over the years the original 'butterfly' skin incisions have been modified in many ways, the aim being to remove less skin. In some centres a linear incision in the groin is recommended. However, the author continues to remove a narrow (1 cm wide) band of skin as this can be grasped with tissue forceps and the entire block of nodes manipulated with ease. If a tissue forceps is applied to fat after using a linear incision the forceps tends to 'cut through'.

It is important to utilize bony landmarks and to ignore natural skin folds, which may be very variable, particularly in obese patients.

The initial incision curving down towards the groin is made from the inferior aspect of the anterior superior iliac spine to a midpoint low over the symphysis pubis, followed by an incision from the anterior superior iliac spine to a point 4 cm below the pubic tubercle with a curve towards the groin fold. A third incision is now made from this last point curving upwards and medially to terminate close to the crural fold (Fig. 12.11). In recent years the author has tended to dispense with the short third incision and to take out a narrow (1-cm) band of skin made with two slightly curving lines. The skin removed from the groin will be minimal, a narrow band less than 1 cm wide, with a narrow releasing incision over the line of the upper part of the saphenous vein.

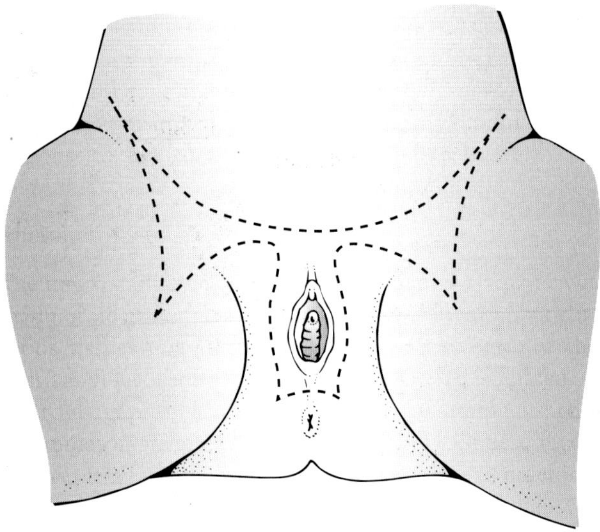

Fig. 12.11 The 'butterfly' incision.

DEFINING THE FASCIAL PLANES IN THE LOWER AND UPPER INCISIONS

The band of skin in the groin is picked up using a Lane's tissue forceps so that the whole block of tissue in the groin can be manoeuvred during the dissection. By putting slight tension with the left hand on the upper edge of the skin incision undercutting can be achieved down to the aponeurosis of the external oblique muscle above the groin. The fascia over the sartorius muscle, which forms the lateral boundary of the femoral triangle, can now be identified in a similar manner. This fascia is now incised longitudinally from the anterior superior iliac spine to the apex of the femoral triangle (Fig. 12.12). Small arteries and veins in the fat and muscle surfaces will be cut during these incisions; they should be meticulously identified, and ligated or diathermied.

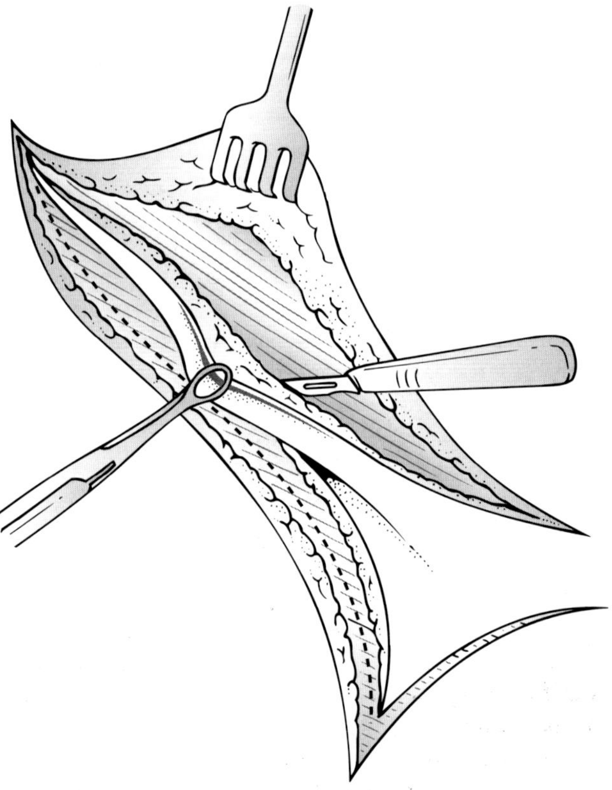

Fig. 12.12 Incising the fat and fascia down to the external oblique aponeurosis and the sartorius muscle.

DIVIDING THE SAPHENOUS VEIN

The saphenous vein is identified in the lower part of the releasing incision. It is isolated where it lies above the fascia lata. It is then divided and ligated at the apex of the releasing incision. At this point the dissection can be deepened down to the fascia over the adductor muscles. The fascia is incised transversely medial to the femoral artery (Fig. 12.13). The medial edge of the incised fascia covering the sartorius muscle is now picked up using two small Spencer Wells clips, and elevated (Fig. 12.14). The strands of the nerve which can now be seen in the soft tissue at the medial side of the sartorius muscle are the branches of the femoral and the genitofemoral nerves. Some of these fibres are now cut as the femoral artery is defined by incising the fascia of the lateral wall of the femoral sheath. The artery should be meticulously cleared from the apex of the femoral triangle to the inguinal ligament. The condensation of fascia lateral to the artery along the inguinal ligament is divided with scissors to leave the external oblique aponeurosis clean.

REMOVING THE GROIN NODES FROM THE FEMORAL VESSELS

As the fascia that forms the femoral sheath is elevated, the artery can be cleared. On the medial side of the femoral artery the femoral vein can be seen; it is cleared from the inguinal ligament distally. The saphenous vein can now be isolated as it enters the femoral vein. When the fascia is lifted and rotated medially by the assistant it has the effect of opening the saphenous opening (the fossa ovalis). The loose cribriform fascia that fills the fossa can be separated and the edges of the opening defined. The saphenous vein is now clamped, cut and ligated as it enters the femoral vein (Fig. 12.15). Thus, by elevating this fascia all nodes and lymphatic tissue lying above the fascia will be automatically removed.

CLEARING THE ADDUCTOR MUSCLES

The whole block of tissue containing the groin nodes is turned medially. On the medial side of the femoral vein the fascia over the adductor muscles is incised longitudinally as close to the vein as possible. Small veins that enter the muscles may require ligating at this point. The releasing incision at the apex of the femoral triangle is now joined and the fascia is stripped from the adductor muscles as far

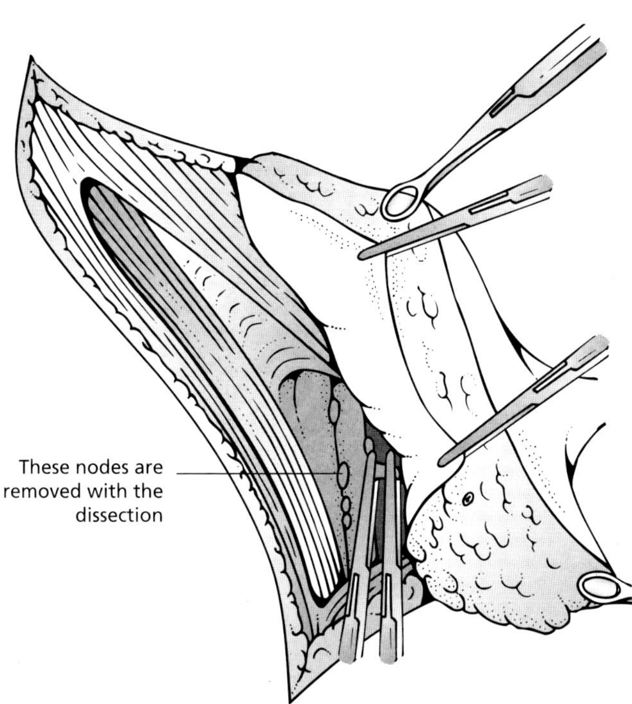

Fig. 12.13 Division of the saphenous vein is carried out in the lower part of the incision which is then carried down onto the fascia over the adductor muscles, which is also divided. This completes the dissection down to the fascia over the external oblique muscles superiorly, the sartorius muscle laterally and the adductor muscles inferomedially.

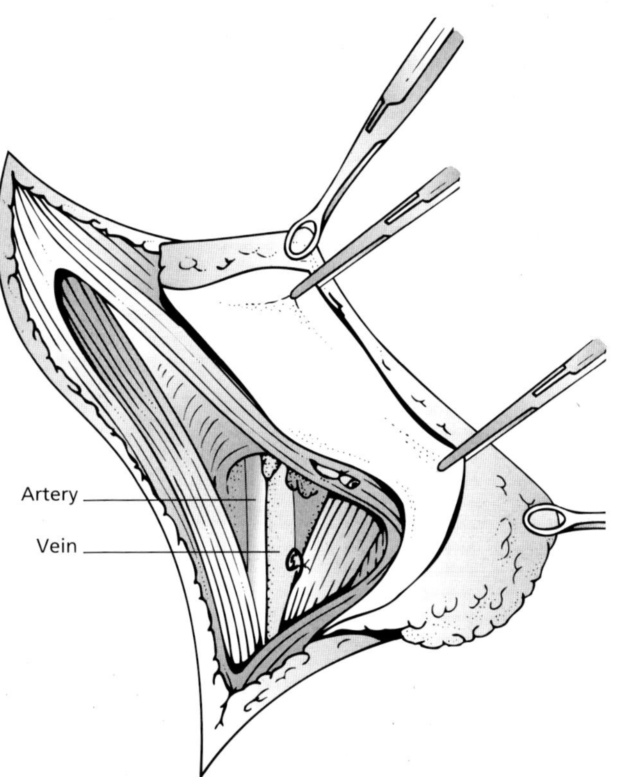

Fig. 12.14 The medial edge of the sartorius fascia is elevated by forceps and drawn medially. This allows the block of tissue containing the lymph nodes to be lifted and dissected from the blood vessels which are lying on the medical side of the sartorius muscle.

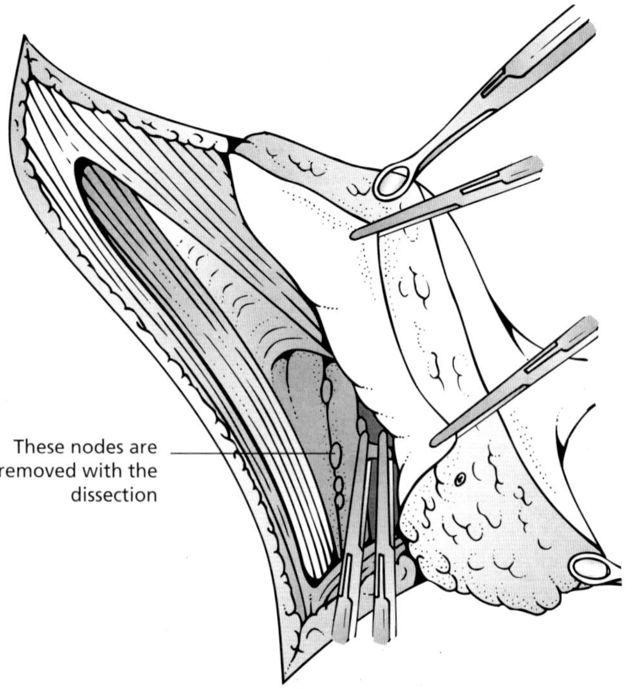

Fig. 12.15 The block of tissue overlying the sartorius fascia is elevated. The femoral artery has been cleaned and the femoral vein exposed. At this point the fossa ovale is visible through which the saphenous vein descends into the femoral vein. The deep femoral nodes which lay close to the fossa ovale can be dissected free and elevated with the block of tissue.

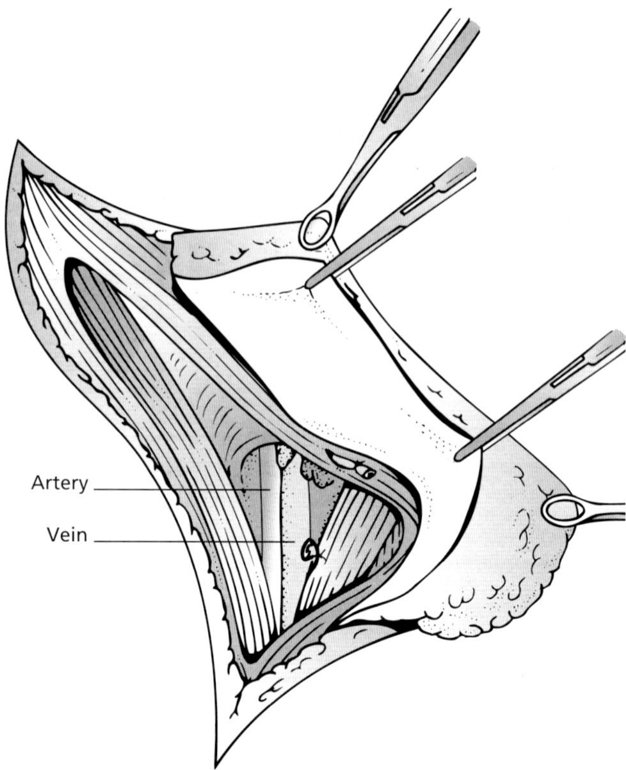

Fig. 12.16 The entire groin contents are elevated and the round ligament is clamped and divided.

medially as the gracilis tendon aponeurosis. In the upper part of this dissection the round ligament is picked up, divided and ligated as it leaves the inguinal canal (Fig. 12.16). The subfascial dissection is then completed through to the pubic symphysis. The entire groin nodes have been removed *en bloc*.

PELVIC NODE DISSECTION

The indications for removing the pelvic nodes are relatively rare. There is a possible case for routine removal in association with large tumours (>4 cm in diameter), but there is a clear indication where the groin nodes are heavily involved and there is evidence of the tumour spreading directly through the femoral canal into the pelvis. This latter indication is a development of the principle of achieving complete margins around the tumour.

If the pelvic nodes are to be dissected they may now be approached by incising through the external oblique muscle approximately 2 cm above the inguinal ligament, beginning above the femoral canal and extending superolaterally for 8 cm (Fig. 12.17). The internal oblique is then incised along the line of its fibres exposing the transversalis fascia and

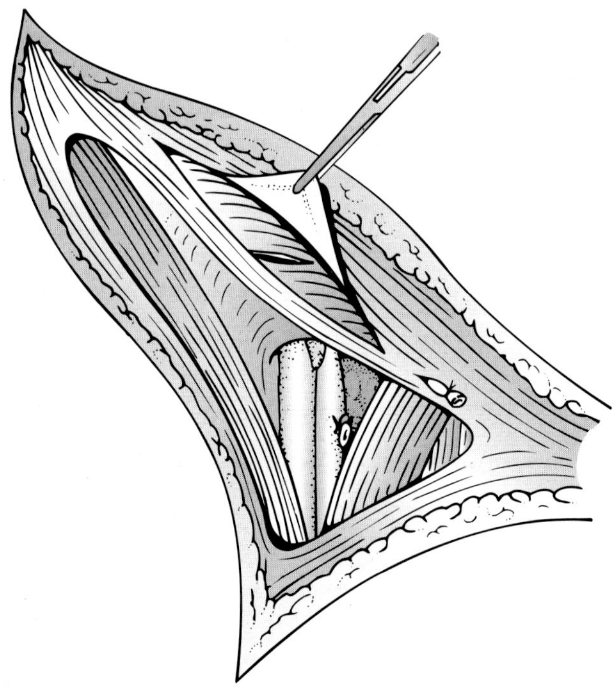

Fig. 12.17 The external oblique aponeurosis is incised superolaterally.

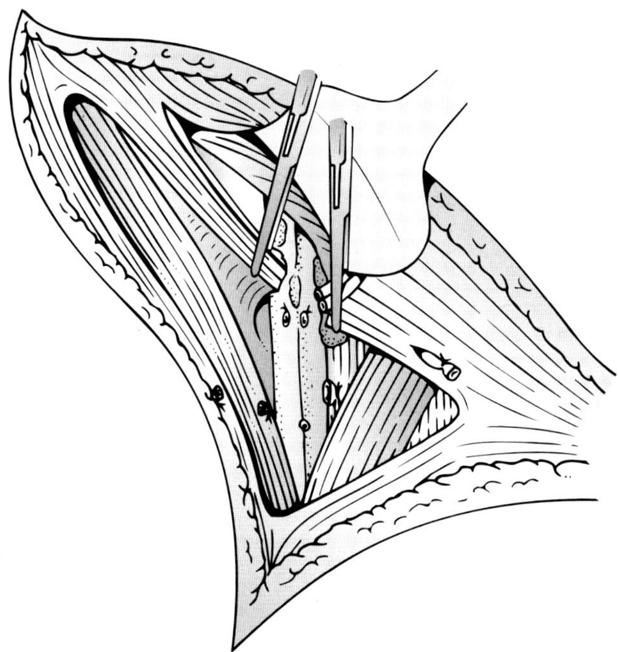

Fig. 12.18 Once the saphenous vein has been divided and ligated close to the femoral vein the fascia can then be dissected free from above the adductor muscles elevating the entire block of tissue and lymph nodes. The final manoeuvre in this dissection is to divide the round ligament at the medial margin of the wound and the whole block of tissue can be removed intact.

peritoneum. Using the fingers the peritoneum is swept from the outer pelvis, exposing the external iliac vessels. The exposure is completed by extending the medial end of the wound down to the femoral canal, applying a large Spencer Wells clip to the inferior epigastric arteries (Fig. 12.18). Through this incision the external iliac vessels can be cleared of nodes up as far as the common iliac vessels, and in direct continuity with the groin node dissection. Although Cloquet's node is said to be constant, the lateral medial external iliac nodes are a more regular feature.

CLOSURE OF THE ABDOMINAL WALL AND INGUINAL LIGAMENT DEFECT

This is achieved by a continuous Dexon or Vicryl suture, beginning with the internal oblique muscles at the medial end of the incision over the femoral canal, travelling laterally, and then returning to the medial end, completing the closure of the external oblique muscles. At this point the femoral canal is reconstructed by suturing the medial part of the external oblique incision to the fascia of the pectineal line, so that the femoral canal admits a fingertip and pressure is not put on the femoral vein.

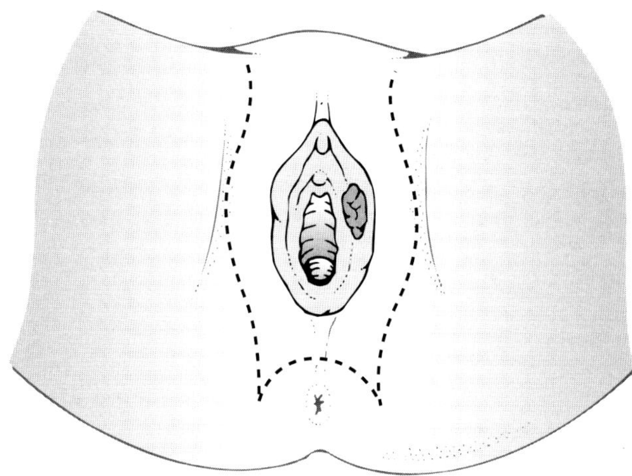

Fig. 12.19 Medial incisions for radical vulvectomy.

DRAINAGE OF THE GROIN AND CLOSURE OF THE SKIN INCISION

Drainage of the space left in the groin is mandatory as up to 300 ml of fluid can collect on each side per day; drainage is carried out by either vacuum or low-pressure continuous-suction drainage through large-diameter drains. Using the modern narrow skin and releasing incisions, closure of the skin presents no problems and can be carried out without tension either using interrupted Dexon, or skin staples for extra speed. The fascia is drawn together with a continuous fine 3.0 Vicryl suture, reducing tension on the skin staples and assisting in achieving an airtight closure. The author feels that the old practice of a sartorius muscle transplant to cover the femoral vessels is not necessary, as the risk of disruption appears to be more theoretical than real.

A similar procedure is now performed on the opposite side.

Radical vulvectomy

The patient is now placed in the lithotomy position. The vulval incision must be varied according to the size and position of the cancer. The basic principle of removal is that a wide margin of normal skin surrounding the cancer must be removed. A margin of 2 cm will markedly reduce the risk of local recurrence. The margin must be adequate both laterally and medially. It is very tempting to pass very close to a cancer that lies close to the urethra or anus. It is in these circumstances that a desire to preserve such structures will increase the risk of local recurrence.

The incision that was carried into the crural fold is now extended inferiorly lateral to the vulva to end alongside the anus, the anus is skirted by a curved incision (Fig. 12.19), and a similar incision is made on the opposite side. The

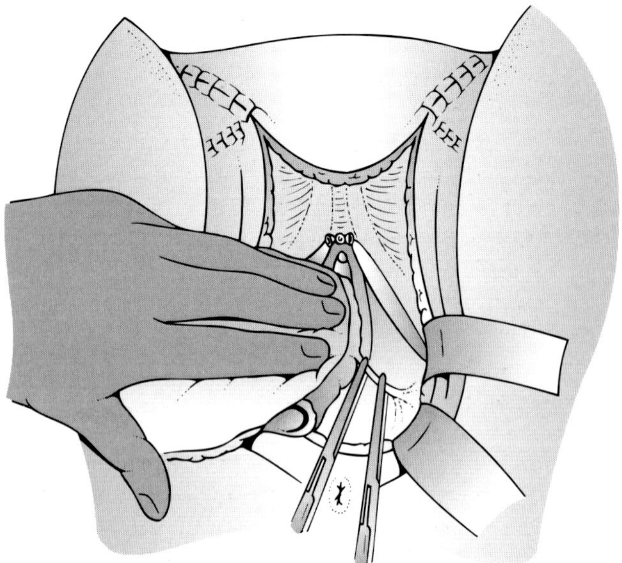

Fig. 12.20 The three main bleeding points on the vulva are best taken care of with square mattress sutures.

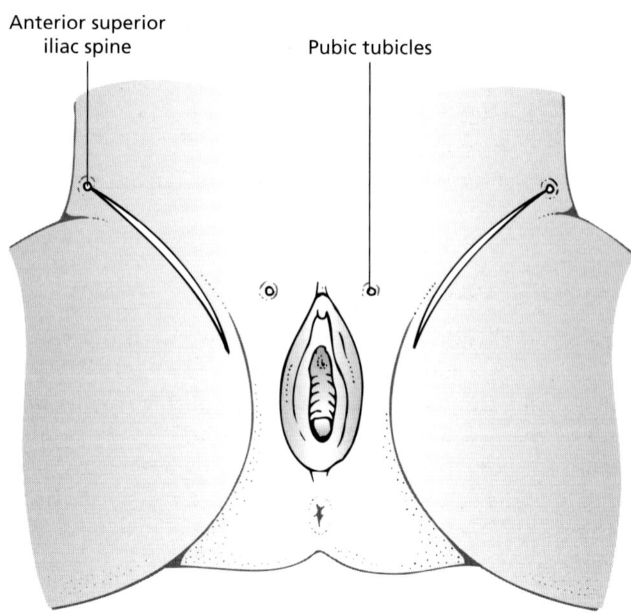

Fig. 12.22 The incision used in the 'triple incision' technique.

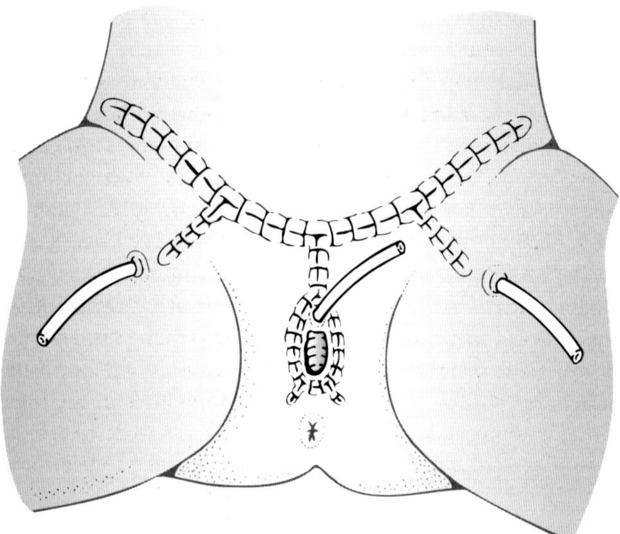

Fig. 12.21 Completed closure of the vulvar wounds.

urethra and vagina are now encircled by the inner incision. If the lesion extends close to the urethra it may be necessary to remove the lower half of it.

The lateral incisions are now extended down to the deep fascia and periosteum, and the entire vulva is removed. Free bleeding occurs at this stage from three main sites: the ends of the two internal pudendal arteries, and the vascular erectile tissue around the base of the clitoris (Fig. 12.20). Square mattress sutures are of great value in dealing with these bleeding points.

Primary closure of these wounds is easily achieved (Fig. 12.21), and the patient leaves the theatre lying flat with suction drains in the groins and a three-way catheter in the bladder.

Variations in technique

It has been suggested for many years that it may be possible to carry out this operation without the need for continuity of tissue between the vulva and groin. Indeed Stoeckel (1930) in some of his early writings commented on the use of separate incisions, as did Bassett (1912). If early carcinoma of the vulva spreads by lymphatic embolization and not by permeation of the lymphatic channels, it is reasonable to perform separate groin node incisions. Since 1985 the author has been using a three-incision technique (Grimshaw *et al.* 1993). The lines of incision are shown in Fig. 12.22. The technique is very simply performed giving the same access to the groins as the 'butterfly' incision. The groin dissection is performed as described above and the dissection is completed by removing the block of tissue at the point where the round ligament appears from the inguinal canal.

The skin may be closed as a Y, or, more recently, by flattening the incision by a straight line closure, using a Vicryl suture to bring the midpoints together, the remainder being apposed using a stapling device. If the skin to be removed is kept to a minimum then the arrow-shaped incision can be closed as a single line. A subcutaneous 3.0 Vicryl suture is also used as described for closure of the 'butterfly' incision.

There is no tension in the wounds and the primary healing rate is excellent. Drainage of the space is essential. It is often found that the wounds are completely healed before drainage has diminished. In these circumstances the patient may have a small lymphatic fistula or develop a tense femoro-inguinal lymphocyst before drainage ceases.

Postoperative care

The epidural catheter is removed at the end of the procedure and the patient is then started on subcutaneous heparin 5000 units twice a day for 10 days or until she is fully mobilized. She is encouraged to begin active movements at a very early stage, i.e. usually on day 2 or 3. It is probably this factor as much as the subcutaneous heparin or antiembolism stockings which has contributed to the reduction of thromboembolic disease in the postoperative period.

Prophylactic antibiotics are not routinely used to supplement the intraoperative regimen, although they should be rapidly prescribed if there is any sign of systemic infection.

Primary healing is now achieved in over 85% of patients. Wound breakdown, however, is still the major complication, and should be treated by meticulous local cleansing with Eusol and hydrogen peroxide. Wound healing after breakdown can be promoted by the use of honey dressings and artificial seawater baths. Silastic foam dressings improved the healing rate after wound breakdown but have been removed from the market because of toxicity risks.

Leg oedema is a frequent problem, which may arise in the postoperative period or may develop slowly in the months following operation. It is more frequently found following groin infection, particularly when associated with cellulitis of the thigh. It is important that any lymphangitis be actively treated with antibiotics. For the patient with established oedema, exercises, massage (both manual and mechanical), appropriate compression stockings and elevation will help to reduce the problem.

Osteitis pubis can be a seriously debilitating complication. In the author's series, four patients out of 515 developed the problem. It is characterized by intense pubic pain, particularly on weight bearing or walking. Often an X-ray and bone scan may not show any evidence of bone damage for a long period after the symptoms begin. The diagnosis should be made on clinical grounds and the patient started on long-term antibiotics suitable for bony infections.

Occasionally, hernias in the groin, especially after pelvic node dissection, and prolapse of the vagina may occur and will require surgical correction.

Radiotherapy for cancer of the vulva

For many decades radiotherapy has struggled to be recognized as a therapeutic modality for cancer of the vulva. A major problem has been the technical difficulties of delivering an effective dose to the vulva and perineum without seriously damaging surrounding skin and causing long-term sequelae. It is now generally accepted that radiation has a small but well-defined role in the following circumstances:

1 as a primary treatment of tumours affecting the anus and urethra with the option of surgical resection and sphincter preservation (Boronow 1973, 1982);
2 as adjunctive therapy for patients with three or more positive groin lymph nodes or where a single node is totally replaced, or there is capsular rupture (Paladini *et al.* 1994);
3 as a brachytherapy technique using implants for small recurrences, particularly around the urethra and anus;
4 as a palliative for the treatment of fungating inoperable tumour;
5 as neo-adjuvant therapy with chemotherapy in a trial situation.

The clearest role for radiotherapy in the treatment of cancer of the vulva is in the adjuvant setting for the patient with involved groin nodes. However, recent work by McCall *et al.* (1995) has highlighted a significant factor that must be taken into account when planning groin and pelvic node radiation fields. They have demonstrated the remarkable variation in the depth of the groin nodes from the skin surface. Traditionally the standard depth of 3 cm is taken when calculating dosages in the groin. These workers showed that the probable reason for the high groin failure rate noted in Gynecologic Oncology Group Protocol #88 was that only 18% of women had all inguinal lymph nodes measured at a depth of 3 cm. More than half of all women in this study would have received less than 60% of the prescribed radiation dose because their nodes were deeper than 5 cm. This valuable reminder has important implications also for the use of radiation as an adjunct to surgery as advocated by Holmsley *et al.* (1986). Clearly, for those patients receiving radiation after removal of the lymph nodes, landmarks such as the femoral vessels would need to be identified in order to maximize the effectiveness of the adjunctive therapy.

Malignant melanoma

The evolution of views on treatment has been fully examined by Dunton *et al.* (1995). Until the early 1980s the standard treatment for malignant melanoma was radical vulvectomy and bilateral inguinal lymphadenectomy regardless of individual features of the tumour. Since then, because of poor survival rates and a realization that melanoma might more logically be treated as it now is on the rest of the skin, the tendency has been to plan treatment with regard to its size, using as criteria the Clark, Chung or Breslow systems. The emphasis is on excision with adequate margins, and there seems no advantage in achieving margins of more than 3 cm, no matter what the size of the lesion. The role of elective lymphadenectomy continues to be debated but in general it is recommended with melanomas of more than 0.75 mm thickness. New techniques to detect clinically occult metastases in the glands are likely to prove of value. As with melanoma elsewhere, the place of adjuvant therapy and immunotherapy is being explored.

Micrographically controlled excision of small vulval tumours

This technique may have a useful place in management of sected vulval tumours, for example basal cell carcinoma, giving good clinical and aesthetic results (Brown *et al.* 1988). It is known that basal cell carcinomas are sometimes difficult to remove adequately by orthodox local excision (Stiller *et al.* 1993).

References

Andreasson, B. & Nyboe, J. (1985) Value of prognostic parameters in squamous cell carcinoma of the vulva. *Gynecologic Oncology* **22**, 341–351.

Bassett, A. (1912) Traitement chirurgical opératoire de l'épithélioma primitif du clitoris. *Revue Chirurgicale Paris* **46**, 456.

Benedet, J.L., Turko, M., Fairey, R.N. & Boyes, D.A. (1979) Squamous carcinoma of the vulva: results of treatment, 1936–1976. *American Journal of Obstetrics and Gynecology* **34**, 201–207.

Boronow, R.C. (1973) Therapeutic alternative to primary exenteration for advanced vulvovaginal cancer. *Gynecologic Oncology* **1**, 223–255.

Boronow, R.C. (1982) Combined therapy as an alternative to exenteration for locally advanced vulvo-vaginal cancer. *Cancer* **49**, 1085–1091.

Brown, M.D., Zachary, C.B., Grekin, R.C. & Swanson, N.A. (1988) Genital tumours: their management by micrographic surgery. *Journal of the American Academy of Dermatology* **18**, 115–122.

Burrows, N.P., Jones, D.H., Hudson, P.M. & Pye, R.J. (1995) Treatment of extramammary Paget's disease by radiotherapy. *British Journal of Dermatology* **132**, 970–972.

Cox, S.M., Kaufman, R.H. & Kaplin, A. (1986) Recurrent carcinoma *in situ* of the vulva in a skin graft. *American Journal of Obstetrics and Gynecology* **155**, 177–179.

Curry, S.L., Wharton, J.T. & Rutledge, F.N. (1980) Positive lymph nodes in vulvar squamous carcinoma. *Gynecological Oncology* **9**, 63–67.

DiSaia, P.J., Creasman, V.V.T. & Rich, W.M. (1979) An alternate approach to early cancer of the vulva. *American Journal of Obstetrics and Gynecology* **133**, 825–830.

Dunton, C.J., Kautzky, M. & Hanau, C. (1995) Malignant melanoma of the vulva: a review. *Obstetrical and Gynecologic Survey* **50**, 739–746.

Fortier, K.J., Clarke-Pearson, D.L., Creasman, W.T. & Johnston, W.M. (1985) Fine-needle aspiration in gynecology: evaluation of extrapelvic lesions in patients with gynecologic malignancy. *Obstetric and Gynecology* **65**, 67–72.

Grimshaw, R.N., Ghazal-Aswad, S. & Monaghan, J.M. (1991) The role of ano-vulvectomy in locally advanced carcinoma of the vulva. *International Journal of Gynecological Cancer* **1**, 15–18.

Grimshaw, R.N., Murdoch, J.B. & Monaghan, J.M. (1993) Radical vulvectomy and bilateral inguinal-femoral lymphadenectomy through separate incisions—experience with 100 cases. *International Journal of Gynecological Cancer* **3**, 18–23.

Hacker, N.L., Berek, J.S., Lagasse, L.D., Nieberg, R.K. & Leuchter, R.S. (1984) Individualization of treatment for stage I squamous cell vulvar carcinoma. *Obstetrics and Gynecology* **63**, 155–162.

Hoffman, J.S., Kumar, N.B. & Morley, G.W. (1985) Prognostic significance of groin lymph node metastases in squamous carcinoma of the vulva. *Obstetrics and Gynecology* **66**, 402–405.

Holmesley, I.A.D., Bundy, B.N., Sedlis, A. & Adcock, L. (1986) Radiation therapy versus pelvic node resection for carcinoma of the vulva with positive groin nodes. *Obstetrics and Gynecology* **68**, 733–740.

Iversen, T. & Aas, M. (1983) Lymph drainage of the vulva. *Gynecological Oncology* **16**, 179–189.

Levenback, C., Burke, T.W., Gershenson, D.M. *et al.* (1994) Intraoperative lymphatic mapping for vulvar cancer. *Obstetrics and Gynecology* **84**, 163.

Levenback, C., Burke, T.W., Morris, M. *et al.* (1995) Potential applications of intraoperative lymphatic mapping in vulvar cancer. *Gynecologic Oncology* **59**, 216–220.

McCall, A.R., Olson, M.C. & Potkul, R.K. (1995) The variation of inguinal lymph node depth in adult women and its importance in planning elective irradiation for vulvar cancer. *Cancer* **75**, 2286–2288.

McDonald, T.W., Morley, G.W., Choo, Y.C. *et al.* (1983) Fine needle aspiration of para-aortic and pelvic lymph nodes showing lymphangiographic abnormalities. *Obstetrics and Gynecology* **61**, 383–388.

Monaghan, J.M. (1985) Management of carcinoma of the vulva. In: *Clinical Gynaecological Oncology* (eds J.S. Shepherd & J.M. Monaghan), pp. 140–167. Blackwell Scientific Publications, Oxford.

Paladini, D., Cross, P., Lopes, A & Monaghan, J.M. (1994) Prognostic significance of lymph node variable in squamous cell carcinoma of the vulva. *Cancer* **74**, 2491–2496.

Parry-Jones, E. (1963) Lymphatics of the vulva. *British Journal of Obstetrics and Gynaecology* **70**, 751–765.

Piver, M.S. & Xynos, F.P. (1983) Pelvic lymphadenectomy in women with carcinoma of the clitoris. *Obstetrics and Gynecology* 1977; **49**, 592–595.

Stiller, M., Klein, W., Dorman, R. & Albom, M. (1993) Bilateral vulvar basal cell carcinomas. *Journal of the American Academy of Dermatology* **28**, 836–838.

Stoeckel, W. (1930) Zur Zentralblatt für Therapie gynäkologie des Vulva karzinoms. *Zentralblatt für Gynäkologie* **1**, 47–71.

Symmonds, R.E. & Webb, M.J. (1981) Pelvic exenteration. In: *Gynecologic Oncology*, Vol. II (ed. M. Coppelson), pp. 896–922. Churchill Livingston, Edinburgh.

Index

Page numbers in *italic* refer to figures